# The Western Herbal Tradition

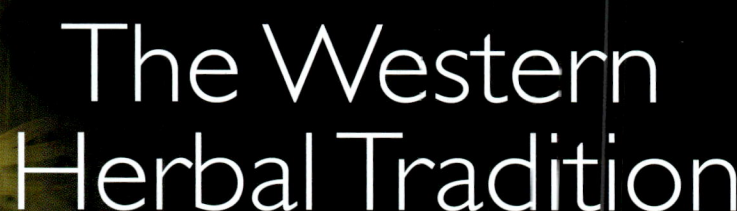

Commissioning Editor: *Claire Wilson*
Development Editor: *Natalie Meylan, Louisa Welch*
Project Manager: *Annie Victor*
Designer: *Kirsteen Wright*

# The Western Herbal Tradition
## 2000 years of medicinal plant knowledge

**Graeme Tobyn** BA FHEA FNIMH
Senior Lecturer in Herbal Medicine,
University of Central Lancashire, Preston, UK

**Alison Denham** BA(Soc) FNIMH
Senior Lecturer in Herbal Medicine,
University of Central Lancashire, Preston, UK Former President, NIMH

**Margaret Whitelegg** BA PhD FNIMH
Former Senior Lecturer in Herbal Medicine,
University of Central Lancashire, Preston, UK Former President, NIMH

Foreword by Sheila Kingsbury

Watercolours by Marije Rowling
Freelance illustrator, painter and teacher, UK

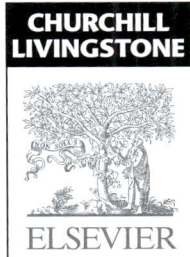

Edinburgh  London  New York  Oxford  Philadelphia  St Louis  Sydney  Toronto  2011

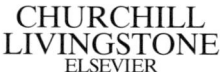

© 2011 Elsevier Ltd All rights reserved.

No part of this publication may be reproduced or transmitted in any form or by any means, electronic or mechanical, including photocopying, recording, or any information storage and retrieval system, without permission in writing from the publisher. Details on how to seek permission, further information about the Publisher's permissions policies and our arrangements with organizations such as the Copyright Clearance Center and the Copyright Licensing Agency, can be found at our website: www.elsevier.com/permissions.

This book and the individual contributions contained in it are protected under copyright by the Publisher (other than as may be noted herein).

ISBN 978-0-443-10344-5

British Library Cataloguing in Publication Data
A catalogue record for this book is available from the British Library

Library of Congress Cataloging in Publication Data
A catalog record for this book is available from the Library of Congress

Notices
Knowledge and best practice in this field are constantly changing. As new research and experience broaden our understanding, changes in research methods, professional practices, or medical treatment may become necessary.

Practitioners and researchers must always rely on their own experience and knowledge in evaluating and using any information, methods, compounds, or experiments described herein. In using such information or methods they should be mindful of their own safety and the safety of others, including parties for whom they have a professional responsibility.

With respect to any drug or pharmaceutical products identified, readers are advised to check the most current information provided (i) on procedures featured or (ii) by the manufacturer of each product to be administered, to verify the recommended dose or formula, the method and duration of administration, and contraindications. It is the responsibility of practitioners, relying on their own experience and knowledge of their patients, to make diagnoses, to determine dosages and the best treatment for each individual patient, and to take all appropriate safety precautions.

To the fullest extent of the law, neither the Publisher nor the authors, contributors, or editors, assume any liability for any injury and/or damage to persons or property as a matter of products liability, negligence or otherwise, or from any use or operation of any methods, products, instructions, or ideas contained in the material herein.

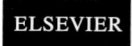

Printed in China

# Contents

| | | |
|---|---|---|
| Foreword | | vii |
| Preface | | ix |
| 1 | The historical sources | 1 |
| 2 | Some observations on the Western herbal tradition | 23 |
| 3 | Origins and proponents of the revival of herbal medicine in 19th century Britain | 29 |
| 4 | A note on Goethe | 37 |
| 5 | Notes on nomenclature, plant descriptions, quality, constituents, safety and dosages | 41 |
| 6 | *Agrimonia eupatoria*, agrimony | 47 |
| 7 | *Alchemilla vulgaris*, lady's mantle | 57 |
| 8 | *Althaea officinalis*, marshmallow; *Malva sylvestris*, common mallow; *Alcea rosea*, hollyhock | 67 |
| 9 | *Apium graveolens*, wild celery | 79 |
| 10 | *Arctium lappa*, burdock | 91 |
| 11 | *Artemisia absinthium*, wormwood | 105 |
| 12 | *Artemisia vulgaris*, mugwort | 123 |
| 13 | *Centaurium erythraea*, centaury | 135 |
| 14 | *Daucus carota*, wild carrot | 145 |
| 15 | *Drimia maritima*, squill | 155 |
| 16 | *Fumaria officinalis*, fumitory | 165 |
| 17 | *Galium aparine*, goosegrass | 173 |
| 18 | *Glechoma hederacea*, ground ivy | 181 |
| 19 | *Hyssopus officinalis*, hyssop | 191 |
| 20 | *Inula helenium*, elecampane | 201 |
| 21 | *Lamium album*, white deadnettle | 211 |
| 22 | *Ocimum basilicum*, basil | 221 |
| 23 | *Paeonia officinalis*, paeony | 231 |
| 24 | *Potentilla erecta*, tormentil | 241 |
| 25 | *Rosa damascena*, damask rose | 253 |
| 26 | *Rubus idaeus*, raspberry | 271 |
| 27 | *Ruta graveolens*, rue | 283 |
| 28 | *Scrophularia nodosa*, figwort | 297 |
| 29 | *Stachys officinalis*, wood betony | 307 |
| 30 | *Tussilago farfara*, coltsfoot | 317 |
| 31 | *Verbena officinalis*, vervain | 327 |
| 32 | *Viola odorata*, sweet violet; *Viola tricolor*, heartsease | 337 |
| Index | | 349 |

# Foreword

The studious explorer of herbal knowledge will revel in the depth and expansive coverage of the plants and their history that are portrayed in this book. I too delight in following the historical trails that illustrate the affects of each age's philosophy and how it impacted medical practice. It is intriguing to see how each player in the historical drama influenced the next generation and beyond as well as how we think about and use each herb. Once you explore the realms of history in regards to each generation's philosophical debates and scientific thinking, you really begin to understand that, essentially, we still grapple with similar debates. Often, what we think is a new idea is actually a related thread of ideas tying us back to past influences. For example, for at least a couple of thousand years now we have been arguing about who is most qualified to advise others on health care and whose expertise we should trust. The political shifts in medical philosophy and power continue to ebb and flow from group to group. Putting our history down more cohesively helps us get a deeper understanding of these shifts and their influences. Graeme Tobyn is no stranger to the realm of historical research on herbal traditions. His book, Culpeper's Herbal, has introduced us to the world of Nicolas Culpeper and his important contributions to Western Herbalism. With his co-authors, he takes us much further back in history with this text, weaving herbs through the last 2000 years and giving context to how they were used throughout that time period.

This book will familiarize the reader with some of the most important historical figures and their roles in the development of Western Herbalism. The authors shine light under many rocks along the way, leaving no virtual stone unturned as the reader is led through Dioscorides' influences and contributions, through Thompsonian era bickering and even lightly treading with Goethe and Steiner in the realm of plant transformation and interconnectivity. What better way to grasp the nature of a plant than to see it within the historical context, thus illustrating the unique plant–human relations that make up our plant medicine. As the authors state 'by doing so we appear to cross a divide between medicine as history and medicine as current …'. As we evolve within the parameters of medicine it becomes vital that we observe with critical awareness the herbal history so that we may move forward in our thinking rather than the proverbial recreation of the wheel. The current practicing herbalist is charged with this assignment to really know the plants in their current transformational state as well as in their historical context, so that they may come to a more true, deeper knowledge of the medicine. In our reductionist haste we are at risk of losing many parts of the story, our grandmother's story, the story of the ages, the philosophers, the scientists and the plants themselves.

Each chapter's coverage of the individual herbs is like having a conference call with all of the historical figures to see how each would have described and used that herb medicinally. For history lovers, especially, lovers of Western Herbal history, this is a dream come true. It is truly exciting to get all of that comparison in one place and see where the agreements and disagreements really stand out. The authors are also generous with the necessary overviews and summaries that make such a text worth having for quick reference as well. I am excited to see the study of the history of Western Herbal tradition rise to a new level, where we have much of the information in one place and we can study the herb and the history in such greater depth. Then, we can come to new, deeply informed understandings of that herb and how we can use it.

The authors do a superb job of filling in the historical information so that we can get a grasp on how one philosophy transitioned into the next. This book does indeed make a contribution 'to the location of herbal medicine in the historical marketplace'. I am sure to use this text in my teachings on the history of herbal medicine and am thankful for the care and toil the authors have put into this work.

Sheila Kingsbury ND, RH (AHG)
Chair, Botanical Medicine
Bastyr University
Seattle, WA, USA

# Preface

In this book we have attempted to outline the transmission of a knowledge of medicinal herbs in the West over 2000 years using both primary sources and their modern translations and editions, and the latest research into plant medicines. It is essentially an outline, since the time span covers long periods in the history of medicine and we could not possibly do justice to the ebb and flow of medical theories, orthodox practice and its alternatives and the development of pharmacy in the course of that time. We have also had to limit the focus in choosing to concentrate on the great, printed herbals of the tradition, and we have not explored the less well known published texts germane to our study, let alone case books and other manuscript evidence. Nevertheless, having taken part of our selection from the second great era of herbal writing among the large folios of the Renaissance and Early Modern periods, it was pleasing to note that we had already singled out the key texts of the Graeco-Roman period cited by the authors of these great herbals. We hope therefore that our readers will feel assured that they are accessing the main current of the herbal tradition passed down the centuries. Equally, we have collected and tried to put into the context of this tradition some 18th, 19th and 20th century medical and herbal texts in order to evaluate the transmission, so far as it exists, in contemporary herbal practice.

As herbal practitioners, still using the herbs described here to treat our patients, we see ourselves as free from the historiographical paradigm within which historians have documented a post-classical decline of medicine from the highest achievement of Graeco-Roman writers and physicians (Touwaide 2005) until the paradigm shift of the Enlightenment. Indeed, the 'Whig' view of history as progress, so prevalent in histories of herbal medicine until a few decades ago, would cast us as hopeless romantics and dangerous dinosaurs in a brave new world of advances in bioscientific knowledge and medical interventions. We trust that our evaluation of the pharmacological constituents of the plants we discuss here, and the inclusion of evidence on the safety and effectiveness of plant medicines, demonstrates that today's herbalists critically evaluate both historical documentation and the latest empirical findings underpinning herbal prescribing.

This book may well be seen as part of a wave of interest in the historical materials we have studied. The historian of medicine Andrew Wear (2000) has paid attention to the transmission of knowledge concerning dandelion as a medicine in his *Knowledge & Practice in English Medicine 1550–1680*, while Michael Adams *et al.* (2009), in a review of European herbals of the 16th and 17th centuries for medicinal herbs to treat rheumatism, comment that 'despite the once wide use of these old herbals produced in many editions for centuries, modern science has barely started to scientifically explore this florilegium'. The authors identify the poor accessibility of these works as a reason for their neglect but assert that 'the scientific examination of historic works can be the base for the 'rediscovery' of long-forgotten remedies and a source of information for a more focused screening for new leads'. We, however, have aimed to explore such sources for remedies whose former indications for use may not be well known although the plants themselves are still very familiar and constitute even today the materia medica of practitioners. In this we have been aided by other recent publications, notably Professor Beck's translation of *Dioscorides De Materia Medica* in 2005, Ann van Arsdall's translation of the *Old English Herbarium* in 2002 and Marion Green's *Trotula* in 2001. Thus we have been fortunate since Graeme's first move to research this study of herbal medicines in March 2002 that these texts have become available.

While we sensed that such a review of the transmission of knowledge of certain herbs might usefully contribute to the literature on herbal medicine, for the precedent that is Mrs Grieve's *A Modern Herbal* published in 1931, compendious as it is, is out of date in relation to plant constituents and lacks an academic referencing, we were also aware of a certain insufficiency of attention to the detail of the tradition in current textbooks on herbal medicine. It is not unusual to find a few lines containing the phrase 'traditionally used for' amid many pages of description and reference to plant assays, in vitro research and animal experimentation. Since herbal medicine has a long tradition, we wanted to contribute critical consideration of its textual provenance to sit alongside the still limited range of scientific investigations that may support clinical use. We have made particular choices of herbs: the plant medicines described here are to be found in the *British Herbal Pharmacopoeia* first published in 1983, and the majority of which are in very common use in the UK and elsewhere in Europe and the USA. However, there is less scientific interest and limited research in these than in those phytomedicines whose evidence base is more accepted and which have been in many cases appropriated for sale in conventional pharmacies as standardized extracts.

Like Catherine O'Sullivan (2005), we too 'are concerned with the place of alternative and complementary medicine within a society dominated by a rational and scientific approach to illness, which privileges the treatment of illness over the health and well-being of the whole person' and we want to draw on our own history as Western herbal practitioners and to stand up among those who 'argue that their knowledge is clinically based, consisting of empirical findings, which are contained in written texts and transmitted through both formal schools and more, informal, personal teacher/student relationships'. Indeed we intend to integrate material from this book into our plans for postgraduate teaching.

A further step is taken by including in some of the monographs the work of Wilhelm Pelikan, who approaches plants through the ideas of Goethe and Rudolf Steiner. In our text it is included as an inspiring example of a rigorous and modern appreciation of healing plants from a spiritual perspective for those interested in such ideas, and for the additional light it can throw on the traditional texts.

That there are three authors to this book was a substantial challenge to management of the research, the composition of the text and agreement on authorial style. Graeme took on the reading of most of the Latin herbals and Ibn Sina in Russian translation; Midge attended specifically to Turner, Gerard, the Latin of Mattioli, Quincy, Miller and the Goethean materials; Alison braved the challenges of the botanical descriptions, the pharmacological constituents and current research, and covered the 19th century texts in particular. All contributed to the authors' biographies. As to the monographs, each of us took nine herbs as final editor and saw through the weaving together of the materials into what we hope are coherent wholes. Each author's monographs were then commented on by the others and revised on the basis of this critical reading. Midge undertook the editing of the manuscript before it was finally submitted. The photographs were taken by Alison.

This book has relied heavily on the library and online resources made available by the Wellcome Medical Library, London. We would like thank the Wellcome Medical Library, the British Library, the Edinburgh Botanic Garden Library, Leeds City Library and the Harris Library, Preston for their help and support. We have been grateful for materials made available online by the Bibliotheque Nationale de France via its Gallica site. Through the SCONUL scheme we were able to use the invaluable resources of the John Rylands Library of the University of Manchester, the J.B. Priestley Library of the University of Bradford and the Brotherton and Edward Boyle Libraries of the University of Leeds. Thanks also go to Janet Barker, Margaret Colquhoun and James Dyson for their encouragement to include the Goethean material. Thanks go to Morag Weatherstone and Sue Goodwin for providing physiomedical source materials and to Jean Dow for use of her dissertation on women physiomedical practitioners submitted in 2004 for the MSc at the Scottish School of Herbal Medicine. Thanks go to Paul Denham for botanical identifications and to Thelma Wightman and Joe Nasr for permission to photograph plants.

The book is written to inform the prescribing of herbal practitioners and thus takes a broad sweep through history. The specialist reader may find errors of fact or interpretation for which we apologise.

*Graeme Tobyn, Alison Denham, Midge Whitelegg*
*Preston 2011*
gwtobyn@uclan.ac.uk
adenham@uclan.ac.uk

## REFERENCES

Adams M, Berset C, Kessler M, Hamburger M 2009 Medicinal herbs for the treatment of rheumatic disorders – a survey of European herbals from the 16th and 17th centuries. Journal of Ethnopharmacology 121:343–359.

O'Sullivan C 2005 Reshaping herbal medicine: knowledge, education and professional culture. Elsevier, London.

Touwaide A 2005 Healers and physicians in ancient and medieval mediterranean cultures. In Yaniv Z. and Bachrach U. (eds) Handbook of medicinal plants. The Haworth Press, London.

Wear A 2000 Knowledge and practice in English medicine 1550–1680 Cambridge University Press, Cambridge.

# CHAPTER 1
# The historical sources

In selecting our range of sources for the Renaissance history of the medicinal use of each of the 27 plants described in this book, we have first consulted what is still the standard work on the history of herbals, Ann R. Arber's *Herbals, their Origins and Evolution: A Chapter in the History of Botany 1470–1670*, first published by Cambridge University Press in 1912. We wish to reflect opinions from a range of European countries. Greece and Italy have representatives already in the classical texts of Dioscorides, Pliny and Galen, and the *Herbarium of Pseudo-Apuleius*. The medieval Salernitan material from southern Italy connects with Arabic sources, represented of course by Ibn Sina but also by Serapio, whose *Liber Aggregatus in Simplicibus Medicinis* (1473) is possibly the earliest herbal to be printed in Europe, and who is referred to not infrequently by our Renaissance sources. Mattioli's commentary from 16th century Italy on Dioscorides' *De Materia Medica* could not be omitted, although we have in places augmented views expressed in this first Latin edition with a later French edition, published a century after the Lyon herbal accredited to Dalechamps, our French representative. Germany's voices come from Hildegard and Fuchs and the Swiss-born Bauhin, while Dodoens speaks for The Netherlands. Macer's herbal too comes from north-west Europe. Along with the English herbals of the period – Turner, Gerard, Parkinson and Culpeper – we have the books of the physicians of Myddfai representing Welsh practice. A notable omission may perhaps be material of Spanish origin, but we have chosen our herbs from the European tradition, whereas a major contribution of Spanish texts has been in describing plants of the New World.

We have benefited from recent translations of Dioscorides, the *Old English Herbarium*, Hildegard's *Physica*, a 15th century version of the Salernitan herbal and a new edition of Turner's herbal, and have drawn on older standards such as W. H. S. Jones' translation of Pliny and a translation of the books of the physicians of Myddfai. For other texts we have made our own translations of the original Latin, French, German and Russian. We have used the translation of Dioscorides by Beck throughout the book and thus have relied on her substantial scholarship.

## MODERN SOURCES

We consulted modern texts because they reflect current usage and have a role in the transmission of knowledge. For each herb, online scientific databases and reference lists in published papers were searched. The search for randomized controlled trials was fruitless in many cases. Points arising from in vitro research are discussed where relevant to themes in the monographs but animal studies on the effectiveness of herbs have not been discussed. The searches were completed in early 2009, and all web addresses given were updated after January 2009.

The primary sources given below are used throughout the book and are not referenced in the text.

## TIMELINE OF AUTHORIAL SOURCES

### Greco-Roman

#### Dioscorides fl. 50–80 AD

Beck LY 2005 Pedanius Dioscorides of Anazarbus: De materia medica. Olms – Weidmann, Hildesheim.
  Osbaldeston T and Wood R 2000 Dioscorides De Materia Medica. Ibidis Press, Johannesburg.

#### Pliny the Elder c. 23–79 AD

Jones WHS (trans) 1949–1962 Pliny Natural History, with an English translation in 10 volumes. William Heinemann, London.
  Pliny C 1601 The Historie of the World. London.

#### Galen of Pergamon c. 130–200 AD

Galen C 1543 De Simplicium Medicamentorum Facultatibus Libri Undecim. Paris.
  Kuhn CG (ed.) 1821–1833 Claudii Galeni opera omnia 20 volumes. C. Cnoblich, Leipzig

#### Pseudo-Apuleius 5th century AD

Hunger FWT (ed.) 1935 The herbal of Pseudo-Apuleius from the ninth century manuscript in the abbey of Monte Cassino. EJ Brill, Leyden.

### Arabic

#### Ibn Sina (Avicenna) c. 980–1037 AD

Abu Ali ibn Sino 2003 Kanon Vrachebnoj Nauki, 10 volumes. Enio, Odessa.

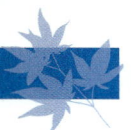

# THE WESTERN HERBAL TRADITION

### Serapio the Younger (Ibn Wafid) 13th century

Serapio 1479 Liber Serapionis Aggregatus in Medicinis Simplicibus. Venice.

## Anglo-Saxon/Late Middle Ages

### The Old English Herbarium c. 1000

Van Arsdall A 2002 Medieval herbal remedies: the Old English Herbarium and Anglo-Saxon medicine. Routledge, London.

### Macer 9–12th century

Macer 1511 Carmen de Virtutibus Herbarum. Paris.

### The Salernitan herbal 12th century

Roberts E, Stearn W (trans) 1984 Livre des Simples Medecines: Codex Bruxellensis IV.1024 A 15th Century French Herbal. De Schutter, Antwerp.

### Hildegard of Bingen 1098–1179

Throop P (trans) 1998 Hildegard von Bingen's Physica. Healing Arts Press, Rochester, VT.

### Physicians of Myddfai 14th and 18th centuries

Pughe J 1861 (1993 reprint) The physicians of Myddvai; Meddygon Myddfai. Llanerch Publishers, Felinfach.

## Renaissance/Early Modern

### Leonhart Fuchs 1501–1566

Fuchs L 1545 De Historia Stirpium. Basileae.
  Meyer F, Trueblood E, Heller J 1999 The Great Herbal of Leonhart Fuchs. Stanford University Press, CA.

### Pietro Andrea Mattioli 1501–1577

Matthioli PA 1554 Petri Andreae Matthioli Medici Senensis Commentarii, in Libros Sex Pedacii Dioscoridis Anazarbei, De Materia Medica 1554. Venice. Online. Available: http://gallica.bnf.fr.
  Matthioli PA 1680 Les Commentaires de M.P. André Matthiole, … sur les six livres de la matière médicinale de Pedacius Dioscoride, … traduits de latin en françois par M. Antoine Du Pinet … augmentez … d'un Traité de chymie en abrégé … par un docteur en médecine. Derniere edition. J.-B. de Ville, Lyons. Online. Available: http://gallica.bnf.fr.

### William Turner 1509/10–1568

Chapman GTL, Tweedle MN (eds) 1995 A New Herball by William Turner, part I, vol 1. Cambridge University Press, Cambridge.
  Chapman GTL, McCombie F, Wesencraft A (eds) 1995 A New Herball by William Turner, parts II & III, vol 2. Cambridge University Press, Cambridge.
  Turner W 1551 A New Herball Steven Mierdman, London. Online. Available: http://library.wellcome.ac.uk/, Early English Books Online (EEBO).

### Rembert Dodoens 1516–1585

Dodoens R 1619 A New Herbal: or Historie of Plants. London. Online. Available: http://library.wellcome.ac.uk/, EEBO.

### Jacques D'Alechamps 1513–1588

D'Alechamps J 1586 Historia Generalis Plantarum. Lugdini.

### Jean Bauhin 1541–1613

Bauhin J 1650 Historia Plantarum Universalis. Ebroduni. Online. Available: http://gallica.bnf.fr.

### John Gerard c.1545–1612

Gerard J 1975 The Herbal or General History of Plants. Dover Publications, New York. Online. Available: http://library.wellcome.ac.uk/, EEBO.

### John Parkinson 1566/7–1650

Parkinson J 1640 Theatrum Botanicum or The Theater of Plants. London. Online. Available: http://library.wellcome.ac.uk/, EEBO.

### Nicholas Culpeper 1616–1654

Culpeper N 1656 The English Physitian. London.
  Culpeper N 1669 Pharmacopoeia Londinensis. London.
  Culpeper N 1995 Culpeper's Complete Herbal. Wordsworth Library, Ware, Herts.

## 18th Century

### John Quincy d. 1722

Quincy J 1724 Pharmacopoeia Officinalis & Extemporanea. London. Also Online. Available: http://library.wellcome.ac.uk/, Eighteenth Century Collections Online (ECCO).

2

## Joseph Miller d. 1748

Miller J 1722 Botanicum Officinale or A Compendious Herbal. E Bell, J Senex, W Taylor, J Osborn, London. Also Online. Available: http://library.wellcome.ac.uk/, ECCO.

## John Hill 1714–1775

Hill J 1755 The Useful Family Herbal. London. Also Online. Available: http://library.wellcome.ac.uk/, ECCO.

## William Cullen 1710–1790

Cullen W 1773 Lectures on Materia Medica. T. Lowndes, London. Online. Available: http://library.wellcome.ac.uk/, ECCO.

# 19th Century American and British

## Albert Isiah Coffin 1790–1866

Coffin AI 1864 Botanic Guide to Health, 49th edn. Haynes, Coffin, London.

## William Fox

Fox W 1920 The Working-man's Model Family Botanic Guide to Health, 22nd edn. W Fox and Sons, Sheffield.

## William Cook 1832–1899

Cook W 1869 (1985 reprint) The Physiomedical Dispensatory. Eclectic Medical Publications, Oregon.

## Finley Ellingwood 1852–1920

Ellingwood F 1919 (1988 reprint) American Materia Medica, Therapeutics and Pharmacognosy. Eclectic Medical Publications, Oregon. Online. Available: http://www.henriettesherbal.com/eclectics/books.html.

# 20th Century texts

## Richard Cranfield Wren

Wren RC 1907 Potter's Cyclopaedia of Botanical Drugs and Preparations. Potter & Clarke, London.

## Richard Hool

Hool RL 1918 Health from British wild herbs. W H Webb, Southport.

## Maud Grieve 1858 to after 1941

Grieve M 1931 (1984 edn) A Modern Herbal. Penguin Books, Harmandsworth.

## Wilhelm Pelikan 1893–1981

Pelikan W 1997 Healing Plants: Insights Through Spiritual Science, vol. 1. Mercury Press, Spring Valley, New York.
    Pelikan W 1962 Heilpflanzenkunde, vol. 2. Verlag am Goetheanum, Dornach.
    Pelikan W 1978 Heilpflanzenkunde, vol. 3. Verlag am Goetheanum, Dornach.

## Rudolf Weiss 1895–1991

Weiss R 1988 Herbal Medicine. Beaconsfield Publishing, Beaconsfield.

## The National Botanic Pharmacopoeia 1921

National Association of Medical Herbalists of Great Britain 1921 The National Botanic Pharmacopoeia, 2nd edn. Woodhouse, Cornthwaite, Bradford.

## Albert Priest and Lilian Priest

Priest A, Priest L 1982 Herbal Medication. LN Fowler, London.

## British Herbal Pharmacopoeia

BHPA Scientific Committee 1983 British Herbal Pharmacopoeia. British Herbal Medicine Association, Keighley, West Yorkshire.

## Thomas Bartram 1913–2009

Bartram T 1995 Encyclopaedia of Herbal Medicine. Grace Publishers, Bournemouth.

# 21st Century texts

## Peter Bradley

Bradley P (ed.) 1992 British Herbal Compendium, vol 1. British Herbal Medicines Association, Bournemouth.
    Bradley P 2006 British Herbal Compendium, vol. 2. British Herbal Medicines Association, Bournemouth.

## Andrew Chevallier

Chevallier A 2001 The Encyclopedia of Medicinal Plants. Dorling Kindersley, London.

## Elizabeth Williamson

Williamson E 2003 Potter's Herbal Cyclopaedia. CW Daniel, London.

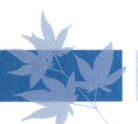

### David Hoffman

Hoffman D 2003 Medical Herbalism: The Science and Practice of Herbal Medicine. Healing Arts Press, Rochester, VT.

### Christopher Menzies-Trull

Menzies-Trull C 2003 Herbal Medicine Keys to Physiomedicalism. Faculty of Physiomedical Herbal Medicine, Newcastle, Staffordshire.

### Simon Mills and Kerry Bone

Mills S, Bone K 2005 The Essential Guide to Herbal Safety. Elsevier, St Louis, Missouri.

### Matthew Wood

Wood M 2008 The Earthwise Herbal: a Complete Guide to Old World Medicinal Plants. North Atlantic Books, Berkeley CA.

## BIOGRAPHIES OF THE EARLIER AUTHORS AND NOTES ON TEXTS

## Dioscorides

Pedanius Dioscorides was born at Anazarbus, which is northeast of Adana in southeastern Turkey. The name Pedanius is a Roman name, suggesting that Dioscorides was a Greek-speaking Roman citizen. He was a physician and probably served in some capacity with the Roman legions in Asia Minor. In his five books of the *De Materia Medica*, the only work now attributed to Dioscorides, over 600 plants, 35 animal products and 90 minerals are discussed, by far the largest treatise on drugs in antiquity, significantly more than in the Hippocratic corpus, and commended and cited in numerous places by Galen. Dioscorides was keen to describe both plants and habitats in his book. It has been argued that he must have travelled widely through the Greek-speaking eastern half of the Roman Empire to gather his knowledge but he will also have depended on reports. In his preface, he claims that while much accurate information was passed on by his forebears, his book surpasses their work, especially in its organization. His entries include a Greek synonym for the plant, its origin, habitat and physical characteristics, the method of preparing it for medicine and a list of therapeutic uses, with some mention of harmful side-effects. Book I (129 entries) deals with aromatics, oils, salves, trees and shrubs, including liquids, gums and fruits; Book II (186 entries) with animal parts, cereals and pot herbs and sharp herbs; Book III (158 entries) with roots, juices, herbs and seeds; Book IV (192 entries) with further roots and herbs; and Book V (162 entries) with wines and minerals. He rejected both an alphabetical listing of medicinal agents, and an ordering by action and opposite action. Instead, he grouped herbs in sequence in the various books according to their broad physiological effects. The altering of his arrangement of plants towards an alphabetical one, which took place perhaps as early as the 3rd century and is evident in the oldest extant version of his treatise, the illustrated Juliana manuscript of 512 AD, shows that Dioscorides' unexplained insight into shared therapeutic effects went unrecognized down the ages. He has much recourse to description by analogy, where one plant resembles another to a certain extent. The botanical descriptions were sometimes very short, which has led to different interpretations and some confusion through the years, with many debates on accuracy of identification, and inevitable errors in translation.

This is the time when Pliny was writing his *Natural History*, and certain parallel passages between this and the *De Materia Medica* confirm the contemporaneity and the shared sources. It has been argued that one of these could be a lost text, that of the notable Roman physician Quintus Sextius Niger, who flourished under the first emperor Augustus. Dioscorides and Pliny appear to have been writing quite independently of one another. The date of writing of *De Materia Medica* is unknown. Dioscorides does quote a number of authors but none of these sources has exact dates. He dedicates the work to Arius of Tarsus, referring to the 'enviable mutual friendship' between Arius and 'the excellent Laecanius Bassus', whom we know to have been Roman proconsul of Asia in 80 AD.

Dioscorides belonged to no definite philosophical school. His method was empiricist and he criticized speculation on the causes of the powers of drugs on the body. He encouraged knowledge based on experience: how a different climate or location affects the strength of the plant; when to gather different parts of a plant and how to store them; and how some retain their medicinal efficacy longer than others.

Dioscorides was a major influence on Galen (2nd century AD), Oribasius (4th century), Alexander of Tralles (6th century), Paul of Aegina (7th century), Aetius of Amida (7th century), Rhazes (9th century) and Ibn Sina (10th century). The earliest translation of Dioscorides into Arabic is ascribed to Istafan ibn-Basil between 800 and 830 and the Arabic Dioscorides remains in circulation today.

### Sources

Beck LY 2005 Pedanius Dioscorides of Anazarbus: De materia medica. Olms – Weidmann, Hildesheim.

Dictionary of scientific biography 1970–80 16 vols. Charles Scribner, New York.

Osbaldeston TA, Wood RPA 2000 Dioscorides de materia medica, being a herbal with many other materials written in Greek in the first century of the common era. Ibidis Press, Johannesburg.

Pavord A 2005 The naming of names: the search for order in the world of plants. Bloomsbury, London.

Riddle J 1985 Dioscorides on pharmacy and medicine. University of Texas, Austin.

Sadak MM 1979 Notes on the introduction and colophon of the Leiden Manuscript of Dioscorides' 'De materia medica'. International Journal of Middle Eastern Studies 10:345–354.

Scarborough J 1984 Early Byzantine pharmacology. Dumbarton Oaks Papers, Symposium on Byzantine Medicine 38:213–232.

Scarborough J, Nutton V 1982 The preface of Dioscorides' materia medica: introduction, translation, and commentary. Transactions and studies of the College of Physicians of Philadelphia 4:187–227.

## Pliny the Elder

Gaius Plinius Secundus was born in Como, Italy around 23 AD and died near Pompeii on 25 August 79 AD during the eruption of Mount Vesuvius, on duty as commander of the fleet based at Misenum. From the age of 12 he was educated in Rome and subsequently entered military command, the main career path open to those of the equestrian order in Roman society. Pliny completed his military service by 57–58 AD. He survived the reign of Nero by retreating to write works of oratory and grammar. He resumed his career after Vespasian became emperor in 69 AD with a series of appointments, including a post as financial regulator of a province. He became counsellor to Vespasian and his son Titus.

Pliny's only extant work is the 37-book *Natural History*, dedicated to Titus in 77 AD, possibly given a final editing by his nephew, Pliny the Younger, only after his death. It was an ambitious project since no encyclopaedia of the whole of nature had previously been attempted. The plan of the work moved from the cosmos to the earth, with its animals, vegetables and minerals. Books 12–19 cover botany, and 20–27 the plant materia medica.

The *Natural History* was written in an uncritical style, covering factual material, yet embracing an all-inclusive method. It proved highly influential in the following centuries, and Pliny's status throughout the Middle Ages equalled that of Aristotle, Galen and Dioscorides. With the development of a critical approach to classical science from the 15th century, Pliny's standing began to suffer, as is evident in the comments of some of our other authors here, and by modern scholarship. On the one hand, Pliny discusses early developments in agricultural and related technological practices alongside dates of introduction into Italy of foreign plants, and gives the earliest surviving history of art. On the other hand, a lack of reliability in quoting or using his many sources and his recounting of myths surrounding a phenomenon without discrimination has left him open to criticisms of lack of originality. Yet his importance in tradition remains considerable.

### Sources

Dictionary of scientific biography 1970–80 16 vols. Charles Scribner, New York.

Jones WHS (trans.) 1949–1962 Pliny Natural History, with an English translation in 10 volumes. William Heinemann, London.

Stannard J 1965 Pliny and Roman botany. Isis 56:420–425.

## Galen

Galen (the forename Claudius seems to have been appended in the Renaissance) was born in Pergamon in 129/130 AD and died between 199 and 215 AD. His stature during his life was so immense, above all owing to the enormous range of his literary works, that after his death he was styled 'divine'. Much is known about Galen's life, since he himself followed an ancient tradition of autobiography. His father Nikon, an architect and geometer, gave private lessons in mathematics to his son at an early age and later arranged for his instruction in philosophy. At age 16 Galen had to pick a career and a significant dream indicated that medicine should be his profession.

Galen undertook his studies in medicine for an unusually extended period of 12 years, first in Pergamon and later in Smyrna, where he also studied Platonic philosophy, before moving on to Corinth and finally Alexandria, then the most famous centre of medical training and research. Galen was seeking to develop his own definitive approach to the practice of medicine. At the age of 28 Galen returned to Pergamon as physician to the gladiators, a post which afforded him the opportunity to make some discoveries in anatomy. Nevertheless, he seems to have found surgery distasteful and his writings contain little on general surgery beyond the repair of injuries or suppurations. He was more interested in the medical treatment of internal diseases and in this his greatest influence was the Hippocratic writings. Thus he adopted the fourfold scheme incorporating the four Empedoclean elements and associated Aristotelian qualities, and the four humours of the Hippocratic text *On the Nature of Man* as a fundamental theoretical basis for medicine.

Galen arrived in Rome in 161 AD, where he speedily set up a medical practice and made an impression by effecting several striking cures of influential patients, although it is interesting to note that Galen had no medical students of his own and he founded no school of medicine. After a brief return to Pergamon, he was summoned to Aquileia by the Empire's two rulers, Marcus Aurelius and Lucius Verus. He became physician to Commodus, the young son

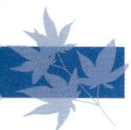

of the Emperor, and spent time in his company in various Italian cities, writing and researching, until 180 AD, when Commodus became Emperor. This close contact with the imperial family, both as physician and as socially prominent personality, continued in Rome for two decades and into the reign of Septimus Severus. In this period Galen lost a large part of his library to a fire in the Temple of Peace in 192 AD. It is not known whether Galen spent his last days in Rome or back home in Pergamon.

Galen's works were translated into Arabic by Hunain ibn Ishaq and others in the 9th century in Baghdad and some challenges to his teachings were made by leading Arab physicians such as Rhazes when their own medical experience contradicted Galen's written view. Other translations were made of philosophical and mathematical works from the Greek and Arabic medicine that developed the philosophical and humoural concepts. Galenism as a medical system was strengthened in the Christian West after 1000 AD by translations from Arabic, notably by Constantine the African in the first instance. The Galenic system, filtered over the centuries by Byzantine and Arab reflection, passed across to Western Europe through such translations.

Developments through the Renaissance and Enlightenment, such as dissections of the human body by Vesalius and Harvey's discovery of the circulation of blood, uncovered the necessarily speculative side of Galen's physiology. Only Galen's reputation as a dietician and as a diagnostician stood firm before the challenges of the Cartesian division between the mind and the body, Newtonian mechanics and the new scientific method. His doctrine of the six non-naturals (diet and lifestyle factors) was the core of conventional rules of medical hygiene until the end of the 19th century, while deeply rooted notions of bad humours and blood purification were commonly shared at the turn of the 20th century.

As far as his therapeutics is concerned, Galen mixed empirical testing of the effects of medicines with speculation on their mode of action, namely the heating, cooling, drying and moistening effects they might have on the body. These actions are still integral to Eastern systems of natural medicine such as Ayurveda and Unani Tibb, while in Western herbal medicine their prevalence diminished after the rise of a mechanical philosophy in the later 17th century. Galen's rational therapeutics are found scattered throughout the massive number of books he wrote, but are principally concentrated in the texts *Mixtures and Properties of Simples*, *Compound Drugs Arranged by Location of Ailment* and *Compound Drugs Arranged by Indication*.

## Sources

Dictionary of scientific biography 1970–80 16 vols. Charles Scribner, New York.

Scarborough J 1984 Early Byzantine pharmacology. Dumbarton Oaks Papers, Symposium on Byzantine Medicine. 38:213–232.

Temkin O 1973 Galenism: rise and decline of a medical philosophy. Cornell University Press, Ithaca.

## Pseudo-Apuleius (Apuleius Platonicus)

The publishing in 1935 of a facsimile copy of *The herbal of Pseudo-Apuleius* from a 9th century Latin manuscript found in the Abbey of Monte Cassino southeast of Rome (codex Casinensis 97) has made available to modern scholars one of the early medieval copies of this text. The herbal is thought to have been written in the 4th or 5th century AD, although whether in Latin or in Greek is not known, and the oldest extant manuscript dates from the 6th century. The author of this herbal is unknown but is certainly not the 1st century Latin writer and student of Platonic philosophy Lucius Apuleius, author of the *Metamorphoses* (also called The Golden Ass). It has been suggested that the name 'Apuleius' was used to suggest Aesculapius, the Roman God of medicine.

The herbal is a prescription book of 132 herbs with pictures to indicate the well-known plants to be used. It was possibly the most practical and most widely used remedy book in the whole of the Middle Ages. Its popularity is evident from the number of manuscripts still in existence.

## Sources

Hunger FWT 1935 The herbal of Pseudo-Apuleius. EJ Brill, Leyden.

Van Arsdall A 2002 Medieval herbal remedies: the Old English Herbarium and Anglo-Saxon medicine. Routledge, London.

## Ibn Sina

Abu Ali Al-Husain ibn Abdallah ibn Sina, known in the medieval West as Avicenna, was born at Afshana near Bukhara in present-day Uzbekistan in 980 AD and died at Hamadan in present-day Iran in 1037. He was known as 'the prince of physicians' and was accorded the epithet 'Galen of Islam'. Like Galen, ibn Sina wrote an autobiography. His major medical textbook, the *Qanun* or *Canon of Medicine*, was the most famous medical textbook of all, both in Arab-speaking countries and in the medieval West.

Ibn Sina was the son of a tax collector. He had memorized the Koran by age 10 then went on to study law, mathematics, physics and astronomy. He turned to medicine aged 16 and was so brilliant that 2 years later he was summoned to treat the Samanid prince Nuh ibn Mansur. He was appointed court physician, which gave him access to the royal library at Bukhara. He twice served as vizier to the Buyid prince at Hamadan in western Iran but had to move a number of times in his life because of political upheavals. He wrote 40 books, half of which dealt with medicine and others on philosophy, science, poetry, music and statecraft.

The *Canon of Medicine* summarized the Hippocratic-Galenic tradition and included Syro-Arab and Indo-Persian practice. He discussed around 760 herbal medicines, which are largely contained in book two of the Canon. The Canon drew on the work of Rhazes (Muhammad ibn Zakariyya al-Razi, died 925 AD), an earlier fellow philosopher-doctor. The Canon was translated into Latin in the 12th century by Gerard of Cremona (d. 1187) with another version by Andrea Alpago (d. 1522). It was used as a textbook of medicine throughout the Middle Ages and continued to be used in the Renaissance alongside Latin translation of Greek works. It was used at the University of Montpellier until 1657 and continues in use today as the vademecum of Unani Tibb medicine.

## Sources

Conrad LI 1995 The Arab-Islamic medical tradition In: Lawrence I. Conrad LI, Neve M, Nutton V, et al (eds) The western medical tradition: 800 BC to AD 1800. Cambridge University Press, Cambridge.

Dictionary of scientific biography 1970–80 16 vols. Charles Scribner, New York.

Nasr SH 1976 Islamic science: an illustrated study. World of Islam Festival Publishing Company, Westerham, Kent.

Shah MH 1966 The general principles of Avicenna's cannon of medicine. Naveed Clinic, Karachi.

Siraisi NG 1987 Avicenna in Renaissance Italy: The canon and medical teaching in Italian universities after 1500. Princeton University Press.

Tschanz DW 2003 Arab roots of European medicine. Heart Views 4:69–80.

Ullmann M 1997 Islamic medicine. Edinburgh University Press, Edinburgh.

## Serapio the Younger, and other texts quoted in the primary sources Averroes, Johannitius, Mesue and Seth

Serapio was styled 'the younger' so as to avoid confusion with Serapio the elder, who was Yuhanna ibn Sarabiyun, one of the last exponents of classical Syriac medical writing and one of the influential authors for the development of medical theory and practice in 9th century Baghdad.

However, the author of *Liber Aggregatus in Medicinis Simplicibus* (Venice 1479) is thought to be Ibn Wafid, who wrote the *Kitab al-Adwiya al-mufrada* (book on simple drugs) which was translated into Latin by Abraham of Tortuso around 1290. Dating of the text is based on its similarity to the *Kitab al-Jami* of Ibn al-Baytar, dubbed chief of botanists in Egypt by the Sultan al-Kamil Muhammed. Ibn al-Baytar wrote this book some time before his death in Damascus in 1248. Fuchs used another translation of the *De Simplicibus Medicinis*, prepared by Otto Brunfels and published in Strasbourg in 1531.

Ullmann points out that the Arabic bibliographers have identified in excess of 100 authors who wrote about materia medica. Many of these works are compilations. Dioscorides is the greatest authority for these compilers, as is evident in our reading of the *Liber Aggregatus*.

Ibn Rushd, Abū al-Walīd Muḥammad ibn Aḥmad ibn Muḥammad, known in the medieval West as Averroes (1126–1198) was born in Cordoba and wrote many texts including commentaries on Aristotle and the Qur'an. Many of his works on philosophy and medicine were translated into Latin.

One of the texts translated by Constantine the African was the Isagogue, an overview of Galenic humoral theory. This was written by Johannitius, Human ibn Ishāq (d. 873 or 877). Human ibn Ishāq, a Nestorian Christian who settled in Baghdad, was the main translator of texts from Greek into Aramaic and Arabic.

John Mesue (777–857), Masawayh Iohannes Aben Mesue, Yūḥannā ibn Masawayh, Abū Zakarīyā', was born into a family of doctors in Gondishapur, western Iran. He was a Nestorian Christian and personal doctor to four caliphs in Baghdad. He wrote a number of monographs on topics including fevers, leprosy, melancholy, dietetics, eye diseases, and medical aphorisms. The name Mesuë, or filius Mesuë, is given to several Latin texts which were not all written by Mesue.

Simeon Seth (fl. 1070–1080) was master of the imperial palace in Constantinople and wrote *Syntagme de Alimentorum Facultatibus*, on the medicinal properties of foods. It was dedicated to the emperor Michael VII, who reigned from 1071 to 1078. He wrote a treatise on smell, taste and touch, and another on urine. An edition of *Syntagme de Alimentorum Facultatibus* in Greek and Latin was published in Basel, Switzerland in 1538.

## Sources

Conrad LI 1995 The Arab–Islamic medical tradition In: Lawrence I. Conrad L I, Neve M, Nutton V, et al (eds) The western medical tradition: 800 BC to AD 1800. Cambridge University Press, Cambridge.

Gutas D 1998 Greek thought, Arabic culture: the Graeco-Arabic translation movement in Baghdad and early 'Abbasid society. Routledge, London.

Meyer F, Trueblood EE, Heller IL 1999 The great herbal of Leonhart Fuchs vol 1, commentary. Stanford University Press, CA.

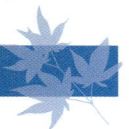

National Library of Medicine 2008 Islamic medical manuscripts. Online. Available: http://www.nlm.nih.gov/hmd/arabic/welcome.html 7 Sept 2009.

Pormann P E 2004 Yuhanna ibn Sarabiyun: further studies into the transmission of his works. Arabic Sciences and Philosophy 14: 233–262.

Riddle J 1985 Dioscorides on pharmacy and medicine. University of Texas, Austin.

Sadak MM 1979 Notes on the introduction and colophon of the Leiden Manuscript of Dioscorides' 'De materia medica'. International Journal of Middle Eastern Studies 10:345–354.

Ullmann M 1997 Islamic medicine. Edinburgh University Press, Edinburgh.

## Medieval medicine

Medieval medicine can be divided into two periods: that of the 6th to 9th centuries AD, dominated by post-Galenic writers, and that from the 10th to the 15th centuries when, though still strongly influenced by Galen, a Christianisation of medicine appears as monasteries became centres of learning and of herbal medicine.

An Old English translation of the *Herbal of Pseudo-Apuleius* was the first illustrated English herbal. Expanded to discuss 185 plants by the inclusion of the treatise on betony *Stachys officinalis* by Antonius Musa, physician to the Roman Emperor Augustus, and by some recipes from the pseudo-Dioscoridean *Ex Herbis Femininis*, it is one of four large medical texts surviving in the vernacular writings of Anglo-Saxon England. These writings are unique in northern Europe, and are the only surviving evidence of medical practice north of the Alps before 1100 AD. They are testimony to the importance of medicine to the Anglo-Saxons.

## Macer's herbal

Macer is the name on the title page of the first herbal printed by moveable type, the *De Viribus Herbarum* of 1477. Our edition dates from 1511. The book is an old Latin poem of over 2000 lines of hexameters which describes the healing powers of 77 plants. It is thought to have been written sometime between 849 and 1112 AD, probably in the 11th century. Details are given of the name of the herb and its temperature plus some recipes with occasional dosages. It was popular in the Middle Ages as the many surviving manuscripts testify. More than 100 of its verses found their way into the Salernitan *Regimen Sanitatis*.

The author, Macer Floridus, is a pseudonym in honour of Aemilius Macer, the Roman poet who died around 16 BC and who may also have composed a botanical work. The real writer is thought by some to be the poet Odo of Meung from the Loire region of France, a layman rather than a monk, and possibly a medical practitioner because of his occasional observations. The work, it is suggested, derives much information from Pliny, or else his material as it appeared in the writings of the Roman botanical writer Gargilius Martialis.

### Sources

Frick G (ed.) 1949 A Middle English translation of Macer Floridus De viribus herbarum. Almqvist & Wiksells, Uppsala.

Flood BP 1977 Pliny and the Medieval 'Macer' medical text. Journal of the History of Medicine, 32:395–402.

## The Salernitan herbal

The School of Salerno is commonly regarded as the earliest university of medieval Europe. At its origin in the second half of the 10th century in a main political and ecclesiastical centre of southern Italy, the doctors practicing there, many of whom were clerics, had already built up a reputation for their practical skills and successful treatments. The school achieved great importance as a centre of medical teaching and practice in the 11–13th centuries, with an established emphasis on practical instruction in contrast to the scholasticism of the later universities. Despite its relative decline after this time, the school continued to exist until 1812. Two famous names connected with the school are those of Constantine the African and Trotula.

Constantine was a Muslim from North Africa who arrived in Salerno perhaps as early as 1065, apparently, according to the account of a Salernitan doctor a century later, as a merchant on a visit to the Lombard prince of Salerno. Finding that they did not have a Latin medical literature, he returned to North Africa and 3 years later came back with a number of medical texts in Arabic, which he proceeded to translate. Constantine was the first important figure in the transmission of Greco-Arabic science to the Latin West. His works show signs of having been written in the Abbey of Monte Cassino, where, having become a Christian, he joined the Benedictine community. He died around 1087.

A group of his translations combined as the *Articella* formed the basis of university medical education throughout the Middle Ages. He translated two compendia: the *Viaticum*, from a work by Ibn al-Jazzar (d. 1009), and the *Pantegni*, his version of the *Kitab al-maliki* of Ali ibn al-Abbas (Haly Abbas, d. 994) and other works, including the Hippocratic *Aphorisms* and *Prognostica* and the treatise on acute diseases, both with the commentaries of Galen. In 1075 Salerno became a Norman duchy, which led to contacts in particular with Paris and, although there are conflicting views on the real nature of the school and the means of transmission of knowledge, the medical school influenced medical practice throughout Europe through commentaries on Galenic and other texts.

Trotula's name has passed down the centuries as that of a woman healer at Salerno who wrote a famous treatise on gynaecology. Recent scholarship has shown that the text is actually composed of three separate works, different in style, content and approach to theory and practice, on cosmetics, conditions of women and treatments of women.

What is considered to be the herbal of the School of Salerno is the manuscript *Circa Instans* of Matthaeus Platearius, possibly the son of Johannes Platearius, who died in 1161. Additions of other medicinal plants were made in the copying of the original manuscript, and later versions also included chapters on food from a 10th century treatise on dietetics by Ishaq Ibn Sulaiman al-Israeli (Isaac Judaeus) translated by Constantine the African as the *Liber Diaetarum universalium et particularium*.

One such later herbal containing these cumulative alterations is the 15th century French manuscript *Livre des Simples Medicines* (Codex Bruxellensis IV 1024), also known as the Secreta Salernitana, Livre des Secres de Salerne, Arboriste, Arbolayre and Grant Herbier en Francoys. It was translated into English as *The Grete Herball*, which was published in London in 1526.

## Sources

Dictionary of scientific biography (1970–80) 16 vols. Charles Scribner, New York.

Garica-Ballester L 1994 Introduction: practical medicine from Salerno to the Black Death. In: Garcia-Ballester L (ed.) Practical medicine from Salerno to the Black Death. Cambridge University Press, Cambridge, pp. 1–29.

Gottfried RS 1986 Doctors and medicine in medieval England 1340–1530. Princeton University Press.

Green M (ed.) 2001 The Trotula. University of Pennsylvania Press, Philadelphia.

Gutas D 1998 Greek thought, Arabic culture: the Graeco-Arabic translation movement in Baghdad and early 'Abbasid society. Routledge, London.

Kristeller PO 1945 The school of Salerno. Bulletin of the History of Medicine 17:138–194.

Nutton V 2003 Book review: Monica H. Green The Trotula: a medical compendium of women's medicine. Medical History 47:136–137.

Roberts E, Stearn W (trans.) 1984 Livre des simples medecines: Codex Bruxellensis IV.1024 a 15th century French herbal. De Schutter, Antwerp.

## Hildegard of Bingen

Hildegard was born in 1098 into an aristocratic family in Bernersheim near Alzey in Rheinhessen. At the age of 8, she joined the Benedictine cloister at nearby Disibodenberg, which had been founded in the 7th century by the Irish monk Disibod. Hildegard became a nun at the age of 16 and was elected abbess in 1136. In 1141, although she had had visions before, these became grander and filled with significance, which she began to describe in her first book *Scivias* (Know The Ways). After 1151 she founded her own convent at Rupertsberg. From 1151 to 1158 she worked on the *Liber Simplicus Medicinae*, comprising nine books on plants, metals, animals, reptiles, diet, stones and humours. She had a deep faith in the value of the parts of God's creation. Her works were not available for many years but indirectly influenced German books of household management. Further editions of her work have been discovered in the 1980s.

The text which we used is a translation of an edition published in 1882 of a 15th century manuscript held in Paris, Cod. 6952 and containing 230 plant medicines.

## Sources

Adamson MW 1995 A reevaluation of Saint Hildegard's physica in light of the latest manuscript finds. In: Schleissner MR (ed.) 1995 Manuscript sources of medieval medicine. Garland, New York, pp 55–80.

Strehlow W, Hertzka G 1988 Hildegard of Bingen's medicine. Bear, Santa Fe, New Mexico.

## The Myddfai physicians

We include another collection of vernacular writings from the British Isles, namely those attributed to the family of healers famous for their cures in the Myddfai region of South Wales.

The English translation of *Meddygon Myddfai* contains three sections: Book 1 is a translation of a Welsh manuscript transcribed at the end of the 14th century, Book 2 is a collection of medical texts handed down in the family and transcribed before 1743, and Book 3 is an account of the legend of LLyn-y-van-vach.

Book 1 formed part of the *Red Book of Hergest* (*LLyfr Coch Hergest*, Jesus MS 111), a substantial collection of Welsh literature and poetry and European material such as Aristotle's advice to Alexander. The texts on medicine are thought to have been transcribed not long after 1382. The scribe was Hywel Fychan ap Hywel Goch of Buellt, working with two assistants, and the compilation was made for Hopcyn ap Tomas (1330 to after 1403), who was a patron of bards and collector of manuscripts. This is a mixture of short treatises compiled for practical purposes of the sort first written in Greek in the 4th century and translated into Latin in the 6th century. There are sections, for instance, on the four elements and humours, the importance of knowledge of the 12 signs of the zodiac, seven enemies of the eye, and fevers and their treatment.

The first paragraph of Book 1 states that it was written by Rhiwallon, physician to Rhys Gryg (d. 1233), king of Deheubarth, Southwest Wales. Rhiwallon had three sons Cadwgan, Gruffudd (Griffith) and Einoin, who became doctors, and Book 2 claims that there was an unbroken descent in Myddfai from Rhiwallon, via his son Einoin to John Jones, surgeon (1697–1793). There are records of medical services being provided by freeholders in Myddfai to the Lord of Llandovery.

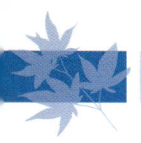

Book 2 is a collection of medical texts collected by Howel the physician, a descendant of Einion, translated from a Welsh version held by John Jones, surgeon. It was copied by William Bona in 1743 and translated into English by John Pughe, surgeon, on behalf of the Welsh Manuscript Society in 1861.

The editors of the text append a story to account for the medical knowledge of the family. The legend of Llyn-y-van-vach which follows was written down in 1841 by William Rees of Tonn near Llandovery using the oral statements of three local people. In the late 1100s a man was looking after cattle near Myddfai when he saw a beautiful woman on the lake. He offered her baked bread, which she refused and then dived under the water. On the second day, he offered her unbaked bread, which was again refused, so his mother suggested moderately baked bread, and on the third day she approached the land and accepted his offer. Then she dived back into the water and reappeared with her sister and her father, who stated that the man could marry her as long as he could distinguish her from her sister. This appeared impossible until one woman moved her foot and he recalled that their sandals were tied in different ways. The father warned that if he struck his bride three times without cause, she would return to the lake, taking back her dowry of cattle, goats and sheep. The couple prospered and had three sons but he struck her unintentionally whilst preparing to go to a christening, then at a wedding feast and lastly at a funeral gathering. She promptly called her cattle and disappeared back into the lake. The sons used to go to the lake in the hope of meeting their mother and one day she appeared and told the eldest son, Rhiwallon, that his mission was to benefit mankind by healing all manner of disorders. She gave him a bag of medical prescriptions and instructions for the preservation of health. His mother appeared again, and while walking back towards their home pointed out herbs which grew nearby and their virtues.

## Sources

Cameron ML 1993 Anglo-Saxon medicine. Cambridge University Press, Cambridge.

Huws D 2000 Medieval Welsh manuscripts. University of Wales Press, Cardiff.

Owen ME 1975 Meddygon Myddfai: a preliminary survey of some Medieval medical writings in Welsh. Studia Celtica 10–11:210–233.

Pughe J 1861, 1993 The physicians of Myddvai; Meddygon Myddfai. Llanerch Publishers, Felinfach.

Thomas PW, Smith DM, Luft D 2007 Rhyddiaith Gymraeg 1350–1425. Online. Available: http://www.rhyddiaithganoloesol.caerdydd.ac.uk 17 May 2008.

Van Arsdall A 2002 Medieval herbal remedies: the Old English Herbarium and Anglo-Saxon medicine. Routledge, London.

Voigts L 1979 Anglo-Saxon plant remedies and the Anglo-Saxons. Isis 70:250–268.

Welsh Biography Online 2007 Hopcyn ap Tomas. Online. Available: http://yba.llgc.org.uk 17 May 2008.

# RENAISSANCE HERBALS

## Leonhart Fuchs

Fuchs was born on 17 January 1501 at Wemding in Bavaria. At the age of 15 he was studying for an arts degree at the University of Erfurt. He went on to take a medical degree at Ingolstadt University and worked as a doctor in Munich before returning to Ingolstadt in 1526 to take up the chair of medicine. Two years later he was called to Ansbach by the fellow protestant Prince Georg, the Margrave of Brandenburg, to set up a protestant university in the town. The plan never materialized but Fuchs remained the Margrave's personal physician, enhancing his reputation by successfully treating sufferers of the sweating sickness (the 'English Sweat') which was sweeping through Germany in 1529. He was then called to Tübingen by Ulrich, Duke of Wurttemberg, to reform its university along humanistic lines, and spent the rest of his life there, as professor of medicine, until his death in 1566.

Fuchs has become known as one of the three founding fathers of German botany, alongside Hieronymus Bock (latinised as Tragus) and Otto Brunfels. All three authors shared a protestant faith. Fuchs founded one of the first German botanical gardens, where he offered botanical study for students. He did not travel to further his studies, being interested rather in native German plants, but he took part in the rapidly developing network of scholars throughout Europe who shared their knowledge and exchanged plants. Religious beliefs were not always accommodated and Fuchs and Mattioli clashed across the religious divide on academic matters.

As a humanist and man of the Renaissance, Fuchs wanted to draw from what he perceived as the original well of knowledge on plants and medicine, the Greeks. In Tübingen, he opposed the continuing use of Avicenna. His first publication in 1530, *Errata Recentiorum Medicorum* (Errors of Recent Doctors), advocated a return to the use of simples rather than the compound mixtures of arcane ingredients in medieval prescribing. His great work is the herbal, *De Historia Stirpium Commentarii Insignes* of 1542, translated into German, Dutch and English. Here Fuchs tried to identify the plants described by classical authors. He covers 400 wild and 100 domesticated plants, all medicinal, drawn mainly from Dioscorides. For each he provided their various names, a description and the place and time that they may be found.

He added the plant's temperament, its degree of heat, cold, dryness and moisture in the system first proposed by Galen, and its medicinal properties according to Dioscorides, Pliny and Galen. This was augmented by statements from Simeon Seth, from more recent sources and current medical practice or occasionally his own comments. Accompanying the text are 512 woodcut illustrations of plants of very high technical quality by Plantin, of Antwerp, which set new standards in book illustration.

## Sources

Fuchs L 1545 (1980 reprint) Holzschnitte die historischen Taschenbücher. Konrad Kölbl, Grünwald bei München.

Kusukawa S 1996 Leonhart Fuchs on the importance of pictures. Journal of the History of Ideas 58:403–427.

Pavord A 2005 The naming of names: the search for order in the world of plants. Bloomsbury, London.

Reeds KM 1976 Renaissance humanism and botany. Annals of Science 33:519–542.

Sangwine E 1978 The private libraries of Tudor doctors. Journal of the History of Medicine and Allied Sciences 33:167–184.

## Pietro Andrea Gregorio Mattioli

Mattioli was born in Siena, Italy on 12 March 1501 and followed his father into medicine, receiving his degree at the University of Padua in 1523. While developing his skills in surgery in Perugia and Rome (some credit him with the first description of syphilitic buboes of the groin), he made direct observations of herbs and plants, and developed a specific interest in the identification of medicinal herbs in Greek and Roman texts. After Rome was sacked in 1527, Mattioli became personal physician to the bishop of Trento until 1539, when he was appointed city physician at Gorizia in northeast Italy.

In 1544 Mattioli published in Venice an Italian version of Dioscorides' *De Materia Medica*, based on a Latin translation from the Greek of Dioscorides by Jean Ruel published in Paris in 1516, with a commentary, the *Di Pedacio Dioscoride Anazarbeo libri cinque dell'istoria e material medicinale, tradotto in lingua volgare italiana da M.P. Andrea Matthioli sanese medico, con amplissime annotationi et censure*, to help doctors and apothecaries identify the herbs described. These medical and botanical aims of the commentary were unusual for the time. The book was immediately successful and made its author famous. Mattioli then published a new version in Latin in 1554, *Commentarii in Libros Sex Pedacii Dioscoridis Anazarbei*, with synonyms of plant names in different languages, a special commentary and accurate illustrations which were reproductions of his own drawings or elaborations of those of other authors, notably Luca Ghini. New editions with commentaries incorporating comments from other botanists and criticizing other authorities made the book a big seller. During his long lifetime, Mattioli added new plant descriptions and depictions to each subsequent edition as new specimens and seeds were received from ambassadors and other contacts outside Europe. His *Commentarii* continued to be printed regularly into the 18th century.

Mattioli was invited to act as physician at the court of the Holy Roman Emperor Ferdinand I and he later served Maximilian II. Such a wealthy patron gave him many contacts, including the ambassador in Constantinople, Ogier Ghiselin de Busbecq, the man responsible for the removal of the Juliana Anicia Codex from Constantiniple. Mattioli consulted this in preparing his 1568 edition. He died of plague in Trento in 1577.

## Sources

Findlen P 1999 The formation of a scientific community: natural history in sixteenth-century Italy. In: Grafton A, Siraisi N (eds) 1999 Natural particulars: nature and the disciplines in Renaissance Europe. MIT Press, Cambridge, MA.

Dictionary of scientific biography 1970–80 16 vols. Charles Scribner, New York.

Pavord A 2005 The naming of names: the search for order in the world of plants. Bloomsbury, London.

## William Turner

Turner was born in Morpeth, Northumberland in around 1508 and educated there. He studied at Pembroke Hall, Cambridge from 1525 and graduated MA in 1533. His education was influenced by humanist ideals and study of the Greek New Testament and Latin texts. In 1538 he published the *Libellus de Re Herbaria*, his only book written in Latin. This was republished in an expanded form in English, the *Names of Herbes* in 1548 and joined the English names of plants to the list of names appearing in the European herbals. Turner was aware that most 16th century medical practitioners, herbalists and apothecaries had no knowledge of Latin and so could not read a herbal like Fuchs' to access detailed observations on the appearance and habitat of medicinal plants. Other herbals written in English, such as Banckes' herbal of 1525 and the *Grete Herball* of 1526, were translations of earlier medieval works.

He left England in 1540, travelling in Germany, France, Switzerland and Italy. He studied under Luca Ghini in Bologna and obtained his MD in medicine either in Bologna or Ferrara, Italy. On his way back he visited Conrad Gesner in Zurich, with whom he was to have a lifelong correspondence, and began to practice medicine in Holland, remaining for 4 years in East Friesland as personal physician to the Earl of Emden. Turner was a fervent Protestant and during his period in exile wrote two books opposing 'Romish' practices, which were banned and publicly burned in 1546.

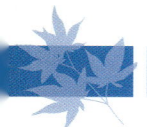

Turner returned to England on the death of Henry VIII in 1547 to practice medicine and divinity and was doctor and chaplain to the Lord Protector, Duke of Somerset at Syon House until 1549 when Somerset was arrested. Turner was appointed Dean of Wells Cathedral in 1551 but when the Catholic Mary I became Queen, Turner once again went into exile, and travelled in Germany between 1553 and 1558. On the succession to the throne of Elizabeth I in 1558, he returned to England and resumed the post of Dean of Wells Cathedral in 1561, where he courted opprobrium for his opposition to priestly vestments. He died in London in 1568 and is buried at St Olave's, Hart Street.

*A New Herball* was published in three parts, the first in London in 1551, the second in Cologne, Germany in 1562 and an addendum in 1568. Turner provided the first clear and systematic survey of English plants, including around 400 woodcuts, mainly those used in Fuch's *De Historia Stirpium*, and detailed observations from his own field studies. The published third part contained a revision of the first two parts.

Turner has been called the 'Father of English Botany' as his education led him to introduce the study of plants in a scientific manner in the English language. Two hundred and thirty-eight native British plants are described and, in common with European writers, he quotes directly from sources such as Galen. The religious and political turmoil of the time led to his work being published in Cologne and it was neither translated nor reprinted until the facsimile edition of 1995.

## Sources

Dictionary of national biography. Oxford University Press, Oxford. Online. Available: http://www.oxforddnb.com.

Chapman GTL, Tweedle MN (eds) 1995 A new herball by William Turner, part I, vol 1. Cambridge University Press, Cambridge.

Chapman GTL, McCombie F, Wesencraft A (eds) 1995 A new herball by William Turner, parts II & III, vol 2. Cambridge University Press, Cambridge.

Pavord A 2005 The naming of names: the search for order in the world of plants. Bloomsbury, London.

Sangwine E 1978 The private libraries of Tudor doctors. Journal of the History of Medicine and Allied Sciences 33:167–184.

## Rembert Dodoens

Rembert van Joenckema was the real name of the author of the *Cruydeboek* of 1554 but he was known to an English readership as Rembert Dodoens, author of *A New Herbal* or *Historie of Plants* translated by Henry Lyte, published in London in 1619. He was born in Mechelen in The Netherlands, now Malines in Belgium, on 29 June 1516 and died at Leiden in The Netherlands on 10 March 1585.

Dodoens graduated as a licentiate in medicine from the catholic University of Louvain, Belgium in 1535. He travelled extensively, as was the custom, through France, Italy and Germany. He worked on a Latin and Greek text of Paul of Aegina published in Basel in 1546.

In 1548 he returned to the place of his birth to work as one of three municipal physicians, and began work on the *Cruydeboek*. It was finished by 1552 and published early in 1554 by Jean Vanderloe of Antwerp. His most important scientific work was the *Stirpium historiae pemptades sex sive libri XXX* of 1583. A translation of this book formed the basis of Gerard's herbal. In 1574, he took up an appointment as physician to the Emperor Maximilian II in Vienna, where Charles de l'Ecluse was in charge of the Imperial Botanic Garden. He remained there as physician to Maximilian's successor, Rudolph II, until 1580, when he attempted to return to Malines but because of political turmoil, he lived in Cologne and then Antwerp.

Dodoens' last appointment in 1582 was in the Faculty of Medicine at the University of Leiden. The famous botanical gardens there were created 2 years after his death in 1585 by Charles de l'Ecluse.

## Sources

Dictionary of scientific biography 1970–80 16 vols. Charles Scribner, New York.

Pavord A 2005 The naming of names: the search for order in the world of plants. Bloomsbury, London.

Reeds KM 1991 Botany in medieval and Renaissance universities. Garland, New York.

Van Meerbeeck PJ 1841, 1980 Recherches historiques et critiques sur la via et les ouvrages de Rembert Dodoens. HES, Utrecht.

## Jean Bauhin

Jean Bauhin, the 'German Pliny', was born in Basel, Switzerland on 12 February 1541, the oldest of seven children. His father was Jean Bauhin, a physician to Margaret of Navarre until exiled from France through religious persecution. His younger brother, Gaspard, compiled the *Pinax theatri botanici* (1623).

Bauhin was educated in Basel with visits to foreign universities, including Montpellier in 1561–1562. There is no evidence that he received an MD from the Montpellier school of medicine in 1562, but in 1563 he established himself in medical practice in Lyon, where he was soon treating plague victims. Driven into exile like his father, in 1568 he moved to Geneva, where he continued in medical practice. He spent a short period teaching in Basel before being appointed physician to Duke Frederick, ruler of Wurttemberg-Montbeliard in 1571.

Bauhin's main interest in his youth was botany, which benefited from the influence of his teacher and friend, Conrad Gesner. Gesner was compiling a *Historia plantarum*, an intended companion to his already famous *Historia animalium*, and up until his death in 1565 he corresponded with Bauhin. Bauhin sent him plant specimens which Bauhin had come across on his travels and accompanied him in 1561 on a novel study of alpine flora in the Rhaetian Alps. Gesner sent Bauhin on to Tübingen to study with Leonhard Fuchs. Somewhere around 1564 Bauhin planted his first garden in Lyon with the collaboration of Jacques D'Alechamps, the recognized author of the anonymous *Historia plantarum generalis* of 1586. Bauhin's own herbal, the *Historia plantarum universalis*, was published posthumously, 6 years after his death at Montbeliard on 26 October 1613.

The full three-volume text was eventually financed and published in 1650–1651. This contained concise and accurate descriptions and synonyms for 5226 plants, mainly from Europe. The number of species covered, a massive increase on the 240 plants described by Brunfels, was only matched by his brother Gaspard's *Pinax*, which contained 6000 plants but was designed as a complete dictionary of plant names rather than as detailed account of each plant.

## Sources

Dictionary of scientific biography 1970–80 16 vols. Charles Scribner, New York.

Dictionnaire historique et biographique de la Suisse 1921–34 8 vols. Neuchatel.

Jorio M (ed) 2002 Dictionnaire historique de la Suisse. Editions Gilles Attinger, Hauterive.

## John Gerard

Gerard was born at or near Nantwich in Cheshire in 1545, educated at a local grammar school, apprenticed at the age of 16 to a barber-surgeon in London and admitted to the Company of Barber-Surgeons on 9th December 1569. He travelled aboard a merchant ship, presumably as its surgeon, around the countries bordering the Baltic sea. This was his only foreign journey and on his return he settled in London, doubtless to work as a barber-surgeon. He moved up the ranks within the Barber-Surgeons' Company and was elected master in 1608.

Gerard's interest in the cultivation of medicinal plants led in 1577 to his becoming superintendent of the gardens of William Cecil, Lord Burleigh, at the Strand in London and at Theobald's in Hertfordshire. He held this position until 1598 and from 1586 until 1603 or 1604 he was curator of the physic garden in Chelsea belonging to the College of Physicians in London. He had his own garden in Holborn and issued a catalogue in 1596 of the 1039 plants he had acquired and cultivated there so had substantial practical knowledge of medicinal plants.

His *Herball* or *Generall Historie of Plantes* was published in 1597. The herbal, occupying 1392 pages plus introduction and index, is divided into three books. Book 1 covers monocotyledons. Book 2 takes up most of the rest of the text in describing of herbs used as food, medicine and perfumes. The final book of 315 pages contains a miscellany of trees, shrubs and other plants used for medicine. His vivid use of words to describe plants, familiar or never before seen by his readers, made his herbal accessible and it was widely distributed thanks to the growing number of booksellers in England at this time.

There is debate over the 1597 version as Gerard recognized in his preface to the *Herball* that there were faults, some due to his 'limited erudition that someone of greater learning might later correct', but he hoped the reader would take well his good intention in publishing. Yet after his death and on account of the herbal his reputation was tarnished with the accusation of plagiarism. The publisher of the herbal, John Norton, had asked Matthias de l'Obel to check the edition before printing and de l'Obel discovered many errors in the text and the naming of the plant illustrations, which he dealt with as best he could. A further concern is the claim that much of Gerard's work was based on a translation by Robert Priest, a London doctor, of Dodoens' *Stirpium historiae pemptades sex*. Priest died in 1596 or 1597, and this claim does not detract from value of the text and will be finally solved by a critical edition of the texts.

The text which we use is the 1633 second edition, revised and edited by Thomas Johnson, which has been regularly reprinted. Johnson was an avid botanist and member of the Society of Apothecaries, and inserted new illustrations from the stock of Plantin, a printer in Antwerp (Museum Plantin-Moretus 2010). Johnson adds his own comments in a structured way, which helps the reader to understand the debate over the identity of plants in pre-Linnean botany. In a legal document concerning a lease to Gerard of a garden adjoining Somerset House by Anne of Denmark, consort of James I, he was described as 'herbarist' to James I. He died in February 1612 and was buried in Holborn.

## Sources

Arber AR 1986 Herbals, their origins and evolution: a chapter in the history of botany 1470–1670, 3rd edn. Cambridge University Press, Cambridge.

Dictionary of national biography. Oxford University Press, Oxford. Online. Available: http://www.oxforddnb.com.

Dictionary of scientific biography 1970–80 16 vols. Charles Scribner, New York.

Harkness DE 2007 The jewel house: Elizabethan London and the scientific revolution. Yale University Press, New Haven.

Museum Plantin-Moretus 2010 Online. Available: http://museum.antwerpen.be/plantin_Moretus/index_eng.html

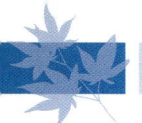

Pavord A 2005 The naming of names: the search for order in the world of plants. Bloomsbury, London.

Sangwine E 1978 The private libraries of Tudor doctors. Journal of the History of Medicine and Allied Sciences 33:167–184.

## John Parkinson

John Parkinson was born 1567 and was apprenticed for 8 years to a London apothecary, Francis Slater, a member of the Grocers' Company. He gained his freedom of that Company in 1593 but felt that the importance of an apothecary's work was not sufficiently recognized. He strongly supported the setting up of a Society of Apothecaries, which was formed in December 1617, and advocated the drawing up of a schedule of all medicines which should be stocked by an apothecary. He was also one of five apothecaries consulted by the College of Physicians during the compilation of the first *Pharmacopoeia Londinensis* (1618). He became apothecary to James I.

He devoted much of his time to tending his garden in Long Acre. In 1629 he published his first work *Paradisi in Sole Paradisus Terrestris* or *A Garden of All Sorts of Pleasant Flowers which our English ayre will permit to be noursed up with a Kitchen Garden and an Orchard*, the first book published on English gardening and which included descriptions of almost a thousand plants.

There had been an intention to add a fourth section on medicinal simples to the three topics of his first book but it took him years to write the monumental *Theatrum Botanicum* of 1640, which describes over 3800 plants in more than 1700 pages. Here Parkinson drew on the plant authorities of his day, including the incorporation of Gaspard Bauhin's synonyms of plants from his *Pinax* and an acknowledged use of the papers of his colleague Matthias de L'Obel. Plants were divided into 17 'tribes', based partly on their medicinal qualities and partly on habitat. Parkinson died in the summer of 1650 and was buried at St Martin-in-the-Fields.

### Sources

Dictionary of national biography. Oxford University Press, Oxford. Online. Available: http://www.oxforddnb.com.

Sangwine E 1978 The private libraries of Tudor doctors, Journal of the History of Medicine and Allied Sciences 33:167–184.

## Nicholas Culpeper

Nicholas Culpeper was born on 18 October 1616, probably in Ockley, Surrey, into the well-established Culpeper family. However, his father, also Nicholas, rector of Ockley, died 19 days before he was born and the family made a settlement on his mother Mary to provide for his future education. Mary took the young Nicholas to live with her father, the Reverend Attersoll, the rector of the parish of St Margaret's in Isfield, where he grew up learning the names of the plants of the surrounding Sussex fields and hedgerows. He attended a free-school in the area and then was admitted to Cambridge University in 1632. It seems by this time that he had fallen in love with the well-born daughter of a wealthy Sussex family and in 1634 he left to elope abroad with her until their parents could be reconciled to the match. On the way to this secret meeting the young woman was struck by lightning and killed.

Culpeper was devastated by this tragedy and did not return to university. He must have shown some interest in medicine because his grandfather then apprenticed him to a Mr White, an apothecary, near Temple Bar, in London, with whom Culpeper began to learn the trade. Just over a year later, White's business failed and Culpeper had to be found another master. Francis Drake in Threadneedle Street agreed to have him alongside his existing apprentice Samuel Leadbetter. When Drake died in February 1639 Leadbetter had just become licensed, and he took Culpeper, who was now deep in the study of medicine, into the business with him.

These were stormy times, with the King and parliament at loggerheads and heading towards civil war. Apothecaries meanwhile were diagnosing and treating those who could not afford doctors and resisting attempts by the College of Physicians to suppress this practice. Although the College of Physicians had few members, they attempted to enforce their monopoly on medical treatment in London. Culpeper himself, between 1642 and 1643, was tried and acquitted of witchcraft and twice Leadbetter was ordered to remove him from his shop. Culpeper was a staunch republican and during this year fought in the battle of Newbury, where he received a musket shot in the chest, a wound which probably hastened his early death at the age of 37 from consumption. In 1640 Culpeper had married 15-year-old Alice Field and through this union came into enough money to leave Leadbetter's shop in 1644 and set himself up as a physician in poor and unfashionable Spitalfields, East London, where he remained until the end of his life, treating the poor and the uneducated.

At the end of the war Culpeper was apparently commissioned to render from Latin into English the Pharmacopoeia of the College of Physicians. He produced *A Physicall Directory* or *A Translation of the London Dispensatory* in 1649, peppered with his own acerbic comments critical of the privilege and avarice of the doctors and with enough information to allow a literate audience to make up the medicines for themselves, thus challenging the monopoly of apothecaries. His strong puritan beliefs had been revolutionized during the civil war – he supported the execution of King Charles in the year of his first publication and he was attacked in print for his rebellious, godless stance and for a book, the pages of which were only 'fit to wipe ones breeches withall'. The translation, however, brought immediate fame and he devoted the remainder of his life to other translations of the leading continental works on medicine of the time, with the purpose of empowering his readers to be able to treat their own ills. He added original works of his own, such as *A Directory for Midwives* and *Semiotica Uranica* or *An Astrological Judgement of Diseases from the Decumbiture of the Sick*, both in 1651, and his herbal *The English Physitian* in 1652, which remains in print today as *Culpeper's Herbal*, as well as annual ephemeredes in the early 1650s.

In subsequent editions of *A Physicall Directory*, Culpeper added a *Key to Galen and Hippocrates, their Method of Physick*, while his translation of the College's new edition of the Pharmacopoeia, *Pharmacopoeia Londinensis* or *A London Dispensatory* of 1653, contained *An Astrologo-physical Discourse*. The book had become a self-help manual of medicine for his readers, through which he sought an end to the monopoly of power by doctors. Culpeper's writings taught the basis of Galenic medicine but rejected the authority of old texts in favour of experiment and observation as a means to proper reasoning in physic. He seems to have been influenced by English Paracelsianism and saw the use of astrology in diagnosing and in identifying the appropriate medicines as the key to the use of his herbal, where almost every medicine described is linked to one of the seven planets and sometimes to the signs of the zodiac.

Culpeper's legacy is stronger as a medical educator than as a physician. His political and religious aims endeared him to the poorer classes, while his revolutionary stance, attacks on privilege and monopoly, and his insistence on the importance of occult practices guaranteed him enemies in print long after his death.

### Sources

Dictionary of national biography. Oxford University Press, Oxford. Online. Available: http://www.oxforddnb.com.

Tobyn G 1997 Culpeper's medicine. Element Books, Shaftesbury, Dorset.

Woolley B 2003 The herbalist: Nicholas Culpeper and the fight for medical freedom. Harper Collins, London.

## THE EIGHTEENTH CENTURY

## John Quincy

John Quincy was an apothecary. He wrote or translated 11 works, the most famous of which were his *Pharmacopoeia Officinalis & Extemporanea* or *A Compleat English Dispensatory*, first published in 1718, and his medical dictionary *Lexicon Physico-medicum* of 1719.

Quincy's *Dispensatory* went through 12 editions before being extensively revised in 1749 by William Lewis, who had translated in English the *Edinburgh Pharmacopoeia* the year before. Lewis' *The New Dispensatory … Intended as a Correction and Improvement of Quincy* was in its turn improved upon, to become *The Edinburgh New Dispensatory* of 1786 and later *The London Dispensatory* of 1811. The first *British Pharmacopoeia* in 1864 was heavily based on *The Edinburgh Dispensatory*. Quincy's translation of Santorio's *Medicina Statica*, for which he was awarded an MD from Edinburgh in 1712, was itself republished as late as 1842.

Quincy's writings reflect his support of contemporary iatrophysical theories based on the mechanics and scientific experiments of his day to promote the good health of humanity. He rejected the Galenic notion of spirits residing in the body and was vehemently against any form of medical quackery or empiricism. Likewise he deprecated the royal touch for scrofula. His *Compleat English Dispensatory* was divided into four parts: a theory of pharmacy and its several processes; a description of the officinal simples with their medicinal virtues and Galenical and chemical preparations; the officinal compositions for apothecaries to dispense; and a number of extemporaneous prescriptions, some of which enjoyed long-lasting popularity, for the treatment of various diseases. Quincy grouped the simples into nervous, stomachics, strengtheners, balsamics, diuretics, diaphoretics, emetics and cathartics, sternutatories, narcotics, coolers, topics and miscellaneous.

His death is dated by his publications and is reckoned to be in 1722.

### Sources

Dictionary of national biography. Oxford University Press, Oxford. Online. Available: http://www.oxforddnb.com.

Howard-Jones N 1951 John Quincy MD apothecary and iatrophysical writer. Journal of the History of Medicine and Allied Sciences, 6:149–175.

## Joseph Miller

Joseph Miller was an apothecary and lecturer in botany at the Chelsea Physick Garden, London. He was appointed Master there in 1738 and continued to work for the Society of Apothecaries, to which the garden belonged, until his death in 1748. In 1722 he published *Botanicum Officinale* or *A Compendious Herbal*. This herbal was heavily drawn upon by Elizabeth Blackwell, author of the *A Curious Herbal* of 1735 for the medicinal properties of the plants she depicted and described, but is otherwise uncelebrated.

### Sources

Madge B 2001 Elizabeth Blackwell – the forgotten herbalist? Health Information and Libraries Journal 18:144–152.

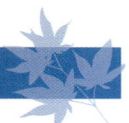

Field H 1820 Memoirs historical and illustrative of the botanick garden at Chelsea. R Gilbert, London.

## William Cullen

William Cullen was born in Hamilton, Scotland on 15 April 1710. His father was an attorney and agent to the Duke of Hamilton and, after university study in Glasgow, he was apprenticed to John Paisley, a Glasgow surgeon apothecary. Cullen went to London in 1729 and the next year was appointed surgeon on a boat bound for the West Indies. He returned north in 1732 and in the years 1734–1736, thanks to a small legacy on the death of his father, Cullen was able to attend classes at the recently founded medical school at the University of Edinburgh, where he became interested in chemistry. He then set up in practice in Hamilton and received the Duke as both patient and then patron.

In order to practice solely as a physician he acquired an MD from Glasgow University in 1740 and moved to Glasgow in 1744. He practiced medicine and lectured on medicine and then from 1747 was appointed to the first independent lectureship in chemistry in Britain. He was appointed professor of chemistry at Edinburgh University in 1755 and this began his illustrious career in Edinburgh, where his private practice also thrived. His courses of lectures continued until his death in early 1790. His lectures in materia medica at Edinburgh were so well received that an unauthorized printing of his lecture notes was made, forcing him to publish them himself in 1773. He was active in the Royal College of Physicians of Edinburgh, of which he was a fellow from 1756 and president from 1773 to 1775, including working on a revision of the Edinburgh pharmacopoeia.

Cullen's lectures endeavoured to develop a systematic approach, showing how signs and symptoms at the bedside related to physiology, and developed a rational basis for prescribing the herbal and chemical medicines of his day. He put the nervous system, then an exciting new area of scientific medicine, at the centre, suggesting that all diseases could be described to some extent as nervous in origin. He introduced the term 'neurosis' into medicine, which through his published works and their translations established the concept across Europe and America.

### Sources

Crellin JK 1971 William Cullen: his calibre as a teacher, and an unpublished introduction to his *A treatise on the material medica*, London, 1773. Medical History 15: 79–87.

Dictionary of national biography. Oxford University Press, Oxford. Online. Available: http://www.oxforddnb.com.

Dictionary of scientific biography 1970–80 16 vols. Charles Scribner, New York.

## John Hill

John Hill, physician and actor, came from Lincolnshire. His father had a Cambridge medical degree and worked as a theologian. Little is known of his early life before London apothecary Edward Angier took him on as an apprentice in 1730–1731. Hill maintained a lifelong interest in botany, which competed throughout with an equal passion for the theatre. Hill ran an apothecary shop near the Strand in London and accepted commissions from wealthy patrons around the country to collect plant specimens while at the same time furthering his acting career.

In 1743 Hill returned to London and to his business and, now settled in Westminster, he became acquainted with significant naturalists and fellows of the Royal Society, while promoting his interest in natural science. This propelled him into a life of prolific writing in the course of which he obtained an MD degree from the University of St Andrews. He edited journals and wrote books on acting and on science among a variety of other topics. His *The Useful Family Herbal* came out in 1754 and was republished the next year along with his *British Herbal*. In 1759 he brought out his *Flora Britannica*, the first Linnaean flora of Britain, and was encouraged by his patron Lord Bute to begin work on his magnum opus, *The Vegetable System*, which ran to 26 volumes by the time of his death in 1775. This brought him international recognition, including his presentation by Linnaeus at the Swedish Court, from where he obtained a knighthood at the end of his life.

Other publications appeared, including *Cautions Against the Immoderate Use of Snuff*, which associated tobacco with cancerous growths. Hill spent much money on producing his various works, some of which he recouped by manufacturing and exporting herbal medicines such as 'tincture of valerian', on the virtues of which he had already published a separate work, and 'essence of water dock'.

Hill continued his links with the theatrical world for a time but he was a controversial figure and made many enemies. He died at his home in Golden Square, London, on 22 November 1775.

### Sources

Dictionary of national biography. Oxford University Press, Oxford. Online. Available: http://www.oxforddnb.com.

# 19TH CENTURY BRITISH

## Albert Isiah Coffin

Coffin was born in Ohio, USA. He practised the methods of Samuel Thomson (1769–1843), who patented a self-help system of herbal medicine which was very popular in pre-civil war America. By 1834 he was a Thomsonian agent in Ohio. He came to Britain in 1839, firstly to London but then lived in Hull, Leeds and then Manchester from 1847. Coffin was a salesman but he was responsible for a medical self-help movement which served to promote the health and well-being of working people, particularly in Northern England. He was in partnership with Thomas Harle, a qualified doctor, in Manchester and also in London from 1850. He published journals and *A Treatise on Midwifery* and *The Diseases of Women and Children* in 1849. *The Botanic Guide to Health* discusses medical theories briefly, and then gives a description of herbs grouped by actions and sections on the treatment of diseases with accounts of successful cases. Coffin was a firm believer in temperance and his book includes practical advice on health and diet. *Skelton's Botanic Recorder* (1855) gives accounts of his public disputes with other herbalists partly because he sought a monopoly on the importation of the American herbs used, and partly because he disagreed with other Thomsonian herbalists, such as John Skelton, who sought to widen the materia medica and to improve the education of herbalists.

The text used is the 49th edition, which is undated but the preface states that the edition has been revised and corrected and that over 40 000 books had been sold. It includes testimonials for the 35th edition in 1864. Coffin died in 1866, so the 49th edition may be a copy of the 35th edition.

### Sources

Coffin AI 1845, 1864 Botanic guide to health. Haynes, Coffin, London.

Haller JS 2000 The people's doctors: Samuel Thomson and the American botanical movement, 1790–1860. Southern Illinois University Press.

Skelton J 1955 Skelton's botanic recorder. Josiah Coplestone, Leeds.

## William Fox

According to the 22nd edition of his book, William Fox established his business in 1840. He is listed in the *White's Directory for Sheffield* of 1852 as herbalist and agent to Dr Coffin. The 19th and 22nd editions were edited by his son Alfred Russell Fox, Botanical Pharmacy, 8 Castle Street, Sheffield. The 24th edition of *The Model Family Botanic Guide* is dated 1932 and states that 250 000 copies had been sold since the first edition. In the introduction, the medical theories of and life of Samuel Thomson are discussed, followed by a description of herbs grouped by actions and sections on the treatment of diseases. It ends with a price list of herbs obtainable from the Botanical Pharmacy.

### Sources

Fox W 1920 The working-man's model family botanic guide to health, 22nd edn. W Fox and Sons, Sheffield.

## William Cook

William Cook was a significant figure in the development of education for herbal practitioners in 19th century America. He had originally been trained as an eclectic at the time before eclecticism and physio-medicalism divided, and taught at the Botanico-Medical College in Cincinatti in the 1850s. The neo-Thomsonians began to describe themselves as physio-medicalists around 1852. In 1859 he set up the Physio-Medical College in Cincinatti, and in 1885 he set up the Chicago Physio-Medical College, which was renamed the College of Medicine and Surgery in 1897. His book, published in 1869, brings together a substantially wider range of herbs than originally used by Thomsonians.

### Sources

Berman A 1956 Neo-Thomsonianism in the United States. Journal of the History of Medicine 11:133–154.

Haller JS 1997 Kindly medicine, physio-medicalism in America 1836–1911. Kent State University Press.

## Finley Ellingwood

Finley Ellingwood was born in Manchester, Indiana on 12 September 1852. He obtained a medical degree from Bennett Medical College in Chicago in 1878. After practising as a physician in Illinois for 6 years, he became Professor of Chemistry in Bennett Medical College from 1884 to 1900 and later Professor of Materia Medica and Therapeutics from 1900 to 1907. He ran a practice in Chicago during this time, wrote several books on eclectic medicine and edited a number of medical journals. He was secretary of the National Eclectic Medical Association from 1902 to 1907. He died in California in 1920.

### Sources

Henrietta's Herbal. Online. Available: http://www.henriettesherbal.com/eclectics/books.html.

http://homepages.rootsweb.ancestry.com/~mhender/BioFinleyEllingwood.html.

## Richard Cranfield Wren

In 1896 Richard Wren became a partner in the company of Potter & Clarke in East London, which had been founded in 1812. *Potter's Cyclopaedia* was designed to provide a concise summary of the names, synonyms, parts used, actions, indications and dosage of medicinal plants.

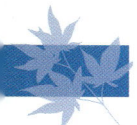

This edition was revised and reprinted 17 times, followed by new editions in 1989 and 2003.

## Richard Hool

Richard Lawrence Hool practised in Bolton, Lancashire. He established a business in 1872 in the Market Hall, which continues to be owned and managed by his descendants today. As a keen botanist he collected herbs in the wild and was President of the Bolton Linnean Medical Botanist Society and an active contributor to the Lancashire branch of the National Association of Medical Herbalists.

## Maud Grieve

Sophie Emma Magdalene Law was born on 4 May 1858, in Islington, London, to James Law, a warehouseman and his wife Sophia Ballisat. She lived in India with her husband William Sommerville Grieve and retired with him to Chalfont St Peter, Buckinghamshire in 1905. At her home there she established a garden for the growing of medicinal and culinary herbs and became the county's representative for the Daughters of Ceres, a movement concerned with increasing the opportunities for women in horticultural jobs, and helped to found the National Herb Growing Association. During World War I she provided comprehensive training in the preparation of medicinal herbs to relieve a shortage of medical supplies. To this end she also issued a series of pamphlets on the cultivation and use of medicinal herbs. After the war she published several booklets and trained former servicemen, some of whom went to British colonies to start herb farms. She was a Fellow of the Royal Horticultural Society and President of the British Guild of Herb Growers.

*A Modern Herbal* was conceived and edited by Hilda Leyel, founder of the Society of Herbalists, based on Grieve's monographs and extended by the editor to include American herbs.

### Sources

Dictionary of national biography. Oxford University Press, Oxford. Online. Available: http://www.oxforddnb.com.

## Wilhelm Pelikan

Wilhelm Pelikan studied chemistry in Vienna and Graz. He heard Rudolf Steiner lecture in Vienna in 1918 and went on to become a private pupil of his. He was head of the Weleda establishment for 40 years, developing a range of anthroposophical medicines, and researching on the efficacy of potentisation, among many other ventures in his full life. He established medicinal herb gardens in the firm's grounds and elsewhere, and was co-editor of the *Weleda Korrespondenzblaetter für Aerzte*. He undertook Goethean study of metals and botany of medicinal plants, producing the books *The Secrets of Metals*, and the three volume *Healing Plants*, the latter offering a remarkably sensitive exploration of the nature of individual plants within their families and their relationship to the human being.

### Source

Berufsverband Anthroposophischer Apoteker in Deutschland 2006 Pioneers in Anthroposophic Pharmacy. Online. Available: http://wwwiaap.org.uk/download/pioneers-in-anthroposophic-pharmacy-june-2006.pdf.

## Rudolf Weiss

Professor Rudolf Fritz Weiss has been referred to as the founding father of modern German phytotherapy. He was born in Berlin and studied botany and medicine at the university there, qualifying as a doctor in 1922. A teaching post in herbal medicine was interrupted by war service as an army doctor, followed by 7 years in Russian captivity as a doctor in prisoner-of-war camp hospitals. He retired from clinical practice in 1961 and devoted his life to scientific development and acceptance of herbal medicine. He was appointed a member of the German Commission E in 1978. He was founder of the Zeitschrift für Phytotherapie and lectured on current advances in the subject at the University of Tübingen.

### Source

Weiss R 1988 Herbal medicine. Beaconsfield Publishing, Beaconsfield.

## The National Botanic Pharmacopoeia

The first edition of the *National Botanic Pharmacopoeia* was brought out in 1905 to meet the needs of students working towards the examination for entry to the National Association of Medical Herbalists (NAHM). The NAMH was founded in the UK in 1868 to promote professional practice and to set education standards. At the end of World War II the Association became the National Institute of Medical Herbalists (NIMH), but remains the oldest professional body of practising herbalists in the world today.

In his introduction, JAS Parkinson stated that one of the aims of the modest work was to bring order out of chaos in the herbal material medica, and through the light of modern scientific methods of research to establish more certainly and constantly the properties and safe applications of medicinal plants.

The second edition of the pharmacopoeia was produced in 1921 with the assistance of Dr Sarah Webb, W Burns Lingard and RC Wren, author of *Potter's Cyclopaedia*. JW Scurrah stated in the preface that all poisonous remedies had been removed from the text, and about 40 non-poisonous herbs added.

## Albert and Lilian Priest

*Herbal Medication* is described as a handbook for clinical students and newly qualified herbal practitioners, and written with the presumption of their adequate knowledge of pre-clinical sciences and of a sound basis of naturopathic and physiomedical philosophy by Albert and Lilian Priest, who drew on over 35 years of experience in the practice of natural therapeutics. Albert Priest had been Vice-Dean of the British College of Naturopathy and Osteopathy and Director of Education of the National Institute of Medical Herbalists and edited the journal *The Herbal Practitioner* from 1945 to 1965. In the foreword the authors expressed thanks to Albert Orbell FNIMH for inculcating in them during clinical training the same therapeutic principles.

## *British Herbal Pharmacopoeia*

The *British Herbal Pharmacopoeia* was published as a consolidated edition in 1983 that brought together sections 1, 2 and 3 published in 1971–1974, which were then published as part 1 in 1976 and part 2 in 1979. In the preface of the 1983 edition, the chairman pays tribute to the vision and dedication of the former chairman F Fletcher Hyde and to the support given over many years by the secretary H Hall. In the preface to the 1974 edition, Fletcher Hyde states that the work required for the monographs was started in 1965 by the eight members and three advisory members of the Scientific Committee of the British Herbal Medicine Association. He states that the therapeutics section was his responsibility with the support of two advisory members and input from herbal practitioners. Fletcher Hyde entered practice in Leicester in 1934 and was Director of Research of the National Institute of Medical Herbalists for over 30 years, and President for 8 years from 1967 to 1975. His papers are held at the Complementary and Alternative Medicine Library and Information Service (CAMLIS Online. Available: http://www.cam.nhs.uk/about/archive/).

## Thomas Bartram

Thomas Bartram was a consulting medical herbalist, well known throughout the herbal world, particularly for his *Encyclopaedia of Herbal Medicine*. He was a fellow of the National Institute of Medical Herbalists and the Royal Society of Health and Health Food Institute. He founded Gerard House, for international innovators in herbal medicine, in 1958. He was editor of the magazine *Grace*.

## Peter Bradley

Peter Bradley was trained in chemistry and is a Fellow of the Royal Society of Chemistry. He prepared documentation on quality, safety and efficacy required during the EC Review of Medicines for herbal medicines with product licences of right granted under the Medicines Act 1968, and this spurred his interest in the constituents of medicinal plants. He has been a member of the ESCOP Scientific Committee for over 20 years (including 14 years as Co-Chairman), and a member of the Board of the British Herbal Medicine Association for over 25 years.

## Andrew Chevallier

Andrew Chevallier is a practising herbalist and fellow and past president of the National Institute of Medical Herbalists. He was instrumental in establishing the first university BSc programme for herbal medicine in the UK and is the author of several books.

## Elizabeth Williamson

Professor Elizabeth Williamson is a registered pharmacist and Director of Pharmacy Practice at the University of Reading. She is a member of the British Pharmacopoeia Commission and Chair of the Expert Advisory Group for Herbal and Complementary Medicines, which advises the Commission on standards for herbal medicine.

## David Hoffman

David Hoffman has been a medical herbalist since 1979. He trained with the National Institute of Medical Herbalists. He was inaugural president of the American Herbalist Guild and has taught phytotherapy widely. He is a teacher, author and consultant in North America.

## Christopher Menzies-Trull

Christopher Menzies-Trull is a physiomedical herbal practitioner, having trained with the National Institute of Medical Herbalists. He completed the course in 1979, the same year as he qualified as a state registered nurse.

## Simon Mills and Kerry Bone

Simon Mills is teaching fellow at the Peninsula College of Medicine and Dentistry. He is a herbal practitioner of many years standing, author and co-author of a number of authoritative texts on herbal medicine. His roles have included President of the National Institute of Medical Herbalists, founder of the College of Practitioners of Phytotherapy, special advisor to the House of Lords Science and Technology Committee's inquiry onto complementary and alternative medicine, and Joint Director of the Centre for Complementary Health Studies at Exeter University. He is Secretary of the European Scientific Cooperative on Phytotherapy, and Member of the Advisory Board of the American Botanical Council.

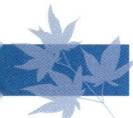

# THE WESTERN HERBAL TRADITION

**Table 1.1** Sources used throughout the book (and therefore not referenced in the text)

| Author or title | Century | Text used |
|---|---|---|
| Bauhin | 17th | Bauhin J 1650 Historia Plantarum Universalis. Ebroduni. |
| Bartram | 20th | Bartram T 1995 Encyclopaedia of Herbal Medicine. Grace Publishers, Bournemouth. |
| Bradley | 21st | Bradley P (ed.) 2006 British Herbal Compendium vol. 2. British Herbal Medicines Association, Bournemouth. |
| British Herbal Pharmacopoeia | 20th | BHPA Scientific Committee 1983 British Herbal Pharmacopoeia. British Herbal Medicine Association, Keighley, West Yorkshire. |
| Chevallier | 21st | Chevallier A 2001 The Encyclopedia of Medicinal Plants. Dorling Kindersley, London. |
| Coffin | 19th | Coffin AI 1864 Botanic Guide to Health, 49th edn. Haynes, Coffin, London. |
| Cook | 19th | Cook W 1869 (1985 reprint) The Physiomedical Dispensatory. Eclectic Medical Publications, Oregon. |
| Cullen | 18th | Cullen W 1773 Lectures on Materia Medica. T. Lowndes, London. Online. Available: http://library.wellcome.ac.uk/ECCO. |
| Culpeper | 17th | Culpeper N 1656 The English Physitian. London. Culpeper N 1995 Culpeper's Complete Herbal. Wordsworth Library, Ware, Herts. |
| D'Alechamps | 16th | D'Alechamps J 1586 Historia Generalis Plantarum. Lugdini. |
| Dioscorides | 1st | Beck LY 2005 Pedanius Dioscorides of Anazarbus: De Materia Medica. Olms–Weidmann, Hildesheim. |
| Dodoens | 16th | Dodoens R 1619 A New Herbal: or Historie of Plants. London. |
| Ellingwood | 19th, 20th | Ellingwood F 1919 (1988 reprint) American Materia Medica, Therapeutics and Pharmacognosy. Eclectic Medical Publications, Oregon. |
| Fox | 19th | Fox W 1920 The Working-Man's Model Family Botanic Guide to Health, 22nd edn. W Fox and Sons, Sheffield. |
| Fuchs | 16th | Fuchs L 1545 De Historia Stirpium. Basileae. |
| Galen | 2nd | Galen C 1543 De Simplicium Medicamentorum Facultatibus Libri Undecim. Paris. |
| Gerard | 17th | Gerard J 1975 The Herbal or General History of Plants. Dover Publications, New York. |
| Grieve | 20th | Grieve M 1931 (1984 edn) A Modern Herbal. Penguin Books, Harmandsworth. |
| Hildegard | 12th | Throop P (trans.) 1998 Hildegard von Bingen's Physica. Healing Arts Press, Rochester, VT. |
| Hill | 18th | Hill J 1755 The Useful Family Herbal. London. |
| Hoffman | 21st | Hoffman D 2003 Medical Herbalism: The Science and Practice of Herbal Medicine. Healing Arts Press, Rochester, VT. |
| Ibn Sina (Avicenna) | 11th | Abu Ali ibn Sino 2003 Kanon Vrachebnoj Nauki.10 vols. Enio, Odessa. |
| Hool | 20th | Hool RL 1918 Health from British wild herbs. W H Webb, Southport. |
| Macer | 11th | Macer 1511 Carmen de Virtutibus Herbarum. Paris. |
| Mattioli | 16th | Matthioli P A 1554 Petri Andreae Matthioli Medici Senensis Commentarii, in Libros Sex Pedacii Dioscoridis Anazarbei, De Materia Medica 1554. Venice. |
| Menzies-Trull | 21st | Menzies-Trull C 2003 Herbal Medicine Keys to Physiomedicalism. Faculty of Physiomedical Herbal Medicine, Newcastle, Staffordshire. |

## The historical sources — Chapter 1

**Table 1.1** *continued*

| Author or title | Century | Text used |
|---|---|---|
| Mills and Bone | 21st | Mills S, Bone K 2005 The Essential Guide to Herbal Safety. Elsevier, St Louis, Missouri. |
| Miller | 18th | Miller J 1722 Botanicum Officinale or A Compendious Herbal. E Bell, J Senex, W Taylor, J Osborn, London. |
| Myddfai physicians | 14th, 18th | Pughe J 1861 (1993 reprint) The Physicians of Myddvai; Medcygon Myddfai. Llanerch Publishers, Felinfach. |
| National Botanic Pharmacopoeia | 20th | National Association of Medical Herbalists of Great Britain 1921 The National Botanic Pharmacopoeia, 2nd edn. Woodhouse, Cornthwaite, Bradford. |
| Old English Herbarium | 10th, 11th | Van Arsdall A 2002 Medieval Herbal Remedies: The Old English Herbarium and Anglo-Saxon Medicine. Routledge, London. |
| Parkinson | 17th | Parkinson J 1640 Theatrum Botanicum: or The Theater of Plants. London |
| Pelikan | 20th | Pelikan W 1997 Healing Plants: Insights Through Spiritual Science, vol. 1. Mercury Press, Spring Valley, New York.<br>Pelikan W 1962 Heilpflanzenkunde, vol.2. Verlag am Goetheanum, Dornach.<br>Pelikan W 1978 Heilpflanzenkunde, vol. 3. Verlag am Goetheanum, Dornach. |
| Pliny | 1st | Jones W H S (trans.) 1949–1962 Pliny Natural History, with an English translation in 10 volumes. William Heinemann, London. |
| Priest and Priest | 20th | Priest A, Priest L 1982 Herbal Medication. LN Fowler, London. |
| Pseudo-Apuleius | 5th | Hunger F W T (ed.) 1935 The herbal of Pseudo-Apuleius from the ninth century manuscript in the abbey of Monte Cassino. EJ Brill, Leyden. |
| Quincy | 18th | Quincy J 1724 Pharmacopoeia Officinalis & Extemporanea. London. |
| Salernitan herbal | 12th | Roberts E, Stearn W (trans.) 1984 Livre des Simples Medecines: Codex Bruxellensis IV.1024 A 15th Century French Herbal. De Schutter, Antwerp. |
| Serapio the Younger | 13th | Serapio 1479 Liber Serapionis Aggregatus in Medicinis Simplicibus. Venice. |
| Turner | 16th | Chapman GTL, Tweedle MN (eds) 1995 A New Herball by William Turner, part I, vol 1. Cambridge University Press, Cambridge.<br>Chapman GTL, McCombie F, Wesencraft A (eds) 1995 A New Herball by William Turner, parts II & III, vol 2. Cambridge University Press, Cambridge. |
| Weiss | 20th | Weiss R 1988 Herbal Medicine. Beaconsfield Publishing, Beaconsfield. |
| Williamson | 21st | Williamson E 2003 Potter's Herbal Cyclopaedia. CW Daniel, London. |
| Wood | 21st | Wood M 2008 The Earthwise Herbal: a Complete Guide to Old World Medicinal Plants. North Atlantic Books, Berkeley CA. |
| Wren | 20th | Wren RC 1907 Potter's Cyclopaedia of Botanical Drugs and Preparations. Potter & Clarke, London. |

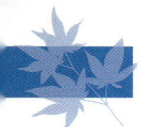

Kerry Bone is a medical herbalist practising in Queensland, Australia. He is an experienced research and industrial chemist. He is co-founder and head of research and development of MediHerb. He is a Fellow of the National Herbalist Association of Australia and of the National Institute of Medical Herbalists in the UK. He is founder and Principal of the Australian College of Phytotherapy. He has written extensively on herbal medicine and lectures internationally.

## Matthew Wood

Matthew Wood lives near Minneapolis in the USA. He has practised as a herbalist since 1982 in traditional western herbalism. He is the author of several books on herbal medicine.

# CHAPTER 2
# Some observations on the Western herbal tradition

We have begun our study of the Western herbal tradition with the *De Materia Medica* (the materials of medicine) of Dioscorides, written around 80 AD and describing over 600 plant medicines. This is appropriate in that he is regarded as the first writer in history to approach medical botany as an applied science and the chief authority on pharmacy for the subsequent 1600 years (Kremer & Urdang 1963; Riddle 1985). The date of his work also provides a neat time period of nearly 2000 years in which we have attempted to discuss a variety of statements on each of our 27 plant medicines. Thus we have omitted Theophrastus, friend and pupil of Aristotle and often named the 'father of botany', who died in 286 BC, and Crateuas of the 1st century BC, who produced the earliest known illustrated herbal. Crateuas and other writers such as Sextus Niger have been cited as sources for both Dioscorides and Pliny, whose Natural History was composed at the same time as *De Materia Medica*. Kremer and Urdang (1963) rule out Theophratus as a source for Dioscorides but his name is mentioned by Pliny.

According to Riddle (1985), Dioscorides deliberately avoided positing an explicit medical theory in which to understand the uses of the plants he described, but he did determine their various actions on the body, such as warming or cooling, mollifying or astringent, bitter, cleansing, diuretic, diaphoretic and so on. These actions or properties were followed by their indications, but only occasionally did he explicitly link the property to the indication. Furthermore, the action of a herb that is specified for a certain condition may not necessarily be substituted by another herb with the same action, for each herb has its own nature and resulting set of indications, but the reader may infer that another herb with the same property could be tested out as a replacement if the original herb is not available. Thus the inclusion of plant actions lifts the pharmacy of Dioscorides above one which contains only simple statements that such and such a herb is good for such and such a condition. Despite this elaboration, the solidly empirical nature of Dioscorides' approach guaranteed his work continued acceptance in the changing course of medicine down the centuries. In fact, *De Materia Medica* never became unknown in any period of our authors, although the extent to which the indications from Dioscorides for any plant discussed here were transmitted by later writers varies from case to case. His work was not so much rediscovered by the medical humanists of the Renaissance; rather there was a massive increase in interest in him as a medical authority. Mattioli's translation and commentary on the *De Materia Medica*, for instance, became the most well-read scientific text published in the 16th century (Findlen 1999).

Pliny, by contrast, discussed plant medicines among the whole range of subjects included in his natural history. His descriptions of the uses of plants included the magical and the superstitious, which were part and parcel of ancient medicine, and which found resonance with the medieval mixture of magic, religion and medicine, but later attracted criticism in the writings of some Renaissance authors. More serious was the accusation levelled against him by the leading authority on Greek medicine at the University of Ferrara, Nicolaus Leoniceno (1428–1524), that he made mistakes in translating and transmitting Greek medical material. Others came to his defence, citing scribal errors and not Pliny's original writings as the source of inaccuracies, or agreeing with Pliny on the basis of their own or others' experience of plants. Nevertheless, a result of these debates was that some medical writers viewed the Greeks as the absolute authority in medicine and that all transmissions by intermediaries, including the Roman and Arabic writers, were full of mistakes (Conrad et al 1995). This provided the initial shaping and propagation of Renaissance medical learning through books (Findlen 1999).

When we come to Galen, the third of our Classical sources, we are faced with a huge volume of writings. Galenic medicine has been explored in many histories of medicine and the reader may consult a key text such as Conrad et al (1995) while the philosophical position of Galen is well contextualized in Hall (1975). For this text we have consulted only his *De Simplicium Medicamentorum Temperamentis ac Facultatibus Libri Undecim* (11 books on the temperaments and powers of simples). This is the text from which those of our Renaissance authors who have directly cited Galen have mainly drawn. The publishing by the Aldine Press in Venice of Galen's collected works in Greek in 1525 and subsequent Latin versions based on the original Greek texts provided access to accurate Galenic opinion on the qualities and substance of herbs and consequently their rational employment in medicine (Conrad et al 1995). We have not consulted Galen's *Methodus Medendi* (Method of healing), where such rational treatment is exemplified, a work which, although used at the medical school in Alexandria in the 5th and 6th centuries AD (Temkin 1973), was unknown to medieval Western Europe and which was not taught to any great extent in European universities even after its publication among Galen's works (Conrad et al 1995).

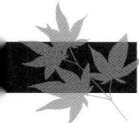

In his book on the temperaments and powers of simples, Galen used a categorization of the qualities of each plant, whether it heats, cools, dries or moistens the body, and the degree of this effect from mild in the first degree to extreme in the fourth degree. In relationship to these were other qualities, to be detected by taste, as pungent, bitter, astringent, bland or sweet, or again in effect by an ability to penetrate into, rarify and thin substances in the body or to condense, thicken or repel them. The passive qualities provided softening, hardening and drying actions. These aspects of Galen's pharmacology posited a theoretical basis for medical treatment where an excess or deficiency of a humour and the degree to which it was out of balance in the body so as to produce a diseased state could be remedied by the administration of a medicine which diminished or restored the humour in exactly the right degree in order to re-establish the balance of health in an individual. The knowledge of these qualities was at once rational and experiential and appeared reliable inasmuch as it could be re-confirmed experimentally, so that it proved to be a most attractive feature of Galen's therapeutics (Temkin 1973).

Galen's assessment of the temperaments of individual plant medicines typically involved assigning an active virtue, either hot or cold, and a passive one, either moist or dry, although sometimes only one quality was assigned on the evidence of the effects of the herb. Those plant medicines with higher degrees of heat inevitably produced an increasingly drying effect as a direct result of the active quality of heat. Bitter herbs were associated with heat because of the perceived action of bitter substances on the body: their sharpness combined with heat allowed them to cut through and break up thick phlegmatic humours, supporting the body's own healing power to remove the now modified encumbrances. Pungent herbs also heated, penetrated and thinned dense material. Indeed all hot herbs were considered to have a cutting power. However, the converse was not as consistently true for herbs with a cooling quality. They were as likely to be drying as they were to be moistening, and a true astringent action was often associated with an active cooling effect. A bland or sweet taste in a cooling herb denoted a moist passive quality.

Degrees of these four qualities correlated with their perceptible impact on the body. The first degree of heat or cold and dryness or moisture represented an imperceptible effect on the body and allowed an extended use as a tonic, while the topical application of medicaments possessing the fourth degree of heat could rapidly inflame the skin, and of cold could soon numb it, so that their applications should be specific, necessary and limited in duration. Ingesting a medicine cold in the fourth degree could kill by putting out the flame of life. Poisons were formally grouped in this last category. The categories in between, the second and third degrees, denoted perceptible and strong effects, respectively.

Culpeper (1669) wrote a short resume of indications for use according to the degree of qualities in a plant medicine. Herbs hot in the first degree matched the temperature of the human body in health and in disease thin humours, expelling them by sweat and insensible transpiration and so treated fevers; they remedied weariness, bred good blood by gently supporting the digestive fire and eased pain by correcting the extreme of heat or cold responsible for the pain. Herbs hot in the second degree were hotter than the human body; they cut and scattered tough humours by their own force and power when nature could not. Those hot in the third and fourth degree were yet more powerful, heating and cutting compacted humours, provoking sweat and resisting poison (the alexipharmic remedies). Herbs cold in the first degree balanced the heat of food and the heat of the bowels and cooled fevers and inflammations. A cool astringent remedy strengthened the retentive faculty of the body and was used to rectify a tendency to vomit. Those cold in the second degree were used to treat an imbalance of choler or yellow bile humour and pacify the inordinate movement of the spirits, resulting in insomnia, or, by closing the pores, stop the escape of the spirits in cases of fainting; topically, such herbs were applied to hot inflammations. Herbs cold in the third degree were more powerful still, while those in the extreme fourth degree represented the narcotics, which stupefied the senses and poisoned the body. A moistening quality smoothed and softened, easing a dry cough for instance, and in the second degree and above remedied a sharpness of humours (as may be inferred in patients who cannot tolerate vinegar, the fruit acids in berries and other sharp foods). Finally drying herbs countered moisture in the body in varying degrees. It may be observed also that strongly heating herbs of the Galenic materia medica could be rationally linked to diuretic and emmenogogic actions but these same actions were also attributed to certain other plants of a milder quality, according to their individual nature. Again, if a herb has the power to close up a wound, then it would be ascribed a drying effect in Galenic pharmacology, no matter how emollient the herb appeared to the sense of taste and touch.

Inevitably herbs act on the body in ways that could not be explained exclusively by recourse to their discernible qualities. The classic case is the purgatives, which were one of the mainstays of removal of excessive quantities of a humour from the body. Galen himself recognized that the action of purgatives was not to be explained through their temperament but rather through the peculiarity of their total substance. Such knowledge is irrational and can be known through experience only. The magnetic property of the lodestone put the mineral magnetite in this category also, where it represented the prototype of all occult forces (Temkin 1958). The effects of the total substance of a thing came under extended consideration in the 16th century as an explanation for new diseases like syphilis and the plague, which eluded understanding by means of

Galen's humoral pathology, and for some new medicines such as cinchona bark, whose effects were not explainable through their sensible qualities (Conrad et al 1995).

In general it may be said that the actions of a given medicine on the body were known from experience and only some effects had a rational explanation according to Galenic pharmacology. Indeed it must be recognized that the irreducible 'substance' of a herb can refer to its material components, or pharmacological constituents as they are described today, and equally to its essence in a more than material sense. The prima materia of the elements which constitute the materiality of objects, and so the elements themselves, cannot be detected by the senses. According to Aristotle they are to be inferred from the four qualities perceptible in each object. Thus the active qualities of heat and cold are observed to work on things to bring them together, the hot combining things of the same kind while destroying that which is foreign, and the cold combining homogeneous and heterogeneous things alike. For example, fire embraces that which is combustible and leaves behind that which is not, while cold freezes and hardens everything together. As to the passive qualities, which are operated on by form, the moist is that which is not determined by its own boundary but is easily adaptable to form, as water is contained in a bucket which otherwise would flow out onto the ground and be entirely dispersed. Dry is the opposite, being determined by its own boundary and not easily fitting into a container, such as a square peg in a round hole (Lloyd 1964). But Empedocles, who originated the concept of all bodies being composed of four elements or 'roots' and who belonged to the Pythagorean tradition impugned by Aristotle, linked each with a supernatural deity. The first element to separate out of the primordial mass, air (ether) he linked with Zeus, while the concentration of a denser substance within is earth, identified with Zeus' consort Hera. As the Earth spins on its axis, water is forced out onto the surface of the globe, which Empedocles dedicated to Hestis, the subject of a Sicilian cult associated with the worship of Persephone, consort of the lord of the underworld. Finally fire, belonging to Hades' realm, shoots up out of the underworld and creates humankind on the surface of the Earth, then continues into the air to crystallise parts of the ether into stars and to create the source of all heat and light, the sun (Kingsley 1996). The opposing pairs of fire–water and air–earth are thus represented by two marriages between gods and goddesses, while the gods of fire and air are brothers, and the females representing water and earth are also related. Thus the inter-relatedness of all the components of life, including its materiality, is open to mythic as well as scientific interpretation.

Returning to the tradition of herbals, we find a fully empirical approach in the *Herbal of Pseudo-Apuleius*, thought to be written around 500 AD, where the entries for each plant follow the formula 'for condition x use the herb in way y'. The method of preparation is galenical, i.e. infusions and decoctions, and some of the most important solvents or vehicles for the plant drugs are, in all the texts mentioned so far, vinegar, wine, oil and honey. A striking factor in the Classical herbals, and continued in Pseudo-Apuleius (for the name Apuleius is thought by some to suggest Aesculapius, the Greek god of medicine) is the frequency of topical use of plant medicine. This is not surprising in view of the fact, according to Salazar (2000), that there was effectively no period in antiquity in which the Greek or Roman armies were not involved in combat and military operation, and the treatment of war wounds is the only sort of medical activity mentioned in the Iliad. Medical practitioners attached to armies on the move were very likely required to source at least some of the wound herbs required from the locality and if one plant was unavailable, another suitable one would have to be substituted (Salazar 2000). Since Dioscorides is thought to have spent time as an army doctor, his classification of plant actions which allows the possibility of substitution may have arisen from the necessities of gathering wound-healing plants while on the move. Again according to Salazar (2000) the texts of antiquity make no real distinction between styptic agents used topically on wounds and prepared as a drink for a gastrointestinal haemorrhage. The same is true of remedies classified as haemostatic and agglutinant (closing up wounds). The books contain many antiinflammatory agents too and, coupled with instructions on the management of inflammation, which may have concerned the permitting of the process to a degree as long as it did not get out of hand, the impression is that inflammation is a process a Greek or Roman doctor felt able to control. On the other hand there was little written on analgesics.

The *Herbal of Pseudo-Apuleius* appears to be the most important of our texts so far for medicine in Latin-reading Medieval Europe up until the 11th century. It was translated into Anglo-Saxon around the year 1000 as the Old English Herbarium. In the introduction to her translation of the text into English, Van Arsdall (2002) sees the Herbarium falling into a common corpus of texts used in a pan-European healing tradition. The approach within this tradition is empirical, practical and innovatory in that adaptation of statements reproduced from southern European sources for practical use in a local (northern) environment were evidently made (Voigts 1979). This is no blind copying of Classical works. Furthermore, the dissemination of knowledge is also oral concerning which centres of healing such as Benedictine monasteries, where the copying of texts was also carried out, played an important role. Illustrations in such medical texts leave much to be desired when compared to Renaissance botanical drawings, but Van Arsdall contends that the texts were not intended to be instructional, but instead they are like cookbooks for experienced cooks. She sees the same form in textbooks of modern herbal medicine, where it is assumed that the reader already has extensive familiarity with the material under discussion and knows, for instance, how to diagnose the conditions for which the remedies will be used, and how to prepare them for use. Nevertheless, the problem of identifying which plant is being discussed is a perennial one, to which the monographs in this book will bear witness. For the northern Europeans, the names of plants, rather than their physical descriptions, became the important link back to the Classical sources, and in lists of names provided for each plant it was usual for the Greek or more often Latin name to be written first. While we have attempted to clarify plant identities in this way, using Greek or Latin names, the extra problem of translation of Arabic names has posed significant problems and we have made the best of what we can with an early printed edition of Serapio and a modern translation of Ibn Sina from Arabic into Russian where Linnaean binomials are provided by the translators and commentators.

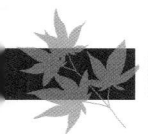

The movement to re-establish the authority of medical theory can be linked to the rise to fame of the medical school of Salerno as a beacon of Greek medicine in Europe from the 11th century. A key factor in this development is Constantine the African, who brought original Arabic medical works and translations of Greek and Roman texts to southern Italy and set about rendering them into Latin. Galenic pharmacological assessment now recombined with empirical medieval medicine and, for instance, in the later version of the Salernitan herbal with which we have worked the temperament of the herb is consistently given, although not always in agreement with Galen's own, alongside ancient and contemporary indications for use. *The Trotula* text on the treatment of women shows the importance the writer accorded the primary differentiation of female patients into those requiring heating medicines and those requiring cooling ones (Green 2002). Macer's herbal also offers the temperament of each plant but these can differ again from the Salernitan entries on the 27 plants reviewed here and reflect other sources. Webster (2008) has commented on a complexity of relationship between late antique and medieval books of knowledge, such as encyclopaedias and bestiaries, which inhibits a clear determination of definitive sources for medieval writings transmitted into the Renaissance. This appears to us to be very true of Hildegard's writings on the plants we are discussing here. Sometimes she agrees with our other sources regarding a plant's temperament, but often her entry is striking in its difference over qualities or uses. Yet her instructions are always very practical, as if the treatments were carried out on a regular basis. McVaugh (1969) comments that, in relation to Galenic pharmacology, medieval physicians 'did make an attempt to describe with increasing precision the sensory stages corresponding to the four degrees, and they did continue to insist on assigning a numerical degree of hot or cold to every medicine in the pharmacopoeia. Indeed, their frequent divergence over the exact intensity of different medicines suggests that they were concerned enough with these medicinal degrees to sometimes reconfirm them independently'. Divergence from Galenic orthodoxy on plant qualities is evident in our monographs.

The Salernitan pharmacopoeia was composed of single plant medicines or 'simples' and a formulary of compound drugs. How were these compounds decided – from empirical use, or through a theoretical evaluation of the qualities of each ingredient? Galen intended a simple combining of herbs, but the formulae of Arabic and medieval European physicians became lengthy and mathematical rules were proposed for measuring the overall heating, cooling, drying and moistening effects of a compound remedy, by Al-Kindi (d. ca. 870) in Baghdad and by Arnald of Villanova (d. 1311) in Montpellier. A second question concerns the variation of qualitative effect on the body if a herb of a certain temperament is given in a range of doses. It is fair to say that this matter is no more decided today concerning the prescribing of mixtures and their individual dosages than it was centuries ago.

With the Renaissance authors we find ourselves on increasingly stable ground regarding textual transmission and the citing of Dioscorides, Pliny and Galen is accurate and consistent. Indeed, the authors of these herbals, apart from Culpeper, appeared largely unaffected by the iconoclastic re-presentation of medical theory and practice that was Paracelsianism, and Galenic orthodoxy was the norm until its decline in the face of the new mechanical philosophy of the latter part of the 17th century. Innovation was making an appearance, however, in the voluminous sections in plant entries discussing the identification of species and the opinions of ancient and contemporary writers. These morphological descriptions and illustrations have been the focus and main interest for many years of a number of studies into Renaissance herbals, most notably Ann R. Arber's *Herbals, their Origins and Evolution: A Chapter in the History of Botany 1470–1670*. If this is the standard work on herbals, it is because botany is a recognized area of historical research. Our concern has rather been to focus on the medicinal virtues and indications of the plants as recorded in the various periods of our authors and to show the transmission of knowledge of the method of healing across two great periods of herbal writing and beyond as far as current practice today. By doing so we appear to cross a divide between medicine as history and medicine as current, partially evidenced practice, and our researches have taken us into a consequently less-travelled terrain. Historiography has moved on from a Whiggish view of progress where what has not survived did not deserve to continue, to a burgeoning in the last 30 years of a social history of medicine, featuring the rise of professional bodies and their power struggles, the accounts of individual physicians and their patients, and a full range of other practitioners, regular and irregular, participating in the medical marketplace (Kassell 2005). Our book is a small contribution to the location of herbal medicine within this historical marketplace and, we hope, a major contribution to a critical awareness among current practising herbalists of their own long textual tradition through a study of the primary sources.

It cannot be doubted that the Classical and Renaissance texts we have consulted were major scientific works of their day, written by leading scientists and physicians, and represent the broad sweep of Classical and Galenic tradition. The earlier 16th century herbals of Fuchs and Turner and the first Latin edition of Mattioli's Commentaries faithfully reproduce the views of Dioscorides, Pliny and Galen. Of the three Mattioli is by far the most disputative. There is some documentation of new uses for plants, as far as they have been tried and tested by later practitioners (Fuchs 'ex recentioribus', for instance), or indeed plants unknown to the Ancients but in regular employment in the 16th and 17th centuries. Dalechamps' Lyon herbal is thorough on some herbs and partial on others, whereas the English translation of Dodoens seems to confirm that it is an early work for the author, and here and there some opinions were altered in his more mature writings. Gerard gives us a very English appreciation of the herbs, mentioning exact and sometimes still familiar locations where they may be found in his day, as well as drawing on earlier materials. Bauhin's three-volume work is the most detailed and encyclopaedic. He draws on numerous sources for his material and is very careful in his presentation of facts and opinions. Equally, Parkinson's large folio herbal is thorough, seemingly reflecting a distillation of earlier writings, including Bauhin's. Culpeper's English Physitian was written for a popular audience and is often a direct lift of Parkinson's material with added astrological detail. When Culpeper has something of his own to say about a plant, his entry is distinctive and quite unlike Parkinson's.

Just as in the case of many aspects of wound treatment in antiquity, later medical practice can at times sound plausible to the modern ear. In a review of a recently discovered 15th century English manuscript on the aetiology, classification, diagnosis and management of ulcers, the authors, a surgeon and a pharmacologist, conclude that, although the details may have changed, the principles and approaches of this treatment remain valid even today (Kirkpatrick & Naylor 1997). On the other hand, occult practices in Renaissance medicine, drawing on neoplatonic and hermetic philosophies and using the ancient analogy of the macrocosm-microcosm, can seem aberrant and retrograde, no matter how attentive the practitioner may have been to the study of nature and natural philosophy. The only example here is that of Nicolas Culpeper, who practised an astrological medicine which, without casting Hippocratic and Galenic medicine aside, nevertheless sought magnetic remedies to treat sympathetically, or 'like by like', any diseased part of the body. The magnetic attraction lay in the correspondence between planetary ruler of the part or organ, and of the plant or other medicine to be used. With this aim, he recorded for over 300 herbs in his English Physitian one of the seven planets as governor. This consistency of application stands in stark contrast with all the other works we have consulted where astrological references are effectively completely absent.

Culpeper's herbal is the last of our texts chronologically to continue the transmission of Greek medicine and its Roman, Arabic, Medieval and Renaissance translators. Bacon's injunction for experimental knowledge only, Cartesian dualism, new scientific discoveries and the rise of a mechanical philosophy dealt the death blow to Galenism as a theory of medicine. The plant entries in the 18th century texts we have consulted are much smaller. There is no need to discuss names or descriptions of herbs since botany is on firmer ground. There are no temperaments of herbs and their actions are explained in other ways. Quincy employs a new physiology of the body to explain the effects of remedies. Miller and Hill provide brief indications limited to more modest claims for what plants can achieve in healing. Cullen is quite sceptical of many traditional uses of herbs and must himself have played a part in cleansing from the Edinburgh Dispensatory the rump of galenicals no longer sold in the apothecaries' shops. However, medical practice lagged far behind the development of biomedical scientific theory. Galen's pharmacology persisted longer than other aspects of his medical science and 'the therapeutic anarchy that followed its destruction made itself felt beyond the middle of the 19th century' (Temkin 1973). By that time a revival of herbal medicine was underway, imported from a new quarter, North America.

## REFERENCES

Arber AR 1986 Herbals, their origins and evolution: a chapter in the history of botany 1470–1670. Cambridge University Press, Cambridge.

Conrad L, Neve M, Nutton V, et al 1995 The Western medical tradition 800 BC to AD 1800, Cambridge University Press, Cambridge.

Culpeper N 1669 A key to Galen and Hypocrates their method of physick. In: Culpeper 1669 Pharmacopoeia Londinensis. London.

Findlen P 1999 The formation of the scientific community: natural history in sixteenth century Italy. In: Grafton A, Siraisi N (eds) 1999 Natural particulars: nature and the disciplines in Renaissance Europe. Massachusetts Institute of Technology, Cambridge

Green M 2001 The Trotula: An English translation of the medieval compendium of women's medicine. University of Pennsylvania Press, Philadelphia.

Hall TS 1975 History of general physiology 600 B.C. to A.D. 1900, vol. 1. University of Chicago Press, Chicago.

Kassell L 2005 Medicine and magic in Elizabethan London. Clarendon Press, Oxford.

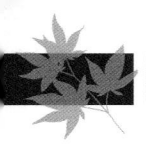

Kingsley P 1996 Ancient philosophy, mystery and magic: Empedocles and the Pythagorean tradition. Clarendon Press, Oxford.

Kirkpatrick J, Naylor I 1997 Ulcer management in medieval England. Journal of Wound Care 6:350–352.

Kremer E, Urdang G 1963 History of pharmacy. 3rd edn. J B Lippincott, Philadelphia.

Lloyd GER 1964 The hot and the cold, the dry and the wet in Greek philosophy. Journal of Hellenic Studies 84:92–106.

McVaugh MR 1969 Quantified medical theory and practice at 14th century Montpellier. Bulletin of the History of Medicine 43:397–413.

Riddle J 1985 Dioscorides on pharmacy and medicine. University of Texas Press, Austin.

Salazar C 2000 The treatment of war wounds in Graeco-Roman antiquity. EJ Brill, Leiden.

Temkin O 1958 Galenicals and Galenism in the history of medicine. In: Galdston I (ed.) 1958 The impact of the antibiotics on medicine and society. Monograph II. International Universities Press, New York.

Temkin O 1973 Galenism: rise and decline of a medical philosophy. Cornell University Press, Ithaca.

Van Arsdall A 2002 Medieval Herbal Remedies: The Old English Herbarium and Anglo-Saxon Medicine. Routledge, London.

Voigts LE 1979 Anglo-Saxon plant remedies and the Anglo-Saxons. Isis 70:250–269.

Webster C 2008 Paracelsus: medicine, magic and mission at the end of time. Yale University Press, New Haven.

# CHAPTER 3
# Origins and proponents of the revival of herbal medicine in 19th century Britain

Around 1978 the study of physiomedicalism was removed from the training course leading to membership of the National Institute of Medical Herbalists. This reflected a desire to modernize herbal medicine, to increase the number of European herbs prescribed and to reduce reliance on American herbs. I will argue that the concepts of physiomedicalism reflect 18th century thinking and thus the wider Western philosophical tradition, so the move towards phytotherapy led to a loss in subtlety of the conceptualization and language used to describe the actions of the medicines. I will briefly consider the lives of Samuel Thomson, Albert Coffin and John Skelton, and the influences from America on British herbal medicine in the 19th and early 20th centuries. This essay raises themes for discussion rather than offering conclusions.

The starting point is a discussion of the influences on Thomsonian herbal medicine which flourished in early 19th century America. The emphasis given to vitalism, reinterpreted through physiomedicalism (Priest & Priest 2000) continues, albeit implicitly, to influence current prescribing, and the self-help approach advocated by Thomson formed part of a wider movement towards self-reliance in healthcare which remains important in current herbal practice.

Thomsonianism is discussed by Haller (2000) and in the autobiography of Thomson (1769–1843) (Thomson 1832a, 1849, Comfort 1869, Fox 1920). Born on a farm in New Hampshire, Thomson describes how as a boy he was taught to collect herbs by a woman named Benton. She would use different herbs until the patient perspired (Thomson 1832b) and this formed the basis of the system of healing which he later developed. A small number of herbs was used to treat common illnesses, in particular childhood and epidemic fevers.

Thomson emphasizes his lack of education and that his knowledge came from experimentation. He claims that experience is the best teacher and his vivid accounts of treatments show a keen observation of patients. He recounts his treatment of his family and then, after 1806, his experiences as he travelled as a herbalist in the towns of New Hampshire and Maine (Thomson 1832a, Estes 1992). Thomson gained a patent for his system in 1813 (Ball 1925), which was sold through 'family rights' and the Friendly Botanic Society (Thomson 1832a, Haller 2000, Estes 1992), with a first edition published in 1822 and a second in 1825 (Thomson 1825). Berman (1951) argues that Thomsonianism was popular in rural communities as doctors were undereducated, with study averaging 13 weeks, and that, under the influence of Benjamin Rush, bloodletting and mercurial treatment persisted longer than in Europe. Other advantages were that treatment could be started immediately, costs would be lower and the self-help ethos was in tune with the democratic spirit of the times (Wallace 1980, Flannery 2002). Self-help in medicine was fundamental to healthcare at the time and manuscript sources show that a wide range of methods was used (Moss 1999).

Thomson (1832a) argues that heat is life and cold is death so bloodletting 'to cool the body' in fever only gave cold the upper hand. The Thomsonian course of treatment is described by Comfort (1869) and depends on the use of herbs alongside steam to 'reanimate.' Remedy No. 1: lobelia *Lobelia inflata* as an emetic to cleanse the stomach and overpower cold followed by No. 2: cayenne *Capsicum annuum* to retain internal heat and cause perspiration, No. 3: astringents to scour the stomach and bowels and No. 4: bitters to correct the bile and restore digestion. No. 5 was a dysentery syrup and No. 6 rheumatic drops containing cayenne and myrrh. Other herbs used are discussed by Haller (2000) and an English edition includes more herbs (Thomson 1849). Estes (1992) sets Thomson in his historical context, and states that 75% of the 63 plant remedies listed in his 1835 edition were listed in the Edinburgh Dispensatory, republished in Philadelphia in 1791. Further accounts are given by Robinson (1830), Stevens (1847) and Colby (2007). Thomson collected herbs in the wild, but made no reference to Native Americans and their knowledge of indigenous herbs. He advocated the use of lobelia *Lobelia inflata* and claimed to have discovered its use as an emetic, but there will have been other sources of information. Another Thomsonian practitioner Mattson (1841) is at pains to disprove this claim stating that lobelia was already used as an emetic alongside vapour baths by the Ma[r]shpee Indians of Martha's Vineyard, Massachusetts (Mashpee Wampanoag Tribe 2009).

The system emphasized the importance of heat. This excerpt from Thomson's Principles (Skelton 1853) gives an impression:

> 29. That medicine that will most readily and safely open obstructions, promote perspiration, and restore a salutary operation of the digestive powers, by exciting and maintaining a due

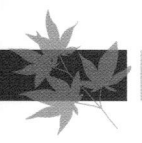

*degree of heat and action through the system, is best suited to every state or form of disease, and must be universally applicable to a diseased state of the human system ...*

*44. The animal body is the machine so constructed, so modified, endowed with such a capacity for life, call it vital principle, or what you please, that heat rarifying and lightening air, stimulating and expanding the lungs, puts the machinery into motion, and pumps the tide of life through the crimson channels.*

To set this in context we need to consider the possible influences on its composition. Skelton (1853) writes that Hippocrates said that the 'type of all disease was one', and Samuel Thomson 'the simple American ploughman. ... discovered the same truth'. Skelton uses the phrases '*Omnium morborum unus*' and '*idem modus est*': 'the type of all disease is one' and 'disease is a unit'. These phrases were the basis of my search which led to *Breaths* (Jones 1923), part of the *Hippocratic corpus*, where it is stated that 'so while diseases are thought to be entirely unlike one another, owing to the difference in their seat, in reality all have but one essence and cause' (Jones 1923). The *Hippocratic corpus* contains books by different authors incorporated together at the medical school of Cos, and the philosophy and identity of the author of *Breaths* is a topic of debate (Jouanna 1999), as it is unusual in ascribing all disease to one cause, namely that air which is breathed in is fundamental to life. Pitman (2004, 2005) takes current concepts in holistic medicine and discusses related texts within the *Hippocratic corpus*.

The proposition that a text of the *Hippocratic corpus* influenced 18th century thought in America is given some support by Coxe (1846) in the commentary on his translation of *Breaths*, titled *On flatus*, 'we here find, in a few words, the doctrine of the unity of disease, as more fully laid down and elaborated by the late Professor Rush ... and as such, taught it in the University of Pennsylvania'. Rush was familiar with the *Hippocratic corpus* and had translated the *Aphorisms of Hippocrates* in his teens (Corner 1948). Estes (1992) argues that while it is unlikely that Thomson had read Hippocrates, the texts would have been discussed in medical writings of the time. He proposes two other Hippocratic texts as possible sources: *The heart* and *The nature of the child*.

Chance then led to a mention of the phrase 'disease is a unit' in Porter (1995) discussing 18th century debate on the nature of the vital force. Through history, there are advocates of treatment which relies on a theoretical framework such as the Dogmatists of ancient Rome, and advocates of treatment with an empirical approach, such as the Empiricists of ancient Rome. In the 18th century these arguments came to a head as a sequel to the startling 17th century advances in the application of mathematics to natural phenomena. For example, the 'mechanical approach' of Quincy, writing in 1712, led to him to argue that 'the material substance of the body was of the same matter and thus subject to the same laws [as] any other part of the material world of much viler Account' (Howard-Jones 1951). Equally there was intense debate about the nature of the soul, the relationship between the soul and the body, the nature of the vital force if considered to exist, and finally the nature of God (French 2003, Porter 2003). Such debates form the backbone of Western thought and I will not enter the argument. Porter (1995) summarizes the views of Stahl (1660–1734), who perceives the soul as a power which guides the tissues, and Haller (1708–1777), who considers the vital force to be an innate property of the tissues. This was based on his physiological experiments in which he demonstrated that irritability, the ability to respond to stimuli, was inherent in tissues. Porter suggests that the views of Haller influenced John Brown, whose ideas were taken up by Benjamin Rush, and this formed the next line of enquiry.

Brown (1735–1788) studied at the Edinburgh School of Medicine under Cullen. In 1780 he began to lecture in Edinburgh on a system of medicine which proposed that disease had only one cause: a variation in the degree of excitement, and that therefore the body could rely only on its inherent natural energy. This argument, Brunonianism, immediately led to major debate as Brown argued that there are no particular cures for particular diseases (Risse 1988). This is not the first time in history that a method of treatment has prioritized one factor at the expense of all others. In ancient Rome, the Methodist sect believed that the choice of remedies should be based only on assessment of whether the body is dry or fluid or in a mixed condition (Edelstein 1967).

Returning to our theme, Benjamin Rush (1745–1813) studied medicine in Edinburgh from 1766 to 1768 and practised medicine in Philadelphia from 1769. He was a signatory of the United States Declaration of Independence (Goodrich 1829) and his lectures at the newly founded medical school in Philadelphia were published from 1789 as volumes of *Medical inquiries and observations*. My contention is that Thomson was influenced by medical texts of the time through a medical student who rented a house on his farm for 7 years from 1790. Dr Bliss was the student of a 'root doctor', and Thomson (1832b) says that he 'spared no pains to give him all the information in his power'. The two men could have discussed such matters in the evenings of the 1790s.

Rush (1805) states '1. Cold. This is universally acknowledged to be a predisposing cause of fever.'; '5. There is but one exciting cause of fever, and that is stimulus. ... this proposition is of great application, inasmuch as it cuts the sinews of the division of disease from their remote causes. Thus it establishes the sameness of a pleurisy, whether it be excited by heat, succeeding cold, or by contagion of the smallpox and measles, or by the miasmata of yellow fever';

# Origins and proponents of the revival of herbal medicine in 19th century Britain

'6. ... Thus fire is a unit, whether it be produced by friction, percussion, electricity, fermentation, or by a piece of wood or coal in a state of inflammation'. The actual conclusions and treatments proposed by Thomson and Rush were utterly opposed but this extensive quotation illustrates the debate of the time. Rush (Corner 1948) describes his anguish as he moved away from the principles of Cullen during the 1780s and, although influenced by Brown, his arguments were much more coherent, and Gross (1861) observes that Rush was actually at great pains to identify diseases and to form diagnoses. Rush appears to have been the source of the physiomedical concept 'to equalize the circulation' as '... the business of medicine is to equalize them in the cure of fever; that is, to abstract the excesses from the blood and restore them to other parts of the body' (Corner 1948). My argument is that physiomedicalism is based on 18th century concepts which were developed in the context of a progression from humoral thinking. This is more explicit in the lectures on Thomsonianism given by Robinson (1830), which he prefaced with a discussion of 18th century concepts of the soul and the vital force and the theories of Cullen, Brown and Rush.

The link between Thomsonianism and Britain was a North American herbalist, Albert Isiah Coffin (1798–1866), who settled in Britain in 1838. Coffin (1864) introduced the Thomsonian herbal system and thus the usage of North American medicinal plants and, revisiting his book, there were the previously unnoticed names of Rush and Brown. Coffin was a Thomsonian agent (Haller 2000) in New York in 1833 and Mississippi in 1834 (Hersey 1834). Coffin was not the only person to introduce the American materia medica and the practice of steaming to Britain. Whitlaw (1829) travelled to North America in 1796 and collected botanic specimens, published a book on herbal medicine and set up vapour bath infirmaries in Britain in the 1830s (Haller 2000). However, Coffin was crucial in increasing the prominence of herbal medicine, particularly in working-class communities. This movement remains a significant, if implicit, influence on current herbal practice in Britain but was built on an already existing traditional practice of herbal medicine (Brown 1982).

Coffin (1864) copied the principles of Thomson without acknowledgment, whereas John Stevens (1847) gives a detailed account of Thomsonian principles and treatment and, according to his brother who practised in Bristol, they also introduced the Thomsonian system (Brown 1982). However, Coffin did acknowledge his debt to Native Americans. He describes how 'our early life was devoted to the study of medicine, as taught and practised in the school' but he developed a severe cough at the age of 16. The next winter it returned with 'bluish-grey and gluey expectoration'. 'The most eminent of the faculty attended us' but his condition deteriorated over the next 3 years such that he was very thin and coughing up blood. 'At this time a tribe of the Seneca Indians encamped in the neighbourhood; one of the women ... saw us and inquired how long we had been in that condition. ... she brought from the fields and woods some of nature's remedies, and in three months, thanks to her aid, we were restored to perfect health; and from that time to the present our lungs have never failed us'.

Coffin arrived in London, moved to Hull, Leeds, then Manchester from 1847 until 1850 when he moved back to London. He set up botanic societies and gave lectures. The Manchester Guardian describes Coffin as touring towns with announcements that he would 'in four lectures, teach every man to be his own doctor' (Miley 1988). There were large attendances: 458 persons sat down to tea in 1847 in the Temperance Hall, Bolton (Miley 1988). Coffin arrived in a Britain in the grips of rapid urbanization, which was associated with numerous political and social movements and with religious nonconformism. The belief in self-reliance allied well with the Thomsonian movement (Flannery 2002, Connor 1995). As an example, Miley (1988) describes James Scolefield, pastor of the Swedenborgian Church, Manchester, who promoted vegetarianism and herbalism, prescribed and sold a cholera mix, and allowed a Chartist Conference to be held there in 1842.

Amongst the herbalists of the time, a central figure in the development of herbal medicine in 19th century Britain was John Skelton. Skelton was originally a shoemaker, a republican and signatory to the People's Charter of 1838 (Jones 1975). Chartism was a widespread working-class movement which collected enormous petitions in 1839 and 1842 in support of six points, including universal male suffrage. Skelton (1853) states that he was born 'over 40 years ago' in Devon where he collected herbs for his grandmother. He moved to Plymouth and recounts how he met John Brenmer in the shoemakers. Brenmer had moved down from Scotland where he had been in the habit of taking pellitory *Parietaria diffusa* for his 'gravel'. Skelton knew where some grew on orchard walls and collected some pellitory and refers to the payment as 'his first doctor's fee'. Miley (1988) gives examples of Skelton's skills as a speaker at Chartist meetings and in 1848 he was contracted by Coffin for 2 years to lecture in the Midlands and the North and encourage the development of botanic societies (Skelton 1852). In 1848, the people of Sheffield are reported to have left 'highly delighted with the intellectual treat'. Skelton settled in Leeds in 1851 but later argued publicly with Coffin who, like Thomson, had arguments with other herbalists in an attempt to keep a monopoly on the supply of herbs to Thomsonian agents. In a discussion of plantain *Plantago* species, Skelton (1852) promoted self-help and the collection of native herbs rather than reliance on imported materials. He refers to his purchase of a 1633 copy of Gerard and to owning copies of herbals, including Dodoens, Hill, Culpeper and Parkinson and books by Cullen, Thornton (1810) and Woodville (1810). Editions of Culpeper had remained in print continuously and a new edition was published in

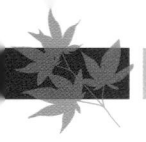

1814 (Parkins 1814). Later, Skelton studied to obtain medical qualifications at St Bartholomew's Hospital, London and was listed in the Medical Directory as qualifying in 1864. His book *The Science and Practice of Medicine* (Skelton 1904) was first published in 1870 and continued in use into the 1920s (Skelton 1930).

Alongside herbal books, other books were published as self-help guides to family medicine and a discussion of two examples helps to set the herbal texts in context. William Buchan (1729–1805) studied medicine at Edinburgh and published *Domestic Medicine, or The Family Physician*, in 1769, which ran to 19 editions in his lifetime. Buchan (1818) gives thorough descriptions, for example of the symptoms of fever, which would enable the lay person to recognize the symptoms of common illnesses. Some advice is thoroughly modern: a light diet and 'what is so likely to abate the heat, attenuate the humours, remove spasms and obstructions, promote perspiration, increase the quantity of urine, and in short produce every salutary effect in an ardent or inflammatory fever, as drinking plentifully of water …'. Taking the example of pleurisy, he proposes many causes but gives an accurate description of the symptoms, the location of the inflammation and course of the disease. The treatment takes many forms, including bleeding and blistering poultices: 'almost every person knows, when a fever is attended with a violent pain of the side, and a quick hard pulse, that bleeding is necessary'. The medicines given include cabbage poultices, 'small doses of purified nitre and camphire,' squill in a pectoral decoction and decoction of Seneca rattlesnake root *Polygala senega* (Turcotte & Kenkel 2009). At the end is an index, a list of over 180 herbs and animal parts with brief descriptions, a list of simples, including herbs and minerals that should be kept to hand, and finally substantial detail on methods of preparation (Buchan 1818).

Another important influence was John Wesley (1703–1791), the founder of Methodism, who travelled many miles annually to preach in the open air (Waller 2003). He opened dispensaries and in 1747 published *Primitive Physic*, which ran to 32 editions. His advice on diet, exercise, cold bathing, moderation of the passions and the correct amount of sleep is thought to be based on the work of, amongst others, George Cheyne (1671–1743), who according to Guerrini (2000) 'transformed the six non-naturals [of Galenic medicine] into the seven deadly sins'. In the late eighteenth century, according to Smith (1985), the six Galenic non-naturals (air, diet, sleep, exercise, evacuations and possessions of the mind) were used to advocate a 'cool regimen', including, for example, moderate exercise, bathing and a 'low' diet of vegetables. Wesley (1828) combined home remedies, advice and prescriptions from current medical publications (Rogal 1978) and other treatments of the time, including calomel, bleeding and electrotherapy (Waller 2003). For pleurisy 'a fever attended with violent pain in the side, and the pulse remarkably hard', Wesley (1828) makes six suggestions, including a decoction of nettles with a poultice of hot boiled nettles. Wesley was influenced by the early Church and believed that through grace, finding God in the heart, people could be content in themselves and help others. This is explored by Madden (2007) but the relevance here is that this approach encourages trust in one's own resources. An advantage of self-help in the late 18th and early 19th century was that the patient would be less likely to be bled and was perhaps less likely to take large amounts of calomel. Another questionable aspect of 18th century medicine is the number of medicines prescribed. The casebook of Samuel Glass 1715–1773 (Clark undated) describes a case of pleurisy in a man who fortunately recovered. He was bled a total of 45 oz of blood over three sessions and had two large blisters applied. He was prescribed two preparations and two cough syrups, with a total of 18 ingredients.

Thomsonian rhetoric emphasized the incongruity that the people with the medical qualifications continued to use outdated methods such as calomel and bleeding, and Thomsonian herbal practitioners quickly sought further education in herbal medicine with a broad medical curriculum and materia medica. Flannery (2002) gives an account of the popularity of Thomsonianism focused on its connection with increasing literacy and education. Education was opposed by Thomson (1832a) and Coffin, who both thought that practitioners should observe patients rather than read books. They would have sympathized with the Methodists in ancient Rome who argued that it is not necessary to learn all the diseases or all about the individual constitution, and that therefore a practitioner could be trained in six months (Edelstein 1967). Alva Curtis (1797–1881), an educational pioneer, who opened the Botanico-Medical College in 1836, split with Thomson over this issue. Many sources argue that it was one of the issues which led practitioners in America to join the Eclectic movement founded by Wooster Beach (Haller 2000). Thomsonianism developed into the physiomedical movement and William Cook (1832–1899) founded a school named the Physio-Medical Institute in 1859 in Cincinatti. Haller (1997) gives a thorough account of the developments within physiomedicalism in America in the second half of the 19th century and recounts the debate between vitalism and materialism. Unfortunately he ascribes part of the demise of physiomedicalism to disagreements between practitioners, which exacerbated the struggle to modernize the curriculum and facilities in physiomedical schools.

However, American practice did influence education and practice in Britain through personal contact between the two countries. For example, in 1914, the President of the National Association of Medical Herbalists, John Marlow, is stated to have studied herbal and Eclectic practice and obtained his diploma from the Ohio University, Cincinatti (Dawes 1914). A significant influence was Dr Sarah Webb (1867–1935), who graduated from the

College of Medicine and Surgery, Chicago. This was set up by Cook and others in 1897 and was a successor to the Chicago Physio-Medical College which Cook had run since 1885 (Haller 1997). She practised in America before marrying William Webb, who practised in Southport, Lancashire. Later, she was Principal of the College of Botanic Medicine in London and published *Diseases of Women* in 1920, *Mother and Child* in 1920 and *Menopause or Change of Life in Women* in 1922 (Dow unpublished). Webb (1916) contributed to the *Standard Guide to Non-Poisonous Herbal Medicine*, which also includes lectures given in Southport in 1916 by a lecturer from the Chicago College. A discussion of developments in the 20th century is outside the scope of this review but, just to give a flavour, Morley (1963) of Doncaster discusses the profound influence on his practice of the writings of Keith (1901) on the vital function, the vix medicatrix naturae, in health and disease. Burns Lingard (1958), who qualified as a member of the National Institute of Medical Herbalists in 1905, gives prescriptions for pleurisy and pneumonia based on pleurisy root *Asclepias tuberosa* and Composition essence, which is a Thomsonian preparation. He states that 'it is my proud boast that in all my 50 years I have never lost a case of pneumonia, pleurisy or influenza ... during the influenza epidemic of 1918–1919 I dispensed over 15 000 bottles of medicine'. The course notes prepared in the late 1950s by Albert Priest (unpublished) drew mainly on Cook's text (1985) written in 1869 and Thurston (1900) but discuss other authors. To explain the basic principles, Priest used quotations from Cook: the vital force is 'the form of energy ordering the movement of matter at the organic level' and Thurston: 'the human organism is a systematic and purposeful aggregation of tissue cells, each developed from bioplasm, through which works the Vital force'. The central theme of physiomedicalism is that where the tissues are too relaxed or too contracted (tense) to respond to the vital force, then changes in function are observed and the normal periodicity of function is disturbed. Symptoms are thus clues to estimate the degree of change from normal function and the underlying trophicity, that is associated changes in the organic tissues. The discussion by Cook (1985) of relaxation, contraction and other actions is a good starting place. The later text of Thurston draws on physiology to emphasise the significance of the circulation of blood to the tissues and the state of equilibrium of the nervous system. This makes for a somewhat laborious text which is usefully explained by Menzies-Trull (2003). There is an associated emphasis on alternatives to remove accumulations, obstruction and poisons. This aspect was emphasized by Skelton (1853): unless caused by an accident, 'disease is obstruction, arising immediately or remotely' which arises from lack of food, air, water, exercise or 'pure blood' and the purpose of herbal medicine is to restore the condition of body.

This essay has concentrated on the social context rather than the therapies. It is a partial account in that no coherent analysis has been attempted of changes in the perception of the body and of the process of healing. Rosenberg (1977) offers a thought-provoking discussion of the changes in healthcare during the 19th century and locates the perception of the value of a treatment within the culture of the time. The combination of changes in society, in public health and life expectancy, in scientific, religious and philosophical thinking in the last 150 years make it difficult to 'get inside the head' of the practitioners of the past. So, why is it relevant to the herbal practitioner of today? My argument is that the language used to express the meaning of the actions allows the modern reader to learn more about the traditional usage of the herbs which we prescribe today. The authors and practitioners visualized the actions of herbs and their influences on the bodily systems without the benefit of the analysis of the compounds within the herbs. In the present day we can use both forms of knowledge. If I make a diagnosis of pleurisy associated with viral infection, which is considered to be a common cause (Kass et al 2007), then the question is how to resolve the infection and ensure that there are no further episodes. Lifestyle would be discussed but prescribing is a solitary art: the modern practitioner now knows that an antiviral herb would be useful – but which one?, which expectorant?, which alterative?, which circulatory stimulant?, would an adaptogen be useful now or later?, would a diaphoretic tea be useful?, what about a local preparation? In my experience, small changes in prescriptions have substantial effects. The language of actions can help the practitioner to make these choices and there could be much deeper discussion of the meaning of the concepts behind the terminology of plant actions. Mills (1991) and Hoffman (2003) have made useful contributions. While one can disagree with some of his conclusions, Wood (1997, 2004) has invigorated the debate in Britain. Herbal practitioners now have an opportunity to reengage with our tradition because so many books that were only available in special collections are available online. By looking back to the 18th and 19th centuries, we find clues to explain the actions of plants, and thus to formulate the correct prescription for the individual patient.

## REFERENCES

Ball JM 1925 Samuel Thomson (1769–1843) and his patented system of medicine. Annals of Medical History 7:144–153.

Berman A 1951 The Thomsonian movement and its relation to American pharmacy and medicine. Bulletin of the History of Medicine 25:405–428.

Brown PS 1982 Herbalists and medical botanists in mid-nineteenth century Britain with special reference to Bristol. Medical History 26:405–420.

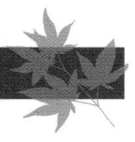

Buchan W 1818 Domestic medicine. W Lewis, London.

Burns Lingard W 1958 Herbal prescriptions from a consultants case book. National Institute of Medical Herbalists, Elland, Yorkshire.

Cameron A [undated] Samuel Glass (1715–1773) ms. Centre for Medical History, University of Exeter. Online. Available: http://www.centres.ex.ac.uk/medhist/news/transcripts/glass.pdf.

Coffin AI 1864 Botanic guide to health, 49th ed. Haynes, Coffin, London.

Colby T 2007 A guide to health: being an exposition of the principles of the Thomsonian system. Kessinger Publishing, Montana.

Comfort JW 1869 The practice of medicine on Thomsonian principles. Lindsay & Blakiston, Philadelphia. Online. Available: http://books.google.com.

Connor JJ 1995 Thomsonian medical books and the culture of dissent in upper Canada. Canadian Bulletin of Medical History 12:289–311.

Cook W 1985 The physiomedical dispensatory. Eclectic Medical Publications, Portland, Oregon. Online. Available: http://www.henriettesherbal.com/eclectic/cook/index.html.

Corner GW (ed.) 1948 The autobiography of Benjamin Rush. American Philosophical Society, Princetown University Press.

Coxe JR 1846 The writings of Hippocrates and Galen. Epitomised from the original Latin translations. Lindsay and Blakiston, Philadelphia. Online. Available: http://oll.libertyfund.org/title/1988/128144.

Dawes A (ed.) 1914 Year book. National Association of Medical Herbalists of Great Britain, Worcester.

Edelstein L 1967 The Methodists. In: Temkin O, Temkin CL (eds) 1967 Ancient medicine, selected papers of Ludwig Edelstein. John Hopkins Press, Baltimore, pp 173–194.

Estes JW 1992 Thomson rewrites Hippocrates. In: Benes P, Benes JM (eds) Medicine and healing. The Dublin Seminar for New England Folklife Annual Proceedings 1990. Boston University, pp 113–132.

Flannery M 2002 The early botanical medical movement as a reflection of life, liberty, and literacy in Jacksonian America. Journal of the Medical Library Association 90:442–454.

Fox W 1920 The working-man's model family botanic guide to health, 22nd edn. W Fox and Sons, Sheffield.

French RK 2003 Medicine before science. Cambridge University Press, Cambridge.

Goodrich CA 1829 Lives of the signers to the Declaration of Independence. William Reed, New York. Online. Available: http://books.google.co.uk.

Gross SD (ed.) 1861 Lives of eminent American physicians and surgeons of the nineteenth century. Lindsay & Blakiston, Philadelphia. Online. Available: http://books.google.co.uk.

Guerrini A 2000 Obesity and depression in the Enlightenment. University of Oklahoma Press, Norman.

Haller JS 1997 Kindly medicine, physio-medicalism in America 1836–1911. Kent State University Press.

Haller JS 2000 The people's doctors: Samuel Thomson and the American botanical movement, 1790–1869. Southern Illinois University Press.

Hersey T 1834 The Thomsonian recorder. Jarvis Pike, Columbus, Ohio. Online. Available: http://books.google.co.uk.

Hoffman D 2003 Medical herbalism: the science and practice of herbal medicine. Healing Arts Press, Rochester, Vermont.

Howard-Jones N 1951 John Quincy, M.D. [d.1722], Apothecary and iatrophysical writer. Journal of the History of Medicine 6:149–175.

Jones WHS 1923 Hippocrates vol 2. Harvard University Press, Cambridge, MA.

Jones D 1975 Chartism and the chartists. St Martin's Press, New York.

Jouanna J 1999 Hippocrates. DeBevoise M B (transl) John Hopkins University Press, Baltimore.

Kass SM, Williams PM, Reamy BV 2007 Pleurisy. American Family Physician 75:1357–1364.

Keith MC 1901 The domestic practice and botanic handbook. M C Keith, Bellville, Ohio.

Madden D 2007 A cheap, safe and natural medicine: religion, medicine and culture in John Wesley's primitive physic. Editions Rodopi B V, Amsterdam.

Mashpee Wampanoag Tribe 2009 Online. Available: http://mashpeewampanoagtribe.com.

Mattson M 1841 The American vegetable practice. DL Hale, Boston.

Menzies-Trull C 2003 Herbal medicine keys to physiomedicalism. Newcastle, Staffordshire.

Miley U 1988 Herbalism and herbal medicine in the 19th and early 20th centuries: with particular reference to North West England. MSc thesis, UMIST U8484.

Mills S 1991 Out of the earth. Viking Arkana, London.

Morley CW 1963 Our physio-medical heritage. The Herbal Practitioner, professional journal for physio-medical-practitioners 15:11–13.

Moss K 1999 Southern folk medicine, 1750–1820. University of South Carolina Press, Columbia, SC.

Parkins (ed.) 1814 The English physician enlarged. B & R Crosby, London. Online. Available: http://books.google.co.uk.

Pitman V 2004 Sources of holism in ancient Greek and Indian medicine. Motilal Barnasidas, Delhi.

Pitman V 2005 the relationship of classical Greek medicine to contemporary Western Herbalism: an exploration of the idea of 'holism'. In: O'Sullivan C (ed.) Reshaping herbal medicine. Elsevier, London.

Porter R 1995 The eighteenth century In: Conrad L I, Neve M, Nutton V, et al (eds) The Western medical tradition. Cambridge University Press, Cambridge.

Porter R 2003 Flesh in the Age of Reason. Penguin Books, London.

Priest AW, Priest LR 2000 Herbal medication. CW Daniel, Saffron Walden, Essex.

Risse GB 1988 Brunonian therapeutics: new wine in old bottles? In: Bynum WF, Porter R (eds) Brunonianism in

Britain and Europe. Wellcome Institute for the History of Medicine, London, pp 46–62.

Robinson S 1830 A course of fifteen lectures on medical botany, denominated Thomson's new theory of medical practice. J Howe, Boston.

Rogal SJ 1978 Pills for the poor: John Wesley's primitive physic. The Yale Journal of Biology and Medicine 51:81–90.

Rosenberg CE 1977 The therapeutic revolution: medicine, meaning, and social change in nineteenth century America. Perspectives in Biology and Medicine 20:485–506.

Rush B 1805 Medical inquiries and observations, 2nd edn, vol 3. J. Conrad, Philadelphia. Online. Available: http://books.google.co.uk.

Skelton J 1852 Dr Skelton's botanic record and family herbal. Current News 3:7.

Skelton J 1853 A plea for the botanic practice of medicine. J Watson, London.

Skelton J 1904 The science and practice of medicine. National Association of Medical Herbalists, London.

Skelton J 1930 Bronchitis. The Medical Herbalist 55:182–195.

Smith G 1985 Prescribing the rules of health: self-help and advice in the late eighteenth century. In: Porter R (ed.) Patients and practitioners. Cambridge University Press, Cambridge, pp 249–282.

Stevens J 1847 Medical reform, or physiology and botanic practice, for the people. John Turner, Birmingham; Whittaker & Co, London. Online. Available: http://books.google.co.uk.

Thomson S 1825 A narrative of the life and medical discoveries of Samuel Thomson; containing an account of his system of practice, and the manner of curing disease with vegetable medicine, upon a plan entirely new, to which is added an introduction to his new guide to health or, botanic family physician, containing the principles upon which the system is founded, with remarks on fevers, steaming, poison. Printed for the author by EG House, Boston.

Thomson S 1832a New guide to health; or, botanic family physician. 3rd edn. Thomson, Samuel, Clark Street. Online. Available: http://books.google.co.uk.

Thomson S 1832b A narrative of the life and medical discoveries of Samuel Thomson: containing an account of his system of practice, and the manner of curing disease with vegetable medicine, upon a plan entirely new; to which is prefixed an introduction to his New guide to health, or Botanic family physician; containing the principles upon which the system is founded, with remarks on fevers, steaming, poison, 8th edn. Pike, Platt, Columbus, Ohio. Online. Available: http://books.google.co.uk.

Thomson S 1849 New guide to health, or botanic physician. Simpkin, Marshall, London. Online. Available: http://books.google.co.uk.

Thornton RJ 1810 A new family herbal. Richard Phillips, London. Available: http://books.google.co.uk.

Thurston JM 1900 The philosophy of physiomedicalism. Nicholson Printing, Richmond, Indiana. Online. Available: http://www.herbological.com/images/downloads/thurston.pdf.

Turcotte C, Kenkel N 2009 Seneca Snakeroot (Polygala senega L.) history and use. Online. Available: http://www.umanitoba.ca/botany/LABS/ECOLOGY/seneca.html.

Wallace DJ 1980 Thomsonians: the people's doctors. Clio Medica 14:169–186.

Waller R 2003 John Wesley. Society for the Promulgation of Christian Knowledge, London.

Webb S 1916 Nervous system and sympathetic nervous system in relation to the abdominal brain. In: Webb W (ed.) 1916 Standard guide to non-poisonous herbal medicine. WH Webb, Southport.

Wesley J 1828 Primitive physic. J Mason, London.

Whitlaw C 1829 New medical discoveries, with a defence of the Linnaean doctrine and a translation of his vegetable materia medica, which now first appears in an English dress. Published by the author, London.

Wood M 1997 The book of herbal wisdom. North Atlantic Books, Berkeley.

Wood M 2004 The practice of traditional Western herbalism: basic organs and systems. North Atlantic Books, Berkeley.

Woodville W 1810 Medical botany, 2nd edn. William Phillips, London. Online. Available: http://books.google.co.uk.

# CHAPTER 4
# A note on Goethe

We have included among the authors the work of Wilhelm Pelikan. His approach is singular in that, based on the ideas of Goethe and Rudolf Steiner, it offers a more esoteric, spiritual, in-depth consideration of the herbs, pursued with rigour, and from a recent perspective.

It could be argued that our old authors would not have 'seen' the plants, nor human beings, nor illness, as we do today. Schmidt, in his preface to Pelikan, suggests the old medieval herbals were written 'out of an old, instinctive vision of the inner human being and the plant world'. He regrets/laments how pharmacology has become a 'science of materials'; it no longer dwells in the relationship between plants and human beings. Our consciousness/way of seeing the world, and indeed our constitutions and diseases, have changed considerably over time. We can no longer achieve that instinctive relationship, it is argued (see, for example, Steiner's (1997) *An outline of esoteric science*), nor should we try. Yet to dismiss the knowledge and in most cases the obviously extensive experience within the old herbals as pre-scientific irrelevance throws out baby, bathwater and bath too, and leaves us with a pharmacology quite unrelated to nature. Paracelsus, on the other hand, scorned slavish copying of old writers and urged a more direct, personal experience, both inner and outer. Pelikan's approach through Goethe's methodology and Steiner's insights building on Goethe's ideas suggest one way to reawaken a living and practical appreciation of the old herbals and forge a way of working with plants through felt experience. We may then begin to rebuild consciously a deeper understanding of plants, human beings in health and illness, and the relationship between them.

Goethe (1749–1832) was one of Germany's foremost poets and playwrights, and for some time the multiskilled administrator for the Duke of Weimar. He was also a scientist, but his science was revolutionary and very different from both the Enlightenment science of his day and from modern science. Rudolf Steiner (1861–1925) was an Austrian philosopher and scientist, and founder of Anthroposophy – a 'science of the spirit extending our knowledge and understanding beyond the foundations laid down by natural science' (Evans & Rodger 1992). Anthroposophical ideas can be applied to all aspects of life; Steiner particularly wrote and lectured on agriculture, education, care of the disabled, art and architecture, medicine and economics.

Goethe felt passionately that the move towards the quantitative science of his day, which promoted only a mechanised view of a material world and relegated quality to the subjective, necessarily and abhorrently diminished experience of nature and limited human faculties in appreciation of it. Zajonc (1998) cites from Goethe's autobiography a response by Goethe to reading Holbach's System of Nature 'But hollow and empty did we feel in this atheistical half-night, in which earth vanished with all its images, heaven with all its stars'. Through meticulous work, supported by his artistic sensibilities he devised a rigorous methodology that allows rich exploration of the qualitative realm and perceived articulation of it, restores life to nature and furnishes a capacity for human beings to forge a consciously intuitive place within it. This is necessarily the briefest outline. For extensive exploration of the many aspects of Goethean Science see works by, for example, Bortoft (1996), Naydler (1996), Seamon & Zajonc (1998) and Hoffman (2007).

When dealing with the living world there are aspects of organic development beyond the material. For Goethe, these are not abstractions to mystical faith but an entirely perceivable goal implicit in the phenomenon itself. Towards this end Goethe introduced the discipline of morphology, which aims to study not the finished forms of phenomena, but the formative forces which produce them. From an in-depth study of the physical through the senses, the underlying creative formative principles of nature, of which the changing physical is a living manifestation, can be perceived. An inner lawfulness can be felt, one can 'see' inner patterns and relationships, things are no longer accidental but differently manifesting parts of a living, creating, non-sense-perceptible whole. Bortoft speaks of the wholeness of the phenomena, 'But the whole comes into presence *within* its parts, and we cannot encounter the whole in the same way that we encounter the parts. We should not think of the whole as if it were a thing' (Bortoft 1998). One eventually experiences an 'apercu', a moment of intuition where one perceives the 'Urphaenomen', the essence (which is not abstract) of a phenomenon from which all aspects of it can be explained. Goethe considered the human being to be the most exact scientific instrument, 'In so far as we make use of our healthy senses, the human being is the most powerful and exact scientific instrument possible' (Naydler 1996), since only human beings have the faculties to penetrate to this depth and 'read' these 'open secrets'. For such qualitative perception, faculties are developed other than the analytic mind, Bortoft says, and beyond the deductive reasoning process. Hoffmann (2007) comments 'A scientific thinking that is mechanical and logical perceives only that dimension of nature that is mechanical and logical'. Barnes (1999) says of 'the deeper levels of reality with which Goethe was concerned – the levels at which the

©2009 Elsevier Ltd, Inc, BV
DOI: 10.1016/B978-0-443-10344-5.00009-4

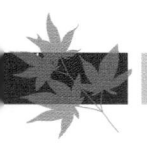

phenomena manifest their own life and being' that 'their practice requires new, transformed human capacities of perception'. He remarks '[Goethe] sensed that the plant, which is constantly in a state of becoming, ever transforming itself, cannot be grasped by a thinking that is static, passive, and only able to separate, define, and identify the phenomena'. But we can develop the cognitive ability and this faculty can be awoken by 'doing', by remaining with the object and developing what Goethe termed a 'delicate empiricism' that allows the inner lawfulness to shine through. Goethe tells us each phenomenon studied opens a new organ of perception. Bortoft (1998) speaks of a different way of thinking, a switch from an analytical, sequential and logical mode to a holistic, non-linear and intuitive, reached 'when the mind functions as an organ of perception instead of the medium of logical thought'. Hoffman (2007) speaks of thinking that 'undergoes … a qualitative transformation, such that it is able to perceive the phenomenon in a 'higher' dimension of itself. Riegner and Wilkes (1998) cite Steiner '[he] argued that, by training one's observational skills and by becoming increasingly aware of one's cognizing activity, the student would be led toward an experience of the 'idea within the reality''. Hoffman (2007) says 'the human artistic faculties are formed into organs of cognition'.

A ready introduction to Goethe's plant study is often demonstrated through the metamorphosis of the leaf. The leaves in Figure 4.1 are all the stem leaves from one plant just after flowering. The leaves will not change shape. All are different, yet if one 'moves through' the shapes a clear flow of movement can be perceived; if one leaf were withheld it could easily be replaced; an 'extra' leaf could be drawn in the sequence. One begins to sense a lawfulness about the plant; the living plant is all of these leaves but not any one in particular. Brady (1998) describes them as 'snapshots of continuous movement'; he says 'The movement under consideration is metamorphosis, which is not the outward alteration of one form into another but the differing outward expressions of an inward idea … The idea is intuited in the object, as a felt potency of growth and, hence, 'life''. Hence we can 'see', remaining with the phenomena, what is not at first available to the senses, intuiting a deeper phenomenon.

Pelikan bases his work on Goethe's methodology and Rudolf Steiner's further development of it. Other authors write with similarly inspiring insight. The works of Grohmann (1989), writing in the 1950s and 1960s, and Kranich (1997) in the 1970s and later, for example, offer a wonderful, meticulously observed, Goethe-inspired study of the plant world, through which one can begin to appreciate (among other aspects) the nature of the plant families and their relationship to one another and the whole; how each family offers a different expression of nature's possibilities; how each variety within the family finds its unique, but related, place within the limits of the family to express some aspect of it and how a lawfulness of expression emerges. One can begin to develop a sense of 'moving through', a 'felt experience' of how each species metamorphoses to explore and express its boundaries and reflect the possibilities within them, and their place within the plant world as a whole. The forces within the plant too are explored. One begins to 'get a feel' for reading their nature; nothing of their expression, from the colour and shape of the flowers, to the nature of their sap, and their constituents is 'accidental'. Kranich takes us on a journey through the families of the water lily, bindweed, cabbage, buttercup, rose, carrot, pea, deadnettle and daisy, exploring their natures and boundaries; the hidden heat in the cabbage family, for example, the changeable water and light nature of the buttercup family, the airy carrot family and the fiery labiates. Pelikan, within the families he covers, reflects the implications within medicines. Reading Pelikan on poppy, for example, the links begin to appear between the shape of the leaves, the early drop of the petals, the unique effect of opium and seeds which can safely be eaten in cakes. Simonis (1981) has a similar approach. Current authors on Goethean plant study are equally exciting, for example Colquhoun & Ahrens (1996), Bockemuehl & Suchantke (1995), Bockemuehl (undated, 2000, 2003) and Hoffman (2007).

Consideration of the role of the elements, earth, water, air and fire/warmth, plays into the plant study on many levels, and while this is a modern re-examination, it nevertheless advances our appreciation of the old texts. Holdrege, in his foreword to Hoffman's (2007) Goethean science of living form; the artistic stages, which the author bases on an elemental approach to foster 'mobility of thought', says 'most of us think of these four elements as substances. Hoffman shows, however, that already the Greeks saw them as ways of knowing … The four elements are qualities, they lead us more deeply into the qualitative features of nature, which have long been considered off-limits to scientific inquiry'. Planetary aspects of plant life are considered too in a number of texts that again help towards further appreciation of plant nature.

The references to Pelikan (and others) in our text are unfortunately necessarily partial, since they refer to complex concepts in anthroposophical medicine. We acknowledge this is appreciably frustrating. We have included them, however, to demonstrate, albeit partially, how a deep appreciation of plants can be applied to healing through a similarly profound consideration of the human being. Pelikan himself details the four-fold and three-fold concepts of the human being; how the four-fold physical, etheric/time/life body, astral body and ego/spiritual body of the human being relate/correspond to the earth/mineral, water/plant, air/animal, warmth/human, respectively, and how the parts of the plant, root, leaf, flower and seed fit into the picture; how the root corresponds to the earth/physical, the leaf the water/etheric,

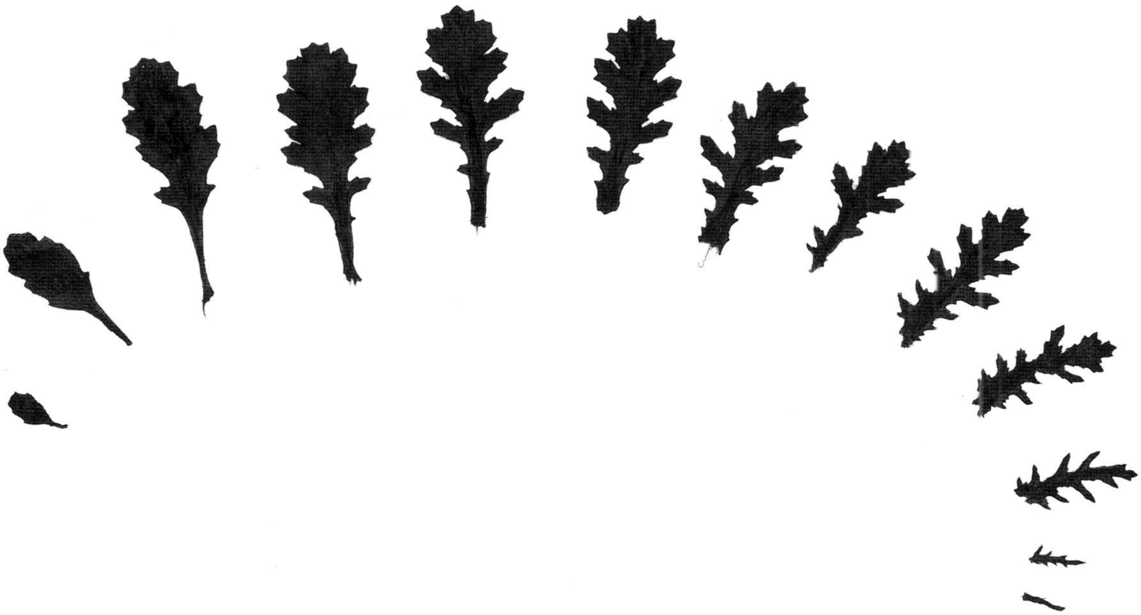

**Figure 4.1** Leaf sequence of *Senecio* spp.

the flower to the air/astral, and the seed the warmth/ego, although only the first two are contained within the plant, the remaining two remain necessarily outside. Then, for the three-fold, how the polarities of the nerve-sense system and metabolic/limb system are balanced by the central rhythmic system, and how these are reflected in roots, flowers and leaves, respectively, and the implications for treatment. For expansion of these ideas readers are referred to anthroposophical texts, particularly Evans & Rodger (1992), Van der Bie & Hueber (2003) and Bott (2004).

Anthroposophical medicine describes itself as an extension of conventional medicine and not an alternative therapy. Steiner was clear that practitioners should first train in orthodox medicine. However, an appreciation of plants and their healing capacities are so profound and can throw such light on the relationship between humans and plants, and past and present implications for healing, we feel our text gains considerably from its inclusion. And so Pelikan's work is offered in the spirit expressed by Schmidt in his preface to the 1988 edition 'We hope, therefore, that this work may prove a major building block in the new approach to pharmaceutics and that it may find its way to all who feel the inner need for such a new science, be they clinicians, teachers, farmers, or simply people who take a loving interest in the plant world and its relationship to the essential human being'.

# REFERENCES

Barnes J 1999 Goethe and the power of rhythm. Adonis Press, New York.

Bockemuehl J (undated) Ein Leitfaden zur Heilpflanzenerkenntnis, vol. 1. Verlag am Goetheanum, Dornach.

Bockemuehl J 2000 Ein Leitfaden zur Heilpflanzenerkenntnis, vol. 2. Verlag am Goetheanum, Dornach.

Bockemuehl J 2003 Ein Leitfaden zur Heilpflanzenerkenntnis vol. 3. Verlag am Goetheanum, Dornach.

Bockemuhl J, Suchantke A 1995 The metamorphosis of plants. Novalis Press, Capetown.

Bortoft H 1996 The wholeness of nature: Goethe's way of science. Floris Books, Edinburgh.

Bortoft H 1998 Counterfeit and authentic wholes: finding a means for dwelling in nature. In: Seamon D, Zajonc A (eds) Goethe's way of science: a phenomenology of nature. State University of New York Press, pp 277–298.

Bott V 2004 An introduction to anthroposophical medicine. Sophia Books, Forest Row.

Brady R 1998 The idea in nature: rereading Goethe's organics. In: Seamon D, Zajonc A (eds) Goethe's way of science: a phenomenology of nature. State University of New York Press, pp 83–111.

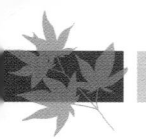

Colquhoun M, Ahrens A 1996 New eyes for plants. Floris Books, Edinburgh.

Evans M, Rodger I 1992 Healing for body, soul and spirit. Floris Books, Edinburgh.

Grohmann G 1989 The plant, vols 1 and 2. Bio-dynamic Farming and Gardening Association Inc, Kimberton.

Hoffmann N 2007 Goethe's science of living form: the artistic stages. Adonis Press, New York.

Kranich EM 1997 Pflanze und Kosmos: Grundlinie einer kosmologischen Botanik. Verlag Freies Geistesleben, Stuttgart.

Naydler J 1996 Goethe on science: an anthology of Goethe's scientific writings. Floris Books, Edinburgh.

Riegner M, Wilkes J 1998 Flowforms and the language of water. In: Seamon D, Zajonc A (eds) Goethe's way of science: a phenomenology of nature. State University of New York Press, pp 233–252.

Seamon D, Zajonc A (eds) 1998 Goethe's way of science: a phenomenology of nature. State University of New York Press.

Simonis WC 1981 Heilpflanzen, 3 vols. Novalis Verlag, Berlin.

Steiner R 1997 An outline of esoteric science. Anthroposophic Press, Great Barrington MA.

Van der Bie G, Huber M 2003 Foundations of anthroposophical medicine. Floris Books, Edinburgh.

Zajonc A 1998 Goethe and the science of his time: an historical introduction. In: Seamon D, Zajonc A (eds) Goethe's way of science: a phenomenology of nature. State University of New York Press, pp 15–30.

# CHAPTER 5
# Notes on nomenclature, plant descriptions, quality, constituents, safety and dosages

## NOMENCLATURE

The binomial nomenclature used follows Farah (2005) where available and additional sources, including the International Plant Names Index (2009) and the Plants Database (USDA 2010). In the text only current binomials are italicized. Pharmaceutical names, Ancient Greek and Latin names, medieval names and pre-Linnean botanical names are in ordinary type. For example, in the chapter on mugwort *Artemisia vulgaris*, Mattioli refers to Artemisia tenuifolia but this is not italicized as it is not a current binomial.

As a source for the naming and identification of the herbs in her translation of *De Materia Medica* by Dioscorides, Beck (2005) mainly uses André (1985), who refers to original sources and scholarship. Beck states that this is a topic which requires substantial further study and we have discussed the identification of a number of the herbs in this book.

Where possible, a binomial is provided for other herbs given by our sources but this is not provided where the identity is unclear. Green (2001) gives a helpful list identifying the herbs given in *The Trotula*, which relies on Hunt (1989). In some cases where there can be confusion over the common name, only the binomial is given. In all cases, the responsibility of the practitioner is to consider the evidence further and use current botanical sources to confirm the identity of herbs when intending to use a recipe given in the book.

## PLANT DESCRIPTIONS

For the plant descriptions, several sources are used, which are not referenced individually. They are Akeroyd (2003), Gibbons & Brough (1996), Grey-Wilson (1994), Podlech (2001), Stace (1991), Sterry (2006), Sutton (1996) and the four volumes of the *Flora Europaea* (Tutin et al 1964, 1968, 1973, 1976). For families we refer to the *Flora Europaea* and Judd et al (1999). Barker (2001) is a useful herbal textbook which groups herbs according to family. Non-technical terms are used where possible so, for example, 'smooth' rather than 'glaucous'. Hickey & King (2000) and Allaby (2006) are references for terminology.

The distribution is broadly given for Europe but readers are referred to the Plants Database of the United States Department of Agriculture (USDA 2010) for distribution maps of wild plants for the USA.

## QUALITY

Dioscorides gave particular attention to the quality of sources of plant materials and information is provided here on related species and other factors relevant to the quality of medicinal plant materials, but cultivation is not discussed.

Local sources of information should be consulted when considering wild collection. Many herbs in this book are included in the substantial quantities of medicinal herbs collected in the wild, especially in eastern Europe and the Balkans (Lange 2004). Herbal products licensed for sale under the European Union Directive on Traditional Herbal Medicinal Products have to show that the herbs are sourced in the light of guidance on good agricultural and collection practice (GACP) (EMEA 2002). The World Health Organization has published Guidelines on GACP (WHO 2003) and the International Standards for Sustainable Wild Collection of Medicinal and Aromatic Plants (ISSC-MAP 2007) is a joint project which provides a framework for standard operating procedures. The Medicinal Plant Specialist Group (2008) coordinates conservation efforts for medicinal plants.

## CONSTITUENTS

The aim of the table of constituents is to include all recent reports and to refer only to original papers. In the search, reference books, online scientific databases and the reference lists of papers were consulted. Readers are referred to the reviews listed, which will include older material and further detail on studies of the pharmacological actions of the herbs. For some herbs we discuss the role of polyphenols (Scalbert et al 2005) and antioxidants (Kohen & Nyska 2002), but have not given a full overview of the topic. The searches for all the monographs were completed in early 2009.

©2009 Elsevier Ltd, Inc, BV
DOI: 10.1016/B978-0-443-10344-5.00010-0

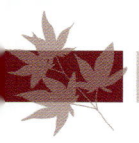

The table of categories of constituents is laid out in the following order: alkaloids; polysaccharides and mucilage; terpenes: monoterpenes, sesquiterpenes, triterpenes and their glycosides; phenylpropanoids: phenolic acids, flavonoids, condensed and hydrolyzable tannins; other compounds.

Examples of named compounds are given in each category after a colon but this list is not exhaustive. Where concentrations are given, they are either given as a total for that category at the beginning of the line or after the named individual compound. Concentrations are given as a percentage of dried plant material. For volatile oils only, concentrations of individual compounds are given as a percentage of the total oil. Concentrations are unreliable as they vary according to the time of year, time of day and situation of the plant. Identification of compounds in plant materials and the calculation of concentration depends on the methodologies used to analyse the compounds (Heinrich et al 2004), and this is an area where significant advances in technique continue to be made (Gray et al 2010).

## SAFETY

Information on safety is provided under three categories: do not use, use caution or monitor. The assumption is that herbal practitioners will use other reference sources where required.

Adverse event reports were sought for each herb up to mid 2009.

For some herbs we have summarized in-vitro studies but only used animal studies where there is a safety concern, such as use in pregnancy. Safety concerns about the usage of herbs during pregnancy and lactation have been inadequately investigated for most herbs, which makes evaluation of the evidence controversial in some cases. This topic is thoroughly reviewed by Bone in Mills & Bone (2005), and their advice is given where available. As he argues, the lack of evidence on the safety of herbal medicines in pregnancy cannot be construed as demonstrating that they are safe, and dosage should be given careful consideration.

## DOSAGES

Dosages are given by the authorial sources in Greek, Roman, Islamic and medieval units, and later in the Apothecaries' system and in the Avoirdupois system. Sometimes authors express weights using the weight of a coin used at the time, such as the Roman denarius (Richardson 2004). The dirham was an Islamic unit of weight based on a coin equivalent to 3 g. The dirham remains a unit of coinage in many countries.

It is useful to convert all units to metric units (Sizes 2006) and Marriott (2006) gives a detailed account of historical weights and measures. The following tables give Greek and Roman weights and measures which we have used, metric units and pre-metric units of weights and measures (Tables 5.1, 5.2 and 5.3).

## Pre-metric units

Although weights and measures throughout Europe were influenced by the Roman system, they varied between countries and provinces until the early 1800s, when most countries followed France in enforcing the metric system, which was established in France between 1799 and 1840. Units in recipes from before the nineteenth century will reflect national and local variation, and may include measures which have since been superseded.

The Avoirdupois system continued in use in Britain until 1971 and remains in use in the USA. There is some variation between the Avoirdupois systems in the two countries, for example the pint is different. The variations between US customary units and British Imperial weights came about because the US system was developed before

**Table 5.1** Ancient Greek and Roman weights and measures

| | Weight* | Rounded |
|---|---|---|
| Obol | 0.568 g | 600 mg |
| Triobolon | 1.794 g | 1800 mg |
| Drachme | 3.411 g | 4 g |
| Holce | 3.411 g | 3.5 g |
| Mina | 436.6 g | 437 g |
| | **Measure** | |
| Cyathos | 0.0456 L | 45 mL |
| Oxybaphon | 0.0684 L | 70 mL |
| Cotyle | 0.274 L | 274 mL |
| Sextarius | 1 Avoirdupois pint (578 mL); 12 cyathi, therefore 540 mL** | |

* As given in Beck (2005), after Berendes. See also Richardson (2004).
** Richardson (2004).

# Notes on nomenclature, plant descriptions, quality, constituents, safety and dosages | Chapter | 5

**Table 5.2** Table of systems of weight (mass)*

| Metric SI units | Avoirdupois (Imperial) | Apothecaries' weights |
|---|---|---|
| Microgram (μg/mcg)<br>1000 mcg = 1 mg | 1 grain** = 65 mg | 1 grain** = 65 mg |
| Milligram (mg)<br>1000 mg = 1 g | | 1 scruple = 20 grains = 1300 mg |
| Gram (g)<br>1000 g = 1 kg | ¼ oz = 7 g<br>½ oz = 14 g<br>1 ounce (oz) = 437.5 grains = 28.3 g (round to 28 g)<br>1 pound (lb) = 7000 grains = 16 oz = 454 g | 1 drachm = 60 grains = 3900 mg<br><br>1 ounce = 480 grains (8 drachms) = 31.2 g (round to 31 g) |

*For each system, read down the column from the smallest unit.
**The grain is the same in both systems. No abbreviation as could be confused with g.

**Table 5.3** Table of systems of measures (volume)*

| Metric SI units | Avoirdupois (Imperial) | Apothecaries' weights (Troy) |
|---|---|---|
| Millilitre (mL) | 1 minim = 0.06 mL<br><br><br>1 fl oz = 480 minims = 28.8 mL (round to 30 mL) | 1 minim = 0.06 mL<br>1 fl scruple = 20 minims<br>1 fl drachm = 60 minims = 3.6 mL<br>1 fl oz = 480 minims = 28.8 mL (round to 30 mL) |
| Litre (L)<br>1000 mL = 1 L | 1 pint = 20 fl oz = 568.5 mL<br>1 quart = 2 pints<br>1 gallon = 8 pints | |

*For each system, read down the column from the smallest unit.

the Imperial system was standardized by the Weights and Measures Act of 1824.

The Apothecaries' system developed from Roman units and was in use in Britain in the preparation of medicines until it was withdrawn in 1858, but continued to be used in the USA. Extra caution in the calculation of dosage is necessary when consulting 19th century and early 20th century texts as the date of writing may be many years earlier than it appears, as later editions were sometimes for the main part reprints of earlier editions.

The Avoirdupois and Apothecaries' systems differ. This can pose problems as in some texts it is not clear whether the units used are expressed in Avoirdupois or Apothecaries' weights and measures. Both systems use the common unit of the grain but the ounce is different in each system. Both systems use the ounce, but the Apothecaries' system also uses the scruple and the drachm. In the Apothecaries' system, prescriptions were commonly written using symbols (Royal Pharmaceutical Society of Great Britain 2010) for scruple, drachm and ounce with the amounts expressed in Roman numerals (Cooper & McLaren 1933, Marriott 2006). If a recipe gives drachms and scruples, then it is fair to expect that the Apothecaries' system was used.

We have used the archaic term 'drachm' as, although the term 'dram' is now used interchangeably with drachm, a

43

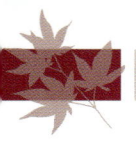

dram was formerly a unit in the Avoirdupois system of 1/16 of an ounce (Cooper & McLaren 1933). Conversion of the drachm to metric units gives an example of rounding and metrication of pre-metric units. Richardson (2004) gives the Greek drachm as 6 obols, which would be 3.4 g, but also gives the Roman drachm as 4.33 g. The drachm is given in Table 5.2 as 3.9 g and, given this variation, the drachm has been rounded in this book to 4 g. The preface to the 1974 edition of the *British Herbal Pharmacopoeia* also gives the drachm as 4 g.

The volumes in the Apothecaries' and Avoirdupois systems are almost identical. A commonly used equivalence in the recent past has been to express the old volume of ½–1 fl drachm as 2–4 mL. One teaspoon is 5 mL but the Imperial teaspoon is 3.5 mL and 1 tablespoon is 15 mL. Williamson (2003) gives a wineglassful as 1½ fl oz, which is 45 mL. However, Sizes (2006) gives a wineglassful as a unit of 2 fl oz in the Apothecaries' system and therefore 60 mL. This is smaller than a modern wineglass, which is at least 125 mL but often much larger. Even in modern texts, caution should be used in establishing whether a recipe is using the US pint or the Avoirdupois (Imperial) pint. In addition, the volume of a cup varies in different countries. Drops vary but can be measured into a 10 mL measuring cylinder to obtain a reproducible measurement of volume.

## Using parts to calculate proportions

If attempting to use a recipe given in the book, the practitioner should express the quantities in metric units using Tables 5.1, 5.2 and 5.3, review the amounts with care and compare with other reference sources both in books and online.

It can be useful to express a recipe as parts and then calculate the weight or measure in metric units. For example, if 1 drachm is the smallest unit, then take 1 part as 4 g. One ounce would then be expressed as 8 parts, therefore 32 g.

Ratios of parts can be expressed as weight/volume (w/v), weight/weight (w/w), volume/volume (v/v), volume/weight (v/w).

In sets of ratios, if each pair is in the ratio 1:3 then the corresponding number in set B (the bottom line) is three times the corresponding number in set A (the top line). Items with the same unit form the set (the horizontal line). The amount of herb in a 5 mL dose of tincture where the ratio is 1:3 (w/v) is:

$$\frac{330 \text{ g}}{1000 \text{ mL}} = \frac{x \text{ g}}{5 \text{ mL}} = \frac{5 \times 330}{1000} = 1.65 \text{ g}$$

The weight of herb in the example is rounded to 330 g. The aim is reproducibility of the preparation based on thorough record-keeping so that the eventual dosage for the final preparation is clear. Calculations should be written out in full as possible sources of error include putting the decimal point in the wrong place, lack of attention to units (leading to incorrect expression of proportions) and incorrect rendering of other units into metric units. Use whole units where possible, e.g. 400 mg rather than 0.4 g (Rees et al 2005).

## REFERENCES

Akeroyd J 2003 The encyclopaedia of wild flowers. Parragon, Bath.

Allaby M (ed) 2006 Oxford dictionary of plant sciences. Oxford University Press, Oxford.

André J 1985 Les noms de plantes dans la Rome antique. Les Belles Lettres, Paris.

Barker J 2001 The Medicinal flora of Britain and northwestern Europe. Wionter Press, West Wickham, Kent.

Beck LY 2005 Pedanius Dioscorides of Anazarbus: De Materia Medica. Olms Weidmann, Hildesheim.

Cooper JW, McLaren AC 1933 Latin for pharmaceutical students. Pitman & Sons, London.

EMEA 2002 Points to consider on good agricultural practice and good collection practice for starting materials of herbal origin. EMEA/HMPWP/31/99 Rev 3. Online. Available: http://www.emea.europa.eu/pdfs/human/hmpc/003199en.pdf 10 Sept 2009.

Farah MH 2005 Accepted scientific names of therapeutic plants. Uppsala Monitoring Centre, World Health Organization, Uppsala, Sweden.

Gibbons B, Brough, P 1996 Wild flowers of Britain & Northern Europe. Chancellor Press, London.

Gray MJ, Chang D, Zhang Y et al 2010 Development of liquid chromatography/mass spectrometry methods for the quantitative analysis of herbal medicine in biological fluids: a review. Biomedical Chromatography 24: 91–103.

Green MH (ed.) 2001 The Trotula. University of Pennsylvania Press, Philadelphia.

Grey-Wilson C 1994 Wild flowers of Britain and Northwest Europe. Dorling Kindersley, London.

Heinrich MM, Barnes J, Gibbons S, Williamson EM 2004 Fundamentals of pharmacognosy and phytotherapy. Churchill Livingstone, Edinburgh.

Hickey M, King C 2000 The Cambridge illustrated glossary of botanical terms. Cambridge University Press, Cambridge.

Hunt T 1989 Plant names of medieval England. DS Brewer, Cambridge.

International Plant Names Index 2009 Online. Available: http://www.ipni.org/index.html.

ISSC-MAP 2007 International standards for sustainable wild collection of medicinal and aromatic plants. Online. Available: http://www.fairwild.org/ 10 Sept 2009.

Judd WS, Campbell C, Stevens P 1999 Plant systematics: a phylogenetic approach. Sinauer Associates, MA.

Kohen R, Nyska A 2002 Invited Review: Oxidation of Biological Systems: Oxidative Stress Phenomena, Antioxidants, Redox Reactions, and Methods for Their Quantification. Toxicologic Pathology 30: 620–650.

Lange D 2004 The German foreign trade in medicinal and aromatic plants during the 1990s. Medicinal Plant Conservation. Medicinal Plant Conservation MPSG Newsletter 9/10, 38–46.

Marriott J 2006 Pharmaceutical compounding and dispensing. Pharmaceutical Press, London.

Medicinal Plant Specialist Group 2008 World Conservation Union (IUCN) Species Survival Commission. Online. Available: http://www.iucn.org/about/work/programmes/species/about_ssc/specialist_groups/directory_specialist_groups/directory_sg_plants/ssc_medicinalplant_home/.

Mills S, Bone K 2005 The essential guide to herbal safety. Churchill Livingstone, St Louis.

Podlech D 2001 Herbs and healing plants of Britain and Europe. Diamond Books, London.

Rees J, Smith I, Smith B 2005 Introduction to pharmaceutical calculations. Pharmaceutical Press, London.

Richardson WF 2004 Numbering and measuring in the classical world. Bristol Phoenix Press, Exeter.

Royal Pharmaceutical Society of Great Britain 2010 Objects in the history of pharmacy. Online. Available: http://www.rpsgb.org.uk/informationresources/museum/resources/informationsheets.html.

Scalbert A, Manach C, Morand C et al 2005 Dietary Polyphenols and the Prevention of Diseases. Critical Reviews in Food Science and Nutrition 45: 287–306.

Sizes 2006 Imperial measure. Online. Available: http://www.sizes.com/units/imperial_sys.htm 20 Nov 2009.

Stace C 1991 New flora of the British Isles. Cambridge University Press, Cambridge.

Sterry P 2006 Complete British wild flowers. HarperCollins, London.

Sutton D 1996 Field guide to the wild flowers of Britain and northern Europe. Kingfisher Books, London.

Tutin TG, Heywood VH, Burges NA, et al 1964 Flora Europaea, vol 1. Cambridge University Press, Cambridge.

Tutin TG, Heywood VH, Burges NA, et al 1968 Flora Europaea, vol 2. Cambridge University Press, Cambridge.

Tutin TG, Heywood VH, Burges NA, et al 1973 Flora Europaea, vol 3. Cambridge University Press, Cambridge.

Tutin TG, Heywood VH, Burges NA, et al 1976 Flora Europaea, vol 4. Cambridge University Press, Cambridge.

USDA 2010 Plants Database. US Department of Agriculture Natural Resources Conservation Service. Online. Available: http://plants.usda.gov/index.html 1 Feb 2010

WHO 2003 WHO guidelines on good agricultural and collection practices. Online. Available: http://whqlibdoc.who.int/publications/2003/9241546271.pdf 10 Sept 2009.

Williamson E 2003 Potter's herbal cyclopaedia. CW Daniel, Saffron Walden.

# CHAPTER 6
# *Agrimonia eupatoria*, agrimony

## DESCRIPTION

### Family: Rosaceae                                                             Part used: aerial parts

*Agrimonia eupatoria* L. is a hardy, herbaceous perennial found throughout Europe in grassland and verges (Tutin et al 1968). *The Flora of Turkey* (Davis 1972) gives two *Agrimonia* species, including *Agrimonia eupatoria*.

Erect, reddish, pubescent stems (50–150 cm high) bear alternate, pinnate, toothed leaves with velvety undersides with small pairs between larger pairs. There is a basal rosette of leaves. Bright yellow flowers with five small petals occur on long, slender spikes from June to September. Small, cone-shaped fruits are enclosed in a characteristic bristled calyx-tube. The hooked bristles enable widespread dispersal of seeds on animal fur. It also spreads vegetatively by stout, woody, deep-lying rhizomes.

**Other species used:** fragrant agrimony *Agrimonia procera* Wallr. syn. *Agrimonia odorata* (Bradley 2006), which is a larger plant with leaves green on both sides, pale yellow flowers and bell-shaped fruits (Sterry 2006, p 84). It has similar constituents but is scented (Carnat et al 1991). *Agrimonia pilosa* is used in China (WHO 1989).

### Quality
Collect during or shortly before flowering (BHMA 1983).

## THE EUPATORION OF DIOSCORIDES

Dioscorides (IV 41) describes agrimony under the title 'eupatorion', by which name it was known until the Linnaean classification of the 18th century. The name is linked with a king of Pontus, Mithridates Eupator, a famous plant collector and author of a botanical text in Greek, who died around 63 BC. Thus Pliny records, 'it hath gotten credit and reputation by a king, as may appear by the name'. Many centuries later Fuchs puts forward the retrospective notion that Mithridates, on discovering the medicinal use of the plant, named it 'hepatorium' because it heals the liver.

Both internal and external uses of agrimony are recorded by Dioscorides in the 1st century AD. The leaves are applied topically in some form of oil or grease to wounds and ulcers that are proving difficult to heal. The powdered herb or seed or both together are taken in wine for dysentery and bloody diarrhoea, for liver disease and for those bitten by reptiles.

Galen, in classifying a rational herbal therapeutics, defines the internal activity of the plant: by virtue of its thin parts – an ability to penetrate thickened residues more usually found in notably pungent or heating herbs – it cuts, scours and cleanses humours obstructing the fine, narrow passages of the liver 'without manifest heat', while its binding power helps to reopen the channels and restore power and strength to that organ. Thus, by its gentle heating and astringing qualities – Galen classifies it as hot and dry in the first degree – agrimony is made a tonic to the liver. This toning effect is extended by later authors, no doubt in recognition of Dioscorides' recommendation of the plant for dysenteries, to the other organs of the alimentary system whose operations draw on the power of that central organ of digestion. Serapio, from the Arabic tradition, tells us that al-Razi has demonstrated by experiment that the benefit to the liver of Dioscorides' eupatorion is not as great as that of wormwood.

In elemental terms, therefore, agrimony imparts a gentle fire to the body. In Aristotelian physics, fire implies heat and light, and the ability to separate out different kinds of substance. It warms and dries. Its power is greater than expected from what the senses can detect of its fiery quality. Its astringency, also moderate, nevertheless provides it with a high ranking among the wound herbs of the herbal tradition.

In the second great age of herbals, during the Renaissance (Stannard 1969), there is much discussion concerning the correct botanical species. Parkinson, for example, identifies several species of agrimony besides the common scentless one. Among these are two species native to Italy: the sweet-smelling *Agrimonia odorata* (now designated *Agrimonia procera* Wallr, aromatic with pale yellow flowers, which is rarer in the UK but has the same European distribution and similar pharmacological constituents as *Agrimonia eupatoria*), which he favours above the common

©2009 Elsevier Ltd, Inc, BV
DOI: 10.1016/B978-0-443-10344-5.00011-2

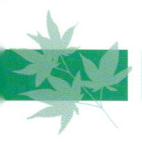

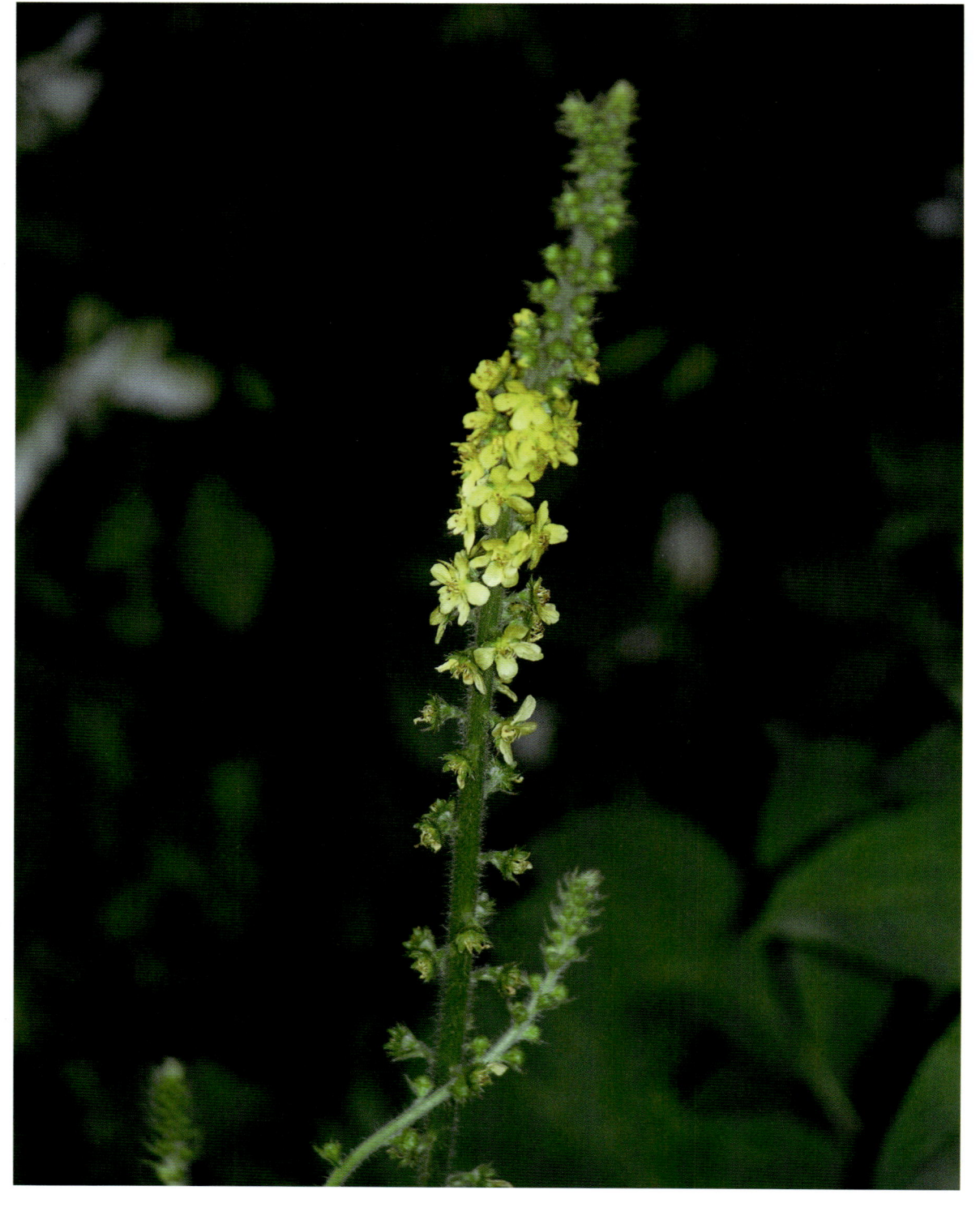

Figure 6.1 *Agrimonia eupatoria*, agrimony (a garden in Yorkshire, June).

sort but recognizes is hard to come by in England; and also a bastard agrimony, although this common name was usually applied in England to the bur-marigold or water agrimony *Bidens tripartita*. While Fuchs maintains that agrimony should be picked in the summer when in flower, Dodoens and Bauhin cite Mesue in insisting that for medicinal use agrimony should be gathered in May before flowering because the root then is very odoriferous. This may be a reference to *Agrimonia procera*. Meanwhile, another 16th century physician, Caesalpinus is reported by Bauhin to have detected no aroma from the plant, on account of which Galen had commended it for those drunk on mandrake, nor any cutting power evident in medicinal usage, and therefore to doubt the identification. Bauhin, however, assures his readers that agrimony is the true eupatorion: 'whoever is a doctor, after this let him use agrimony confidently, if he wishes to use eupatorium'.

In the 20th century Grieve states that agrimony is subject to considerable variation of form and suggests that the common sort can also be aromatic and that as a consequence the distinction between *Agrimonia eupatoria* and *Agrimonia procera* is scarcely maintained by the botanists of her day. She mentions the aromatic plant gathered early in the season as an ingredient of a blood-cleansing 'spring drink' and maintains that the fragrance of common agrimony is retained in the dried aerial plant, which may explain its popularity in France as a tisane.

Concerning another species, the hemp agrimony *Eupatorium cannabinum*, Parkinson writes 'all the apothecaries of our land, especially of London nowadays, do use the first kind of agrimony as the most assured eupatorium of Dioscorides. Howsoever in former times, both we and they beyond the seas did usually take the *Eupatorium cannabinum*, which they called Eupatorium vulgare, for the true kind'. This former time beyond the sea is discussed by Mattioli, who criticizes 'almost the whole throng of apothecaries' for a replacement, or just as often a mixing, of Dioscorides' agrimony with that of Ibn Sina's hemp agrimony. Mesue's eupatorium is a third kind, the tops of which, soaked in white wine and diluted, Italian women give to their children, Mattioli affirms, as a successful remedy for worms. Grieve suggests later that the water and hemp agrimonies, although not actually related botanically to common agrimony, were given the same name by the older herbalists because of their similar qualities. Dalechamps refers to the 'officinal' eupatorion as sold in apothecary shops, while his entry of 'common agrimony' depicts and describes hemp agrimony, 'the eupatorion of Avicenna', which is often substituted for officinal agrimony because it has been observed to have greater powers and benefit for the liver.

By and large then, Renaissance authors of herbals are satisfied with the identification of the true eupatorion of Dioscorides. Nevertheless, a confusion has been handed down through medieval texts over the centuries even as far as our own period with Grieve, who suggested that the name agrimony is derived from argemone, 'a word given by the Greeks to plants which were healing to the eyes' (also Ducourthial 2003). Fernie (1897), one of Grieve's sources, states that the name agrimony is 'derived from the Greek, and means 'shining' because the herb is thought to cure cataract of the eye'. Pliny and Dioscorides already differentiate these two herbs, but a later illustrated manuscript of the Dioscorides text appears to depict agrimony without rosette, under the name argemone. In the herbal of pseudo-Apuleius, agrimonia is misspelled as argimonia and the first listed use is for defects or pain in the eyes. A similar entry is transmitted in medieval texts such as the Old English Herbarium and the Salernitan herbal: the fresh herb – or, if not available, the dried herb soaked in hot water for a day – well crushed and placed on the eyes, is stated to be profitable for eye pains and bruises, discolouration and swelling.

The Herbal of Pseudo-Apuleius offers several uses for agrimony: the same application for the eyes could be laid on ulcerous sores, gashes caused by blows from a wooden club or iron weapon and infected wounds in order to open them up for cleansing, while the fresh herb pounded in vinegar could be used on warts. Internally, at a dose of 9 g of herb in two cups of wine (the Salernitan dose is slightly smaller), the Dioscoridean application for snake bite is repeated, as is the use in fluxes, but a sore abdomen or spleen replaces the classical indication of liver dysfunction. The *Old English Herbarium* repeats these, with the omission of the use in fluxes. The plant is called garclive in Anglo-Saxon. Grieve cites Chaucer on 'egrimoyne' used with mugwort and vinegar for a bad back and all wounds.

Hildegard, however, writes of quite different uses for the plant. While continuing the medieval notion that agrimony heals the eyes, in this case from clouded vision, it is also applied to those who have lost understanding and knowledge, when the head should be shaved and washed with a decoction of agrimony. The bilious or those with a cold stomach and intestinal mucus should drink the herb in wine. Head catarrh is remedied with a complete regime, including pills made from agrimony, fennel, galangal, female fern and celandine. A bathing regime for skin eruptions due to lust or (sexual) incontinence is also described, where agrimony *Agrimonia eupatoria*, hyssop *Hyssopus officinalis*, asarum *Asarum europaeum* and menstrual blood are added to the bath.

The Galenic qualities of agrimony and its classical indications are restored in Renaissance herbals from Fuchs onwards, alongside new uses for the herb and also the root, and a new preparation of a distilled water. A decoction of the herb in wine is found to be useful for the urinary tract, helping to correct foul or bloody urine, and strangury, or the inability to pass urine except painfully and drop by drop. Abdominal colic (from Mesue), worms in the digestive tract and obstructions of the liver and spleen (which are usually taken to mean jaundice and malaria) are treated using herb and root. Coughs are

**49**

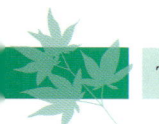

relieved as the cleansing power of the plant works on phlegm-filled lungs. A warm decoction is to be taken before the fit of an ague or malaria to prevent the attack and gradually to cure the disease. For Culpeper, agrimony acts as a tonic in the sense of its ability to help correct all imbalances of qualities in the body. He writes: 'It is a most admirable remedy for such whose livers are annoyed either by heat or cold. The liver is the former of blood, the blood the nourisher of the body, and agrimony a strengthener of the liver'. Culpeper recommends a dose of 1 drachm (4 g).

## A WOUND HERB

The topical use of agrimony, usually applied in wine or vinegar, also continues to be greatly esteemed, evidenced by its inclusion in a preparation for a new kind of wound. Fernie (1897) tells us that 'this herb formed an ingredient of the genuine arquebusade water, as prepared against wounds inflicted by an arquebus, or hand-gun, and it was mentioned by Philip de Comines in his account of the

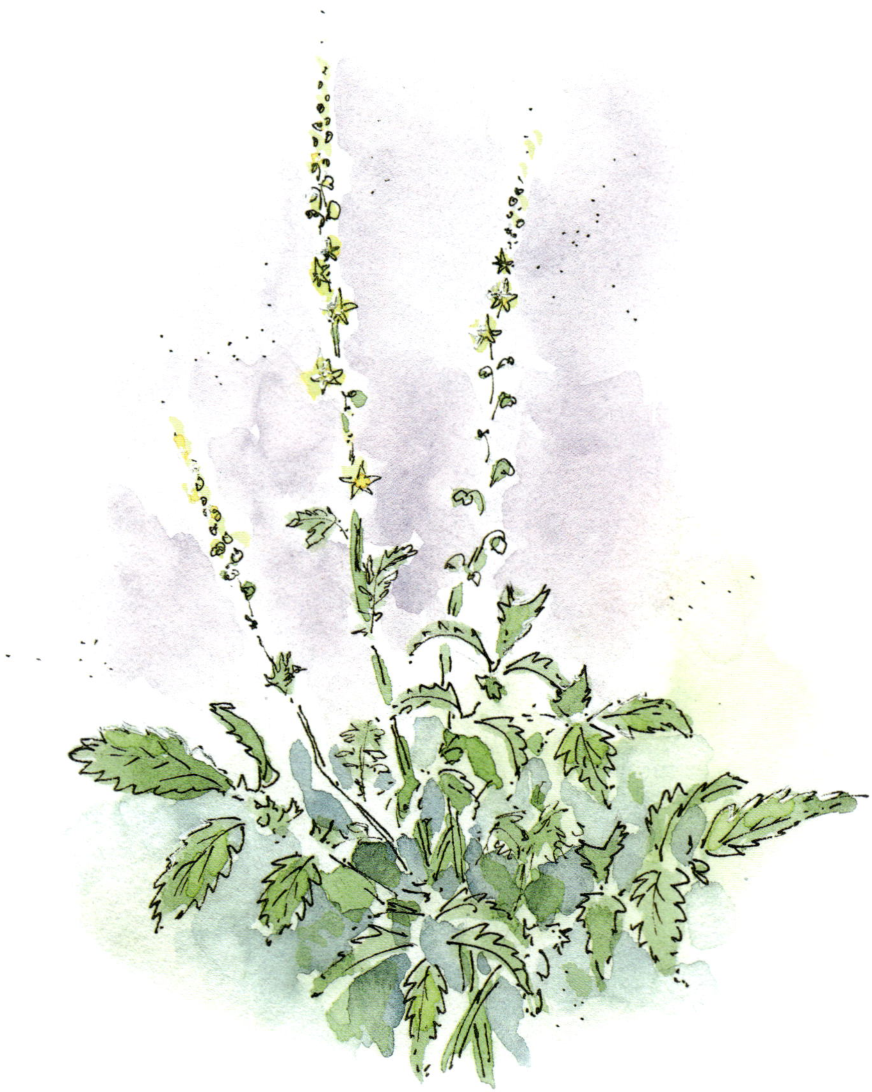

**Figure 6.2** *Agrimonia eupatoria*, agrimony.

battle of Morat, 1476. When the Yeomen of the Guard were first formed in England (1485), half were armed with bows and arrows, whilst the other half carried arquebuses. In France the 'eau de arquebusade' is still applied for sprains and bruises, being 'carefully made from many aromatic herbs'. The value placed on the herb naturally led it to be listed in the *London Dispensatory of the Royal College of Physicians* (1618) and later in the *Edinburgh Dispensatory*.

Other topical uses come from the Arabic writer Mesue: to draw thorns, splinters and nails, for abscesses in the ear canal and to restrict the seeping of blood into the skin (ecchymoses), to reduce the swelling and pain of fractures and to strengthen sub-luxated joints. A fistula might be cured by placing the powder of three roots of agrimony into it.

In the early 18th century, Quincy reports that country people use the bruised herb or its juice for bruising and fresh wounds, while physicians employ it in the treatment of dropsy (presumably portal hypertension) and cachexic states. He quotes Etmuller on its ability to take away swelling and inflammation of the scrotum. Miller emphasizes its use in strangury and for 'bloody water' and refers to Riviere's extolling of the powdered leaf for incontinence of urine. Quincy notes that the herb is available in few shops but that barber-surgeons make frequent use of it in fomentations, to dissolve hard tumours or to disperse and absorb oedematous swellings and superfluous moisture.

In the latter part of the century, however, when medical practitioners are making increasing use of mineral compounds and imported and exotic plants, agrimony is dropped by mainstream medicine. Cullen reports in 1773 that of the eight vegetable astringents in the *London Dispensatory*, chief among these being agrimony, it and four others had now been omitted 'not from any noxious quality, but only from their not being used in present practice'. Rose *Rosa* species, cinquefoil *Potentilla* species and tormentil *Potentilla erecta* are retained because of their fragrance or on account of their greater astringent power (tormentil is classified by Culpeper as heating in the first degree but drying in the third, and it contains up to four times as much tannin as does agrimony).

## AGRIMONY OUT OF THE MAINSTREAM

Use of agrimony is continued, however, by some practitioners. Green, in his *Universal Herbal* of 1832, records that 'its root appears to possess the properties of Peruvian bark *Cinchona pubescens* in a very considerable degree, without manifesting any of its inconvenient qualities', and if taken in large doses, either in decoction or powder, 'seldom fails to cure the ague', as Culpeper had already suggested. Hill, in mid-18th century, uses agrimony for treating jaundice, another old use. His prescription states 6 oz of the crown of the root in a quart of boiling water, sweetened with honey, and half a pint of the infusion drunk three times daily.

Coffin, writing in 1349, finds Culpeper at fault 'as he oftimes is, for he ascribes such abundance of good properties that if half be true, humans would scarcely require any other medicine'. Coffin struggles to accept the sheer number of herbs in Culpeper's writings which he claims can open obstructions of the liver and spleen. Yet, regarding agrimony, he refers to Hooper's description of the herb as a valuable astringent which, by the testimony of Clomel, 'was successful in enlargement of the liver' in two cases. To this binding effect can be added a diuretic action and, according to Gray's supplement to the Pharmacopoeia, a vermifuge. Coffin also lists the use of agrimony, in combination with other herbs, for dropsy and jaundice, and it is given freely to children suffering measles, scarlet fever and chicken pox. Coffin's indications for agrimony in exanthemata later appear also in the National Botanic Pharmacopoeia. The National Botanic Pharmacopoeia classifies the herb as an astringent tonic and diuretic, useful also for coughs, diarrhoea and relaxed bowels as an infusion with raspberry leaf *Rubus idaeus* and sugar, jaundice and other liver problems. Grieve specifies a fluid extract preparation, to be prescribed at a dose of 10–60 drops. Coffin's prescription for jaundice is to use 1 oz of each of barberry bark *Berberis vulgaris*, centaury *Centaurium erythraea*, bog bean *Menyanthes trifoliata*, agrimony and raspberry leaf *Rubus idaeus* decocted in a quart of water. After straining, 1/2 oz of cayenne pepper is added, along with mountain flax *Linum catharticum* if the patient is constipated, and a wineglassful (60 mL) of the mixture taken three or four times daily. After 3–4 days, the patient receives a vapour bath. If his jaundice is not relieved, a standard lobelia *Lobelia inflata* emetic is given and the bath repeated.

Hool summarizes the actions of agrimony promoted by the new botanic practitioners of Victorian England: tonic, stimulant, astringent, stomachic, hepatic, diuretic and diaphoretic. Hool emphasizes the use of agrimony in digestive problems, notably dyspepsia and biliousness, namely vomiting before and after meals, sour and watery eructations, sick headache, debility and a tendency to jaundice. He adds diabetes to the list, and not on account of its diuretic effects. The indication may come from the earlier Robinson (1868), who adds incontinence of urine and recommends the herb be boiled in milk for these two conditions. Robinson repeats older uses, such as the seed for bloody flux, a hot infusion before the fit of an ague, and uses for lungs, skin and blood, mentions agrimony's fame as a vulnerary and regards few herbs as effective in haemoptysis, haematuria and disorders of the liver. He contributes a use with alum and honey internally for tape worms. Wren affirms the tonic effect of agrimony, promoting assimilation of food, reducing a cough and astringing relaxed bowels with a 1:10 infusion taken frequently.

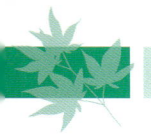

Agrimony may be largely out of favour in mainstream medicine in Europe in the 1800s but in America, where it is also native, it is in use by the growing number of herbalists in practice. Cook classifies agrimony as a mild stimulating astringent, causing no irritation but toning the mucous membranes of the body and with application to skin and kidneys, for which latter it is highly regarded by some, including one doctor who considered it very useful for childhood enuresis. As an astringent, it can treat diarrhoea, leucorrhoea and blood loss from uterus, bowel or lungs. The dose to be employed, of an infusion of 1 oz of the herb steeped in a pint of boiling water (commonly 25 g to 500 mL of water) for an hour, is 2 fl oz (50 mL) every hour or two. A preparation much stronger than this can also be used cold. It is, by popular reputation, useful in chronic coughs with excessive expectoration and is employed as a gargle for aphthous ulcers and sore throats, and as a wash for ophthalmia from various causes. Cook cannot confirm its usefulness in jaundice, asthma, scrofula and obstructed menstruation and concludes 'From having once been valued beyond its deserts, it naturally has fallen to a reputation below its real merits – for it deserves much regard in its proper place'. He also provides one example of use of the root of agrimony, as a warm decoction given freely for calculous difficulties.

Ellingwood classes agrimony among the general renal stimulants, for 'all authors agree … that its influence is most direct upon the kidneys, correcting imperfect elimination through these organs'. He details the specific symptomatology of kidney or bladder pain and inflammation, foul-smelling urine with sediment, renal congestion and general irritability of the urinary organs. In addition, he states its particular employment also in incontinence of urine with coughing or sneezing in the elderly, for bronchial or pulmonary cough with thick, profuse secretions, and for dysuria with dysmenorrhoea in women. In this last presentation, agrimony will have a beneficially soothing effect on the nervous system. He adds 'we would be inclined to combine macrotys *Cimicifuga racemosa* or gelsemium *Gelsemium sempervirens* and pulsatilla *Pulsatilla vulgaris* with agrimony, but the old doctors believed the latter remedy would cover the entire group of symptoms'.

## ASTRINGENCY

Recent authors identify agrimony as a topical astringent for wounds, ulcers and sore throats and an astringent, bitter tonic, indicated for gastrointestinal and urinary problems such as indigestion, diarrhoea and colitis, urinary tract infections, enuresis and incontinence and kidney and bladder gravel. Because of its gentleness it is particularly suitable for children and the elderly. These indications are largely represented in the British Herbal Pharmacopoeia (1983): a mild astringent for diarrhoea in children, mucous colitis and grumbling appendicitis; a diuretic for cystitis and kidney stones; and external use as a gargle for acute sore throat and chronic nasopharyngeal catarrh. Agrimony has also been used in France for venous insufficiency and heavy legs, and for haemorrhoids.

Among the German authors, Schulz et al (1998) suggest agrimony only for mild, transient forms of diarrhoea and inflammations of the oropharyngeal mucosa, while Weiss specifies its use in chronic cholecystopathies with gastric subacidity, but requiring consistent use for some time to achieve success. Williamson references research indicating anti-diabetic activity, lending weight to the claim of Hool and Robinson 100 years earlier. Hoffmann offers it as a herb of choice in early-stage appendicitis and mentions human trials in which beneficial effects on chronic gastroduodenitis and cutaneous porphyria were found. In the latter, 20 patients, aged 27–66, with non-acute porphyria (Pătraşcu et al 1984), took infusions three to four times per day for 15 days with no other treatment. The skin eruptions improved with less hyperpigmentation and serum iron levels and urinary porphyrins decreased. Participants also had improved appetite and less dyspepsia. Hoffmann also refers to agrimony's long tradition of use as a spring tonic (which appears to go back only to Grieve) and Bartram gives a prescription for this: equal parts agrimony, raspberry leaves *Rubus idaeus*, lemon balm *Melissa officinalis* and nettles *Urtica dioica*. Priest and Priest classify agrimony as a gently stimulating tonic with gastrointestinal emphasis. It benefits the elderly by restoring debilitated conditions and can help with rheumatism and arthritis, urinary incontinence, a relaxed bowel and leucorrhoea in females. An additional indication is liver atrophy. Menzies-Trull refers to respiratory conditions: asthma, bronchitis and tuberculosis. He also quotes uses dating back to Culpeper and earlier: gout, dysentery, malaria, leucorrhoea. These physiomedical authors expect agrimony to be prescribed with other indicated herbs for the conditions listed.

Wood offers other indications for agrimony with reference to the plant's use as one of the 38 remedies discovered by Dr Bach, in this case for those who hide their worries behind a brave face. Wood suggests it is indicated for those under work-related tension and problems between employer and employee, or who hold their breath to suppress pain or 'who are tortured to capture the breath' in conditions such as whooping cough, bronchitis and asthma.

Astringent herbs like agrimony are traditionally used to treat diarrhoea, and are thought to influence the digestive tract membrane, to limit loss of fluid, to reduce permeability of the gut wall and to decrease secretions. The intensity of action in the gastrointestinal tract (measured as binding potency) is not directly associated with the intensity of the sense of astringency in the mouth

(Okuda 2005), but the indications for agrimony in such documents as the *Commission E Monographs* (Blumenthal 1998) from Germany is limited to what could be achieved with its moderate content of tannins: mild, non-specific, acute diarrhoea; inflammation of oral and pharyngeal mucosa, and topically for mild, superficial inflammation of the skin. This is to be effected by an average daily dose of 3 g of the dried aerial parts or equivalent preparations.

It may be that the action of agrimony actually depends more on a broad range of polyphenols rather than just tannins. In-vitro studies have attempted to show a link between antioxidant activity and concentration of polyphenols, including phenolic acids, flavonoids, condensed and hydrolysable tannins. The role of antioxidants in foods and herbal medicines has been investigated as it is argued that components in the diet may protect the body against cell damage caused by excess reactive oxygen species (Rice-Evans et al 1997). Tringali (2001) argues that flavonoids in the diet may be of especial significance in protection of cell membranes from lipid peroxidation, thus protecting cells from damage.

Studies on agrimony suggest it has a range of antioxidant constituents. Correia et al (2007) found strong antioxidant activity and associated this activity with total polyphenolic content. Venskutonis et al (2007) found that radical scavenging capacity varied depending on the solvent and was highest in more polar solvents. Ivanova et al (2005) investigated infusions (1 : 200) of 21 Bulgarian medicinal plants for total phenolic content and antioxidant activity. *Agrimonia eupatoria* was amongst seven plants shown to have high phenolic content and high antioxidant activity. *Origanum vulgare* and *Melissa officinalis* showed highest antioxidant activity, and Heilerová et al (2003) also found that aqueous extracts of *Origanum vulgare*, gathered wild in Slovakia, and cultivated *Melissa officinalis* Citra exhibited significantly higher antioxidant activity than wild-crafted *Agrimonia eupatoria*.

The drying quality of agrimony recorded in classical texts thus has a link with the current phytotherapeutic indications of the herb, but, removed from its Galenic therapeutic context, there is nothing to support the idea of the plant's fire, of its warmth and light. However, Pelikan's focus is on the connection between agrimony's reported silica content and its quality of light: 'from a short rootstock, the plant, held in closely, soars upward in a straight line … and the richly flowered floral spike becomes the principal organ … the small flowers are a warm glowing golden yellow. A delicate aromatic scent, somewhat like turpentine, is emitted by the root and by leaf and stem glands, enveloping the plant. Light and dryness seem to have given it form.'

Pelikan lists the plant's chemical constituents as tannins, bitter principles, volatile oil and niacinamide, while the ash contains much silica. He credits the plant's tannins for the main traditional indications. Elsewhere Pelikan discusses how tannins can be perceived as a tool fashioned by the astral nature of the plant as a medium of communication between the astral and etheric. Being thus associated with the astral nature – the flowering, air aspect – of a plant may account, Pelikan explains, for some properties of tannins: their particular occurrence in plants with abundant flowering processes, and especially plants producing flowers 'against' a strong etheric, or watery, influence as in marsh and water-based plants. It explains the desire of tannin solutions to absorb air, the element belonging to the astral sphere and their ability to make animal substances resist putrefaction and maintain their form. Pelikan cites the traditional use of agrimony for haemorrhages, badly healing wounds, varices, diarrhoea and digestive disorders.

Its silica content, through its relationship to skin and light, disposes agrimony towards chronic skin conditions and pulmonary TB. The properties and roles of silica are broad-ranging but Pelikan does comment that 'in the organic sphere, silica is able to follow the paths of protein synthesis from changeable and unformed to a defined shape; it can be the vehicle and tool of those particular form principles. It 'takes its actions along metabolic pathways to the very regions of the body where live principles become lifeless' and where the form principle takes effect in the enveloping structures of organs, skin and bone. In 'silica plants' one may frequently see a form principle going right into the smallest detail.'

It would seem that agrimony has had a consistent use as a topical herb for a variety of conditions and was held in high esteem as a wound herb. Internally there are reports of its use for conditions of the gastrointestinal tract, respiratory and urinary systems. While Dioscorides gave it as a treatment for diarrhoea and dysentery, Galen elaborated a more complex use for the liver due to its gently heating and drying qualities and its use for treating liver conditions was reported in 19th century England, while Weiss more recently recorded its use in chronic gall bladder problems associated with gastric subacidity. In 19th century America during the same period it was popular for treating productive coughs and phlegm on the chest, and was a remedy for the urinary system, not only as a tonic astringent but to treat dysuria, irritability and congestion of the kidneys. Agrimony is suitable for childhood exanthemas and also for the elderly, for stress incontinence, cachexia and as a general tonic. It is likely that agrimony will not be prescribed on its own, but with other relevant herbs.

## RECOMMENDATIONS

- Wounds of all kinds, sprains, bruises, joint pains, swellings, aphthous ulcers and sore throat.

- Liver disease, portal hypertension, jaundice, chronic gall bladder disease with associated gastric subacidity.
- Diarrhoea and bloody diarrhoea, colitis, dyspepsia, nausea and vomiting, inflammation of stomach and duodenum.
- Urinary tract infections and urinary calculi, stress incontinence and cachexia in the elderly.
- Exanthemas in children, such as measles, German measles and chicken pox.
- Leucorrhoea, menorrhagia and dysmenorrhoea.
- Tonic for the elderly, especially in the presence of the above conditions or with arthritic and rheumatic symptoms.
- Further research into the suggested usefulness of agrimony in diabetes mellitus is needed.

Dosage: The *British Herbal Pharmacopoeia* recommends 2–4 g three times a day of dried aerial parts.

## CONSTITUENTS

Reviews: Barnes et al (2007), Bisset & Wichtl (2001), Bradley (2006), Williamson (2003).

### Volatile oil

Total 0.2% only found in *Agrimonia procera* (Bisset & Wichtl 2001).

### Triterpenes

Triterpene glycosides: euscapic acid, esters of euscapic acid and tormentic acid (commercial) (Bilia et al 1993).

### Phenolic acids

Total 2.3% (12 compounds): mainly p-hydroxybenzoic acid, protocatechuic acid, vanillic acid, salicylic acid (wild, Poland, Shabana et al 2003).

### Flavonoids

Tiliroside (Correia et al 2006).

### Flavonol glycosides

Total 0.3%, quercetin glycosides: (collected, nine sites, Serbia) (Gorunovic et al 1989).
Total 0.9%, quercetin glycosides: hyperoside 0.4%, rutin, quercitrin, isoquercitrin (flowering tops, wild, seven sites, France) (Carnat et al 1991).
Quercetin glycosides: hyperoside, isoquercitrin; kaempferol glycosides (wild, Portugal) (Correia et al 2006).
Kaempferol glycosides (Bilia et al 1993).

### Flavone glycosides

Total 0.3%, luteolin glycosides, apigenin glycosides (Shabana et al 2003).
Apigenin 6-C-glucoside (isovitexin) (Correia et al 2006).

### Isoflavonoids

Daidzein, biochanin A (leaves, commercial, Czech Republic) (Bajer et al 2007).

### Tannins

Total 7.4% (Carnat et al 1991); total 10.1% (Shabana et al 2003).

### Condensed tannins

Catechin tannins 7.1%; leucoanthocyanins 6.9% (decoction) (Gorunovic et al 1989).
Catechin and epicatechin type oligomers, in particular procyanidin dimers (type B), trimers and tetramers (45% aqueous-ethanol solution) (Correia et al 2006).

### Hydrolyzable tannins

A small proportion of ellagitannins is cited by Bradley (2006) but there is a lack of more recent studies. This is important as agrimoniin, an ellagitannin oligomer found in root of *Agrimonia pilosa* (Miyamoto et al 1985), has been found to have a range of activities (Okuda et al 1989). More recently, agrimoniin was found in vitro to inhibit human neutrophil elastase and thus could have an antiinflammatory activity in psoriasis (Hrenn et al 2006). Agrimoniin is found in other Rosaceae such as *Potentilla erecta* and *Alchemilla vulgaris*.

## RECOMMENDATIONS ON SAFETY

- Use caution where there is constipation. Side-effects of nausea or constipation possible with excess doses and strengths.

## REFERENCES

Bajer T, Adam M, Galla L, et al 2007 Comparison of various extraction techniques for isolation and determination of isoflavonoids in plants. Journal of Separation Science 30:122–127.

Barnes J, Anderson LA, Phillipson JD 2007 Herbal medicines, 3rd edn. Pharmaceutical Press, London.

BHMA 1983 British herbal pharmacopoeia. British Herbal Medicine Association, Keighley.

Bilia AR, Palme E, Catalano S 1993 Constituents and biological assay of *Agrimonia eupatoria*. Fitoterapia 64:549–550.

Bisset NG, Wichtl M (eds) 2001 Herbal drugs and phytopharmaceuticals, 2nd edn. Medpharm, Stuttgart.

Blumenthal M (ed.) 1998 The complete German Commission E monographs. American Botanical Council, Texas.

Bradley PR 2006 British herbal compendium, vol 2. British Herbal Medicine Association, Bournemouth.

Carnat A, Lamaison JL, Petitjean-Freytet C 1991 L'aigrimoine étudé. Plantes Medicinales et Phytotherapeutique 25:202–211.

Correia H, González-Paramás A, Amaral MT, et al 2006 Polyphenolic profile characterization of *Agrimonia eupatoria* L. by HPLC with different detection devices. Biomedical Chromatography 20:88–94.

Correia HS, Batista MT, Dinis TC 2007 The activity of an extract and fraction of *Agrimonia eupatoria* L. against reactive species. Biofactors 29:91–104.

Davis PH (ed.) 1972 Flora of Turkey, vol 4. Edinburgh University Press, Edinburgh.

Ducourthial G 2003 Flore magique et astrologique de l'antiquite. Belin, Paris.

Fernie WT 1897 Herbal simples approved for modern uses of cure. Boericke & Tafel, Philadelphia. Online. Available: http://www.gutenberg.org.

Gorunovic M, Stosic D, Lukic P 1989 Le valeur de l'aigremoine comme plante medicinale. Herba Hungarica 28:45–49.

Heilerová L, Bučková M, Tarapčik P, et al 2003 Comparison of antioxidant activity data for aqueous extracts of lemon balm (*Melissa officinalis* L.), oregano (*Origanum vulgare* L.), thyme (*Thymus vulgaris* L.), and agrimony (*Agrimonia eupatoria* L.) obtained by conventional methods and the DNA-based biosensor. Czech Journal of Food Sciences 21:78–84.

Hrenn A, Steinbrecher T, Labahn A, et al 2006 Plant phenolics inhibit neutrophil elastase. Planta Medica 72:1127–1131.

Ivanova, D, Gerova, D, Chervenkov, T, et al 2005 Polyphenols and antioxidant capacity of Bulgarian medicinal plants. Journal of Ethnopharmacology 96:145–150.

Miyamoto K, Koshiura R, Ikeya Y et al 1985 Isolation of Agrimoniin, an antitumour constituent, from the roots of *Agrimonia pilosa* Ledeb. Chem Pharmaceut Bull 33:3977–3981.

Okuda T, Yoshida T, Hatano T 1989 Ellagitannins as active constituents of medicinal plants. Planta Medica 55:117–122.

Okuda T 2005 Systematics and health effects of chemically distinct tannins in medicinal plants. Phytochemistry 66:2012–2031.

Pătrașcu V, Chebac- Pătrașcu I, Gheorgiu G 1984 Favourable therapeutic results in cutaneous porphyria obtained with *Agrimonia eupatoria*. Dermato-venerologia 29:153–157.

Rice-Evans C, Miller N, Pagana G 1997 Antioxidant properties of phenolic compounds. Trends in Plant Science 2:152–159.

Robinson M 1868 The new family herbal and botanic physician. William Nicholson, London.

Schulz V, Häensel R, Tyler VE 1998 Rational phytotherapy. Springer-Verlag, Berlin.

Shabana MH, Węglarz Z, Geszprych A, et al 2003 Phenolic constitutents of agrimony. Herba Polonica 49:24–28.

Stannard J 1969 The herbal as a medical document. Bulletin of the History of Medicine 43:212.

Sterry P 2006 Complete British wild flowers. Harper Collins, London.

Tringali C 2001 Bioactive compounds from natural sources: isolation, characterisation and biological properties. Taylor & Francis, London.

Tutin TG, Heywood VH, Burges NA, et al 1968 Flora Europaea, vol 2. Cambridge University Press, Cambridge.

Venskutonis PR, Škėmaitė M, Ragažinskienė O 2007 Radical scavenging capacity of *Agrimonia eupatoria* and *Agrimonia procera*. Fitoterapia 78:166–168.

Williamson E 2003 Potter's herbal cyclopaedia. CW Daniel, Saffron Walden.

WHO 1989 Medicinal plants in China. World Health Organization, Manila.

# CHAPTER 7
# *Alchemilla vulgaris*, lady's mantle

## DESCRIPTION

**Family: Rosaceae**  **Part used: leaves, aerial parts**

Estimates of the number of species within the genus *Alchemilla* vary but there are at least 250 (Gehrke et al 2008). The many closely related species are distinguished by leaf shape and degree of hairiness (Gibbons & Brough 1996). The *Flora of Turkey* (Davis 1972) gives 50 *Alchemilla* species not including *Alchemilla vulgaris* but including *Alchemilla mollis*.

*Alchemilla vulgaris* is a herbaceous perennial found throughout Europe, especially on upland grassland and verges. Thin round green stems (up to 60 cm but usually less) bear bright green, palmately lobed leaves with toothed edges. There is a basal rosette and tufts of leaves encircle the stem at the apices. Tiny yellowy-green flowers occur in dense, terminal compound cymes with four sepals and stamens but no petals. The seed is an achene. The rhizome is woody and the plant spreads vegetatively and by seed. Characteristic water droplets are exuded by the leaves when air humidity is high.

*Alchemilla vulgaris* is an aggregate species divided into 12 sections of apomictic microspecies that are clones arising from seed produced by asexual reproduction (Sepp et al 2000). The microspecies are often not distinct morphologically and vary genetically where the microspecies is widespread (Sepp et al 2000). As microspecies hybridize, there are different opinions on the extent to which this has resulted in new species and thus as to the number of species in the genus. Stace (1991) distinguishes 15 species that are native or have been introduced to the UK. A study of 23 widespread microspecies in Estonia found that the best characteristic for distinguishing species is the degree and type of hairiness (Sepp & Paal 1998).

Some authors, such as Bisset & Wichtl (2001), refer to *Alchemilla xanthochlora*, which is distinguished in the *Flora Europaea* (Tutin et al 1968) by its densely hairy stems and petioles. The *European Pharmacopoeia* of 2000 referred to *Alchemilla xanthochlora* Rothm but the 2003 version refers to *Alchemilla vulgaris* L. sensu latiore (Bradley 2006). Where available we have used the list of accepted scientific names and synonyms published by the Uppsala Monitoring Centre (2005), but *Alchemilla* is not included. We have therefore used *Alchemilla vulgaris* in accordance with Bradley (2006) and recent reviews of the genus such as Gehrke et al (2008).

**Other species used:** *Alchemilla alpina* has palmately lobed leaves, with white silky hairs on the underside.

### Quality

The existence of endemic microspecies makes it possible mistakenly to collect endemic species rather than the widespread species, and herbalists should refer to sources on the local distribution of wild flowers when planning wild collection. For example, a survey of upper Teesdale and Weardale (northern UK) found both Scandinavian species, which may be relicts left after the Ice Age, and a mountain species, *Alchemilla monticola*, which is widespread in Europe but only found in the UK in certain road-side localities in Teesdale (Bradshaw 1962).

The plant commonly found in gardens is *Alchemilla mollis* (Buser) Rothm, which is a native of the Carpathians. It is larger with paler green leaves and dense, stiff hairs. It is a species rather than a garden variety, and, as lady's mantle is considered a generally safe plant, there is no evidence to suggest that this cannot be used.

## WHICH ALCHEMILLA: THE DEBATE

The origins of the tradition for lady's mantle are not as clearly definable as for many herbs. The plant goes under many names – lady's mantle, lion's foot, lion's paw, greater sanicle, padelyon, syndaw, synnaw, bear's foot, nine hooks, stellaria, leontopidium, leontopodion – but the leontopodion of Dioscorides carries a description quite different from lady's mantle, and is another species altogether, leontopetalon, *Leontice leontopetalum*. Chevallier of our modern authors writes how two preparations are recommended in Andres de Laguna's 1590 translation of Dioscorides for lady's mantle. Indeed the herb is there in Laguna's text, appended to the entry for aster atticus, but with reference to Beck's translation of Dioscorides where there is no such addition, and in comparison with

THE WESTERN HERBAL TRADITION

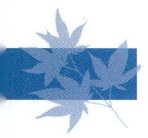

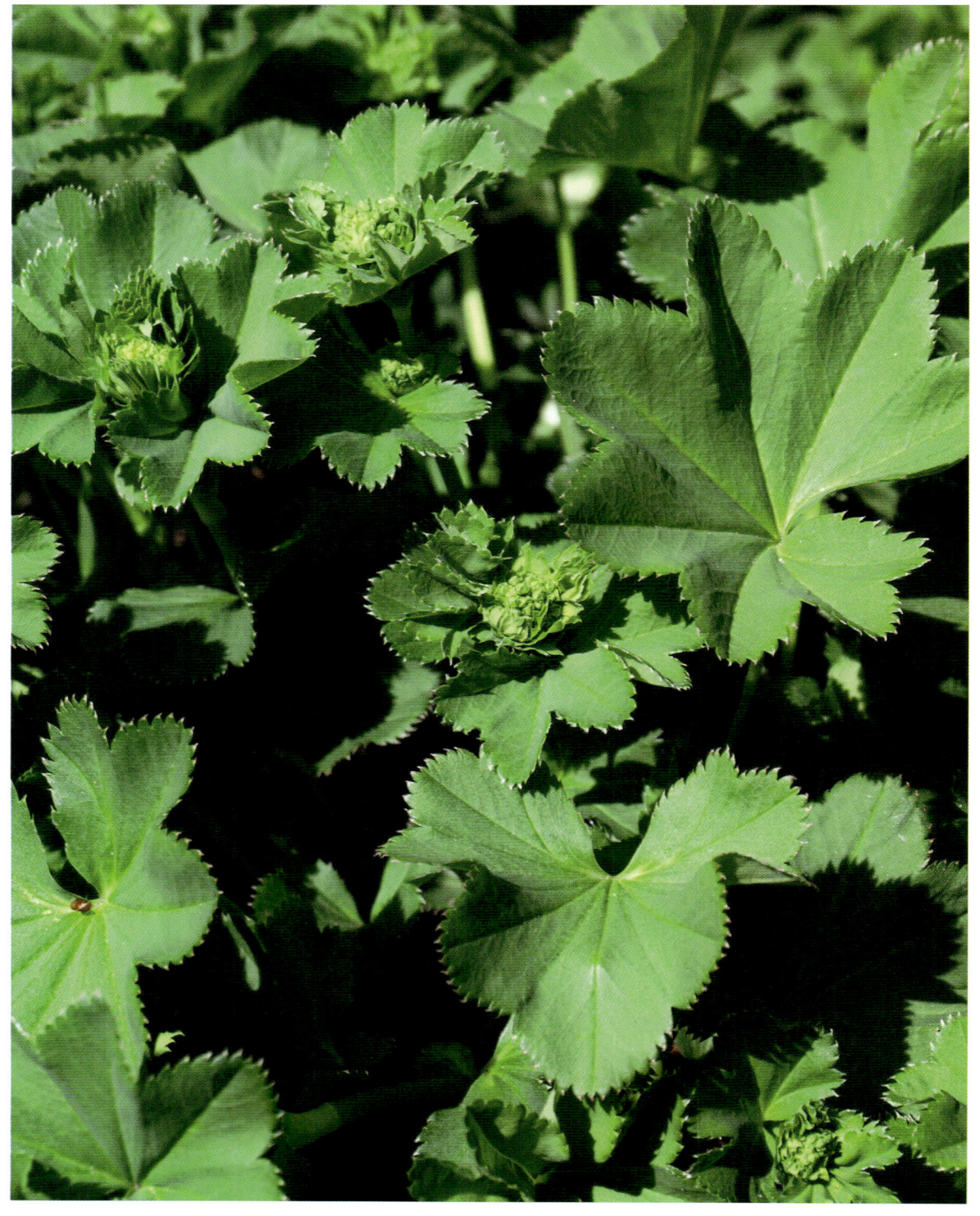

**Figure 7.1** *Alchemilla vulgaris*, lady's mantle (a garden in Yorkshire, May).

Mattioli's 1554 and later manuscripts (see below), where a very similar addendum appears in exactly the same place, beginning 'and this puts me in mind of a plant called Stellaria which I would not want to leave out', we may assume that the text is not from Dioscorides at all, but a later addition. Galen has no mention of the plant. Pliny writes in book 26 of leontopodion how it binds the belly, but purges choler, like rhubarb, which purges, yet binds; taken to the weight of two Roman denarii, in mead or honeyed water; and the seed taken in drink, 'it is said', causes strange visions and fantastical dreams. Bauhin finds two other references in Pliny to the same plant – the powdered seed with polenta in water draws out anything stuck in the flesh, and the same plant, when applied, draws out arrow tips; the plant also counters the deceptions of magic. Bauhin says he agrees with Dalechamps here that Pliny is discussing a different species from the leontopidion of Dioscorides. It is clearly not the same plant since none of the applications match in the least, but nor is it necessarily lady's mantle. The Renaissance authors, other than Bauhin and, according to Bauhin, Dalechamps, carry no reference to Pliny for this herb, and that is unusual where there is an entry in Pliny. Their citings are rather of 'later writers', so the question whether this herb of Pliny's is lady's mantle remains unanswered.

Apuleius refers to the herb pes leonis, leontopodion in Greek, and mentions two further names, aeopes and phastifylon, neither of which are repeated in other texts. It grows in fields, ditches and 'near where swallows live'. He suggests only one use for the plant and this information is repeated, again with no additional text, in the 13th century Salernitan herbal under leontopodion or pie de lion. The Salernitan version says that a married man who is unable to have intercourse with his wife should gather the plant of seven branches when the moon is waning, cook it in water, wash his whole body with it; on the first night he should make a fumigation of Aristolochia in front of his bedroom then go to his wife, and 'he will do his duty'. Further magical use is found in the Old English Herbarium: 'if someone has the condition of being under an evil spell, you can untie them from it: take 5 of the plants we call lion's foot without their roots, while the moon is waning, and wash the person with it. Lead the person out of the house in the early evening and fumigate him with the birthwort plant. When going outside the person must not look back; in this way you can undo the conditions'. Bauhin comments on Apuleius, saying that Galen and later doctors do not mention leontopodium. What Apuleius calls leontopodium is obviously leontopetalon and Bauhin concludes that magical use of lady's mantle is a confusion with the leontopetalon plant, the 'lion's foot', which was used as an amulet for lovers, although Dioscorides does not carry this magical use.

We can find no reference to lady's mantle among the Arabic writers, nor do the Renaissance authors refer to the Arabic writers for this herb, although this is a custom they readily exercise given the opportunity. I can find no reference to the plant in our copy of Hildegard, and I could find no mention in the Myddfai text nor *The Trotula* (Green 2001).

## WOUND AND WOMEN'S HERB

The first broad coverage falls in the Renaissance. The earliest clearly identifiable reference appears to be in Jerome Bock, alias Hieronymus Tragus, who first, according to Grieve, appended the name lady's mantle to the plant in the early 1500s. Bock's text, however, actually says 'others call it our lady's mantle', so it appears he did not coin the name himself, even if he might have been the first to introduce it as such. The lady in this case is the Virgin Mary, it is 'Our Lady's mantle', 'Unser Frauen Mantel' in German. The name alchemilla is attributed by a number of sources to its being prized by the alchemists for the dew on its leaves and the excrescence from the leaf veins, which could 'fix Mercury' according to Parkinson, yet he continues, 'but these idle fancies are now quite worne out, as I thinke'. There is little contention among the Renaissance authors and all repeat more or less the same virtues. They all praise its properties highly. Mattioli says these properties are 'strong'. 'It is accounted as one of the most singular wound herbes that is', says Parkinson, and this is one of the principal uses of the plant. A few authors, among them Parkinson, Dalechamps and Mattioli, say the Germans particularly appreciate this application and 'extol it with exceeding great praise' (Parkinson), giving it both internally and externally for this purpose; 'and [they] never dress any wound either inward or outward, but they give of the decoction hereof to drinke: and either wash the wound with the said decoction, or dip tents therein and put them thereunto'. Fuchs writes of these uses how the decoction as a wash will close up all wounds, or a soaked linen cloth is applied to the same purpose; how the decoction closes up internal wounds too and indeed its power to agglutinate is so 'amazingly great', it can heal abdominal hernias or ruptures, 'especially in boys'. Its leaves and roots are strongly astringent and drying, he says, 'later writers say in the second degree'. Dalechamps makes the same reference to hernias in children using the dried powder (of the root) or the distilled water in a decoction of the same alchemilla, 'so great is its agglutinating power'.

Dodoens and others refer to inflamed wounds and swellings; how lady's mantle will remove inflammation, cool heat, stop blood loss and ease pain. Bauhin says the herb and root can be added to wound drinks, powders, plasters and ointments; Parkinson, repeated by Culpeper, that it will even heal wounds which are fistulous and hollow; it will seal wounds promptly and effectively; 'but for fresh or green wounds or cuts, it so quickly healeth them up, that it suffereth not any quitture [purulent discharge] to grow therein, but consolidateth the lippes of the wound, yet not suffering any corruption to remain behinde'. He extends it too to bruises from falls. De Laguna adds its use for fractures in infants and older children.

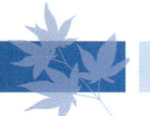

The herb achieves this reputation since its leaves are strongly astringent and drying, according to Fuchs, and others. 'Later writers', Fuchs writes, 'say in the second degree'. Culpeper, in the *Pharmacopoeia Londinensis*, designates the leaves hot and dry in the second degree, 'some say third'. 'They are less heating than healing', says Dalechamps. Such astringent qualities also recommend it

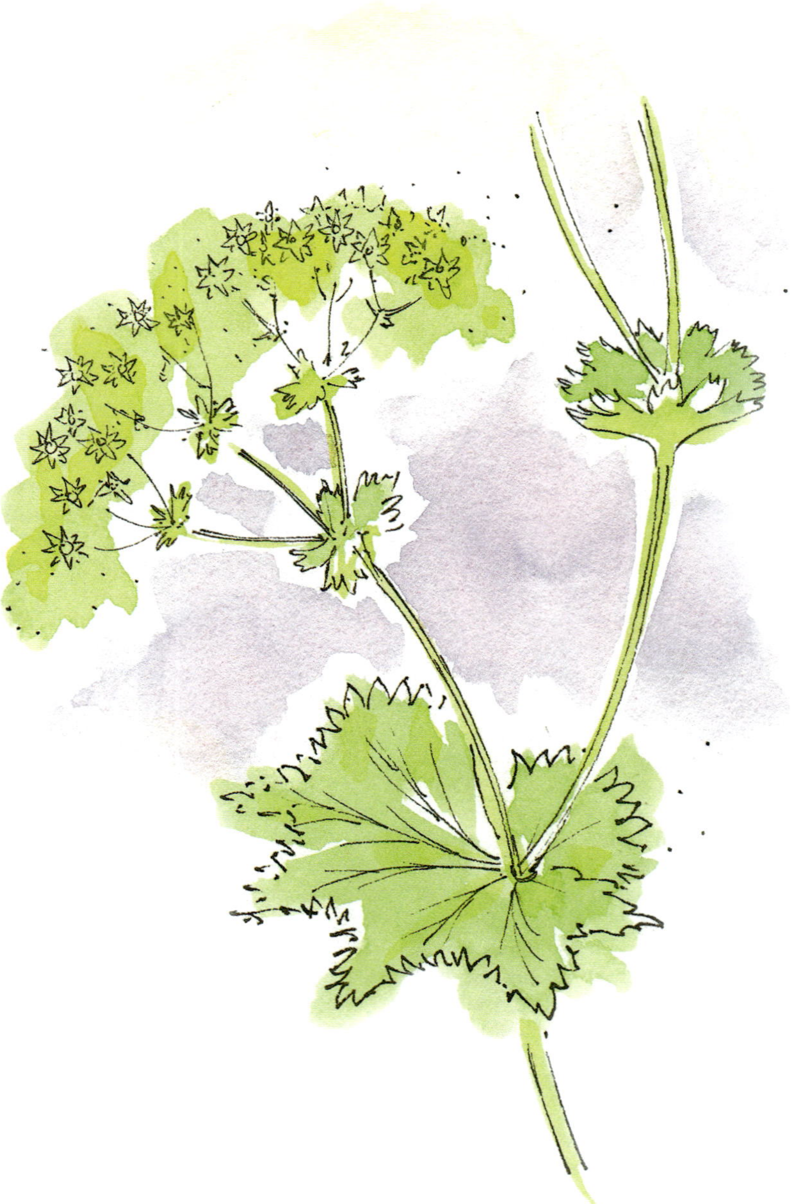

**Figure 7.2** *Alchemilla vulgaris*, lady's mantle.

among these Renaissance authors for stopping vomiting and fluxes of all kinds.

It is then taken up for women's use, as its name implies, for a number of purposes. Culpeper designates it a herb of Venus. Having praised its virtues for fluxes of all kinds, no broad mention is made of its use in menorrhagia in particular, yet this is its main modern application. Perhaps this action is simply understood from its earlier context of stopping blood loss and fluxes. Attention is drawn rather to its facility for stopping leucorrhoea, the distilled water used internally or externally as a douche. This facility is so marked, it draws further (and very alike) observation from Dalechamps and Mattioli. Dalechamps writes that the distilled water injected into the vagina stops leucorrhoea to such a degree that a daily injection can help to distinguish 'corrupted from uncorrupted things by its strong constriction of the place'; the more quickly and efficaciously if the woman sits in a decoction. Mattioli writes similarly. De Laguna's text avoids the euphemisms and spells it out, an observation cited by Chevallier of our modern authors, 'lady's mantle astringes the female parts for those who want to appear virginal'. It was obviously a very popular remedy since de Laguna designates it 'sold a thousand times'. Such a use is clearly deemed not worthy of inclusion by Dodoens, Culpeper, Gerard, Parkinson, Fuchs nor Bauhin, since it appears in none of their texts.

They do all carry, however, the recommendation that the herb, both drunk and externally applied, will reduce the size of large and/or sagging breasts and make them firmer. Dalechamps suggests for this purpose that it be mixed with dried roses, alum, horsetail and hypocysthis. De Laguna comments that thus those girls who had lost that which they thought they would never get back are aided by this saintly herb, since there is not a product of nature without a reason.

Then we find an old approach to failure to conceive and miscarriage – that the womb in some cases is too cold, moist and slippery, and thus allows the foetus to slip out. Parkinson speaks of 'too much humidity of the matrice and fluxe of moist humours thereunto, causing the seeds not to abide but to passe away without fruite'. This herb, according a number of our Renaissance authors, remedies that condition. Parkinson says it 'will reduce their bodies to so good and conformable an estate, that they shall thereby be made more fit and able to retaine the conception, and beare out their children'. Bauhin simply says the herb facilitates conception by drying up superfluous moisture. A number of the authors suggest more or less the same regimen: that the herb should be taken for 15 to 20 days to aid conception; the powder in wine or soup, one spoonful per day, says Dalechamps; it should be the distilled water taken internally, Parkinson says and in addition a woman should sit in a bath of the decocted herb.

## STILL VALUED

By the 18th century, writers still appear to value lady's mantle highly. Miller prized it among the 'principal vulnerary' herbs, as 'drying and binding, incrassating and consolidating'. He cites its great capacity to stop inward bleeding, immoderate flux of menses, leucorrhoea, for wounds, prescribed in 'traumatic apozems' (decoction or infusion) and for flagging breasts, although his language is very delicate here: 'to bring them to a greater firmness and a smaller compass'.

Quincy commends it as a 'most noble vulnerary'. He is not expansive on its virtues but concisely appreciative, saying it will 'consolidate, astringe and thicken the blood, which makes it also prescribed in haemorrhages and other fluxes'. The use of the herb for miscarriage and fertility has disappeared altogether. Moreover, Quincy's comment that a water used to be distilled from the flowers may suggest its general use was not necessarily widespread, or at least not as popular as in the past. However, given that it is the flowers he speaks of here, and they are not substantial, it could rather refer to the preference for more material doses and strengths of composition in the 18th century. Lady's mantle, understandably, falls in Quincy's 'Of Balsamics' section under category 3 'Of Vulneraries'. He explains the manner of effectiveness of such herbs: these are balsamics, which are not only softening and adhesive but by their 'disposition to motion' and their particular shaping, tend to abrade and carry with them any particles they meet with. Hence such medicines cleanse and heal, 'that is they incarnate or fill up with new flesh, all ulcerations and foulnesses occasion'd thereby, both internal and external'. Such medicine will be able to preserve its primary properties, until it reaches its place of action, as is required for all balsamics. When there, its adhesive quality, 'which consists in the comparative largeness of a surface and flexibility of its component parts' allows it to adhere, slough off and carry away any exudates, and then, by the same property, will stick to the wound, and will fill and nourish it until healed. A similar process happens on external application: 'by the warmth of their parts they rarify and by their adhesive quality they join with, and take off along with them in every dressing, what is thrown upon the place to which they are apply'd, until a more convenient matter is supplied; which it forwards, in adhering to and incarnating the eroded cavities'.

Hill describes lady's mantle or 'Archimilla' as 'a very pretty little plant'. Although Miller says the leaves are chiefly used, Hill tells us the root is the part most valuable, either decocted fresh, or dried and powdered. It is strange that he barely mentions its use for wounds, the only reference on this point being 'for all other bleedings', following its use for overflowings of the menses and for bloody fluxes. He notes its use for diarrhoea 'good against common purgings'. Then he turns its use for firming breasts to very practical account: 'the good women of the North of England apply the leaves to their breasts to make them recover their form after they have been swelled with milk, hence the name, he says, 'ladies mantle'.

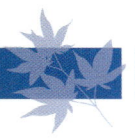

No reference is made to the herb in Fox, Cook, Ellingwood, Hool, nor more recently in Priest & Priest.

Grieve introduces the tannins to account for its astringent and styptic qualities. She summarizes, via Culpeper, the earlier uses as a binding and drying herb for wounds, implying perhaps little use of the herb as a vulnerary in her day. Modern usage, she says, is for excessive menstruation, taken internally as an infusion, 1 oz to 1 pint in teacupful doses as required, and the same used externally as a douche. She covers use of the root, 'considered by some the most valuable part of the plant', for stopping bleedings and diarrhoea, as decoction or dried powder. Is this reference perhaps to Hill or to more contemporary writers? There is a reference too, in Grieve, to Swedish use of the tincture of the leaves for spasmodic or convulsive diseases. Such a reference is also made in the *National botanic pharmacopoeia*, attributed to having been recorded by Dr Marlow. Grieve continues that the herb placed under the pillow at night promotes quiet sleep, but this singular use appears to come from Fernie's confusion of this plant with parsley piert *Alchemilla arvensis*.

Through the literature thus far lady's mantle has been relatively limited to uses mainly from its astringing and related properties, but Maria Treben (1982) appears to have valued the herb for a considerably wider number of applications. Her list includes diabetes, ulcers, miscarriage, uterine prolapse, hernia, muscle weakness, multiple sclerosis, anaemia, partum praeparator, abdominal disorders, wound fever, inflammations of the abdomen and obesity. She adds too that it is heart strengthening and has a reputation in Austria for use in cardiac muscle disorders. This seems to be a more recent claim, although Williamson, later, refers to the flavonoids which, as well as inhibiting elastase and trypsin in vitro, confer angioprotective effects. Wood too includes in his specific indications a capacity to strengthen heart muscles, walls and atria, and its use for arteriosclerosis, although he offers no specific discussion of its effects on the cardiovascular system. As a women's herb, Treben notes its use in both conception and the opposite end of the childbirth journey as partum praeparator. She says that in antiquity, lady's mantle was regarded as a holy plant, and cites 'Father Kuenzle, the well-known Swiss herbalist', who said 'Every pregnant woman should drink large quantities of Lady's Mantle in the last 8–10 days before giving birth ... If this gift of providence were more widely known, there would be fewer widowers and fewer children without mothers'. The recommendation in some current texts is to avoid in pregnancy. Weiss too refers to wider uses in the past than are found in our literature, for metabolic diseases and as a blood purifier. He concludes, however, that all these claims seem unjustified and limits his indications to constitutional leucorrhoea due to lack of real information on the plant's actions.

In the British Herbal Pharmacopoeia, use is restricted to the dried aerial parts, indicated for some of the traditional uses: diarrhoea, dysentery, passive haemorrhage and menorrhagia, with specific indications for acute diarrhoea and epidemic diarrhoea of infants. Topically it is indicated for leucorrhoea and pruritus vulvae, itching of the vulva. This latter is the first indication for use for vulval itch in our literature; unless it is perhaps a reference back to the astringing of the female genitalia considered by Dalechamps, Mattioli and de Laguna. Other uses as a women's herb, and indeed its past fame as a wound herb, have disappeared altogether.

Lady's mantle still appears in modern texts and for the most part within the bounds of traditional use, based largely round its astringent, styptic and vulnerary actions. In its application to women's health, the approaches to the herb extend, in some texts, more towards an alterative, or at least an amphoteric, action, an all-round 'women's herb', and while still a herb associated with drying and astringent qualities, it will nevertheless address both menorrhagia and scanty periods alike: it is both emmenagogue and styptic (Hoffman), it improves regulation of the cycle (Chevallier) and it is a uterine tonic (Menzies Trull). Brooke (1992) has a comprehensive list: painful periods, infertility, heavy periods, post-partum haemorrhage, uterine tonic, thrush, pelvic inflammatory disease, fibroids, menopausal flooding, sweating in menopause and wounds. Chevallier mentions endometriosis too, and Hoffman and Wood a role in menopause.

The astringent effects on the gastrointestinal system are appreciated in a number of texts, both for checking diarrhoea and healing oral mucosa; and application for wounds is not ignored. Wood emphasizes its capacity to restore tone through its drying and strengthening action, to heal torn tissue, and he suggests broader applications in this respect, for example for torn eardrums, rectal tear, uterine prolapse and pelvic floor atony. Wood makes a case for its specific use for 'pale sensitive women with prominent blue veins'. Both Wood and Menzies Trull reprise its use for toning breasts, and there may be a very modern connection here since research has demonstrated some effect when used in anticellulite creams, as well as antioxidant and antiinflammatory activity.

## RESEARCH

There have been a number of in vitro studies suggesting that plants which contain polyphenols, such as flavonoids, coumarins, hydrolysable and condensed tannins, have a range of antiinflammatory actions. Some examples relevant to lady's mantle are of interest. An in vitro study in France of 16 tinctures found an association between the concentration of phenolic compounds and antioxidant and antiinflammatory action. *Alchemilla vulgaris* was second to meadowsweet *Filipendula ulmaria*, in activity (Trouillas et al 2003). An in vitro study on antioxidant action found that the water extract was more effective that the methanol extract (Hamad et al 2007). A study of infusions (1:200) made from 23 Bulgarian medicinal plants found that *Alchemilla vulgaris* had the highest antioxidant action and again there was a strong correlation between polyphenol concentration and antioxidant activity (Kiselova et al 2006). Many plants in the Rosaceae family contain polyphenols and tannins. In a study of 24 wild collected plants in Siberia, 6 of the 10 most antioxidant plants were Rosaceae. A range of in vitro methods was used, and concentration of tannins rather than flavonoids was shown to correlate with antioxidant activity (Oktyabrsky et al 2009).

It is argued that this may support the claim that plants containing polyphenols can be useful externally, for example to resist aging of the skin. Skin aging has been associated with loss of elastin, a protein in the dermis, and it is argued that inhibition of elastase may decrease skin aging and therefore wrinkles. A plant product containing extracts of *Alchemilla vulgaris* and other herbs was found to inhibit human leukocyte elastase in vitro. The level of inhibition was associated with the concentration of tannins and image analysis of skin after use of a cream containing 5% of the compound found a decrease in wrinkles (Benaiges et al 1998).

Lady's mantle's effect on heavy periods has also been researched. An open study in Romania in the 1970s on 341 girls aged 11 to 17 investigated the fluid extract of *Alchemilla vulgaris* (5.8% tannins, 2.2% flavonoid glycosides) for reduction of excessive menstrual flow. The dose was 50–60 drops, three to five times per day. The participants were monitored for up to 6 years. Excessive flow stopped in three to five days, and volume of flow was reduced when used 10–15 days before the period (Petcu et al, cited in Bradley 2006).

Pelikan looks further at the plant to take us closer to its application. As a member of the rose family the plant has inherent harmony of form, but the emphasis is at the watery/etheric end of the type. The leaf, the watery/etheric member of the plant, Pelikan says, has become the principal organ. It takes on the flower role as far as it can. It obviously cannot secrete nectar as a flower can, but the water it secretes at the ends of the leaf veins might be seen to approach this effect. Pelikan expresses this activity very poetically: 'The fluid organism of this plant may be said to be compressed by the light-borne forces of the morning, stepping outside its boundaries. Thus at a lower level, in a (sic) cruder form, something occurs which in the flower develops as the higher function of nectar production when the astral sphere, coming from the outside, takes hold of the etheric organisation, "squeezing" it and causing it to release nectar from its glands.' At the same time dew drops gather on the hairy leaves in the humidity of the morning air. This is the 'water of heaven', he points out, so sought after by the alchemists. When the flower does grow, it is formed from the more leaf-like principles – the epicalyx and calyx, rather than producing regular petals, and it takes the leaf with it 'unchallenged' – there is little metamorphosis in these stem leaves imposed by the flower, the leaf principle remains strong. The flower remains golden green, a leaf colour, although it does have a flower's scent. Pelikan suggests that in lady's mantle the leaf principle and floral principle fuse and this interpenetration provides the signature, the key to its application. 'The human counterpart to it may be found in rhythmic processes; not in the sphere of the heart and lung, however, but in the rhythmic organ placed in the metabolic region, ... the uterus'. Thus lady's mantle is a help in childbirth and is styptic. Then follows a lovely image of maternal recovery – the etheric body is the body chiefly responsible for growth and so is vastly dominant in pregnancy. Lady's mantle then is key to restoring balance: 'With its help the mother's astral body, which during pregnancy has largely withdrawn from the organs of birth, having to yield to tremendously powerful growth processes, is able to incorporate itself again healthily, restoring these organs to the maternal organism.'

## RECOMMENDATIONS

- There seems little doubt of lady's mantle's excellence as a wound herb. There may be a case for taking it internally as well as an external application. Thus infusion of the leaves, possibly decoction of the root, or distilled water of the leaves as application for wounds of all kinds, minor burns, and skin conditions other than very dry ones.
- Internally for diarrhoea and vomiting, though use of any tannin based preparation should never be long term because of threat of malabsorption.
- For a range of women's conditions, particularly menorrhagia and leucorrhoea; the herb may well be of use in endometriosis, fibroids and incompetent cervix.
- External application to tone breasts after breast feeding, or for cosmetic purposes; possibly internal consumption too.
- Possible cosmetic role to combat aging skin, but this needs further investigation.

Dosage: The *British Herbal Pharmacopoeia* recommends 2–4 g three times a day of dried aerial parts.

## RECOMMENDATIONS ON SAFETY

No safety concerns are documented.

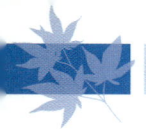

## CONSTITUENTS

Reviews: Bisset & Wichtl (2001), Bradley (2006), Williamson (2003).

### Triterpenes

*Alchemilla vulgaris, Alchemilla alpina, Alchemilla faroënsis* (endemic cross between the former), oleanolic acid, ursolic acid, tormentic acid, euscopic acid (wild, Iceland) (Olafsdottir et al 2001).

### Flavonoids

Total 0.39% (leaves, Russia) (Oktyabrsky et al 2009).
Flavonols: quercetin glucosides, a kaempferol glycoside (in flower, Italy) (D'Agostino et al 1998).
Flavonol: quercitin 3-arabinopyranoside (*Alchemilla xanthochlora*, wild France) (Fraisse et al 2000).
No flavonoids found, which could reflect habitat (Iceland) (Olafsdottir et al 2001).

### Tannins

Total 0.6% (leaves, Russia) (Oktyabrsky et al 2009).
Phenolic compounds 0.62%; tannins 0.21% (commercial, France) (Trouillas et al 2003).

### Hydrolyzable tannins

Ellagitannins: pedunculagin (monomer) 1.2%, agrimoniin (dimer) 3.5–3.8%, laevigatin F (dimer) 0.9% (commercial and cultivated, Germany) (Geiger et al 1994).
*Alchemilla mollis*: total 2% (1:5 decoction); total 1.7% (tincture, 50% ethanol) (commercial, Germany) (Schimmer & Lindenbaum 1995).

## REFERENCES

Benaiges A, Marcet P, Armengol R, et al 1998 Study of the refirming effect of a plant complex. International Journal of Cosmetic Science 20:223–233.

Bisset NG, Wichtl M (eds) 2001 Herbal drugs and phytopharmaceuticals, 2nd edn. Medpharm, Stuttgart.

Bradley PR 2006 British herbal compendium, vol 2. British Herbal Medicine Association, Bournemouth.

Bradshaw ME 1962 The distribution and status of the five species of the *Alchemilla vulgaris* L. aggregate in Upper Teesdale. Journal of Ecology 50: 681–706.

Brooke E 1992 A woman's book of herbs. The Women's Press, London.

Davis PH (ed.) 1972 Flora of Turkey, vol 4. Edinburgh University Press, Edinburgh.

D'Agostino M, Dini I, Ramundo E, et al 1998 Flavonoid glycosides of *Alchemilla vulgaris* L. Phytotherapy Research 12:S162–S163.

De Laguna A 1590 Pedacio Dioscorides Anazarbeo, acerca de la material medicinal, y de los venenos mortiferos, traduzido de lengua griega en la vulgar castellana illustrado y con claras y substantiales annotations, y con las figuras de innumeras plantas exquisitas y raras por el doctor Andres de laguna, medical de Julio III, Pont. Maxi. Online. Available: http://gallica.bnf.fr.

Fraisse D, Heitz A, Carnat A, et al 2000 Quercetin 3-arabinopyranoside, a major flavonoid compound from *Alchemilla xanthochlora*. Fitoterapia 71:463–464.

Gehrke B, Bräuchler C, Romoleroux K, et al 2008 Molecular phylogenetics of *Alchemilla, Aphanes* and *Lachemilla* (Rosaceae) inferred from plastid and nuclear intron and spacer DNA sequences, with comments on generic classification. Molecular Phylogenetics and Evolution 47:1030–1044.

Geiger C, Scholz E, Rimpler H 1994 Ellagitannins from *Alchemilla xanthochlora* and *Potentilla erecta*. Planta Medica 60:384–385.

Gibbons B, Brough P 1996 Wild flowers of Britain & Northern Europe. Chancellor Press, London.

Green MH (ed) 2001 The Trotula. University of Pennsylvania Press, Philadelphia.

Hamad I, Erol-Dayi O, Pekmez M, et al 2007 Free radical scavenging activity and protective effects of *Alchemilla vulgaris* L. Journal of Biotechnology 131:S40–S41.

Kiselova Y, Ivanova D, Chervenkov T, et al 2006 Correlation between the in vitro antioxidant activity and polyphenol content of aqueous extracts from Bulgarian herbs. Phytotherapy Research 20:961–965.

Oktyabrsky O, Vysochina G, Muzyka N, et al 2009 Assessment of anti-oxidant activity of plant extracts using microbial test systems. Journal of Applied Microbiology 106:1175–1183.

Olafsdottir ES, Omarsdottir S, Jaroszewski JW 2001 Constituents of three Icelandic *Alchemilla* species. Biochemical Systematics and Ecology 29:959–962.

Schimmer O, Lindenbaum M 1995 Tannins with antimutagenic properties in the herb of *Alchemilla* species and *Potentilla anserina*. Planta Medica 61:141–145.

Sepp S, Paal J 1998 Taxonomic continuum of *Alchemilla* (Rosaceae) in Estonia. Nordic Journal of Botany 18:519–535.

Sepp S, Bobrova VK, Troitsky AK, et al 2000 Genetic polymorphism detected with RAPD analysis and morphological variability in some microspecies of apomictic *Alchemilla*. Annales Botanici Fennici 37:105–123.

Stace C 1991 New flora of the British Isles. Cambridge University Press, Cambridge.

Treben M 1982 Health through God's pharmacy. Ennsthaller, Steyr, Austria.

Trouillas P, Calliste C-A, Allais D-P, et al 2003 Antioxidant, anti-inflammatory and antiproliferative properties of sixteen water plant extracts used in the Limousin countryside as herbal teas. Food Chemistry 80:399–407.

Tutin TG, Heywood VH, Burges NA, et al 1968 Flora Europaea, vol 2. Cambridge University Press, Cambridge.

Uppsala Monitoring Centre 2005 Accepted scientific names of therapeutic plants and their synonyms. WHO Collaborating Centre for International Drug Monitoring, Sweden.

Williamson E 2003 Potter's Herbal Cyclopaedia. CW Daniel, Saffron Walden.

# CHAPTER 8

# *Althaea officinalis*, marshmallow; *Malva sylvestris*, common mallow; *Alcea rosea*, hollyhock

## DESCRIPTION

**Family: Malvaceae**　　　　　　　　　　　　　　　　**Part used: root, leaf and flower**

*Althaea officinalis* L. is a herbaceous perennial, native to Britain, found wild in ditches near the coast and as a garden escape elsewhere (Stace 1991). The *Flora of Turkey* (Davis 1967) gives four *Althaea* species, including *Althaea officinalis*.

Erect, stiff, velvety stems (to 150 cm high) bear alternate, velvety leaves with three to five shallow lobes, folded like a fan. Pale pink flowers with five broad petals occur in axillary clusters from May to September. The fruit is a ring of nutlets in the base of the persistent calyx.

**Other Malvaceae species used:** common mallow *Malva sylvestris*, a perennial, with pinky-purple veined flowers, found throughout Europe (Gibbons & Brough 1996) and dwarf mallow *Malva neglecta*, a prostrate annual with pale pink, veined flowers (Grey-Wilson 1994). The biennial garden plant hollyhock *Alcea rosea*, is also used (Podlech 1996).

### Quality

Root should be collected from 2-year-old plants, in autumn (Mills 2003) and leaves just before flowering for highest mucilage (Bisset & Wichtl 2001).

Adulteration with other Malvaceae species is possible (Bisset & Wichtl 2001).

Both the common mallow (II 18) and the marshmallow (III 146) are described in Dioscorides. The common mallow (moloche, meaning softening in the same way that mallow is linked to the word mellow) is more edible when grown in a garden than the one gathered in the wild, but in any case is bad for the stomach as a regular article of the diet. Dodoens gives the reason for this as softening and loosening the stomach, presumably reducing that organ's ability to retain food long enough to concoct or digest it. He describes the garden mallow as hollyhock but recognizes that, as a medicine, the wild common mallow is the stronger. The more palatable garden variety is recommended by Dioscorides to ease the bowels and help the intestines, especially if the stems are used, and a decoction can be given as an enema for gnawing pains of the intestines, uterus and anus. Ibn Sina states that the flowers of common mallow are prepared as a drink or in an ointment with olive oil for ulcerations of the intestines and in external use to help abrasions. It is also beneficial for pains around the bladder, when the seed is used, mixed with wild fenugreek seed, or according to some, wild lotus, and given in wine. Ibn Sina includes the kidneys and suggests ulceration as the cause of pain, while Turner writes of abscesses of kidneys and bladder, over which organs a plaster made of the seeds with oil of roses should be laid.

Cooked as a broth they help all deadly poisons as long as those who take the broth keep vomiting it up again. It is also beneficial for those bitten by poisonous spiders. Mallows also encourage the production of breast milk. Ibn Sina adds that the leaves and flowers soothe a cough from a hot, dry chest, while its seeds also help to remove roughness from the windpipe.

Externally the leaves chewed and applied with salt help lachrymal fistulas and abscesses, according to Turner, but to cicatrize these wounds they must be used without salt once the healing process has started. Ibn Sina notes that mallow will help new flesh to grow in these places. It is good for wasp and bee stings, and for poisonous spider bites, and provides immunity to stings if the ground leaves in olive oil are smeared on the body. It will similarly benefit burns and erysipelas. Using urine instead of olive oil, it is a treatment for dandruff and scurf. A decoction of the plant can be used as an emollient sitz bath to soften the uterus.

In Dioscorides, the entry for marshmallow appears in a separate book from that of mallows, despite its description as a kind of wild mallow. Its Greek name 'althaia' is derived from the words 'althos', a medicine, and 'althaiein', to heal. Thus it can treat many diseases and is very useful. Fuchs records medicinal uses of marshmallow predating

©2009 Elsevier Ltd, Inc, BV
DOI: 10.1016/B978-0-443-10344-5.00013-6

# THE WESTERN HERBAL TRADITION

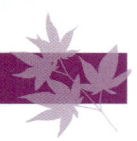

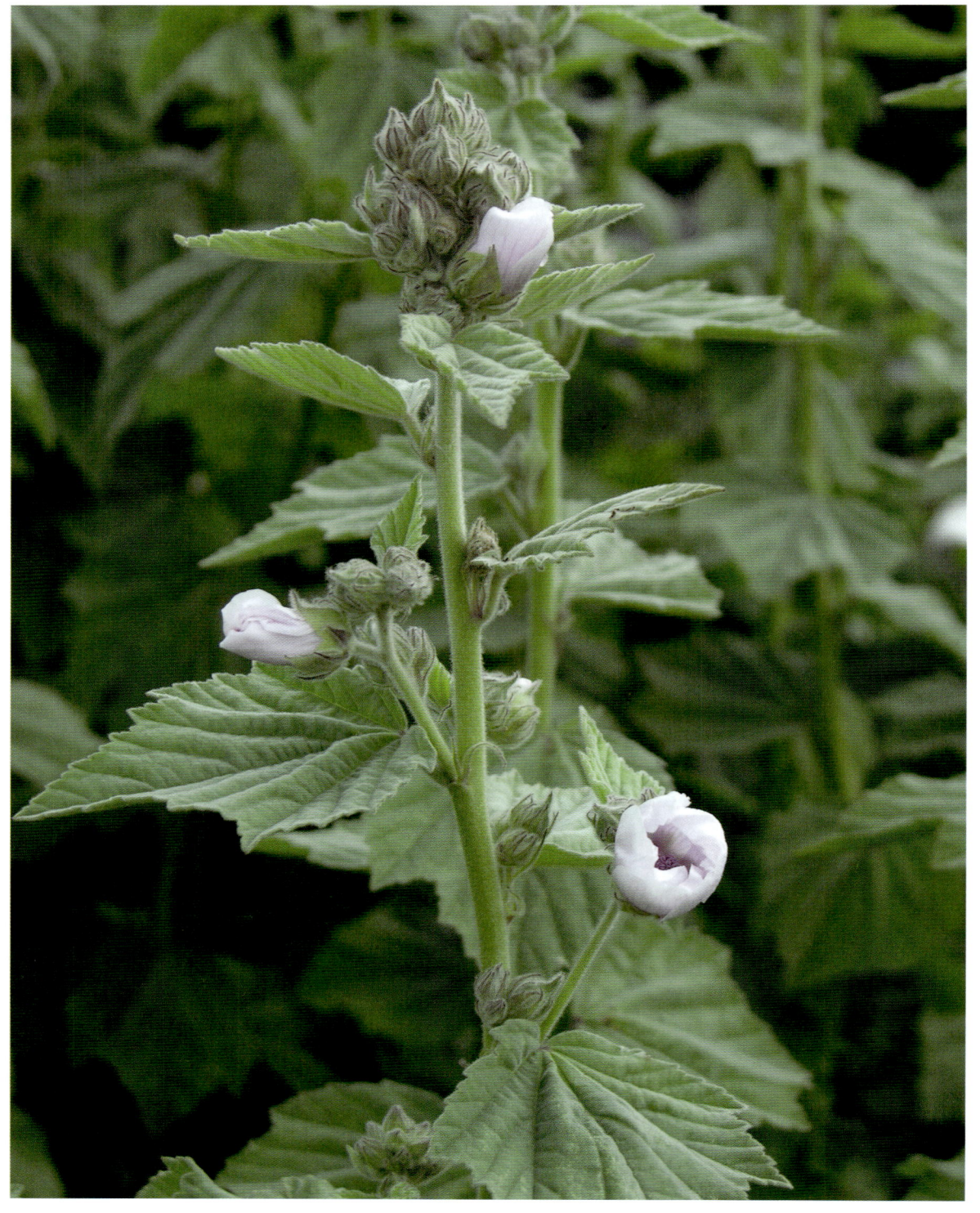

**Figure 8.1** *Althaea officinalis*, common marshmallow (an allotment in Horsforth, Yorkshire, July).

Dioscorides when he cites Hippocrates and Theophrastus. Hippocrates recommends marshmallow for wounds and bruises: the decocted root is given to the wounded as a drink to quench thirst arising through loss of blood. It is also applied with honey and resin to haemorrhages, dislocations and swollen muscles. It treats dysentery and lung problems such as wheezing and shortness of breath, and comforts muscles and sinews. Theophrastus notes that if meats are cooked with marshmallows, the pieces will be joined together. As a medicine, marshmallow in wine is good for ruptures and coughs, while topically, in oil, it is applied to ulcers.

Dioscorides notes that the root is clammy and when pounded and mixed with water and left outside it thickens the water. The decoction of this mucilaginous root in wine is drunk for dysentery, difficult micturition and urinary stones. A French translation of Mattioli's Commentaries recommends the seed for kidney stones and gives a dose of approximately 6 g, saying 'it breaks kidney stones and evicts them, removing all difficulty of urine and easing its pains'. It can also be used for hip pains, ruptures and 'tremblings'. The seed can equally be used for dysentery and for the vomiting of blood and excessive discharges from the bowels; for bee and other insect stings. Boiled with vinegar and used as a mouthwash, it helps toothache.

The root, seed and leaves of marshmallow are also used externally, bruised on their own or boiled in wine or hydromel, i.e. honey-water, for wounds, swellings and suppurations, parotitis or mumps, inflammations of the breasts, disorders of the anus (which Dodoens renders as chaps or fissures), bruises and flatulence. Distension of the nerves is also listed. This can mean muscle tension, for Pliny mentions muscle cramps and cricks in the neck and Dodoens writes of 'tremblings of the sinews'. Riviere in his *Practice of Physick* (Culpeper et al 1655) tells us that in arthritis 'the parts pained are membranes, tendons, nerves and all the nervous parts that are near the joints, which are stretched by the humour which flows into them, or by their sharpness are pricked and twitched'. Marshmallow root applied topically brings wounds to a head, disperses purulent discharge and causes cicatrisation. The leaves mixed with oil can be laid to bites and burns. The powdered seed rubbed onto the skin with vinegar and exposed to the sun cleans the skin of dull-white spots – probably psoriasis, particularly when exposure to the sun is specified. Rubbed on with wood sorrel prevents hurt from poisonous beasts.

Dioscorides adds that a pessary can be made from marshmallow, by boiling and mixing with pig fat or turpentine, and inserted for inflammation and closures of the womb. The decoction is used to bring out the afterbirth.

Pliny gives similar descriptions of some of these uses of mallows without differentiating between the garden and the two wild species. He notes that these herbs were highly praised, that the fresh plant is the most effective form, and that less than 50 mL of the fresh juice daily would render a person free of all diseases. This dose becomes a spoonful in Parkinson in the 17th century, repeated by the Victorian Robinson (1868), who then credits it to Pliny. The benefits of marshmallow, says Pliny, extend even to the place where they grow, since they fatten any ground on which they are sown.

Pliny covers a range of uses of the mallows similar to that of Dioscorides: they are diuretics, counter-poisons and wound herbs, dissolving pustules without breaking the skin or leaving an ulcer, drawing thorns from the flesh and treating burns, the stings of scorpions and the bites of shrews. They cleanse enlarged glands and scrofula and are mixed with honey for cankers in the mouth, or the fresh plant is decocted and used as a wash for tetters (any kind of raised skin lesions), ringworm and dandruff and spreading scabs on the head (the plant to be putrified and resolved in chamber-lie for these last uses, apparently; Parkinson instead prefers the juice boiled in oil) and loose teeth. Additional indications are phlegm and rheum, presumably caused by a certain altered form of the phlegm humour, which is best treated by softening demulcents. This action is augmented when marshmallow is decocted in milk and Pliny recommends such a liquid is taken after supper for 5 days to cure a cough. However, it is not stated whether the cough is dry or productive. Some specific doses of the juice or decoction of fresh mallow root are recorded by Pliny: 135 and 180 mL doses, respectively, for melancholy and madness. Epilepsy can also be helped but Culpeper has Pliny recommending it as especially good for this disease.

Gynaecological practices, too, are mentioned by Pliny: wise midwives regularly give the juice of mallows in wine to women in labour or, if the woman sits on mallows 'under her [birthing] stool' she will deliver speedily. To facilitate conception, a handful of leaves with oil and wine can be used to ensure regular menses. The powdered seed of one plant spread on a woman's pudenda will make her insatiable for sexual union. Three marshmallow roots bound to her will do the same, while one root tied with black wool will prevent evil accidents to her breasts. A uterine injection or douche is beneficial for tumours (fibroids?).

Galen writes that marshmallows have a digesting and loosening action, diminishing phlegmons or purulent inflammations under the skin, mitigating pain and concocting hard pustules. The root and seed are the equal of the fresh herb in treating these things. They are formed of thin parts and are more drying and cleansing than they appear to be. This astringent action makes the root useful for dysentery, diarrhoea and vomiting blood, and complements Pliny's use of mallows in enemas for bloody diarrhoea and as a drink for nausea and retching. Also, the seed breaks kidney stones. For Galen, who allows the names malva and althaea to be used interchangeably, the mallows convey a softening, digesting action. But he notes that the watery nature of the garden mallow weakens its power compared to wild mallows, which are more drying and cutting, and he indicates its medicinal use is to soften the stomach and treat pain there. He allows wild mallow root to replace that of marshmallow and speaks of its leaves as having a binding or astringent action.

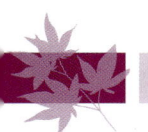

Mattioli quotes Galen from the second book of his *On the Faculties of Foods* (*De Alimentorum Facultatibus*) regarding an experiment to prove the heating effect of wild mallows and marshmallows. He first compares mallows and lettuces, noting that each have garden and wild varieties. It is also well known to all that lettuce is cooling, whereas 'there is something glutinous mixed in the juice of mallow which lettuce is lacking. But it clearly lacks the cooling quality [of lettuce] which can be seen before tasting it. If you make a cataplasm out of each herb and put them on something weakened by heat like erysipelas, in a way in which men have been accustomed to do frequently, beating the leaves extremely diligently into tiny pieces until they are reduced most precisely to smoothness; for then you know that lettuce clearly cools, while malva possesses a certain heat, moderate and as if tepid'. Clearly, while a major action of mallows is to digest accumulations of purulent material, the lettuce is understood to have a more beneficial healing effect on the hot erysipelas because it has the right temperature, namely a colder quality, which conforms to the Galenic principle of therapeutics whereby a humoral imbalance manifesting signs of qualities in excess are treated by medicines of the opposite qualities.

The *Herbal of Apuleius* also records the common mallows and marshmallows. *Malva sylvestris* seems to have two entries, as astula regia and as erratica, which may also refer to marshmallow. The powdered root of astula is taken in

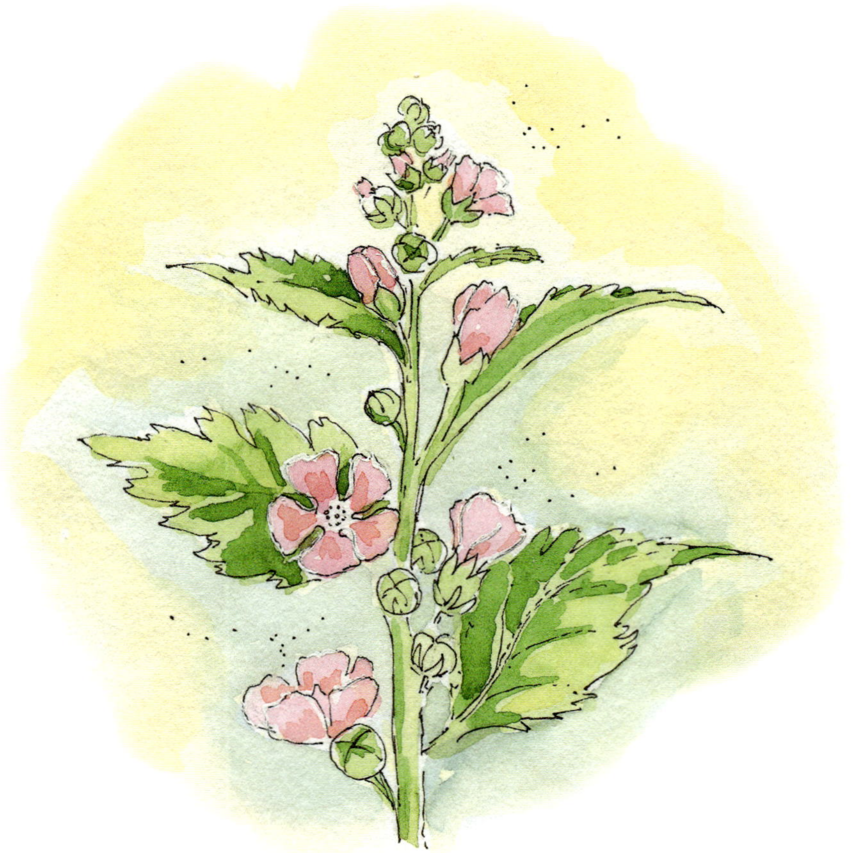

**Figure 8.2** *Althaea officinalis*, common marshmallow.

wine for dysentery and its seed is mixed with very sharp vinegar to astringe the belly and rectify fluxes. A reduced decoction of the root of erratica drunk on an empty stomach for 3 days will remove bladder pains, or the herb in fat can be applied to nerve pain or cooked in oil and laid on with a cloth for pains in the sides. The root can be roasted and applied to close a fresh wound or for swellings in the groin. Apuleius calls marshmallow altea, or malbavisca or hibiscus. Mattioli tells us that malva visca is its Italian name and hibiscus, from Dioscorides' hebiskos, its Roman name. It is found in damp places and is used for gout, the herb pounded into fat and applied to effect a cure in 3 days; any accumulation of diseased matter growing on the body, for which a decoction with fenugreek and crushed linseed applied to the affected area or added to a bath will disperse all hardness and heal; finally intestinal pain, where the same decoction applied to the belly has been tried and found effective, again in 3 days. The first two only of these indications appear in Macer's herbal of the medieval period concerning the mallow that grows in fields and hot places. Shredded with tallow and applied to gout, 'he shall be whole in 3 days'. Mixed with linseed and moistened with vinegar – fenugreek may have been harder to come by in Northern Europe – it can be applied to a patient's side to counter 'wicked gatherings' of humours.

The Salernitan herbal brings us back to Galenic pharmacology and equates mauve, malviscus or wild mallow, with the 'twice-as good' bismauve or marshmallow, in terms of heating and drying qualities, notwithstanding its power to soften and convey a moistening quality. A differentiated cold and moist type is identified as dwarf mallow. Some of the indications already discussed have been included here: intestinal pain, hardness in the body and use of the ointment, notably to ripen abscesses. The root is decocted in water until all the liquid has boiled away, leaving a sticky substance and this applied to the abscess will also work. The classical indication of cough is here treated with the seed and this medicine is also nutritious and benefits those who have become thin. The seed boiled in oil is also given to soften dandruff of the scalp. Hildegard follows suit, by differentiating the hot and dry marshmallow, whose only indication is for fevers when it is pounded in vinegar and left overnight to be taken the following morning on an empty stomach, from the cold and damp mallow, not fit to be eaten raw because 'it would be poison, because it is slimy and has thick, poisonous humours, which it imparts to a person'. Instead, the young shoots cooked and pureed with lard can help digestion in a weak stomach if taken moderately. Both common and marshmallows may be used externally for headache, particularly that arising from melancholy brought on by fever, combined with twice as much sage *Salvia officinalis* and sprinkled with olive oil before plastering on the head and tied with a cloth each day for 3 days. The dew to be found on mallow leaves during or at the end of a clear, calm night is used to moisten the eyes and eyelids in order to clear the vision. The use of mallows in fevers is not recorded in our classical authors but finds an echo in the *Red Book* of the physicians of Myddfai, where the recipes specify, simply, mallows in combination with other herbs for intermittent fevers, as well as for haemorrhoids and abdominal complaints and the spoonful of juice each morning to preserve constant health.

## CONTROVERSY OVER THE TEMPERAMENT OF MALLOWS

If the medieval texts transmitted only a limited part of the classical teaching on the uses of mallows, what of the Arabic texts of Ibn Sina and Serapio? As we might expect, the statements of Dioscorides, Pliny and Galen are extensively preserved in Ibn Sina's entries for mallows and marshmallows. He specifies a mallow ointment for joint pains as well as muscle tension and 'trembling of the limbs' and notes that the 'gum' of marshmallow quenches thirst. He suggests the application of the leaves in cases of pleurisy or lung inflammation. Marshmallow is temperately hot and drying, but Galen's statement that the garden species has a more watery nature, and that mallows in general are unexpectedly drying in action despite appearances to the contrary, not least the clamminess of marshmallow root and the garden mallow in general, leads to attributions of cold and moist qualities to the garden mallow within Ibn Sina's scheme, with the recognition that the wild variety is drier than this.

This attribution of different qualities to some species is also found in Serapio, who lists the classical actions and indications of malva and althaea in separate entries, although 'malvaviscus' and 'bismalva' are mentioned as wild forms of Malva. The potential for confusion here is realized and criticized by William Turner among our 16th century writers, but not by the earlier Fuchs and Mattioli, since the former attributes the classical indications only to althaea or marshmallow while the latter quotes only the actions of Theophrastus and Galen on the same species. Turner writes 'Galen and the Arabians agree not in the complexion of the mallow, for Galen giveth a warm quality unto mallows' and he quotes Galen's experiment in the treatment of erysipelas, a condition caused by an excess of heat. While Turner discusses both the mallow (moloche) and the marshmallow (althaea), and describes the classical actions and indications of both, he refers to Serapio's citation of Mesue for the origin of the attribution of mallow's cold and moist qualities. We have not found this citation in the texts examined but it would identify the source of this attribution of qualities of mallows in both Ibn Sina and, via the translations from Arabic texts of Constantine the African, the Salernitan herbal.

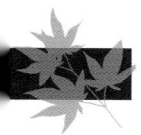

Turner goes on to differentiate the garden mallow into the 'tree mallow of the great bigness that it groweth to' and the lesser kind, 'our common hollyhock', as distinct from the wild or marshmallow, called althaea or even aristalthaea because of its 'excellent working'. Mattioli also discusses the tree mallow – mentioned in Theophrastus – and records seeing one on the shores of the river Benaci near Grignani in a monastery, where the monks' tending of the bush allowed it to become a tree.

As to actions, Turner considers the mallow to soften the belly and remove all hardness from the body. The marshmallow, particularly its root boiled in water until the liquid has evaporated and the remaining sticky substance applied, is better than other mallows at ripening purulent matter; or the root can be crushed, mixed with fat and applied to hot abscesses, to bring the infected matter to a head. An ointment can be made with oil and wax. A decoction of the seed of either marsh or common mallows helps a dry cough – Pliny recommends it for the same boiled in milk and taken for 5 days after supper and Fuchs adds that this decoction speedily heals even stubborn coughs. The seeds placed in a sachet and boiled in oil help soften scurfiness.

In the Lyons herbal of Dalechamps and the French translation of Mattioli's commentaries, little is given in addition to restating the classical sources on mallows. Dalechamps emphasizes that marshmallows clear crude, sticky phlegm by urine and mitigate severe pains on urination, whether occurring at the beginning, end or in the middle of urination, signifying kidney and especially bladder stones. He says the plant is to be found in damp fertile places, meadows and ditches. Bauhin says the same, noting that it flowers in July and August and, quoting Brunfels, is good for asthma. An addition to Mattioli's description of malva includes the eating of the cooked leaves for hoarseness, and the little shoots in salad to stimulate appetite, while the roots, dried and soaked for a whole day in water, wrapped in paper and cooked in warm cinders then dried again, are 'very remarkable for rubbing teeth and making them white, for they get rid of all dirt'.

Dodoens is full of clarity on the species he is discussing. Garden mallow is the hollyhock or 'beyond the sea rose' (Rosa ultramarina). The common mallow and the dwarf mallow, mentioned above in relation to the Salernitan herbal, are his wild mallows and a separate category exists for marshmallow. He also differentiates a small wild mallow, like the marshmallow, only leaves a little rounder and smaller, flowers pale, stalks not as long or upright, but trailing along the ground, the root likewise round and thick. Mallows nourish more than lettuce; they are of a digestive and softening nature and temperate in heat and moisture, while the marshmallow is temperate in heat and dry in the first degree. Thus Dodoens surpasses Ibn Sina on the temperament of mallows by considering all except the marshmallow as moist in quality. As a medicine, the wild mallow is stronger than the garden variety. Likewise, marshmallow root is more efficacious than marshmallow leaf and is mainly used for the range of indications for mallows. New introductions are limited to vehicles and methods for delivering the herbal medicines: the wild mallows applied by themselves or pounded into pig fat are better for softening, ripening and dissolving all kinds of hot and cold swellings; the roots roasted in the embers and hot ashes are pounded and used as a plaster for ulcerations and soreness of women's breasts.

Gerard tells us that 'the common marshmallow groweth very plentifully in the marshes both on the Kentish and Essex shore alongst the river of Thames, about Woolwich, Erith, Greenhyth, Gravesend, Tilburie, Lee, Colchester Harwich and in most salt marshes about London. Being planted in gardens it prospereth well and continueth long'. Marshmallow, he writes with reference to Galen, is moderately hot but drier than other mallows, and its seed and root are drier still. Its roots are to be gathered in March or September, and the leaves and seed are also employed for the cited indications. However, he reckons that the leaves are particularly useful in kidney and bladder stones to help them descend and pass more easily, while a decoction of the roots helps bloody diarrhoea but not because of a drying action: rather than any astringency, and contrary to Galen, it is because they mitigate the associated pain. In order to stop the flux, they must be mixed with astringent remedies such as bistort *Polygonum bistorta* or tormentil *Potentilla erecta*. Another recipe combines marshmallow root with mallow and violet leaves *Viola odorata*, powdered fenugreek *Trigonella foenum-graecum* and linseed *Linum usitatissimum*, black bryony root *Tamus communis* and some fat in a poultice applied very warm to soften and mollify abscesses and hard swellings of the womb and joints, peri-anal tears, green wounds and old ulcers.

Parkinson describes three types of mallows: the now 'little used' malva with entire leaves; the more deeply jagged leaves of alcea, the hollyhock; and the soft leaves of althaea. In reference to the Greek name moloche for mallows he quotes Martial on the benefits of the herb for emptying the bowels and advises boiled marshmallow and hollyhock leaves in salads. The leaves or root boiled in wine or water, with parsley or fennel to open the body, eliminate choleric humours and ease the pain of constipation, for which an enema may also be used. Seed, leaf or root is decocted for hot lung diseases like ulcers, phthisis or consumption and pleurisy, but he requires that this medicine must be taken for some time to be effective. The herb can be given as a syrup or conserve. Externally, wild mallows are better for softening, ripening and dissolving all kinds of hot and cold swellings, particularly a poultice of the leaves with bean or barley flour and oil of roses for hardness and swelling of the liver, spleen and genitals. The feet may be bathed in a decoction of leaves or root or flowers for defluxions of catarrh from the head which rise out of an overheated stomach, while the flowers boiled in oil or honeywater and alum act as a gargle for throat affections.

Under mallows Culpeper describes marshmallow but not the common mallows, since they are well known to his readers. He uses a number of Parkinson's recommendations for mallows but produces a fuller list of indications, adding new uses for the dried root in hoarseness and boiled in milk for whooping cough, and by quoting, for instance, Hippocrates on treatment of the wounded and Pliny on the protective effect of the juice and its employment in epilepsy, and its help for a speedy delivery in labour. He also restates the medieval combination of a mucilage of marshmallow root with powdered linseed and fenugreek as an emollient and anodyne for use as plasters and ointments and in pastilles. He comments further under marshmallow root in his translation of the *Pharmacopoeia Londinensis* on boiling a handful of common mallow leaves with the same quantity of marshmallow root if a fever accompanies the disease, recalling Hildegard's main indication for these herbs. In the same text, Culpeper lists marshmallow as hot in the first degree and dry in the second, and mallows as cold and moist in the first degree, thus combining the evaluations of both Galen and Ibn Sina and emphasizing the difference in qualities between these species. Both plants, however, are assigned to Venus, suggesting an emollient, anodyne and easing effect. Culpeper also describes a cure made with mallows:

> *You may remember not long since there was a raging disease called the bloody flux. The College of Physicians, not knowing what to make of it, called it 'the plague in the guts' for their wits were at* ne plus ultra *about it. My son was taken with the same disease and the excoriation of his bowels was exceeding great. Myself being in the country was sent up for. The only thing I gave him was mallows bruised and boiled in his milk and drink. In two days – the blessings of God being upon it – it cured him and I here, to show my thankfulness to God in communicating it to his creatures, leave it to posterity.*

## 18TH AND 19TH CENTURY SPECIES PREFERENCES

Quincy includes the mallows under emollient medicines for use in conditions where there is evidence of sharpness and acrimony in the symptoms, which could be understood as acidity of the digestion or irritation of the urinary system. His comments demonstrate the diminishing use of common mallow, and the preference for the root of marshmallow. Mallows, he writes, are like marshmallows but not as good and are used very little, except by mothers for their children's gripes, when it is put into their food. However, a decoction of marshmallow root is given for dysentery, colic, urinary obstruction, helping to expel gravel and treat strangury and the heat of urine. Quincy also lists gonorrhoea but as symptomatic treatment only, and the inclusion of marshmallows in enemas and cataplasms. Hill restates Pliny on the greater power of the fresh plant, although the dried is also effective, and advises choosing a plant with leaves only and no stem, i.e. gathered in spring. He wants a strong decoction of marshmallow root taken in quantity for bowel and urinary conditions while the leaves can be decocted for use in enemas. He also names the common mallow (malva) and the weaker vervain mallow (alcea), whose root and leaves could be used. For Cullen, mallows are inferior in degree compared to marshmallows but both are demulcent and externally emollient.

Coffin, the immigrant 'lecturer on medical botany' from America who spearheaded the Victorian revival of botanic medicine in England, writes not of marshmallow but the weaker hollyhock, 'the flowers of which I use medicinally, for healing the throat and stomach, when sore or after an inflammation'. A tea of the flowers heals inflammation of the mucous membrane or lining of the stomach, while the pulverized leaves may be applied as a poultice. He gives a recipe for a conserve of hollyhock flowers, to which is added cayenne pepper *Capsicum annuum*, ginger *Zingiber officinale*, poplar bark *Populus tremuloides*, sugar and cloves *Syzygium aromaticum*, which is good for a cough. Coffin's fellow American Cook, writing a couple of decades later, focuses instead on the common mallow *Malva sylvestris* and the dwarf mallow *Malva rotundifolia*, an infusion of the leaves used in kidney and urinary complaints with agrimony added, and for bowel problems, including dysentery. He accords the plant slight nervine tonic properties. Marshmallow is naturalized on US marshes, he tells us, and its mucilage is soothing to all mucous membranes and acts like all mucilaginous plants as a moderate diuretic: it should be given as an infusion or decoction mixed with other herbs 'more permanent in nature'. Internally marshmallow can be used for a range of disease conditions of the respiratory, digestive and urinary organs, while externally the root boiled in milk is the basis for an external poultice for inflamed eyes, itchy skin, sores, bruises and burns. A syrup can be made by macerating 1½ oz of root in 1 pint of water for 12 hours before adding 2 lbs of sugar to the strained liquor as it heats. The syrup can easily ferment but is an elegant demulcent for coughs, especially if ½ oz lobelia herb *Lobelia inflata* is mixed into the syrup. Alternatively, a more antispasmodic effect is obtained and the syrup better preserved if 2 fl oz of a tincture of black cohosh *Cimicifuga racemosa* is added.

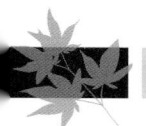

Back in England, Robinson, writing in the 1860s, largely copies or paraphrases Culpeper on the mallows, leaving out some statements such as Dioscorides' provocation of vomiting in cases of poisoning, but scurrilously paraphrasing Culpeper's words above, so that it sounds like his own son who was taken ill. Robinson provides indications not found in Culpeper for a decoction of marshmallow root: where the natural mucus has been abraided from the coats of the intestines (re-interpreting Culpeper's strong indication of efficacy in 'excoriations in the guts, or the bloody flux, by qualifying the violence of sharp, fretting humours, easing the pains, and healing the soreness); in catarrhs from thin rheums … in cases where the lochia have been too thin and sharp after childbirth'.

Fernie (1897), writing at the end of the century, demonstrates his erudition by mentioning the references to mallows in Pythagoras, Plato, Cicero, Horace and the book of Job: 'The root is sweet and very mucilaginous, containing more than half its weight of saccharine viscous mucilage. It is, therefore, emollient, demulcent, pain-soothing and lubricating, serving to subdue heat and irritation, whilst if applied externally, diminishing the painful soreness of inflamed parts. It is for these reasons much employed in domestic poultices and in decoction as a medicine for pulmonary catarrhs, hoarseness and irritative diarrhoea or dysentery. Also the decoction acts well as a bland soothing collyrium for bathing inflamed eyes'. The decoction is to be prepared by adding 4 oz of dried root to 5 pints of water and boiling down to 3 pints and straining through calico. The syrup provides a healthy stimulation to the kidneys and is prepared by macerating the roots in cold water, before heating the liquid to melt the added sugar and so form the syrup. The flowers and leaves may also be used as infusions.

The National Botanic Pharmacopoeia in the 20th century describes marshmallow as a demulcent, diuretic and expectorant with topical uses for swellings, pain and inflammation, abscesses, sores and ulcers. When a fomentation of the leaves is applied on hot flannels, as hot as the patient can stand, 'very few cases of inflammation do not yield to this treatment'. A 'very popular remedy' for neuralgic pains, gum or breast abscesses, is composed of marshmallow leaves, poppies *Papaver* species and chamomile flowers *Matricaria recutita*, sometimes with hops H*umulus lupulus* and some cayenne *Capsicum annuum* added, onto which is poured a pint of boiling water and half as much of boiling vinegar. The patient is to inhale the hot vapour until the liquid is cool enough to be applied as a fomentation to the part affected. For internal use a decoction of the root is advised as being the more powerful, to relieve difficulty of breathing and soothe coughing spasms, having 'extensive use' in inflammation of the kidneys or bladder, for the stone and gravel and where difficulty is experienced in the passing of urine. A decoction of the powdered root in milk is 'a most effectual remedy' for haemorrhage from the urinary organs and the same preparation may be used for dysentery in adults or children, recalling Culpeper's own example, for it is beneficial in all inflamed conditions of the mucous surfaces but acts without any astringency. A syrup is recommended for lung complaints and for administration to children, and an ointment made from the fresh root is included in the book's list of preparations. The hollyhock is also included in the materia medica section, whose flowers made into a conserve with honey or vinegar are considered valuable for coughs and urinary complaints.

Wren mentions marshmallow with other remedies for bronchitis as well as for cough, limits urinary indications to painful cystitis (and, surprisingly, gonorrhoea, following Cook and Fox). We find here the National Botanic Pharmacopoeia's hot fomentation for topical inflammations into a poultice with slippery elm powder added. Grieve draws the indications for mallows from Fernie (1897), the National Botanic Pharmacopoeia and Wren, with one or two from Robinson, or rather Culpeper. Fernie's decoction of the dried root produces a liquid that is not too thick and viscid. Wren's poultice treats 'the most obstinate inflammation' and prevents mortification (thus the common name mortification root for marshmallow). A poultice of the fresh root mixed with bread is better than the ointment.

We can see that over time both *Althaea officinalis*, perhaps more emphasized in Britain where it grows well, and *Malva* species have been used, perhaps in particular *Malva sylvestris* (Heinrich et al 2004) in Europe. Similar constituents have been isolated from related species (Gudej & Bieganowska 1990). A study of *Malva sylvestris* and *Alcea rosea* hollyhock found that the concentration of mucilage was highest in hollyhock flowers and the authors recommend their use in demulcent teas (Classen & Blaschek 1998). Aerial parts of *Malva neglecta* were found to have relatively high levels of polysaccharides (Pakravan et al 2007) and this herb is used for stomach ache and heartburn in Turkey and the leaves are used a vegetable (Gürbüz et al 2005).

Marshmallow contains high molecular weight polysaccharides which form a colloidal suspension in water (Franz 1989). Polysaccharides are composed of characteristic repeating oligosaccharide units and the viscosity of the gel formed varies in different plants. In marshmallow the polysaccharides are highly branched and hydrophilic, and form a mucus-like suspension. This mucilage is used for its demulcent action to soothe the digestive system and the respiratory tract, in urinary tract infections and externally in 'drawing' preparations (Mills & Bone 2000). A study of the preparation of aqueous extracts prepared using various methods found that a crude mucilage fairly free of starch could be prepared in an extraction time of 6 hours at temperatures up to 30°C (Blaschek & Franz 1986).

Cough can be difficult to diagnose and treat (Morice 2002). Demulcent preparations in water are used as antitussives and dry cough is the main indication for the root given by Mills (2003). The recommended dose is 500 mg to 3 g as a cold macerate, up to a total of 15 g of root per day. The medullary cough reflex depends on vagal receptors in the tracheobronchial wall which are sensitive to irritants and excess mucus (Porth & Matfin 2009) but Eccles (2009) argues that cough in response to irritation is a more complex conscious mechanism. As mucilages are not absorbed and remain in the digestive tract, it is thought that the protective layer formed by the colloid reduces irritation of receptors in the mucous membrane of the pharynx and thus the cough reflex (Schulz et al 1998, Ziment 2002). However, Mills (1991) argues that there could be a sedative effect on the cough reflex via vagal receptors in the digestive tract. Morice (2002) argues that cough is often associated with oesophageal reflux and in this case demulcents could be the treatment of choice.

Randomized controlled trials of cough are difficult to assess as it is thought that the placebo component is substantial (Eccles 2002). A randomized controlled study in the USA on a product including Chinese liquorice *Glycyrrhiza uralensis*, slippery elm *Ulmus rubra* and marshmallow root *Althaea officinalis*, with four other herbs, found that it is was effective in reducing sore throat and associated difficulties in swallowing. Sixty adults took a teabag four times a day for about 7 days. (Brinckmann et al 2003). A recent randomized controlled trial in Iran on people with hypertension who had developed a cough associated with ACE inhibitors found that there was a significant reduction in severity of cough. Sixty-three adults took 40 mg root daily as 20 drops of extract for 4 weeks (Rouhi & Ganji 2007). This is interesting as cough can be a troublesome side-effect of this type of medication, which is widely recommended for effective treatment of hypertension.

Whatever the effectiveness or mechanism of action of demulcent herbs, they have the advantage over opioid-based cough suppressants that they are neither sedative nor addictive. Honey also contains colloids and a recent randomized, partially double-blinded controlled trial in the USA found that honey was useful for children with nocturnal cough. One hundred and five participants, aged 2–18, took one dose of buckwheat honey (Paul et al 2007).

The British Herbal Pharmacopoeia recommends marshmallow root internally as a demulcent and diuretic for gastritis, gastric or peptic ulceration and enteritis, and specifically for gastric and duodenal ulcer, respiratory catarrh with irritating cough and cystitis. Externally, the root may be used for inflammation of the mouth and pharynx and for varicose and thrombotic ulcers. Again, ESCOP and Commission E uses are more limited than those given in the British Herbal Pharmacopoeia, which also describes the preference for marshmallow leaf preparations as an expectorant in bronchitis and respiratory catarrh, specifically associated with digestive weakness. It is also indicated there for cystitis, urethritis, urinary gravel and calculus. Externally it is employed for abscess, boils and ulcers. Generally, the leaf, flower or root of marshmallow may be used for pain in functional digestive disorders, cough and constipation. Topically it has an emollient and softening action, a soothing antipruritic and trophic protector in fissures, grazes, cracks, insect stings, and for aggravating conditions of the buccal cavity and pharynx.

Rudolf Weiss limits his recommendations to 'the most important and best uses for each plant' discussed. He prefers the mucilaginous root of marshmallow to the less mucilaginous leaves, while hollyhock flowers, although they also contain mucilage and tannin, he deems superfluous, adding colour but little action to cough tea mixtures. The flowers and leaves of common and dwarf mallows can be used topically as compresses in acute eczemas and as a gargle but are little used internally. Thus a cold water infusion of marshmallow root extracts the mucilage (as would Fernie's (1897) method for a syrup), and acts as a demulcent herb for acute cough and for exacerbation of chronic bronchitis. The starch is also useful in gargles so a hot tea can be made for gargling by briefly boiling the chopped root.

Priest & Priest are in line with Weiss in advising a cold water infusion of marshmallow root, but in combination with an infusion of marigold *Calendula officinalis* and golden seal *Hydrastis canadensis* for conditions of the digestive and urinary tracts. Topical applications include the poultice with slippery elm, here for inflamed and gangrenous wounds, abscesses, boils and ulcers and a compress of the decocted root for inflamed haemorrhoids and ophthalmia. The ointment made up with 5% of the powdered root treats bedsores, and a dressing of a paste of the root with linseed oil is applied to burns and scalds. An infusion with myrrh *Commiphora molmol* acts as a gargle for inflammations of the mouth and throat.

A number of combinations involving marshmallow are proposed by Menzies-Trull: with pectoral and expectorant herbs for lung conditions; with lobelia herb and antispasmodics in whooping cough; with meadowsweet *Filipendula ulmaria* and comfrey leaf *Symphytum officinale* for gastritis and with cornsilk *Zea mays* or couch grass *Agropyron repens* for urinary problems. He suggests a decoction or tincture of marshmallow root.

Pelikan comments on the mallow family that most remain herbaceous and shrubby, with bright coloured blooms that have something splendid about them but at the same time something mild and gentle 'they glow but they don't blaze', and they mainly do not have a scent. The leafy region pushes into the flowering region, and the latter shows an inclination to bind itself with the leaf region, and lead down into it. He notes the mucilage forming tendency that suffuses the whole plant, while a lot of the parts also tend to form threads or fibres, and that as a general rule a lot of good fibre plants carry a mucilage process. The mucilage process might thus be associated with overcoming woodiness, since woody fibres would be brittle. In forming mucilage, the process is one of holding fast the life element, water. It is the mucilage process, preventing the hardening carbon process, that mainly contributes the healing capacity of the herb, Pelikan says. It is used internally and externally to ease and soften inflammations. Marshmallow as a syrup has a loosening, calming effect on the whole digestive tract and will regulate mucilage secretion there. The interpenetration of leaf and flower in a rhythmic manner suggests that an effect on the metabolic processes in the rhythmic system might be expected. In inflammation and cough reaction, he says, the astral is cramped, and through this plant it is freed. He adds that mallows are good for sleeplessness since they counter the tendency to poor capacity of the astral to free itself from the physical etheric body, to thus allow sleep.

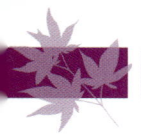

A 'salty' aspect is commented on by Wood as an explanation of marshmallow's emollient action in softening and breaking up hard tissue, for water follows salt. Marshmallow, of course, is a herb of salt marshes. He recommends it for atrophic and irritable tissue states, to soothe the dried out, overheated mucous membranes of smokers and for bronchitis, asthma and emphysema. It will protect the tissues of those undergoing chemotherapy.

## RECOMMENDATIONS

- Our preference here is for the 'twice-as-good' marshmallow, the focus of writers from Quincy to Grieve, rather than the common mallow and on its root in preference to its leaves. There is every reason to follow Pliny in using fresh root preparations such as a specific tincture (dose 2–5 mL) or a freshly prepared ointment (5% powdered root in base) or syrup (BPC 1949 2–10 mL). The infusion (2–5 g) should be made by maceration of the root in cold water, then strained and warmed.
- Gastro-intestinal tract: constipation (a sufficiently large dose); bloody diarrhoea – inflammatory bowel disease and colitis; bilious presentations (with cooling bitters); acid indigestion.
- Urinary: dysuria in urinary tract infections, with urinary antiseptic herbs; urinary stones.
- Respiratory: dry coughs, respiratory catarrh or acute bouts of coughing (syrup); to allay cough as a side-effect of ACE inhibitors.
- Topically: skin inflammation, ulceration, stings and bites, gum and mouth irritations and toothache as ointment, cold maceration or infusion, or a hot poultice of the leaves as required. Relief of pain: inflamed joints, neuralgia, parotitis (mumps), anal fissures, breast inflammation and cysts and pleurisy.
- Daily dosage: for both the root and the leaf, the *British Herbal Pharmacopoeia* recommends 2–5 g three times a day of dried plant material.

## CONSTITUENTS

Reviews: leaf and root (Barnes et al 2007), leaf and root (Bisset & Wichtl 2001), root (Bradley 1992), leaf (Bradley 2006), root (Mills 2003), Williamson (2003), root (WHO 2002).

### Polysaccharides

Root, total mucilage about 11%, pectin 11%, sucrose 10%, starch 37% (Bradley 1992).
Root, neutral polysaccharides 10%, acidic polysaccharides 80%: galacturonic acid 24%, glucuronic acid 22%, rhamnose 35%, arabinose, zylose, mannose, galactose, glucose (Blaschek & Franz 1986).
Leaf, total mucilage about 10% (Bradley 2006).
Leaf, acidic polysaccharide with characteristic oligosaccharide units containing monosaccharides: rhamnose 35%, glucuronic acid 28%, galacturonic acid 31% (fresh, cultivated, Japan) (Shimizu & Tomoda 1985, Tomoda et al 1981).
Leaf, var. *robusta*, acidic polysaccharide: 4-O-methylglucuronoxylan; neutral polysaccharide: glucan (cultivated, Czech Republic) (Kardošová & Machová 2006).

### Phenolic acids

Root, phenolic acids: caffeic acid, p-coumaric acid, ferulic acid, p-hydroxybenzoic acid, salicylic acid, vanillic acid, syringic acid, p-hydroxyphenylacetic acid (cultivated, Poland) (Gudej 1991).

### Coumarins

Root, coumarins: scopoletin (Gudej 1991).

### Flavonoids

Root, flavones: glycosides of hypolaetin, isoscutellarein (cultivation, Poland) (Gudej 1991).
Leaf, tiliroside.
Leaf, flavones: glycosides of hypolaetin, quercetin, kaempferol (cultivation, Poland) (Gudej & Bieganowska 1990)
Flowers, tiliroside.
Flowers, flavones: glycosides of hypolaetin, kaempferol, dihydrokaempferol (Dzido et al 1991).

### Other

Root, starch 37%, pectin 11%, sucrose 10% (Bradley 1992).

## RECOMMENDATIONS ON SAFETY

1. Marshmallow is considered safe in pregnancy and lactation, and no warnings or adverse events were found (Mills & Bone 2005).
2. Monitor long-term usage where the patient is taking other medicines.
   The advice of Commission E that absorption of other medicines may be reduced by use of marshmallow is repeated by later authors but is likely to be minor (Mills & Bone 2005). Consumption of gel fibre has been shown to reduce the rate of gastric emptying and thus rate of uptake of paracetamol, which is used as a measure of rate of gastric emptying (Willems et al 2001). There is widespread addition of pectin and gums to processed foods and widespread usage of other gel-forming mucilages such as psyllium husks *Plantago psyllium* as a bulk laxative (Singh 2007). Psyllium forms a much more viscous gel than marshmallow and this concern appears theoretical and unlikely to be a problem at the recommended dosage.

## REFERENCES

Barnes J, Anderson LA, Phillipson JD 2007 Herbal medicines, 3rd edn. Pharmaceutical Press, London.

Bisset NG, Wichtl M (eds) 2001 Herbal drugs and phytopharmaceuticals, 2nd edn. Medpharm, Stuttgart.

Blaschek W, Franz G 1986 A convenient method for the quantitative determination of mucilage polysaccharides in Althaea Radix. Planta Medica 52:S537.

Bradley PR (ed) 1992 British herbal compendium, vol 1. British Herbal Medicine Association, Bournemouth.

Bradley PR 2006 British herbal compendium, vol 2. British Herbal Medicine Association, Bournemouth.

Brinckmann J, Sigwart H, van Houten TL 2003 Safety and efficacy of a traditional herbal medicine (Throat Coat) in symptomatic temporary relief of pain in patients with acute pharyngitis: a multicenter, prospective, randomized, double-blinded, placebo-controlled study. Journal of Alternative and Complementary Medicine 9:285–298.

Classen B, Blaschek W 1998 High molecular weight acidic polysaccharides from *Malva sylvestris* and *Alcea rosea*. Planta Medica 64:640–644.

Culpeper N, Cole A, Rowland W 1655 The practice of physick … being chiefly a translation of the works of … Lazarus Riverius. Peter Cole, London.

Davis PH (ed.) 1967 Flora of Turkey, vol 2. Edinburgh University Press, Edinburgh.

Dzido TH, Soczewinski E, Gudej J 1991 Computer-aided optimization of high-performance liquid chromatographic analysis of flavonoids from some species of the genus *Althaea*. Journal of Chromatography 550:71–76.

Eccles R 2002 The powerful placebo in cough studies? Pulmonary Pharmacology & Therapeutics 15:303–308.

Eccles R 2009 Central mechanisms IV: conscious control of cough and the placebo effect. Handbook of Experimental Pharmacology 187:241–262.

Fernie WT 1897 Herbal simples approved for modern uses of cure. Boericke & Tafel, Philadelphia. Online. Available: http://www.gutenberg.org.

Franz G 1989 Polysaccharides in pharmacy: current applications and future concepts. Planta medica 55:493–497.

Gibbons B, Brough P 1996 Wild flowers of Britain & Northern Europe. Chancellor Press London.

Grey-Wilson C 1994 Wild flowers of Britain and Northwest Europe. Dorling Kindersley, London.

Gudej J 1991 Flavonoids, phenolic acids and coumarins from the roots of *Althaea officinalis*. Planta Medica 57:284–285.

Gudej J, Bieganowska L 1990 Chromatographic investigations of flavonoid compounds in the leaves and flowers of some species of the genus *Althaea*. Chromatographia 30:333–336.

Gürbüz I, Özkan AM, Yesilada E 2005 Anti-ulcerogenic activity of some plants used in folk medicine of Pinarbasi (Kayseri, Turkey). Journal of Ethnopharmacology 101:313–318.

Heinrich M, Barnes J, Gibbons S, et al 2004 Fundamentals of pharmacognosy and phytotherapy. Churchill Livingstone, Edinburgh.

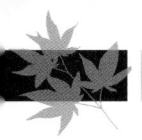

Kardošová A, Machová E 2006 Antioxidant activity of medicinal plant polysaccharides. Fitoterapia 77:367–373.

Mills S 1991 Out of the earth. Viking Arkana, London.

Mills S 2003 ESCOP Monographs: the scientific foundation for herbal medicinal products, 2nd edn. Thieme Medical Publishers, Stuttgart.

Mills S, Bone K 2000 Principles and practice of phytotherapy. Churchill Livingstone, London.

Mills S, Bone K 2005 The essential guide to herbal safety. Churchill Livingstone, St Louis.

Morice AH 2002 Epidemiology of cough. Pulmonary Pharmacology and Therapeutics 15:253–259.

Pakravan M, Abedinzadeh H, Safaeepur J 2007 Comparative studies of mucilage cells in different organs in some species of *Malva*, *Althaea* and *Alcea*. Pakistan Journal of Biological Sciences 10:2603–2605.

Paul IM, Beiler J, McMonagle A, et al 2007 Effect of honey, dextromethorphan, and no treatment on nocturnal cough and sleep quality for coughing children and their parents. Archives of Pediatrics and Adolescent Medicine 161:1140–1146.

Podlech D 1996 Herbs and healing plants of Britain and Europe. Diamond Books, London.

Porth C, Matfin G 2009 Pathophysiology, 8th edn. Lippincott Williams & Wilkins, Philadelphia.

Robinson M 1868 The new family herbal and botanic physician. William Nicholson, London.

Rouhi H, Ganji F 2007 Effect of Althaea officinalis on cough associated with ACE inhibitors. Pakistan Journal of Nutrition 6:256–258.

Schulz V, Hänsel R, Tyler VE 1998 Rational phytotherapy. Springer-Verlag, Berlin.

Shimizu N, Tomoda M 1985 Carbon-13 nuclear magnetic resonance spectra of alditol-form oligosaccharides having the fundamental structural units of the Malvaceae plant mucilages and a related polysaccharide. Chemical and Pharmaceutical Bulletin 33:5539–5542.

Singh B 2007 Psyllium as therapeutic and drug delivery agent. International Journal of Pharmaceutics 4(334):1–14.

Stace C 1991 New flora of the British Isles. Cambridge University Press, Cambridge.

Tomoda M, Shimizu N, Suzuki H, et al 1981 Plant mucilages XXVIII. Isolation and characterization of a mucilage, 'Althaea-mucilage OL,' from the leaves of *Althaea* officinalis. Chemical and Pharmaceutical Bulletin 29:2277–2282.

WHO 2002 WHO monographs on selected medicinal plants, vol 2.

World Health Organisation, Geneva.

Willems M, Quartero AO, Numans ME 2001 How useful is paracetamol absorption as a marker of gastric emptying? A systematic literature study. Digestive Diseases and Sciences 46:2256–2262.

Williamson E 2003 Potter's herbal cyclopaedia. C W Daniel, Saffron Walden.

Ziment I 2002 Herbal antitussives. Pulmonary Pharmacology and Therapeutics 15:327–333.

# CHAPTER 9
# *Apium graveolens*, wild celery

## DESCRIPTION

### Family: Apiaceae     Part used: seeds, root and herb

Six *Apium* species are found in Europe, usually in coastal areas. *Apium graveolens* is also found in other areas as an escape from cultivation. *Apium graveolens* is a biennial with a characteristic smell of celery often found on coastal grassland and field edges. The *Flora of Turkey* (Davis 1972) gives two *Apium* species, including *Apium graveolens*.

Upright solid, grooved smooth stems (to 1 m) bear shiny, pinnate, lobed leaves with a sheathed petiole, and toothed, sheathed, compound basal leaves. White flowers occur in summer in terminal or axillary umbels (4–12 rays, 3–6 cm) which are unstalked or short-stalked. There are no bracts (Tutin 1980). The seeds (1.5 mm) are broadly oval with prominent ridges (Bisset & Wichtl 2001).

### Quality

Celery *Apium graveolens* L. var. *dulce* (Mill.) Pers. is a common vegetable. Stems (blanched petioles) are eaten fresh or cooked. Milder tasting forms were selected in France and Italy from the 1500s (Vaughan & Geissler 1997) and it was in use as a food in Britain by the 1700s (Sturtevant 1886). The root of celeriac *Apium graveolens* var. *rapaceum* (Mill.), celeriac, is eaten as a vegetable.

The studies of the constituents are on various parts of the cultivated plant, and seed of the cultivated variety may be the commercial source plant material.

## COMPLEXITIES OF IDENTIFICATION

Introducing this herb, many herbals speak of the wild celery, a rather bitter herb 'having a poisonous acrimony' says Cullen, and relate it to the better tasting garden variety we serve on our tables. Sturtevant (1886), speaking of its botanical origins, says it originated from *Apium graveolens* L., 'a plant of marshy places'. It is supposed, he says, to be 'the selinon of the Odyssey, the selinon heleion of Hippocrates, the *Eleioselinon* of Theophrastus and Dioscorides and the helioselinon of Pliny and Palladius'. However, he suggests too there is little evidence of its use as a food among the ancients and that if it were planted at all it was for medicinal use only and more likely collected from the wild. It seems cultivation for the table began in Italy in the 1600s and was gradually introduced into France and England by 1700. Sturtevant records a reference to the name celery from a 9th century source in a Strabo poem 'Hortulus', 'where he gives the medicinal uses of Apium and in line 335 uses the word as follows *Passio tum celeri cedit devicta medelae*; the disease then to celery yields, conquered by the remedy, as it may be liberally construed, yet the word *celeri* here may be translated quick-acting, and this suggests that our word *celery* was derived from medicinal uses'.

Tracing the history of celery through older sources, however, is not an uncomplicated exercise. The difficulties of identification are no less surrounding earlier uses of celery than of many other members of the Apiaciae family. This time the confusion is with parsley. Selinon in Greek referred to a number of parsley-type plants. The Latin translation was commonly apium, and epithets were added to distinguish variety, e.g. selinon kepaion, eleoselinon, petroselinon, oreoselinon and hipposelinon. The Greek meaning of selinon as 'joys in marshes' (from Homer), Dalechamps suggests, should be better interpreted 'lunaticum' as Pena says because of a fear-inducing effect from eating it, since it does not always grow in marshes. In the Renaissance herbals a considerable amount of space is allotted to discussion of which selinon is which in the ancient texts and who thinks so. While, by the time of the Renaissance, parsley and celery have their individual entries, there appears no distinctly common separation, reflecting clear agreement of the individual actions of each. Oreoselinon and hipposelinon represent the further reaches of debate about mountain parsley, rock parsley (petro- means rock but is not petroselinon). Macedonian parsley, lovage and

THE WESTERN HERBAL TRADITION

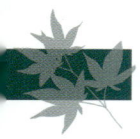

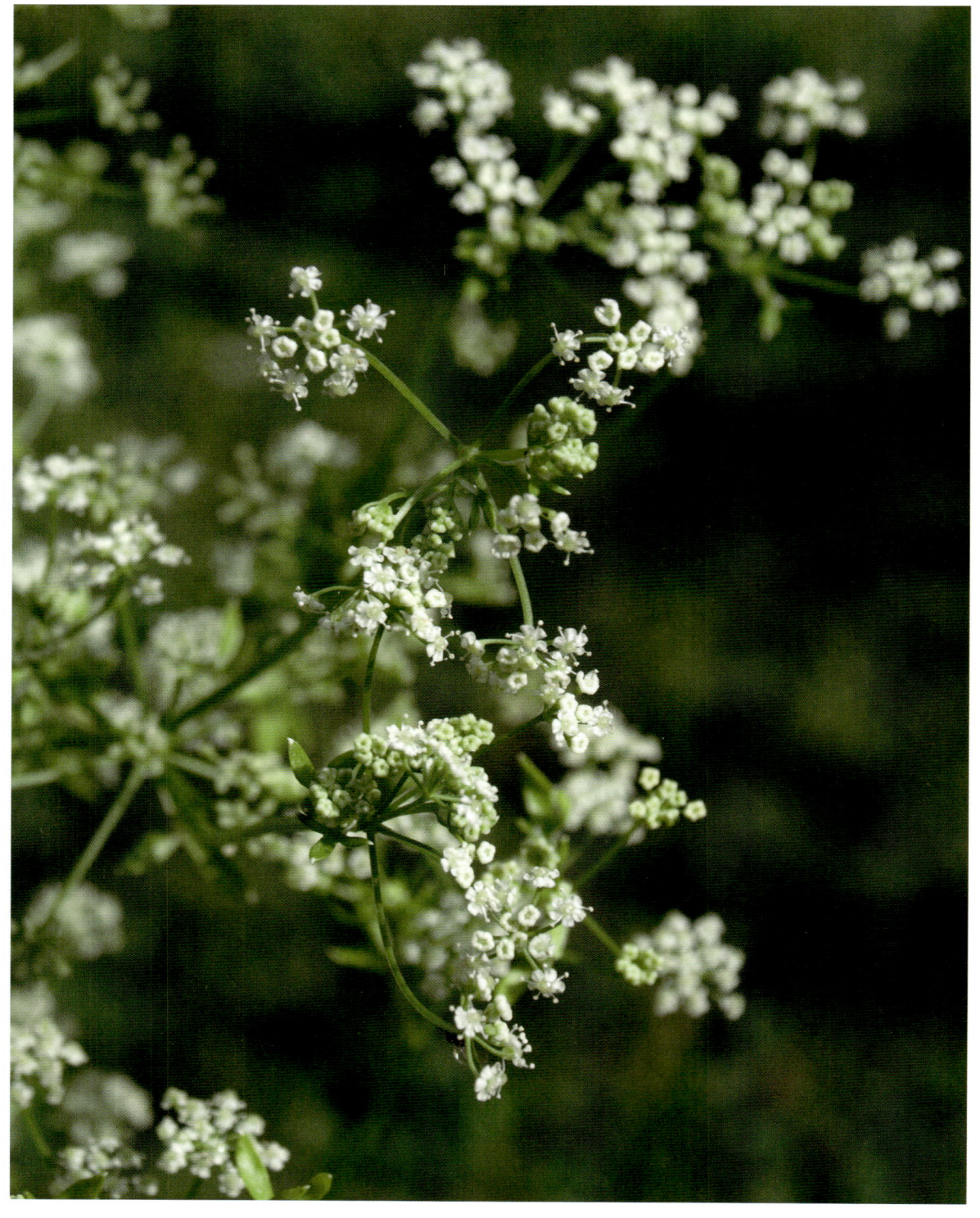

**Figure 9.1** *Apium graveolens*, wild celery (Yorkshire, July).

others, and can thankfully be abandoned here, but the kepaion, eleoselion and petroselinon issue perhaps needs some examination, if only to throw some light on later discrepancies.

It is impossible to discern exactly the apium of the ancients. Galen wrote about selinon, apium and petroselinum, according to the 1543 translation, but these heads may rather reflect the author's grouping. Pliny describes parsley in his Natural History (1949–62), although the editor Jones says this could also be celery, and covers eleoselinum, marsh celery (good for bites of spiders and in wine as emmenagogue), a few entries later. It was Dioscorides who distinguished between selinon kepaion, eleoselinon and petroselinon. Beck interprets Dioscorides' selinon kepaion (III 64) as '*Apium graveolens* L.', garden celery, and eleoselinon as '*A. graveolens* var. *silvestre* L.', marsh celery; petroselinon is '*Petroselinon hortense* Hoffm.', parsley. This distinction is quite at odds with at least some of the Renaissance interpreters. Gerard introduces *parsley* as selinon kepaion, apium hortense, 'the Apothecaries and common Herbarists name it Petroselinum', French du Persil, usually distinguished de jardin (German is Petersilie). Water parsley or smallage, he says, is eleoselinon in Greek, in shops 'Apium with no addition', French de l'ache, Latin palustre [marsh] apium (German Eppich). Dodoens records the same distinction. Parkinson similarly has kepaion as parsley and eleoselinon as smallage, although with two versions for this latter – the 'ordinary smallage', apium palustre, which is 'much more unpleasant and bitter in taste than garden parsley, not to be endured to be eaten alone', and sweet selinum or smallage, apium dulce 'with a warming and comfortable relish'. Fuchs' text on selinon refers, confusingly, to both persil de jardin and l'ache. Mattioli makes no distinction of entry but both he and Dalechamps declare firmly that experts of their time consider the cultivated apium (sativum) of the ancients to be garden parsley, petroselinum, and Mattioli adds that in his day 'that which completes the duty of apium in the shops is no other than palupadium or apium palustre, called eleoselinon by Dioscorides'.

Dioscorides (after Beck) concludes his entry on selinon kepaion and eleoselinon (garden celery and marsh celery) 'The marsh celery which grows in moist places and which is larger than garden celery, also can accomplish the same cures as garden celery'. If this is correct then celery is quite separate from parsley; if Gerard et al are right about kepaion being parsley, then quite a different thing is being said here.

There is no more light shed through the Arabic text of Ibn Sina, which refers to three kinds of 'karafs' – mountain, wild and garden – and it is not clear whether this is a reference to celery or to parsley. 'That which grows in or near water is stronger than the garden, though of like force.' Though he helpfully adds that karafs differs according to the country in which it is found.

Another problem too rears its head with Beck's text on celery. The translation begins: 'The garden celery; this herb is suitable for all the things for which coriander is also suitable …' No other text in our collection, other than de Cleene and Lejeune (2003) mentions this at all, which is odd since the later reference to the marsh and garden variety (or parsley) is repeated by quite a few.

For completeness Beck's translation for coriander, apium and petroselinum of Dioscorides are summarized here, to allow interpretation of later citing.

Coriander (III 63), korion, *Coriandrum sativum* is cooling; for erysipelas and shingles it is used as a plaster made with bread or barley groats; for pustules painful at night, testicular inflammations, and carbuncles it is applied with honey and raisins; and with bruised corn, to dissolve scrofulous swellings of the glands and tumours. The seed drunk with grape-syrup is used for intestinal worms and to promote semen production, but only a little should be taken since 'it dangerously disturbs the thinking process'. Likewise it should not be taken continuously. Inflamed surface tumours are treated with the juice with white lead or litharge, and with vinegar and unguent of roses.

Selinon kepaion (III 64) *Apium graveolens* var. Silvestre L., garden celery and marsh celery. can be used as coriander; it is useful applied for eye inflammations with bread or barley groats; for heart burn and to relax breasts swollen with clots of milk; it is diuretic raw or cooked. '[I]ts decoction and the decoction of its roots' taken internally, counters poisons and is emetic and antidiarrhoeic. The seed is more diuretic and eases flatulence and can be mixed with other herbs as analgesic, against poisonous bites and as a cough remedy.

The marsh celery does the same as the garden celery.

Petroselinon (III 66) *Petroselinon hortense* Hoffm., parsley is diuretic and provokes menses; it can be drunk to help the stomach, gases in the colon, pains in the side, and for the kidneys and bladder. It is suitable for mixing with diuretics and antidotes.

Pliny has more to add, although not without introducing some controversy on his own part. He refers, like Dioscorides, to application with bread or polenta (or fomentation of hot decoction) for the eyes; it is the leaves, he says, which are applied for hardness of the breasts; sick fish are revived with the fresh plant (some later writers repeat this only under parsley). Eating it, he continues, renders men and women sterile. He cites Chrissypus and Dionysius that celery is harmful to the eyes ('an enemy to clarity of sight' interprets Fuchs) and to people suffering from epilepsy. Our translation of Fuchs' version of this latter is 'in the puerperium those eating too much of this food become epileptic', while that of Mattioli reads that it is those who suckle at the breast of a woman who eats celery in childbirth who will become epileptic. Parkinson complains that Pliny has 'erred much' in this reference to epilepsy and that others, including the Arabic writers, followed his wrong lead; that few would believe these things of smallage, let alone of parsley. A number of authors do follow Pliny in this, most forcefully sometimes. For instance Serapio quotes Mesue that karafs is bad for people with epilepsy. Dalechamps cites Ibn Sina too, who says karafs is harmful and arouses fits in those with epilepsy. Seth writes similarly. Bauhin adds that this has been found 'in clear experiment'. This latter claim is encouraging suggesting that this advice is from a practitioner's own experience, but then Gerard's entry on smallage has a remarkably familiar ring about it 'the seed is good for those things for which that of Garden Parsley is; yet is not the use thereof so safe, for it hurteth those that are troubled with the falling sickenesse, as by evident proofes it is very well known'. Turner hedges his bets on epilepsy, claiming that 'divers practitioners' claim this is the case 'as they report'. The association, however, obviously had some practical outcome since Mattioli says 'for which reason it is not surprising if our (doctors) today forbid apium to epileptics'. Yet on quite the contrary track Dalechamps and Culpeper, this latter under parsley, quote Galen as praising celery in his advice for a child with epilepsy.

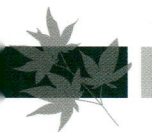

## FOLKLORE

Another reference in Pliny opens up the wide folklore of the plant. It should not be eaten as a food, he says, since

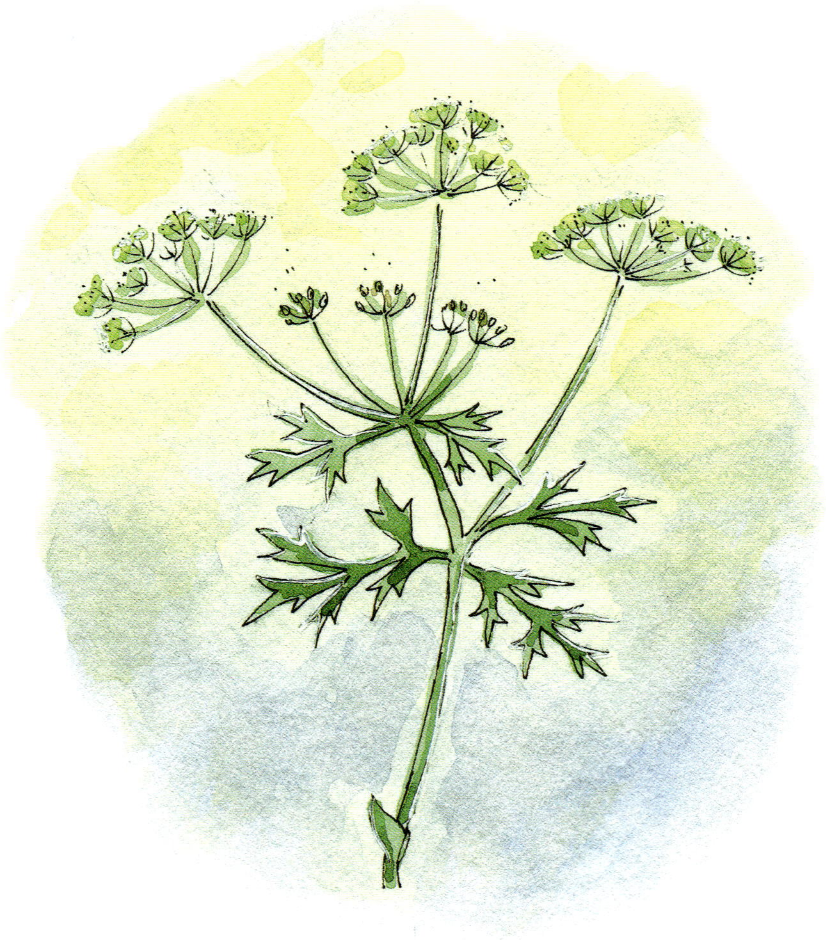

**Figure 9.2** *Apium graveolens*, wild celery.

it is only for use at funeral banquets for the dead. De Cleene and Lejeune's (2003) text contains a considerable entry on celery/parsley (again together) and their links with more hidden forces. In Greek and Roman times celery was a plant dedicated to Hades/Pluto, the god of the Underworld. As such it was eaten at funeral meals, strewn on graves and wreathed around the dead – 'The Greek expression 'deisthai selinon' (to need celery) meant that there had just been a death'. The Isthmean games, held in honour of Neptune/Poseidon (again with associations to the Underworld), and the Nemean games in honour of Zeus were celebrated by 'wreathing the victors with celery' – a double symbolism of death and victory. In wider European lore both parsley and celery were believed to ward off evil spirits, and parsley has a long history of association with the devil – witness the reputed care in choosing the time of planting (preferably Good Friday), the rituals of sowing and (not) transplanting, and its supposed journey to hell and back several times before it will grow.

## THE HOT AND DRY THEME

Galen writes of apium that it is hot and dry in the third degree and so hot that it excites urine and menses. Menses are not mentioned by Dioscorides under kepaion or eleoselinon. It dissipates flatus, Galen adds, the seed more than the herb. Ibn Sina defines it only as hot in the first degree and dry in the second, although it still resolves wind, opens obstructions, causes sweating and eases pain. Culpeper appraises celery as hotter and drier than parsley, so perhaps this indicates Ibn Sina may be writing of parsley here. The wild karafs, Ibn Sina says, ulcerates and causes pain. The jam made from it suits people of a hot nature. It helps cracked nails due to cold, baldness and warts. The facility of ulceration is deployed in the form of bandages to help lichen/herpes and wounds while they have not closed up (Pliny reports this as a spreading disease new to Italy, which begins on the chin, but is painless and not dangerous (Jones 1956). It is thought today to be a form of fungal sycosis (Grmek et al 1993) but has been linked to herpes by other commentators). Garden karafs is one of the ingredients in bandages for pain in the eye and hot swellings of the breast. Karafs helps the liver and spleen but the seeds, if not fried, cause nausea and vomiting. He says that some affirm that all kinds of karafs are helpful to the stomach but quotes Rufus in disagreeing that they sometimes attract to the stomach evil, sharp humours. Raw karafs, he adds, stays a long time in the stomach and provokes nausea. He cites Galen as recommending eating it with lettuce 'as if it tempers the coldness of the lettuce'. It is also good to take after food. The seeds are good for dropsy – they clean the liver and warm it. It causes urination, and mountain karafs breaks stones.

Hildegard considers celery as hot, but adds that it is more green than dry.

This hot, dry theme, together with Dioscorides' recommendations, is taken up by the Renaissance writers and appears variously under parsley and/or celery. Smallage is generally commended as 'stronger' and 'more medicinal' than parsley, although Turner exhorts his readers to prefer parsley. Most, including Dodoens, agree the seed is stronger, although some, as Mesue, commend the root as stronger than the seed. Being strongly hot and dry, it will open and thin, cause diuresis and provoke menses. Culpeper's recommendations are typical, and almost word for word follow Parkinson's 'vertues': (as a herb of Mercury) smallage is 'hotter and drier and much more medicinal than Parsley, for it opens obstructions of the liver and spleen, rarefies thick phlegm and cleanses it and the blood withal. It provokes urine and women's courses, is singularly good against yellow jaundice, tertian and quartan agues if juice thereof be taken but especially made up into a syrup. The juice also put to honey of roses and barley water is very good to gargle the mouth and throat of those that have sores and ulcers'. This lotion, (or 'the juice with honey and beane floure' is Gerard's version') also cleanses and heals all other foul ulcers and cankers elsewhere as a wash. The seed especially expels wind, kills worms and helps stinking breath'. He recommends the root as very good to open obstructions, more so than the herb. Indeed both parsley and apium are counted among the five great opening herbs. Bauhin adds that the distilled water is ascribed by common people to have a peculiar action against dropsy. Fuchs expands with wider recommendations, appearing only under parsley in some other writers, including Culpeper, that it is grateful to the mouth and stomach, provokes urine and the seed in wine or the root in old wine breaks bladder stones. The seeds are diuretic, emmenagogue and cleanse the afterbirth. It can be used as a broth for hardness of the ears (Culpeper says juice with wine dropped into ears) while a decoction of the seeds applied in egg white will remove bruises. Seth suggests further it is difficult to digest, therefore should be taken with food, although it slightly settles the stomach. It not only cleanses the kidney and bladder, he says, but opens obstructions in the veins and arteries too. The seed prevents drunkenness. Gerard tells us in addition that the leaves boiled in hogs' grease and made into the form of a 'pultis', 'take away the paine of felons and whitlows in the fingers and ripen and heale them'. Also Bauhin clarifies that on external ulcers and corrupt wounds with honey it resists putrefaction and represses the stench. The entry in Dodoens mentions only remedying sores, especially of the mouth and throat under smallage/smallach, and otherwise refers the reader, as Turner does, to parsley, which then follows Dioscorides' 'kepaion' exactly. The translation of Dodoens which we used is from the French version translated by Charles de l'Ecluse with Dodoens' cooperation, hence this title will reflect their identification of celery. Culpeper too covers Dioscorides' kepaion under parsley, adding its use by nurses for children with wind, and for the elderly similarly, and various other uses as Fuchs above concerning ears and bruises.

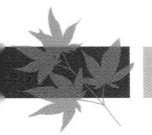

Thus we find little clarity on specific species but a reasonably close consensus on wider applications.

## A HORMONAL HERB?

However, the mainly broad agreement of these authors, apart from the debate on Pliny's errors, on the principal actions of the herb, be it parsley or smallage, fades somewhat on considering a more hormonal context as a galactagogue, aphrodisiac and fertility/antifertility herb. There is similarly no consensus among contemporary authors, and the mediaeval traditions shed little more light. We have seen Dioscorides recommend celery (or more possibly parsley) for relief of breasts swollen with clots of milk and some later authors repeating this, however none of our Renaissance authors otherwise suggest celery is good for promoting the flow of milk. Is Dioscorides' commendation perhaps ambiguous here – will it stop the clotting and hence allow free flow, or will it reduce the clots by reducing the amount of milk? Indeed Seth, quoted by Fuchs, says nursing mothers should not use it for it diminishes milk. Similarly, Serapio cites Constantine the African that celery excites the libido in men and women and therefore is prohibited to those breastfeeding children, since, he says, increase in libido reduces milk. Ibn Sina too has this theme – 'some affirm that karafs breeds lust and it must not be eaten by nursing mothers because it spoils their milk'. Both Menzies-Trull and Bartram of modern authors class celery as galactogogue, although neither accounts clearly for this action.

Both celery and parsley have a reputation for aphrodisiac qualities – De Cleene and Lejeune's (2003) text refers to enduring and widespread folk-lore to this effect, reflected in local names for celery such as Geilwurz (horny herb) or Stehsalat (erection salad). They cite a 15th century German medicine handbook advising on this use: 'Then if you want your wife to love you above all other men, take some celery juice crushed and blended with honey and apply it to the member and testicles, that will make her love none other above you'. However, in our texts, specific mention of this facility appears seldom. Bartram, Williamson (as 'reputed'), and Menzies Trull are rare modern references in this regard, although as, again, it occurs in other Apiaciae – see, for example, wild carrot – there is at least some tradition here.

As abortifacient there is more support but here, it seems, it is more a question of degree. There is clearly agreement on celery's 'provoking the menses' as we have seen. Riddle (1997) too tells us celery seed appears in a recipe for oral contraception from Egypt's 19th dynasty c. 1500 BC, and is occasionally found in anti-fertility recipes from Hippocrates to the Middle Ages, although modern trials, he says, have proved inconclusive. Pliny records it making both men and women sterile, yet Dioscorides says celery acts like coriander, which furthers production of semen. Ibn Sina says karafs causes menses and is harmful for pregnant women – inserting karafs into the vagina will drive out the foetus. All kinds and all parts of karafs clean the kidneys, bladder and womb, but if karafs is eaten continually it fills the womb with a sharp moisture.

*The Trotula* (Green 2001) records wild celery useful ('all diuretic substances are good for her') for deficient menses and paucity of menses, yet it nevertheless reappears 'on Regimen of Pregnant Women' for use, with other herbs, if the belly is distended for windiness for 'it will take away windiness and (danger of) miscarriage if taken as needed', and yet later another part of the text includes celery in a mixture, with wild carrot, sweet flag, dog rose and others, that 'makes women fruitful'. As with wild carrot, can we argue here for the unspecifiable 'tonic' effect on the uterus? Some modern authors, including Chevallier, advise against the use of celery in pregnancy, but not all do so, for example Hoffman has no caution. Wood makes his point strongly '… the plant, like many members of the Apiaciae family, is abortifacient. Even the vegetable eaten in large quantities, can sometimes have this effect – I have known this to occur'. Use in pregnancy is contraindicated in Brinker (1998) 'due to the emmenagogue and abortifacient (empirical) effects and uterine stimulant activity by the seeds and their volatile oil (in vitro or in animals)'. However Mills and Bone are far more reassuring on celery warning rather against parsley: 'other misinformation stems from a confusion of phytochemistry. For example it is often stated in texts that celery fruit (seeds) is contraindicated during pregnancy because it contains significant amounts of apiol, when in fact this is not the case. Parsley is rich in apiol. However pregnant women are typically not instructed to avoid parsley salads during pregnancy.' If Beck's headings are correct, then Dioscorides bears this out, and it is only parsley which provokes menses, not celery.

## LATER USES

By the 18th century celery or smallage is clearly identified as apium and eleoselinum, and the root still referred to as one of the five great opening herbs. Its main traditional uses persisted: 'aperient and discussive, attenuating viscid humours to pass them off by urine, cleansing the liver and good in jaundice' according to Quincy. He classes it as a detergent, class 4 of the Balsamics which soften, restore, heat and cleanse. Miller includes too its use for stone and gravel, dropsie and removing female obstructions, adding too that it is 'one of the herbs eaten in spring to sweeten and purify the blood and help the scurvy'. It appears, however, to be more of a 'home' remedy at this time, as presumably more of the cultivated plant was available by then, rather than largely more sought through the apothecaries, since Quincy suggests 'There needs no trouble to reduce it into any medicinal forms because it is so convenient and agreeable in sallets', and Miller records 'the only official preparation taking its name from smallage is the unguentum (ointment) ex apio'.

On the other side of the Atlantic, Cook and Ellingwood write only on parsley.

## A NERVINE?

Mrs Grieve has a remarkably small entry for smallage. She records the smaller proportion of apiol than in parsley and lists its indications as carminative, stimulant, diuretic tonic and nervine, suggesting it promotes restfulness and sleep and is useful in hysteria, particularly used with skullcap *Scutellaria lateriflora* for nervous cases with loss of tone. This nervine application is somewhat of a departure from our Renaissance and 18th century literature. Dioscorides has mentioned its being profitable for mixing with analgesics, yet this was by no means a focus of those who cited him. From the more local tradition the Myddfai texts speak of celery as a remedy for irritability: 'if a man be irritable of mind, let him drink of the juice of apium (celery) frequently, as it will relieve him of his irritability and produce joy'. They also reprise earlier uses of celery as, for example, with rue and betony for strangury and retention of urine, additionally as an approved remedy for a pain 'pound wild celery and put in some blessed distillation or brandy, strain and add some molten boars lard thereto – mix it well and anoint the painful part therewith', and as a plaster with rue for swelling resulting from a blow. Barker (2001) refers to the tradition of use 'much prescribed for melancholy', although with no reference, and the De Cleene and Lejeune's text specifies such a use in the Middle Ages, although in our literature evidence through the references is thin to say the least. On the other hand, Hildegard suggests that it is not good eaten raw because it gives bad humours; cooked it will lead to healthy humours. Nevertheless, she warns, whatever way it is eaten it can induce an unsettled mind in a person since 'vital energy sometimes harms him'. This use against melancholy, however, is borne out by later literature, where reference to antispasmodic, nervine and sedative applications, mainly through the volatile oils, feature alongside the familiar diuretic and carminative.

## ARTHRITIS AND MODERN USE

Interestingly Hildegard carries one of the few references in the traditional literature to celery for arthritic problems. She recommends it for those tortured by 'gicht', gout, a reference the editor interprets as including at that time gout, arthritis, rheumatism, lumbago and sciatica. She suggests a recipe of pulverized celery seed, a third part of rue, nutmeg less than rue, cloves less than nutmeg, saxifrage less than clove – reduce to a powder If eaten frequently with or without food, it is the best remedy against the complaint and the gicht will cease.

The *British Herbal Pharmacopoeia* (1983) records celery's action as antirheumatic, sedative, urinary antiseptic; indications are rheumatism, arthritis, gout, inflammation of the urinary tract. It is potentiated by dandelion *Taraxacum officinale*.

The chief use of celery in modern literature is for arthritic complaints: gout, rheumatism and arthritis, relying partly on its diuretic nature. Menzies Trull defines it as a 'uric acid solvent diuretic'. It is potentiated by dandelion root, he says, and Barker (2001) anecdotally confirms this from his own experience. Evidence of its antiinflammatory properties are recorded by Mills and Bone. Its sedative nature must enhance the effect too. The specific indications for rheumatic complaints appear in 19th century literature: Fernie (1897) asserts 'Let me fearlessly say that rheumatism is impossible on this diet'. Wood sums up its mode of action – 'Celery is indicated for arthritis, inflammation, heat, dryness, aches, pains and irritability of the tissues … Like many salty emollients it penetrates into calcified or hard deposits, breaks them up, brings back material into the blood stream and out through the kidneys, while increasing the flow of water through cartilage and joint, which is essential for their feeding'.

It has been argued that the some plants traditionally used by herbalists have an antioxidant action that could be linked with an antiinflammatory action. In vitro, six constituents, including the phthalides sedanolide and senkyunolide, showed antiinflammatory activity measured by inhibition of COX-1 and COX-2 (Momin & Nair 2002). The same study found that apigenin had an antioxidant action. A study of 13 essential oils associated the antioxidant activity of celery seed oil with limonene (Wei & Shibamoto 2007). A prescription for osteoarthritis based on a survey of current usage amongst medical herbalists had eight herbs, including *Apium graveolens*, which all contained flavonoids and were shown to be antioxidant (Pendry et al 2005). However, a study of foods and herbs in Turkey found that the highest concentrations of the flavone apigenin (see below) were in honey and in nettles *Urtica dioica* (Karakaya & El 1999), so it is hard to say whether the flavonoids in celery seeds taken at

85

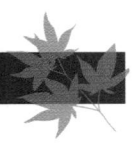

medicinal doses are significant. However, as Pendry et al (2005) argue, the action of a prescription depends on the synergistic action of many constituents.

Pelikan draws together many of the celery themes; as a member of the Apiaciae it is subject to the centripetal, followed by centrifugal impulse that permeates the family; it is hence too a plant of air (see wild carrot for wider discussion in this respect). But what happens to a plant of air when it has an affinity with water as 'marsh' celery? Pelikan locates celery after the hydrocotyles vulgaris and asiatica, where water has more or less an upper hand, and water hemlock where the airy advances greatly into the water, thus producing a poisonous plant. There is a balance in celery leaves between the rounded watery and the finely divided airy form, and to the whole is added a 'salty' leaning from its original wild location as a plant of salt marshes and seashore. The 'downward' and 'upward' impulse he relates to its ancient linking with the underworld as plant of the dead and its victorious crowning of the winners of the Isthmean and Nemean games, from a time when people had a more intuitive inner picture/imagination of outer nature: 'a plant of death, of the grave and mourning … a plant for gaiety. These are two aspects of its nature'. He adds a further link: 'Near Selinunt stood the temple of a chthonic underworld god called Apius to whom celery was dedicated'. Consequently one might expect an effect on the astral/air organization in its relation to the watery etheric. 'Lactation is reduced', he says, 'swollen breasts grow smaller' (cf Dioscorides). He mentions too angina, chronic lung catarrh and cough generally, retention of urine, disorders of bladder and kidney and for stones and gravel, dropsy, gout and rheumatic conditions – many as actions not far removed from those found through the qualities hot and dry in the third degree. Pelikan makes a final point which ties in possibly with Menzies Trull's uric acid solvent diuretic, 'an umbellifer which is also a salt plant can stimulate de-salting processes. This explains the action on salt deposits anywhere in the organism, even the skin'.

The external applications of tradition are gone, but celery still carries its historical uses through to modern recommendation. New applications are now added of course, for example Chevallier, as in the *British Herbal Pharmacopoeia*, refers to its use in lowering blood pressure and as urinary anti-septic, Hoffman to antispasmodic and nervine, Mills and Bone to antiinflammatory, Barker (2001) to anti-rheumatic, Menzies-Trull and Wood to anti-neoplastic.

## RECOMMENDATIONS

- Traditional confusion between celery and parsley obliges some caution in the light of modern information regarding their relative apiol content. However, later mention, once distinguished, confirms an amount of earlier practice.
- It is clearly diuretic with direct application to urinary system conditions, cystitis, gravel and the like.
- Extended effects from its urinary applications speak for its use in rheumatism, gout and arthritis. Some diuresis in high blood pressure might be appended here.
- As a carminative it should ease digestion and rid wind.
- The reputation of the root as one of the five great opening herbs should not be ignored and hence its use in plethoric or obese states.
- There is some traditional reference to easing irritability.
- External application might be considered for mouth ulcers, skin ulcers and whitlows.
- As a precaution it may be wise not to overeat in pregnancy. An effect on the menses appears through the literature, but the tradition is too confused to recommend, for example, the seeds to cleanse the afterbirth, if the effect on breast milk is to suppress it. Dioscorides is clear about relieving breasts blocked with milk, although whether root, herb or seed is not specified.

Dosage: according to the *British Herbal Pharmacopoeia*, 500 mg to 2 g three times a day of dried fruits.

## CONSTITUENTS

Reviews: Barnes et al (2007), Bisset & Wichtl (2001), Mills & Bone (2005), Williamson (2003).

### Volatile oils (seeds unless stated)

Total 2.45%, monoterpenes: limonene 58%; phthalides: sedanolide 7%; sesquiterpenes: beta-selinine 8% (cultivated, Egypt) (Halim et al 1990).
    monoterpenes: limonene 51%; phthalides: 3-n-butylphthalide 7%; sesquiterpenes: beta-selinene 19% (Jagan Mohan Rao et al 2000).
    monoterpenes: alpha-myrcene 32.2%, limonene 16.6%, alpha-pinene 9.6%; sesquiterpenes: humulene and beta-caryophyllene 13.3% (isomers) (leaves, China) (Deng et al 2003).

5 sesquiterpene glucosides (celerioside A–E), 6 aromatic compound glucosides (commercial, Japan) (K tajima et al 2003).
monoterpenes 91–98%: limonene 4–53%, myrcene 12–32%, γ-terpinene 4–49%; sesquiterpenes 1.1–4.9%: beta-caryophyllene (fresh vegetable, 4 cultivars, cultivated, Italy) (Tirillini et al 2004).

### Phthalides

Sedanolide, senkyunolide-N, senkyunolide-J (commercial, USA) (Momin & Nair 2002).
Phthalide glycosides (commercial, Japan) (Kitajima et al 2003).
Total 2.3% (leaves), 0.46% (stalks): sedanenolide, trans- and cis-sedanolides, 3-n-butylphthalide (fresh vegetable, market, Japan) (Kurobayashi 2006).
Phthalides are 12-carbon lactones and mainly account for the characteristic odour of celery. Changes in odour in cooked celery were associated with increased concentration of other compounds, including sotolon, beta-damascenone and beta-ionone, which mask the 'green spicy' note of the phthalides (Kurobayashi 2006).

### Furanocourmarins

Var. *rapaceum*, celeriac, total 0.45%: psoralen, 8-methoxypsoralen, 5-methoxypsoralen (fresh vegetable, market, Finland) (Järvenpää et al 1997).

### Flavonoids

Flavone glycosides: luteolin, apigenin and chrysoeriol glycosides and malonyl derivatives of these glycosides (fresh celery stems and seeds, USA) (Lin et al 2007).

## RECOMMENDATIONS ON SAFETY

1. Monitor patients taking thyroxine.
   Adverse drug report: two women, aged 49 and 55, stabilized on thyroxine, started celery seed tablets for arthritis and it was found that their thyroxine (T4) levels reduced substantially and then improved again after stopping the tablets (product not reported, Australia) (Moses 2001).
2. There is no evidence against the use of celery seed in pregnancy but it is to be used with caution while breastfeeding (Mills & Bone 2005).
3. Do not prescribe for patients with celery allergy, birch or other pollen allergies, nut or kiwi fruit allergy (Food Standards Agency 2009); use caution in atopy and contact dermatitis.

In recent years there has been an increasing incidence of conditions associated with allergy such as hay fever, asthma and eczema (Brown & Reynolds 2006) and studies have sought to identify possible food allergens. Celery has been identified as a significant allergen and, since November 2005, celery is one of 12 foods which must be shown clearly on the ingredient list of pre-packed food (Food Standards Agency 2009).

Allergy to celery as a food is associated with an immediate reaction such as pruritus, sore lips and angio-edema, or with delayed-type hypersensitivity such as exacerbation of atopic eczema. It can also cause occupational contact dermatitis in people who work with celery. Symptoms can be intense, as is shown in a study of 20 patients with celery allergy and pollen allergies who were referred to a specialist centre in France: symptoms were attacks of urticaria and angio-oedema (17/20), respiratory complaints (8/20) and systemic anaphylaxis with vascular collapse (3/20) (Pauli et al 1985). These patients ate celeriac salad, and it may be that the incidence of allergy to celery is higher where celeriac is commonly eaten as a vegetable.

In a case-control study of 1537 adults in Germany, participants with a positive test for allergen-specific IgE antibodies to aeroallergens were matched with participants with negative test results. All participants were then given skin prick tests for various aeroallergens and 10 food allergens and it was found that 25% of all participants were sensitized to at least one food allergen, including hazelnut 18%, celery 15% and peanut 11% (Schäfer et al 2001). This shows that allergies are quite common in the general population. The next study estimated the incidence of reactions in a population of 314 patients in Europe with atopic eczema in remission. The incidence of clear positive reactions ranged from 9% for celery to 39% for *Dermatophagoides pteronyssinus* (dust mites) in atopy patch tests using 200 compounds (Darsow et al 2004).

Both immediate and delayed-type hypersensitivity are associated with consumption of certain proteins, and there is an association between allergy to celery and sensitization to birch pollen aeroallergen (Bohle 2007). People who are allergic to birch pollen also develop hypersensitivity to certain foods, including celery, carrot, apple and hazelnuts (Bohle 2004) as IgE antibodies specific for the main birch pollen allergy cross-react with homologous proteins (Bohle 2007). In a case-control study of 274 people who were allergic to pollen (birch, grass or mugwort), 23% had a positive IgE assay for celery, whereas there were no positive tests in the 55 non-allergic controls (Bircher et al 1994). The major celery allergen Api g 1 is a homologue of the major birch pollen allergen Bet v 1 (Schirmer et al 2005). Immediate-type reactions, referred to as oral allergy syndrome (OAS), are deactivated by heat as the IgE reaction depends on the conformation of the protein (Bohle 2007). However, it has been shown that the T-cell-mediated late-phase reactions, such as deterioration in atopic eczema, are not affected by heat as the reaction is to short peptides (Bohle 2007). A study on people with birch pollen allergy who experienced OAS and the exacerbation of atopic dermatitis on consumption of fresh apple, celery, or carrot retested the population with double-blind, placebo-controlled food challenges with cooked apple, celery or carrot. This did not induce OAS but caused atopic eczema to worsen (Bohle et al 2006).

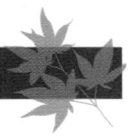

4. Do not use externally when patients use sunbeds

Phytophotodermatitis is a light-sensitive contact dermatitis that occurs when skin which is exposed to sunlight (UVA 320–380 nm) comes into contact with an irritant substance and a red, oedematous rash, sometimes with blisters, develops usually 1–2 days after exposure (Deleo 2004). Furocoumarins have been identified as phototoxic irritants and mainly occur in the Citrus and Apiaceae families with high concentrations found in celery, celeriac and parsnips (Peroutka et al 2007). The furocoumarins are linear coumarins that contain a lactone group and the main ones are psoralen, bergapten (5-methoxypsoralen) and xanthotoxin (8-methoxypsoralen) (Bruneton 1999). These compounds are used orally in combination with ultraviolet light in phototherapy for psoriasis and vitiligo, but their use has been associated with increased incidence of carcinomas (Eisenbrand 2007).

Reactions to furocoumarins in celery occur in greenhouse workers or people working in the grocer trade (Seligman et al 1987). A recent report reviewed the implications of furocoumarins in food because of the increasing use of parsnips, especially in baby foods. It estimated that the oral availability of furocoumarins from food is lower than when taken as part of PUVA therapy, and that the average daily furocoumarin intake in the UK is 0.02 mg/kg body weight (1.2 mg per person) whereas the lowest phototoxic dose is 10 times higher at 0.23 mg/kg (Eisenbrand 2007). As furocoumarins are a normal part of the diet, it seems unreasonable to reduce the use of celery seed. However, the risk of phytophotodermatitis would be relevant if celery seed was used externally in a patient who uses sunbeds.

## REFERENCES

Barker J 2001 The medicinal flora of Britain and Northwestern Europe. Winter Press, West Wickham, Kent.

Barnes J, Anderson LA, Phillipson JD 2007 Herbal medicines, 3rd edn. Pharmaceutical Press, London.

Bircher AJ, Van Melle G, Haller E, et al 1994 IgE to food allergens are highly prevalent in patients allergic to pollens, with and without symptoms of food allergy. Clinical and Experimental Allergy 24:367–374.

Bisset NG, Wichtl M (eds) 2001 Herbal drugs and phytopharmaceuticals, 2nd edn. Medpharm, Stuttgart.

Bohle B 2004 T lymphocytes and food allergy. Molecular Nutrition & Food Research 48:424–433.

Bohle B 2007 The impact of pollen-related food allergens on pollen allergy. Allergy 62:3–10.

Bohle B, Zwölfer B, Heratizadeh A, et al 2006 Cooking birch pollen-related food: divergent consequences for IgE- and T cell-mediated reactivity in vitro and in vivo. Journal of Allergy and Clinical Immunology 118:242–249.

Brinker F 1998 Herb contraindications and drug interactions. Eclectic Medical Publications, Sandy, Oregon.

Brown S, Reynolds NJ 2006 Atopic and non-atopic eczema. British Medical Journal 332:584–588.

Bruneton J 1999 Pharmacognosy, phytochemistry, medicinal plants, 2nd edn. Intercept, London.

Darsow U, Laifaoui J, Kerschenlohr K 2004 The prevalence of positive reactions in the atopy patch test with aeroallergens and food allergens in subjects with atopic eczema: a European multicenter study. Allergy 59:1318–1325.

Davis PH (ed) 1972 Flora of Turkey, vol 4. Edinburgh University Press, Edinburgh.

De Cleene M, Lejeune MC 2003 Compendium of symbolic and ritual plants in Europe. Man and Culture Publishers, Ghent.

Deleo VA 2004 Photocontact dermatitis. Dermatolologic Therapy 17:279–288.

Deng C, Song G, Zheng X, et al 2003 Analysis of the volatile constituents of *Apium graveolens* L. and *Oenanthe* L. by gas chromatography – mass spectrometry, using headspace solid-phase microextraction. Chromatographia 57:805–809.

Eisenbrand G 2007 Toxicological assessment of furocoumarins in foodstuffs. Molecular Nutrition & Food Research 51:367–373.

Fernie WT 1897 Herbal simples approved for modern uses of cure. Boericke & Tafel, Philadelphia. Online. Available: http://www.gutenberg.org.

Food Standards Agency 2009 Celery allergy. Online. Available: http://www.eatwell.gov 15 Mar 2009.

Green MH (ed) 2001 The Trotula. University of Pennsylvania Press, Philadelphia.

Grmek M, Fantini B, Shugaar A 1993 Western medical thought from antiquity to the Middle Ages. Gius. Laterzo & Figli Spa, Rome.

Halim AF, Mashaly M, Salama M, et al 1990 Analysis of celery fruit oil and investigation of the effect of storage. Egyptian Journal of Pharmaceutical Sciences 31:107–113.

Jagan Mohan Rao L, Nagalakshmi S, Pura Naik J et al 2000 Studies on chemical and technological aspects of celery (*Apium graveolens* L.) seed. Journal of Food Science and Technology 37:631–635.

Järvenpää EP, Jestoi MN, Huopalahti R 1997 Quantitative determination of phototoxic furocoumarins in celeriac (*Apium graveolens* L. var. *rapeceum*) using supercritical fluid extraction and high performance liquid chromatography. Phytochemical Analysis 8:250–256.

Jones WHS 1956 Pliny natural history, vol VII. William Heinemann, London.

Karakaya S, El SN 1999 Quercetin, luteolin, apigenin and kaempferol contents of some foods. Food Chemistry 66:289–292.

Kitajima J, Ishikawa T, Satoh M 2003 Polar constituents of celery seed. Phytochemistry 64:1003–1011.

Kurobayashi Y, Kouno E, Fujita A, et al 2006 Potent odorants characterize the aroma quality of leaves and stalks in raw and boiled celery. Bioscience, Biotechnology, and Biochemistry 70:958–965.

Lin L-Z, Lu S, Harnly J 2007 Detection and quantification of glycosylated flavonoid malonates in celery, Chinese celery, and celery seed by LC-DAD-ESI/MS. Journal of Agricultural and Food Chemistry 55:1321–1326.

Mills S, Bone K 2005 The essential guide to herbal safety. Churchill Livingstone, St Louis.

Momin RA, Nair MG 2002 Antioxidant, cyclooxygenase and topoisomerase inhibitory compounds from *Apium graveolens* L. seeds. Phytomedicine 9:312–318.

Moses G 2001 Thyroxine interacts with celery seed tablets? Australian Prescriber 24:6–7.

Pauli G, Bessot JC, Dietemann-Molard A, et al 1985 Celery sensitivity: clinical and immunological correlations with pollen allergy. Clinical Allergy 15:273–279.

Pendry B, Busia K, Bell CM 2005 Phytochemical evaluation of selected antioxidant-containing medicinal plants for use in the preparation of a herbal formula – a preliminary study. Chemistry & Biodiversity 2:917–922.

Peroutka R, Schulzova V, Botek P, et al 2007 Analysis of furanocoumarins in vegetables (Apiaceae) and citrus fruits (Rutaceae). Journal of the Science of Food and Agriculture 87:2152–2163.

Riddle JM 1997 Eve's herbs. Harvard University Press, Cambridge.

Schäfer T, Böhler E, Ruhdorfer S, et al 2001 Epidemiology of food allergy/food intolerance in adults: associations with other manifestations of atopy. Allergy 56:1172–1179.

Schirmer T, Hoffmann-Sommergrube K, Susani M, et al 2005 Crystal structure of the major celery allergen Api g 1: molecular analysis of cross-reactivity. Journal of Molecular Biology 351:1101–1109.

Seligman PJ, Mathias CG, O'Malley MA, et al 1987 Phytophotodermatitis from celery among grocery store workers. Archives of Dermatology 123:1478–1482.

Sturtevant EL 1886 History of celery. The American Naturalist 20:599–606.

Tirillini B, Pellegrino R, Pagiotti R, et al 2004 Volatile compounds in different cultivars of *Apium graveolens* L. Italina Journal of Food Science 16:477–482.

Tutin TG 1980 Umbellifers of the British Isles. Botanical Society of the British Isles, London.

Vaughan JG, Geissler CA 1997 The new Oxford book of food plants. Oxford University Press, Oxford.

Wei A, Shibamoto T 2007 Antioxidant activities and volatile constituents of various essential oils. Journal of Agricultural and Food Chemistry 55:1737–1742.

Williamson E 2003 Potter's Herbal Cyclopaedia. CW Daniel, Saffron Walden.

# CHAPTER 10
# *Arctium lappa*, burdock

## DESCRIPTION

**Family: Asteraceae**                                      **Part used: root, seed, leaf**

*Arctium lappa* L. is a robust biennial, found throughout Europe on roadsides, verges and scrub land. The *Flora of Turkey* (Davis 1975) gives three *Arctium* species, not including *Arctium lappa* but including *Arctium minus*.

Stout, downy, striated, branched stems (to 1 m) bear alternate, entire leaves which are large (to 50 cm long) and wide with a heart-shaped base and white down underneath. The petioles (leaf-stalks) are solid. The spherical, purple flowerheads are stalked and surrounded by dense clusters of scale-like hooked bracts. The egg-shaped seeds are achenes and surrounded by a pappus of yellowish free hairs and characteristic stiff hooked scales derived from the bracts. The ribbed seeds are dispersed by animals as the scales stick firmly to fur.

Lesser burdock *Arctium minus* Bernh. is very similar but smaller (to 50 cm). Basal leaves are smaller and narrower with hollow leaf stalks (Stace 1991). The purple flowerheads occur in clusters and project beyond the surrounding spiny bracts. The seed is not ribbed. *Arctium minus* has three subspecies and a fertile cross with *Arctium lappa* (Stace 1991) and there are many variants (Keil 2006). The photographed specimen may be a cross as it as over 1 m tall but had hollow petioles.

Both species are used interchangeably (Bradley 1992). Greater burdock seeds are widely used in traditional Chinese medicine (WHO 1989, Lü et al 2007). The root is cultivated in Japan and Taiwan as a vegetable cv. Gobo and sold in large pieces, 80 cm long. Inulin content decreases with storage (Ishimaru et al 2004).

### Quality

The root is harvested in autumn or spring, and should be sliced and dried quickly as it is prone to spoiling.

A third of commercial seed samples purchased in China were adulterated with fruits of four other Asteracea species, e.g. *Arctium tomentosum* and one Leguminosae (Kang et al 1999). De Smet et al (1993) include *Arctium tomentosum* as acceptable for medicinal use.

When collecting the seed, care should be taken to avoid contact with the eyes as tiny barbed needles in the burs can injure the cornea (De Smet et al 1993).

Cases have occurred in the 1970s of contamination of burdock root with root of *Atropa belladonna*, which led to anticholinergic poisoning (De Smet et al 1993).

---

Burdock is a name familiar to me since my childhood, not that I was able to recognize the plant as I passed it, which would be often, since in England burdock grows freely in the wild almost everywhere today, and observed by Culpeper; and with a preference for damp earth and waste ground like ditches, by old buildings and roadsides and about towns and villages; so common in fact, says Grieve, that it was not often considered worth cultivating. No, for me it was the strange but pleasant, bitter-sweet taste of a dandelion and burdock drink that I remember. Only later have I come to learn that both dandelion and burdock are herbal alternatives, bitter and diuretic with a cooling effect according to Galenic pharmacological classification. In this regard they complement each other very well.

Burdock was once considered one of the best blood purifiers, according to Grieve. The British Pharmaceutical *Codex* (1934), however, states that burdock is rarely used in medicine but was formerly employed as a diuretic and diaphoretic (at a dose of 1–6 g, in a 1:20 decoction). In its pharmacological index among the appendices there is no listing of an 'alterative' action (although emmenogogue and tonic actions are there), a term which herbalists still use today, as Bartram notes, and interchangeable with 'blood cleanser' or 'depurative'. But what do they mean? What does an alterative alter? One definition is 'those medicines which in particular doses effect a gradual cure by correcting the general diseased habit of body without producing a very visible effect – such as purging, vomiting, or sweating – are generally called alteratives, such as bitter teas and aperient draughts' (Simmonite & Culpeper 1957). This statement is from the pen of WJ Simmonite, a Victorian herbalist and astrologer, rather than from Culpeper

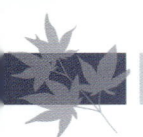

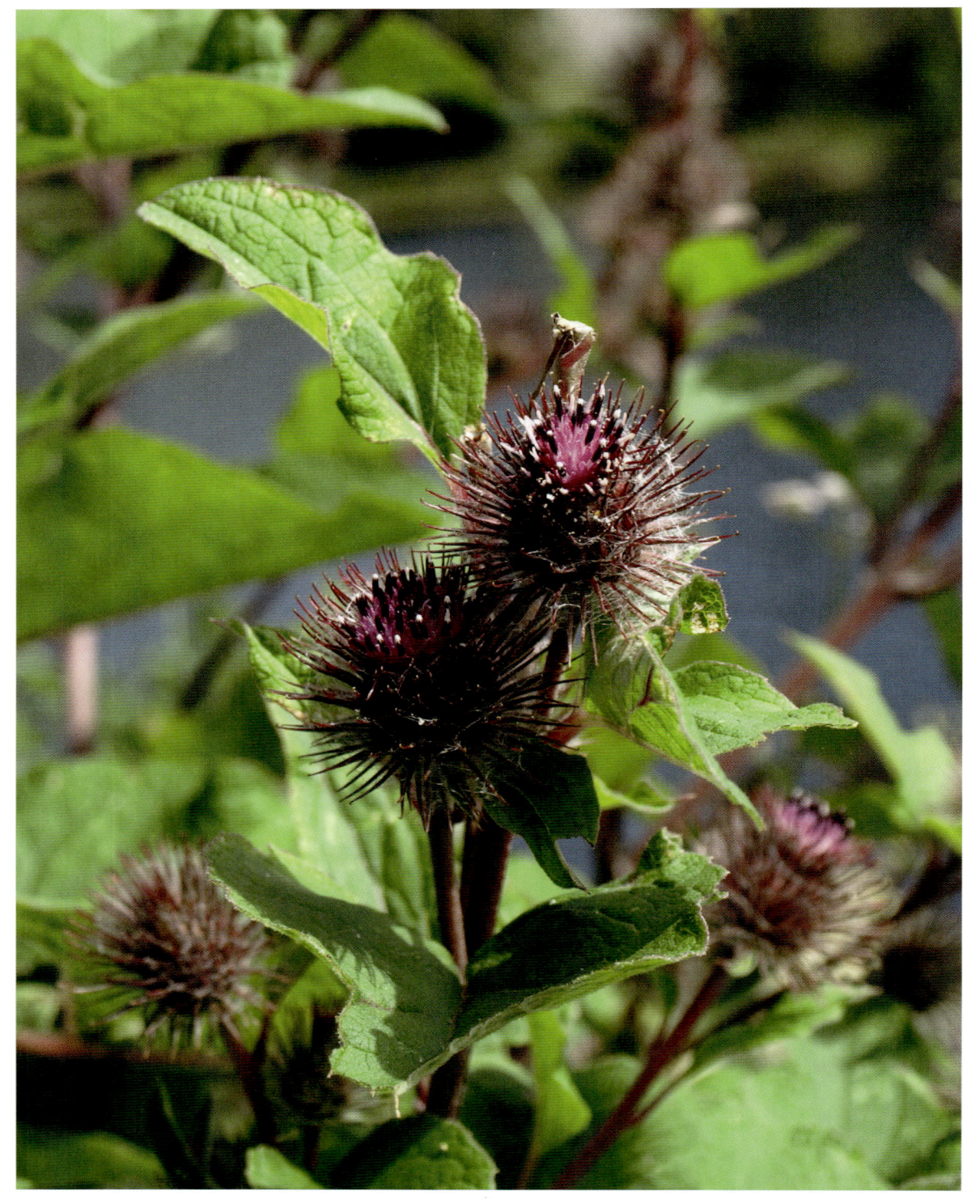

**Figure 10.1** *Arctium* sp., burdock (Farnley reservoir, Yorkshire, July).

since the word 'alterative' is not used by him. The therapeutic strategy of gradual resolution of the patient's condition through a cleansing action suggested by this definition is often the mode of treatment offered today by many professional herbalists: a gentler approach which has replaced the vomits and cathartics of the Galenic tradition, and their more modern counterparts such as lobelia, *Lobelia inflata*, and mountain flax, *Linum catharticum*, which were used by some herbalists until as recently as 50 years ago.

An alterative medicine is elsewhere defined as a herb which promotes the elimination of metabolic waste products, for example uric acid (Priest & Priest). Chevallier writes of a depurative action found with herbs such as burdock, which encourages removal of waste products. Bartram in his entry for alteratives cites Blakiston's Medical Dictionary: 'medicines that alter the process of nutrition, restoring in some unknown way the normal functions of an organ or system … re-establishing healthy nutritive processes'. This definition seems to hark back to concepts of tissue nourishment found in physiomedicalism. Bartram continues 'they are blood cleansers that favourably change the character of the blood and lymph to detoxify and promote renewal of body tissue. The term has been superseded by the word 'adaptogen'. Bartram seems to recognize the problematic nature of claims of detoxification of body fluids in a time when physiomedical or humoral concepts of disease are no longer current. Elsewhere he defines adaptogen as 'a substance that helps the body to adapt to a new strain or stress by stimulating the body's own defensive mechanism. Natural substances in the form of plant medicines offer a gentle alternative to fast-acting synthetic chemical medicine in releasing the body's own source of energy to sustain the immune system'. Can a herbal alterative be restyled an adaptogen? Does a herb which works on elimination via the bile, urine or sweat stimulate an immune response in so doing? Mention of the immune system adds a modern gloss to a much older therapeutic idea, but it is worth adding that species of *Echinacea* now have an evidence base for managing the common cold and viral infections, but were once classified as 'stimulating alteratives' before being restyled 'immunomodulators'.

Hoffmann states that alterative herbs 'gradually restore proper function to the body and increase overall health and vitality … alteratives seem to alter the body's metabolic processes to improve tissues' ability to deal with a range of body functions from nutrition to elimination'. This action is not understood and appears unclear, he says, citing the concept of blood cleansing as meaningless, but is undeniably of value in the holistic approach to health. Such herbs may work on elimination of wastes via kidneys, liver, lungs or skin; by stimulating digestive function; or as immunomodulators. 'Others simply work!' He lists a number of alteratives for each system of the body, and their secondary actions, which probably make more sense to those sceptical of the concept of an alterative action. Thus, whether or not burdock is a primary alterative herb targeting the digestion and skin, it has bitter, hepatic and diuretic actions.

In their chapter on skin diseases, Mills & Bone (2000) prefer to list burdock as 'one of the plant remedies traditionally used as alteratives'. Indications for such herbs are dermatological: furunculosis, eczema, some cases of acne and urticaria, and most other skin diseases, as part of a wider prescription. The use of alterative herbs for joint disease, connective tissue disease and detoxification regimes constitute other 'traditional indications'. Under diuretics, Mills & Bone classify herbs which remove uric acid from the body separately from those possessing a purely diuretic action (although this term has been challenged by Tyler (1999) who prefers the term 'aquaretic' since research has not established the equivalence of these herbal medicines to chemical diuretics) but may share the indications of the latter, including dysuria and oliguria linked to infections and stones, nocturnal enuresis and other functional disturbances of urination, arthritis and skin disorders. Burdock is specifically cited by Mills & Bone as one of five herbs which research has shown to produce, when given internally as infusions, a moderate solvent action on stones formed from urates. An alkalinizing effect on the urine or a possible urinary antiseptic action is proposed as the underlying cause of this benefit.

Burdock is also included in a herbal formula used in a small-scale survey concerning the management of osteoarthritis (Hamblin et al 2004). The fact that alterative herbs are used in the herbal treatment of skin and rheumatic problems implies a belief that this action promotes improvement and healing by flushing out a range of metabolic waste products from joint spaces and stimulating the drainage of lymph and the removal of extracellular materials from skin lesions. A positive statement to this effect is made by Quincy, who affirms that all authors consider burdock seeds to be extremely diuretic and that 'some reckon them effectual in carrying off by those discharges what is very much the occasion of arthritic pains, when 'tis once deposited upon the joints'. Miller from the same period wants the root to be taken internally for pains in the limbs and for gout, while the leaves boiled in milk are applied topically as a cataplasm at the same time.

These 18th century statements provide a foundation for the development of burdock as an alterative diuretic with particular use in arthritic conditions among herbalists and herbal physicians of the 19th century. Coffin writes of an antiscorbutic rather than alterative action of burdock, along with slight aperient and tonic effects. He advises burdock seed as a diuretic and, given in an infusion with the leaves of raspberry *Rubus idaeus* to children, it soothes and tranquillizes the system. The leaves are used for rheumatism and gout, leprosy (presumably copied from older texts – the word lepra in Greek means a scaly condition of the skin), kidney obstructions (which may mean oliguria rather than parenchymal disease) and to cleanse the system after mercury treatment for venereal disease. Externally, the leaves are applied to burns, scalds, and scrofulous swellings – uses also mentioned in Quincy – or wrapped about the feet to reduce a fever. Cook, on the other hand, emphasizes the root, as a relaxant and demulcent alterative medicine producing a slow and mild effect on the kidneys, skin and bowels especially where there is irritability. A mixture of 2 oz of the root decocted in 2 pints of water boiled down to 1 pint and given freely but in small doses, for 'half a pint taken three times a day as some advise would be ridiculous', requires several weeks to produce beneficial effects. A compound syrup of the root is also used. The crushed seeds, Cook continues, are more prompt but also more temporary in their diuretic action, soothing dysuria accompanied by mucus and grey sediment in the urine and irritation of the bladder. The seed is also good for the skin, restoring its natural oils where eruptions cause dryness. Cook relates his own use of a warm infusion of the seeds in typhoid cases and to abate the nausea of lobelia. Fox equates burdock with sarsaparilla in the treatment of rheumatism, skin conditions and enlarged glands and lumps in the neck. The root may be combined variously with dock *Rumex crispus*, slippery elm *Ulmus fulva*, fumitory *Fumaria officinalis*, bittersweet *Solanum dulcamara*, sanicle *Sanicula europaea* and cleavers *Galium aparine* in the treatment of enlarged glands, with marshmallow ointment applied topically. He advises a strong decoction of the seed as a nervine for convulsions, fits, spasms and epilepsy, and as a diuretic for inflammations of the kidneys and bladder. Hool provides the measures for such a decoction: 1 oz burdock seed in 1½ pints of water reduced to 1 pint and given in half-teacup doses before meals. He recommends this for all affections of the kidneys and adds a laxative effect to its diuretic and tonic actions. He affirms that burdock has cured many cases of eczema and he recommends an excellent mixture of 1 oz each of burdock and centaury *Centaurium erythraea*, ½ oz each of dock *Rumex crispus* and fumitory *Fumaria officinalis* and 1 teaspoon of cayenne

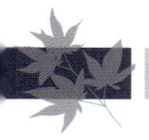

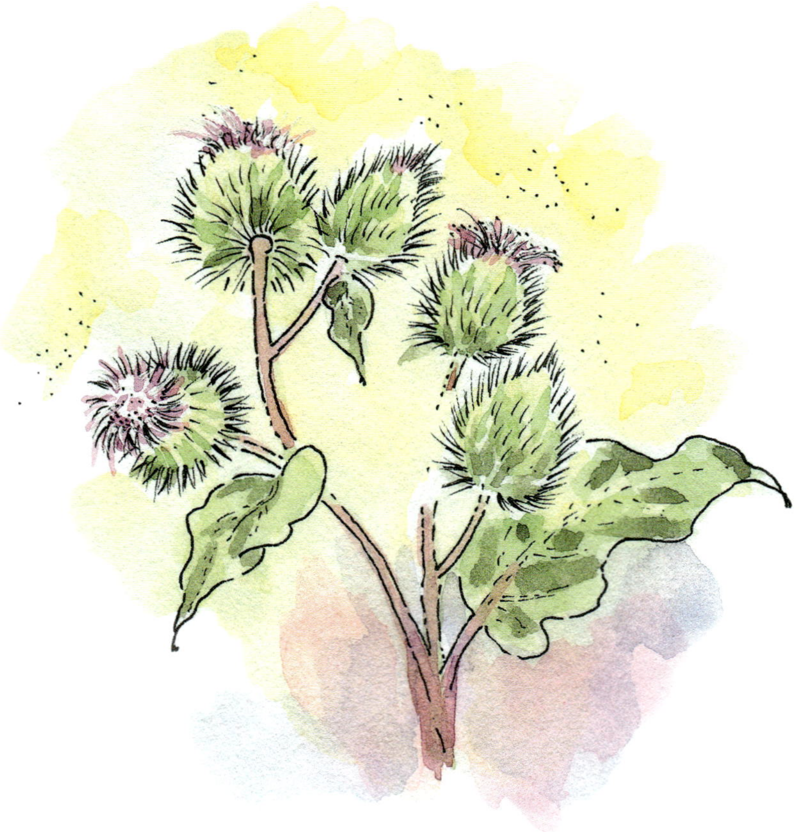

**Figure 10.2** *Arctium* sp., burdock.

pepper *Capsicum annuum*, the total to be simmered in 3 pints of water for 10 minutes. A wineglassful (60 mL) of the cooled, strained liquid is taken three times daily. A second formula for eczema is also included by Hool as a change, in which 1 oz meadowsweet *Filipendula ulmaria* replaces the centaury and ½ oz bogbean *Menyanthes trifoliata* substitutes for dock, using 1 oz burdock seed and no cayenne.

Wren maintains burdock's reputation as a great blood cleanser, an alterative with diuretic and diaphoretic actions, which can be used on its own or in combination, as a decoction of root or seed in the measure provided by Hool. The National Botanic Pharmacopoeia of the same period omits the diaphoretic action, recommends an infusion of the seeds instead, especially in cases of dropsy with co-existing derangement of the nervous system, and includes use of the leaves internally as a tonic for the stomach and externally for inflammations of the skin. Grieve presents a collection of these various indications from her Victorian and Edwardian forebears but adds little that is new. She cites Culpeper's entry on burdock, and Henslow on the mixing of burdock seed with saxifrage (literally, 'stone-breaker' in Latin) and stony seeds or fruit such as ivy berries, gromel seed or crushed date-stones as a remedy for urinary stones seemingly based on the doctrine of signatures. Finally she draws on Gerard for the suggestion of burdock for the table, as a delicate vegetable composed of the stalks of the plant, cut before the flower is open and with the rind stripped off, to be eaten raw in salad or boiled like asparagus. It will have a slight laxative effect, she tells us, while omitting Gerard's observations that it affords pleasant and good nourishment, stirs up lust and increases seed. Fluid extracts of the root and seed are available, she records, with dosage ranges of ½–2 drachms (2–7 mL) and 10–30 drops, respectively.

## BURDOCK IN EARLIER TEXTS

These authors show that the concept of an alterative action for greater burdock can be traced back as far as Quincy, but the plant was known to the Ancients, so what does Culpeper have to report on its medicinal virtues if the term 'alterative' was unknown to him? Actually, Culpeper does write of cleansing medicines. In his *Key to Galen and Hypocrates, their Method of Physic* (1669) he contrasts the more gentle Greek 'rhytics' (actually misspelled from the Greek 'rhyptikos') for external use with the internally administered cathartics. These topical cleansers are of an earthy quality, although they may be hot or cold, and sweet, salty or bitter to the taste. Taken orally, the cathartics purge certain humours from the body as they themselves are voided. Similarly, when applied topically, the rhyptics cleanse foul ulcers by carrying away discharge or thick matter as they themselves are removed. Culpeper distinguishes this cleansing action from the effect of topical discussive medicines which, by their heat when laid on, attempt to thin and disperse an aggregation of matter such as fluid or blood. Other cleansing medicines are designed to remove damaged flesh to facilitate healing. Before the application of cleansing medicines, internal cathartics are prescribed in cases of plethora or cachexy, and generally the need for remedies to reduce inflammation or ease pain is assessed for concomitant administration.

Burdock, however, does not seem to be one of these external cleansers. In his translation of the dispensatory of the London College of Physicians, Culpeper has to append the indications of root and leaf in different sections according to the original layout of the list of medicines by the college authors. Thus the root is temperately hot and dry in the first degree and Culpeper cites Dioscorides and Apuleius on its indications for internal administration: for spitting blood, the bites of mad dogs and toothache, for wind, leucorrhoea (the Myddfai physicians mention lesser burdock for excessive menstruation) and incontinence, and to strengthen the back. The leaves are cold and dry in the first degree and are diuretic and help bladder and joint pains. These indications appear unchanged in his herbal, for Culpeper reproduces Parkinson's list of uses for Bardana or burdock in both texts, adding only the mention of his special application of the leaf for the womb and its associated astrological ruler, Venus.

Dioscorides (IV 106) calls burdock 'arkion', sometimes 'prosopis or prosopion' (from 'prosopon', meaning face). He describes it as having leaves similar to those of the round gourd but larger, tougher darker and rough. The plant is without a stalk and the root is large and white. The root may be taken internally at a dose of one drachm (4 g) together with pine nuts for those who spit blood or suffer from abscesses. Externally the ground root is plastered onto twisted joints to ease pain, while the leaves are used with benefit on old ulcers. The previous entry in Dioscorides (IV 105) describes 'arction', which Beck identifies as bearwort (*Inula candida*, *Celsia orientalis* or *Celsia acaulis*). It is described as having leaves like those of mullein except rougher and rounder, a soft, white, sweet root, a long, soft stem and seed like small cumin (thus presumably ridged or ribbed). The root and fruit boiled in wine eases toothache when held in the mouth, and heals burns and chilblains when the part is washed with it. The decoction is also drunk for hip disease and difficult urination.

If Beck is right that these are quite different plants – and the very bitter taste of burdock leaves should allow no mistake, although the inulin-laden root may taste bittersweet – then it appears that they have been confused in the later interpretation of Dioscorides. Our Renaissance version of Galen is clearly referring to bearwort when it is stated that the root and seed of 'arctium' boiled in wine mitigates toothache and heals burns and chilblains. This arctium is also named Lappa minor, and a Lappa major, 'the other Arctium' or bardana, also called prosopis, is then discussed in the same chapter, its leaves being used to heal old ulcers because of a dry quality and mildly astringent and digesting action. Thus an entirely different plant, the bearwort of Beck, becomes the lesser burdock or Lappa minor in an interpretation of Galen. Culpeper is thus mistaken in listing toothache among the indications of true burdock root. Even the Linnaean binomials *Arctium lappa* and *Arctium minus* for the greater and lesser burdocks seem to reflect a lack of clarity over the Dioscoridean statements on burdock, although Grieve attempts to rationalize the binomial: *Arctium lappa* comes from Arktos, a bear in Greek, which is a reference to the roughness of the burrs, she says, while Lappa is from a Latin verb meaning to seize, or else from the Celtic Llap meaning a hand. The English name unites dock, meaning large-leaved, with burr (Latin burra, a lock of wool), for sheep wool can often be found tangled in the hooked burrs, and this is how the seed is dispersed, by hitching a ride on animals or humans.

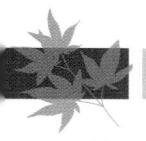

Apuleius discusses the uses of 'prosepis' or 'personatia' (from the Latin persona meaning face): the juice in wine drunk counters snake bites and the leaves rubbed into the skin of a febrile patient drives away the fever; the leaves steeped in warm water then rubbed with salt and fat, a little pitch and vinegar is applied on a cloth to a suppurating or cancerous wound. The root with salt is rubbed into a mad dog bite to speedily heal it, or roots and stems from a plant growing in a dry place treats an old wound full of humours when applied. For burns to the skin and for internal pains 1 cyathos (45 mL) of the juice with 2 cyathi of honey is drunk. Finally, an elaboration on Dioscorides, a drachm (4 g) mixed with pine nuts and a head of mulberries is mixed with wine to form pastilles used for healing those who bring up blood. It is clear that Apuleius is relating the indications of the arkion of Dioscorides and in so doing he extends the indications for the herb. Treating burns, as we have seen, is an indication of bearwort but the instruction of Apuleius is to drink the juice with honey rather than apply it, although the latter makes more sense. Moreover, when these recommendations pass into the Old English Herbarium, there is no mention there of treating burns, and the juice of 'personacia' or burdock with honey is indicated for pain in the abdomen only. The wound full of humours is now described as a wound 'still wet' and treatment is with the root only, mixed with hawthorn leaves *Crataegus monogyna* and applied. Finally, there is no mention of the use from Dioscorides in those who bring up blood.

From these sources is obtained the use of burdock in fevers that appears in Coffin and later texts as a diaphoretic action. Miller recounts that the common people apply the leaves to the feet and wrists in fevers, while physicians and apothecaries specify the root as sudorific and alexipharmic (protecting the heart from poison) and make it an ingredient of the official 'aqua theriacalis'. Burdock leaf is also included, he says, in the unguentum populum for burns and inflammations.

## THE AUTHORITY OF APULEIUS

Is burdock's place in the formula for this ointment based on empirical knowledge of the plant's action or on a misreading of Dioscorides? For once, the authority of Apuleius appears equal with that of the triumvirate of Dioscorides, Pliny and Galen when we turn to the Renaissance writers on burdock. Fuchs, Dalechamps and Bauhin cite him fully. Fuchs indeed avoids citing Pliny at all, gives Dioscorides in full, and Galen on the quality and actions of personatia or bardana. The plant is found everywhere, he tells us – thus providing, we may think, ample opportunity for empirical experiment of reputed uses such as burns – especially at the edges of meadows and fields. Fuchs then cites Apuleius, whose entry is more substantial in terms of uses, but his text has several alterations and accretions too: the juice in honey is now diuretic and used for bladder pain, for burns the rubbed leaf is applied with egg white, and, also among the indications of bearwort, the powdered seed in wine taken for 40 days 'miraculously' heals hip pains (see discussion under ground ivy, Chapter 18). The treatment of snake bites is made by scarification of the wound, then the bruised leaves are applied while 2 denarii (8 g) in weight of the roots are taken in wine, according to Fuch's citing of Columella, who also recommends an ointment of the leaves topically, or the root, for scrofula (see the discussion under figwort Chapter 28).

Meanwhile, Mattioli is more intent on establishing correct species and confirms that the 'personata' of Pliny (bk 25, ch 9), named arkion in Greek, is the Lappa major available in the Italian pharmacies of his day. Pliny also mentions a second large-leaved plant which he calls 'persolata', from the leaves of which, says Mattioli, 'our country people make hats with which they protect themselves from the rays of the sun, while they reap the corn or thresh it in the heat of the dog days'. The same use is conveyed in the Greek and Latin names for burdock, namely prosopis and personata, meaning face, whose 'leaves are the largest of all herbs and exceeding those of the gourd by far' in the opinion of Mattioli, with clear reference back to Dioscorides. Fuchs also explains the name 'personatia' with regard to the theatre and to the use by actors of the large leaves to disguise their faces when the drama requires it.

In Turner, burdock is the great bur, or arkion, personata, or the lappa major of apothecaries, but not persolata. It is found commonly about towns and villages, along ditches and highways, dunghills and other vile places. He only quotes Dioscorides on its uses, omitting any mention of abscesses. The translator of Dodoens gives the plant the name Clote Burre. Dodoens describes the greater and lesser burdocks, stating that the latter is dealt with by Dioscorides in a separate place, and called 'xanthion' in Greek and ditch burre or louse burre in English. Beck identifies the xanthion of Dioscorides (IV 136) as *Xanthium strumarium* L., the broad-leaved burweed. Ignoring this mistaken identity, we find that Dodoens records the majority of uses of greater burdock from Dioscorides and Apuleius as transmitted by Fuchs above. However, it is to the lesser burdock that he credits a healing action on scrofula, specifying the seeds crushed and applied not only to these strumas but to disperse any oedema due to cold humours, for he reckons the lesser burdock hotter in quality than the greater. Furthermore, the juice of lesser burdock, he says, drunk with wine also treats poisonous bites and urinary gravel and stones. The same mistaken link between lesser burdock and the xanthium of Dioscorides is made even in the early 18th century, by Miller and by Quincy, who say, however, that the plant is not used, although it appears in the new catalogue of the Royal College of Physicians.

If Dodoens adds another level of confusion over identity of species in the case of lesser burdock, then Dalechamps becomes another contributor by pointing out that burdock is the arkion of Dioscorides and the personata of Pliny, which all authors recognize, but it is the 'arction' of Galen also, because the prickly heads resemble the heads of shaggy, hairy bears ('arctos' in Greek). Dalechamps' actions for burdock match those of Fuchs, including the citing of Columella, but with the addition of a confection of the root for stones and dysentery. However, the seed is more effective for stones, he notes, and both preparations stir up lust. It may be that what Dodoens attributed to lesser burdock in the Low Countries regarding the treatment of kidney or urinary stones, Dalechamps attributes to the seed or confection of the root of greater burdock in Southern France.

Burdock as a diuretic, one of its modern actions, can thus be dated back to Fuchs, and even before him because the Salernitan herbal proposes that a drink made from the stems of the plant makes a person urinate frequently. This appears in the Salernitan text alongside only two of the uses recorded by Apuleius and does not seem to be derived from the Arabic writers since we find no entry for burdock in Ibn Sina nor Serapio, nor any reference to these authors in relation to burdock in the later herbals. Macer does not describe burdock. An anti-lithic action, evidenced by some modern research, is recorded for the juice of lesser burdock by Dodoens, but this too has a medieval precedent. Hildegard considers that burdock contains some injurious heat and is harmful except to those suffering from the stone. In this case the leaves, for the root is useless she says, should be cooked in the finest wine and the liquid once strained should be taken warm before or after a meal. We may conclude, therefore, that the diuretic and anti-lithic actions of burdock come from empirical medical practice in the medieval period than from a blind copying of ancient texts.

When we turn to Gerard, we find additional uses not mentioned by the preceding authors. Admittedly, he initially sticks close to the latest of the citations above, namely Dalechamps, copying the indications of Dioscorides and Columella, which go back to Fuchs, and taking the confusion of arkion with arction one step further by repeating the indication for bearwort from Dioscorides, which have increased to include strangury. He affirms, however, that it is the stems of the Clot Burre, peeled and boiled in meat broth or eaten raw with salt and pepper, which 'increaseth seed and stirreth up lust', as well as providing good nourishment, especially if the kernel of a pineapple is added! The root pounded and added to ale is good for a windy or cold stomach, while the large leaves can carry a mixture of equal parts of the treacle of Andromachus (the famous plague remedy of the ancients called Theriac and in Gerard's time Venice treacle) and egg whites beaten in a mortar then wrapped around a gouty joint to assuage the exquisite pain of the attack. The root pounded and strained with malmsey treats incontinence, leucorrhoea in women and strengthens the back if egg yolks, powdered acorns and nutmeg are mixed with it and the draught is taken morning and night.

Bauhin too brings something new in his entry for personata or Lappa major. Having cited Apuleius, Dioscorides, Pliny and Galen, and stated a diuretic action which helps kidney stones, he cites Holerius on an emulsion made from the root or 2 drachms (8 g) of the dried flowers of burdock painted onto the chest in cases of pleuritis, and Virtemberg on the use of the leaves applied to the head to ease its pains. This treatment also has an effect on the womb, for it will draw the womb towards the head, or if the leaves are applied to the feet, the womb will be drawn down. This is a special remedy for prolapse of the womb or its suffocation (causing changes in breathing and other emotional and physical responses accredited to the displacement upwards of the womb, which Hippocratic physicians thought could 'wander' around the body, interfering with normal functioning of the parts) and is the use of burdock leaf for the womb that Culpeper acknowledges from Mizaldus in the *Pharmacopoeia Londinensis* (1669): 'if a wise man have but the using of it'. In *The English Physitian*, Culpeper suggests that the leaves can be applied to the belly also, to keep the womb in place and so prevent miscarriage, while in his *Directory for Midwives* (1651), in a chapter on 'the falling out [prolapse] of the womb' he gives instructions for 'my own magnetick cure':

> Take a common Bur-leaf (you may keep them dry all the year, if you please) and apply to her head, and that will draw the womb upward. In the fits of the mother (i.e. suffocation above) put it under the soles of her feet and it will

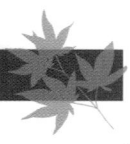

*draw it downwards. Bur-seed beaten into powder will do the like, they command the womb which way you please, and by orderly usage of it will cure any disease of it. 'Tis a plant of venus and is best gathered when she is angular and strong in her hour, and the moon applying to her. [If] it will not readily go up, by reason of carelessness in not using the remedy time enough, you may bathe it as you were told'.*

One of our students has related to us a similar treatment which she witnessed in the North of Scotland. During lambing, a ewe suffered prolapse of the womb. The farmer added burdock leaves to her feed and the womb was restored to its proper place. If this is evidence of an empirical use of burdock, then it is in keeping with the medieval rather than Galenic origins or the main modern uses of the plant, namely as a diuretic and anti-lithic. Its alterative action in the internal treatment of arthritic and skin conditions such as eczema, psoriasis and other chronic conditions is also recorded only after the demise of Galenism.

## MODERN USES AND ESSIAC

When we turn to modern sources, we may imagine that the internal use of burdock for boils echoes the old topical use. However, an antimicrobial action would be desirable to support this action, and this has been linked to polyacetylenes found in fresh burdock root, whereas the classical authors wanted the leaves to be applied topically. Weiss considers the root the most important part of the plant for medicinal use but does not consider its action to be very great and recommends its use only in combination with other herbs. This could include cystitis, as listed by other authors. An oil made from the root can be used, says Weiss, to stimulate hair growth in alopecia and for dry seborrhoea. Mills and Bone also discuss only the root. Wood and Menzies-Trull include the seeds as well, perhaps following the recommendation by Priest & Priest of the seeds, especially in skin conditions. Pelikan highlights the fact that it is only the flower heads of burdock, and its fruit or seed, which display the thistle aspect of the plant. The leaves and root, on the other hand, are rich in mucilage, which he regards as evidence of their 'struggle against spiny hardness'. Here we have an image to link with the several recommendations for the use of burdock in dry skin conditions. Wood notes that burdock root is bitter, sweet and oily, so well suited to dry and atrophic states with constipation and poor emulsification of dietary fats and oils, and in general it helps those persons suffering from long, chronic illness. Pelikan states that burdock shows great vitality in overcoming poor soil conditions.

Owing to the bitterness of the plant burdock is credited by Williamson with laxative and appetite-stimulating effects. For the same reason Menzies-Trull adds central nervous system stimulation, and lists also circulatory and lymphatic stimulant and anti-fungal actions. Hoffmann sees an enhanced indication in rheumatic complaints associated with psoriasis, presumably psoriatic arthropathy. Priest & Priest want the root to be prescribed with ginger *Zingiber officinale* for rheumatism and gout, and with golden seal *Hydrastis candensis* for a tonic effect in vaginal laxity, a use which recalls the old indications of leucorrhoea and menorrhagia. The *British Herbal Pharmacopoeia* suggests combinations of burdock root and curled dock root *Rumex crispus* or red clover flowers *Trifolium pratense* in skin disease, and while the herb has a separate entry from the root, its actions are noted as similar to lappa root, with specific indications as use as poultice for boils and abscesses.

Burdock is the main herb in Essiac tea which is amongst the many products used in the hope of treating and preventing reoccurrence of cancers (Kulp et al 2006, Boon et al 2007). Herbalists customarily use alteratives in the care of patients with cancer (Yance & Valentine 1999), and burdock is considered the alterative par excellence. Essiac was developed in Canada by Rene Caisse after her aunt became ill with cancer (History of Essiac 2007). Rene Caisse was a nurse and treated patients with cancer at the clinic in Ontario which she set up and ran from 1934 until 1942. The preparation was recommended by a miner's wife who had been treated for a breast tumour by a Native American in the early 20th century.

The four original herbs in Essiac are burdock root *Arctium lappa*, small pieces (32 parts by weight), sheep sorrel *Rumex acetosella*, powder, (16 parts), slippery elm bark *Ulmus fulva*, powder (4 parts) and turkey rhubarb root *Rheum palmatum*, powder (1 part). The dried herbs are mixed together and batches can be made using 1 cup (8 fl oz) of dried herb in 2 gallons of distilled water. (The US fluid ounce is slightly larger than the imperial fluid ounce). The recipe is made up taking one part as 5 g, making a total of 265 g in 1800 mL of water. The water is brought to a rolling boil in a pan with the lid on, and then the dried herbs are added, the water is brought back to the boil and boiled for 10 minutes. The mixture should be stirred and the pan left undisturbed overnight. After reheating to steaming hot, the mixture is allowed to cool slightly before it is strained through a cloth. Portions of 30 mL, the quantity of one dose, may be frozen for taking when required in 60 mL of hot water, once daily at bed time on an empty stomach. Food should not be eaten within an hour either before or after taking the tea. The yield from 1800 mL was in one experiment 1600 mL, which gave a dose of just over 3 g of dried burdock in 30 mL. There has been debate concerning the herbs employed and their proportions in the Essiac mixture. An affidavit given by Mary McPherson, who worked with Rene Caisse, proposes slightly different proportions (Essiac Info 2009). Turkey rhubarb does not grow in North America and the original herbs are said to have grown wild, which has led to the suggestion it might have replaced a species of *Polygonum* (Essiac Info 2009). The formula given by Bartram suggests continuing the mixture for 32 days, then every third day. Bartram's formulation differs very slightly in the quantities and he intends the formula for cancers of the stomach and intestines only.

Essiac and similar formulations such as Flor-essence are now widely available (Cancer Research UK 2008, Medline Plus 2008). Flor-essence has the same four ingredients plus four more, including red clover, and, for the sake of clarity, this review does not refer to any studies on Flor-essence although there has been substantial investigation of its use in Russia in gastrointestinal disease (Tamayo et al 2000). There have been some unpublished studies on Essiac (Kaegi 1998) but the only randomized controlled trial investigated quality of life (Zick et al 2006). This is not relevant as Essiac is generally taken with the intention of influencing the progression of the disease.

Natural compounds have been shown in vitro to inhibit various stages in cancer (Boik 2001) and, given the widespread usage of Essiac, it is worth discussing whether it could promote remission in cancer and whether it is safe. A useful review of the herbs in Essiac was undertaken by Tamayo et al (2000), although we can find no evidence to support their statement that there are isoflavonoids in burdock root. In vitro investigations on burdock and Essiac are now reviewed to see whether they provide any support for the use of Essiac. Conflicting points of view are expressed and an array of in vitro studies are used in the literature to support the use of Essiac, but the discussion illustrates the problems in relying on in vitro evidence to support claims for efficacy (Houghton et al 2007).

Studies on burdock have shown antioxidant and anti-inflammatory activity and it is argued that this is associated with anticancer activity (Leonard et al 2006). A recent study found a strong correlation between total polyphenol concentration in burdock root, seed and leaf and antioxidant activity (Trolox assay) (Ferracane et al 2010). The seeds showed greatest antioxidant activity whereas the root had hardly any activity. This study is useful as all three parts were assayed using the same methodology at the same time. In contrast, an in vitro study on burdock root found antioxidant actions: scavenging of free radicals (DPPH assay) and inhibition of oxidation of linoleic acid (Duh 1998). Comparison of aqueous extracts from peeled and unpeeled root showed that antioxidant activity (DPPH assay) was greater in unpeeled roots, and this appeared to be associated with the concentration of chlorogenic acid, which is a phenolic acid found in many herbs and foods and is not particular to burdock (Chen et al 2004).

Three further studies investigated the antioxidant activity of Essiac. It was found to scavenge effectively hydroxyl (Fenton reaction) and superoxide radicals (xanthine/xanthine oxidase assay), and prevent hydroxyl radical-induced lipid peroxidation (Leonard et al 2006). A criticism of this study is the high concentration of Essiac used as the preparation was a 1:2 Essiac tea. Essiac showed significant antioxidant activity (ABTS assay) (Seely et al 2007). In the third study, Essiac showed both antioxidant (TEAC assay) and proinflammatory actions such as induction of tumour necrosis factor-alpha (TNF-alpha), interleukin-1 beta (IL-1 beta) and cyclooxygenase-2 (COX-2) (Cheung et al 2005).

Essiac uses burdock root. However, let us turn to the in vitro studies on the lignan arctigenin (aglycone of arctiin), which is found in burdock seed, as these studies are mentioned in reviews of Essiac. They are only relevant to use of the seed as arctigenin is found only at very low concentration in the root. To illustrate the complexity of in vitro methods, the following examples are given. Some studies can be compared as they use one model to measure anti-inflammatory activity. Inhibition of lipopolysaccharide (LPS) induced nitric oxide production by a murine macrophage RAW 264.7 cell line is used as a measure of inflammatory activity. Excess nitric oxide production by nitric oxide synthase (iNOS) occurs in macrophages in response to proinflammatory stimulation such as IL-1 beta, TNF-alpha and LPS (Park et al 2007). Lignans, in particular diarctigenin and lappao-F, were shown to inhibit this process (Park et al 2007). In a study using this model, arctigenin inhibited nitric oxide production and secretion of the proinflammatory cytokines TNF-alpha and IL-6 in a dose-dependent manner. Arctigenin was found to inhibit expression and activity of iNOS, but not to inhibit COX-2 expression and activity (Zhao et al 2009).

Another team also found inhibition of induction of iNOS using the same mechanism and associated this with the concentration of arctigenin in the seed. They found this inhibition was caused by inhibition of nuclear factor kappa B, which is activated in inflammatory responses to viral and bacterial infection and is involved in the production of iNOS and TNF-alpha. The same team also found that arctigenin inhibited mitogen-activated protein kinase and argue that this shows that arctigenin inhibits cellular responses to extracellular signals such as gene transcription. This results in inhibition of activator protein-1, which is associated with cell proliferation, differentiation and apoptosis. Inhibition of activator protein-1 is thought to result in reduction in production of TNF-alpha m-RNA in cells exposed to LPS and thus reduction in TNF-alpha production by macrophages (Cho et al 2004). The detail is given here to demonstrate the complexity of in vitro methods and thus the risk in making claims based on any one study. To conclude, antioxidant activity in burdock is associated with overall concentration of polyphenols and is highest in the seeds, but also found in leaves and root.

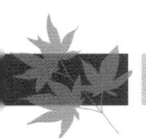

If this finding is linked with the concentration of lignans, then the seeds are the most useful part.

Another line of enquiry has been to investigate the effects of burdock and Essiac on cancer processes. For example, an in vitro study using the LNCaP prostate cancer cell line found that proliferation was inhibited by Essiac (Ottenweller et al 2004). Another study using LNCaP cells found that growth was inhibited by the lignans lappaol A, C and F isolated from burdock seeds and the authors argue that this could support the use of Essiac (Ming et al 2004). However, it would actually support the use of burdock seed not of the root. A further study found no antiproliferative activity for Essiac in prostate cancer (Eberding et al 2007), whereas dose-dependent inhibition of seven cancer cell lines was shown by Seely et al (2007).

In contrast, Essiac at a range of concentrations was shown to actually stimulate cell proliferation relative to untreated controls in four breast cancer cell lines, both oestrogen receptor positive and oestrogen receptor negative (Kulp et al 2006). The authors discuss their methodology to consider why these results differ from other studies. For example, they note the high levels of Essiac extract used in another study which found an antiproliferative activity in breast cancer cells (MCF-7) (Tai et al 2004). In a further study, a metabolite of arctiin formed in the gut showed a proliferative effect on the growth of MCF-7 breast cancer cells, but inhibited estradiol-mediated proliferation of the same cells to a similar degree as tamoxifen (Xie et al 2003). In this study, the metabolite of arctiin appears to have had opposing actions depending on the presence of oestradiol. This interesting research again demonstrates the complexity of in vitro research and the danger of extrapolating the results of any one study to the living body in order to support the use of any medicinal plant.

As the lignans are found in the seeds, studies on arctigenin are not applicable to the use of Essiac, and most studies on the antiproliferative activity of burdock seeds are on the activity of arctigenin (Awale et al 2006, Matsumoto et al 2006). This raises the question of which part of burdock should be used but it also asks whether any in vitro study supports the oral use of burdock. In many cases, we do not know about the absorption of the constituents of herbs. However, in the case of arctigenin there is evidence from pharmacokinetic studies on the uptake and absorption of lignans to show that it is not absorbed into the body. The lignan content and activity of linseed *Linum usissitatum* has been investigated (Mills 2003) and is relevant to burdock. The main lignan in linseed is secoisolariciresinol, which has been found to be transformed by bacteria in the proximal colon to enterodiol and enterolactone, which are then absorbed into the body. The same team found that incubation of arctiin with a human faecal suspension for 9 days led to the formation of six metabolites, and the enterolactones formed were enantiomers of those produced by linseed (Xie et al 2003). In this study, the breakdown of arctiin was gradual and it could be argued that it supports the usage in Russia for gastrointestinal conditions referred to by Tamayo et al (2000) as the metabolites may have local effects in the gut.

The above studies seem neither to support nor oppose the use of burdock or Essiac in cancer. The study on breast cancer cells (Kulp et al 2006) could be important but one can conclude that this finding is not associated with lignans, which are considered to be phytoestrogens as the lignan level is low in burdock root. In addition, it is thought that lignans in the diet may reduce oestrogen levels in postmenopausal women (Sturgeon et al 2008) and be protective against hormone-dependent cancers (Wang 2002). The absorption of lignan metabolites has been studied extensively and the concentration in the blood depends on the diet, bacterial metabolism and conjugation in the intestinal wall and liver but none of these factors explain interindividual variation in blood concentration of enterolactone (Lampe et al 2006). If lignans are sought in the diet then oilseeds especially linseed and sesame seeds and wholegrain cereals are important sources. Arctigenin may have unique actions but otherwise dietary recommendations are more important in this regard than the use of burdock as a herbal medicine.

We found no adverse drug reports on Essiac and, although some reviews make exaggerated claims for the possible effectiveness of Essiac based on in vitro studies, maybe the main conclusion is that appraisal of the traditional evidence for use of burdock as an alterative is of equal value in supporting the use of Essiac.

## RECOMMENDATIONS

- As herbal alterative (however viable that term may be considered) for chronic skin conditions such as eczema, dermatitis, psoriasis and furunculosis. (A specific picture of a chronic skin condition combined with impaired nutrition and weak circulation, as stated by Bone (2003), is not unreasonable.)
- As a component of treatment for arthritic or rheumatic complaints.
- As a bitter tonic for poor appetite and dyspeptic symptoms including mild colic, flatulence and irregular bowel habit (infectious diarrhoea or constipation).
- As a diuretic and anti-lithic for cystitis, urinary gravel and stones and resulting oliguria, and functional problems of urination such as enuresis.
- As an astringent for cases of leucorrhoea and laxity of the womb, and possibly for haemoptysis, where the diagnosis is established and the cause understood.

- For topical use, especially of the leaf. The fresh leaf itself, or an ointment made from it, could be used on sprained or painful joints, wounds, ulcers and boils.
- More research is required before prolapse or threatened miscarriage could be added to the list, but since the former is considered to need surgical intervention and the latter a preposterous suggestion, it is unlikely that further evidence will be forthcoming.
- Pharmacological and in vitro evidence for preferred use of the seed in cancers would need both further human trials to establish real effects, although the seed was traditionally used alongside root and leaf, and the availability of *Arctium lappa* semen from suppliers to the profession.

Dosage: strong decoction: 500 mL per day of the 1:20 decoction of the root.

For non-acute conditions, the smaller dose recommended in the *British Herbal Pharmacopoeia* of 2–6 g three times a day of dried root, in decoction or as equivalent liquid preparations, can be advised, although the habit of many practitioners is to give much smaller amounts for fear of a healing crisis through excessive 'detoxification'.

## CONSTITUENTS

Reviews: root, leaf, Barnes et al (2007), Bardanae root, Bisset & Wichtl (2001), Bradley (2006), Mills & Bone (2005), Williamson (2003).

### Polysaccharides

Root, total 5.2%: mainly inulin-type fructofuranan (cv Herkules, commercial, Slovakia) (Kardošová et al 2003). Inulin is a storage polysaccharide mainly composed of fructose and extracted commercially from tubers of Jerusalem artichoke, *Helianthus tuberosus* (Tófano et al 2007). It is not absorbed and would be insignificant in dried root as concentration falls with storage (Ishimaru et al 2004).
Leaf, neutral polysaccharide 0.9% (Kardošová & Machová 2006).

### Volatile oil

Total 0.1%: sesquiterpenes and sesquiterpene lactones (root, leaf) (Bradley 1992).

### Phenolic acids

Root, total 2.9%: caffeic acid, chlorogenic acid (caffeoylquinic acid), cynarin; Leaf, total 15.3%; Seeds, total 45.8% (organic cultivation, Italy) (Ferracane et al 2010).
Root, total 0.2 to 0.8%: chlorogenic acid and two caffeoylquinic acid derivatives (13 cultivars and fresh roots, Japan) (Wang et al 2001).
Root, hydroxycinnamoylquinic acids; dicaffeoylquinic acid; three dicaffeoylsuccinoylquinic acids; tricaffeoylsuccinoylquinic acid derivatives (fresh cv Gobo, market, Japan) (Maruta et al 1995).
Root, 24 hydroxycinnamoylquinic acids; four monocaffeoylchlorogenic acids; six dicaffeoylquinic acids; two tricaffeoylquinic acids; di- and trisuccinoylquinic acids (fresh, market, USA) (Lin & Harnly 2008).
Peeling the root reduces the content of phenolic compounds, in particular chlorogenic acid (Chen et al 2004).

### Flavonoids

Root, flavone: luteolin; flavonol: quercetin and glycoside: quercitrin (organic cultivation, Italy) (Ferracane et al 2009).
Leaf, flavone: luteolin; flavonol: quercetin and glycosides: quercitrin, rutin (organic cultivation, Italy) (Ferracane et al 2009).

### Lignans

Fruits (seeds), arctiin 49% (aglycone: arctigenin) (glucoside arctiin): (commercial, China) (Wang et al 2005) (note that this concentration is 10 times higher than those given below).
Seeds: arctiin, arctigenin, lappaol A & C & F, matareisinol, arctignan E (organic cultivation, Italy) (Ferracane et al 2009).
Seeds, arctiin 5.5%, arctigenin 2.6% (Lü et al 2007).
Seeds, diarctigenin, lappaol C & D & F, isolappaol C (commercial, Korea) (Park et al 2007).
Seeds, arctigenin, nordihydroguariaretic acid, secoisolariciresinol, sesamin (commercial, Japan) (Awale et al 2006).
Root, leaf: very little arctigenin (organic cultivation, Italy) (Ferracane et al 2009).
Leaf, very little lignans (cultivated, China) (Liu et al 2005).

### Polyacetylenes

Root, two polyacetylenes (fresh, cv Shirohada-sakigake, Japan) (Takasugi et al 1987).

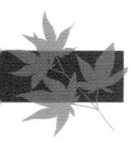

## RECOMMENDATIONS ON SAFETY

1. Do not use burdock externally if the patient has a history of allergic contact dermatitis or allergy to Asteraceae (Compositae). (See Chapter 20 elecampane, *Inula helenium*.)
A report from Spain found that three people developed red exudative dermatitis after using burdock root plasters (Rodriguez et al 1995).
2. The use of Essiac in patients with cancer has not been shown to pose any risks (see above).
3. There is no evidence against the use of burdock in pregnancy and it is considered compatible with breastfeeding (Mills & Bone 2005).

## REFERENCES

Awale S, Lu J, Kalauni SK, et al 2006 Identification of arctigenin as an antitumor agent having the ability to eliminate the tolerance of cancer cells to nutrient starvation. Cancer Research 66:1751–1757.

Barnes J, Anderson LA, Phillipson JD 2007 Herbal Medicines, 3rd edn. Pharmaceutical Press, London.

Bisset NG, Wichtl M (eds) 2001 Herbal drugs and phytopharmaceuticals, 2nd edn. Medpharm, Stuttgart.

Boik J 2001 Natural compounds in cancer therapy. Oregon Medical Press, Portland, Oregon.

Bone K 2003 A clinical guide to blending liquid herbs: herbal formulations for the individual patient. Churchill Livingstone, Edinburgh.

Boon HS, Olatunde F, Zick SM 2007 Trends in complementary/alternative medicine use by breast cancer survivors: comparing survey data from 1998 and 2005. BMC Womens Health 7:4. Online. Available: http://www.pubmedcentral.nih.gov/articlerender.fcgi?tool=pubmed&pubmedid=17397542 16 April 2008.

Bradley PR (ed.) 1992 British herbal compendium, vol 1. British Herbal Medicine Association, Bournemouth.

Bradley PR 2006 British herbal compendium, vol 2. British Herbal Medicine Association, Bournemouth.

The British Pharmaceutical Codex 1934. The Pharmaceutical Press, London.

Cancer Research UK 2008 Essiac. Online. Available: http://www.cancerhelp.org.uk/help/default.asp?page=24499.

Chen FA, Wu AB, Chen CY 2004 The influence of different treatments on the free radical scavenging activity of burdock and variations of its active components. Food Chemistry 86:479–484.

Cheung S, Lim KT, Tai J 2005 Antioxidant and anti-inflammatory properties of ESSIAC and Flor-Essence. Oncology Reports 14:1345–1350.

Cho MK, Jang YP, Kim YC et al 2004 Arctigenin, a phenylpropanoid dibenzylbutyrolactone lignan, inhibits MAP kinases and AP-1 activation via potent MKK inhibition: the role in TNF-alpha inhibition. International Immunopharmacology 4:1419–1429.

Culpeper N 1651 A directory for midwives Peter Cole, London.

Culpeper N 1669 Pharmacopoeia Londinensis. London.

Davis PH (ed) 1975 Flora of Turkey, vol 5. Edinburgh University Press, Edinburgh.

De Smet PAGM, Keller K, Hänsel R et al 1993 Adverse effects of herbal drugs, vol 2. Springer-Verlag, Berlin.

Duh PD 1998 Antioxidant activity of burdock (*Arctium lappa* Linné): its scavenging effect on free-radical and active oxygen. Journal of the American Oil Chemists' Society 75:455–461.

Eberding A, Madera C, Xie S, et al 2007 Evaluation of the antiproliferative effects of Essiac on in vitro and in vivo models of prostate cancer compared to paclitaxel. Nutrition and Cancer 58:188–196.

Essiac Info 2009. Online. Available: http://www.healthfreedom.info/essiac_info.htm 22 June 2009.

Ferracane R, Graziani G, Gallo M, et al 2010 Metabolic profile of the bioactive compounds of burdock (*Arctium lappa*) seeds, roots and leaves. Journal of Pharmaceutical and Biomedical Analysis, 51:399–404.

Hamblin L, Laird A, Parkes E, et al 2004 Herbs used by well-established medical herbalists in the UK in the management of osteoarthritis: a small-scale survey. European Journal of Herbal Medicine 6:5–13.

History of Essiac 2007 Who was Rene Caisse? Online. Available: http://www.essiacinfo.org/caisse.html.

Houghton PJ, Howes MJ, Lee CC, et al 2007 Uses and abuses of in vitro tests in ethnopharmacology: visualizing an elephant. Journal of Ethnopharmacology 110:391–400.

Ishimaru M, Kagoroku K, Chachin K 2004 Effects of the storage conditions of burdock (*Arctium lappa* L.) root on the quality of heat-processed burdock sticks. Scientia Horticulturae 101:1–10.

Kaegi E 1998 Unconventional therapies for cancer: 1. Essiac. The task force on alternative therapies of the Canadian Breast Cancer Research Initiative. Canadian Medical Association Journal 58:897–902.

Kang TG, Kawamura T, Noro Y, et al 1999 Pharmacognostical evaluation of Arctii Fructus (2): adulteration on the Chinese commercial samples. Natural Medicines 53:206–208.

Kardošová A, Ebringerová A, Alfldi J, et al 2003 A biologically active fructan from the roots of *Arctium lappa* L., var. Herkules. International Journal of Biological Macromolecules 33:135–140.

Kardošová A, Machová E 2006 Antioxidant activity of medicinal plant polysaccharides. Fitoterapia 77:367–373.

Keil DJ 2006 Flora of North America, vol 19. Asteraceae, Arctium. Online. Available: http://www.efloras.org/florataxon.aspx?flora_id=1&taxon_id=102484.

Kulp KS, Montgomery JL, Nelson DO, et al 2006 Essiac and Flor-Essence herbal tonics stimulate the in vitro growth of human breast cancer cells. Breast Cancer Research & Treatment 98:249–259.

Lampe JW, Atkinson C, Hullar MAJ 2006 Assessing exposure to lignans and their metabolites in humans. Journal of AOAC International 89:1174–1181.

Leonard SS, Keil D, Mehlman T, et al 2006 Essiac tea: scavenging of reactive oxygen species and effects on DNA damage. Journal of Ethnopharmacology 103:288–296.

Lin LZ, Harnly JM 2008 Identification of hydroxycinnamoylquinic acids of arnica flowers and burdock roots using a standarized LC-DAD-ESI/MS profiling method. Journal of Agricultural and Food Chemistry 56:10105–10114.

Liu S, Chen K, Schliemann W, et al 2005 Isolation and identification of arctiin and arctigenin in leaves of burdock (*Arctium lappa* L.) by polyamide column chromatography in combination with HPLC-ESI/MS. Phytochemical Analysis 16:86–89.

Lü W, Chen Y, Zhang Y, et al 2007 Microemulsion electrokinetic chromatography for the separation of arctiin and arctigenin in Fructus Arctii and its herbal preparations. Journal of Chromatography B 860:127–133.

Maruta Y, Kawabata J, Niki R 1995 Antioxidative caffeoyl-quinic acid derivatives in the roots of burdock (*Arctium lappa* L.). Journal of Agricultural and Food Chemistry 43:2590–2595.

Matsumoto T, Hosono-Nishiyama K, Yamada H 2006 Antiproliferative and apoptotic effects of butyrolactone lignans from *Arctium lappa* on leukemic cells. Planta Medica 72:276–278.

Medline Plus 2008 Essiac. Online. Available: http://www.nlm.nih.gov/medlineplus/druginfo/natural/patient-essiac.html 15 April 2009.

Mills S 2003 ESCOP Monographs: the scientific foundation for herbal medicinal products, 2nd edn. Thieme Medical Publishers, Stuttgart.

Mills S, Bone K 2000 Principles and practice of phytotherapy. Elsevier, Edinburgh.

Mills S, Bone K 2005 The essential guide to herbal safety. Churchill Livingstone, St Louis.

Ming DS, Guns ES, Eberding A, et al 2004 Isolation and characterization of compounds with anti-prostate cancer activity from *Arctium lappa* L. using bioactivity-guided fractionation. Pharmaceutical Biology 42:44–48.

Ottenweller J, Putt K, Blumenthal EJ, et al 2004 Inhibition of prostate cancer-cell proliferation by Essiac. Journal of Alternative and Complementary Medicine 10:687–691.

Park SY, Hong SS, Han XH, et al 2007 Lignans from *Arctium lappa* and their inhibition of LPS-induced nitric oxide production. Chemical & Pharmaceutical Bulletin 55:150–152.

Rodriguez P, Blanco J, Juste S 1995 Allergic contact dermatitis due to burdock (*Arctium lappa*). Contact Dermatitis 33:134–135.

Seely D, Kennedy DA, Myers SP, et al 2007 In vitro analysis of the herbal compound Essiac. Anticancer Research 27:3875–3882.

Simmonite W, Culpeper N 1957 The Simmonite-Culpeper herbal remedies. W Foulsham & Co. London.

Stace C 1991 New flora of the British Isles. Cambridge University Press, Cambridge.

Sturgeon SR, Heersink JL, Volpe SL, et al 2008 Effect of dietary flaxseed on serum levels of estrogens and androgens in postmenopausal women. Nutrition and Cancer 60:612–618.

Tai J, Cheung S, Wong S, et al 2004 In vitro comparison of Essiac and Flor-Essence on human tumor cell lines. Oncology Reports 11:471–476.

Takasugi M, Kawashima S, Katsui N, et al 1987 Two polyacetylenic phytoalexins from *Arctium lappa*. Phytochemistry 26:2957–2958.

Tamayo C, Richardson MA, Diamond S, et al 2000. The chemistry and biological activity of herbs used in Flor-Essence(TM) herbal tonic and Essiac(TM). Phytotherapy Research 14:1–14.

Tófano J, Toneli CL, Mürr FEX, et al 2007 Optimization of a physical concentration process for inulin. Journal of Food Engineering 80:832–838.

Tyler V, Robbers J 1999 Tyler's herbs of choice. Haworth Press, Binghamton, NY.

Wang LQ 2002 Mammalian phytoestrogens: enterodiol and enterolactone. Journal of Chromatography B 777:289–309.

Wang R, Ayano H, Furumoto T, et al 2001 Variation of the content of chlorogenic acid derivatives among cultivars and market items of burdock (*Arctium lappa* L.). Nippon Shokuhin Kagaku Kogaku Kaishi 48:857–862.

Wang X, Li F, Sun Q, et al 2005 Application of preparative high-speed counter-current chromatography for separation and purification of arctiin from Fructus Arctii. Journal of Chromatography A 1063:247–251.

Williamson E 2003 Potter's herbal cyclopaedia. CW Daniel, Saffron Walden.

WHO 1989 Medicinal Plants in China. World Health Organization, Manila.

Yance D, Valentine A 1999 Herbal medicine, healing & cancer. McGraw-Hill, Lincolnwood, Illinois.

Xie L-H, Ahn E-M, Akao T, et al 2003. Transformation of arctiin to estrogenic and antiestrogenic substances by human intestinal bacteria. Chemical and Pharmaceutical Bulletin 51:378–384.

Zhao F, Wang L, Liu K 2009 In vitro anti-inflammatory effects of arctigenin, a lignan from *Arctium lappa* L., through inhibition on iNOS pathway. Journal of Ethnopharmacology 122:457–462.

Zick SM, Sen A, Feng Y 2006 Trial of Essiac to ascertain its effect in women with breast cancer (TEA-BC). Journal of Alternative and Complementary Medicine 12:971–980.

# CHAPTER 11
# *Artemisia absinthium*, wormwood

## DESCRIPTION

**Family: Asteraceae**  **Part used: leaves, flowering tops**

*Artemisia absinthium* L. is a hardy perennial sub-shrub, native to temperate Eurasia and North Africa and cultivated in gardens. The *Flora of Turkey* (Davis 1975) gives 22 *Artemisia* species, including *Artemisia absinthium, Artemisia vulgaris, Artemisia santonicum* and *Artemisia abrotanum*.

Erect, woody stems (over 1 m) bear alternate, much divided, silvery leaves with silky soft hairs on each side. Tiny, rayless yellowy-green flowers occur in late summer in loose panicles which arise from the woody stems. It has a distinctive fragrance, thrives in sunny positions in poor soils and can become very woody.

A similar species, native to Britain, is sea wormwood *Artemisia maritima* L. (syn. *Seriphidium maritima* (L.) Poljakov), which is widespread on coasts in Britain and northern Europe. It is smaller (to 60 cm) with strongly scented woolly divided leaves with blunt, narrow segments. Oval yellow-orange florets occur in August to October.

**Other species used:** Mugwort *Artemisia vulgaris* L., Roman wormwood *Artemisia pontica* L., tarragon *Artemisia dracunculus* L., southernwood *Artemisia abrotanum* L. (Bown 1995). Southernwood *Artemisia abrotanum* has many woody stems with finely divided leaves and rarely flowers. It is widely grown in gardens and is found as a garden escape.

### Quality

Although plant material has been found to be more bitter in September, the herb should be collected by July as the leaves deteriorate in quality during flowering. It would be possible to harvest from some plants in July and then harvest the flowering stems later in the year.

Members of the genus contain similar volatile oils (Lopes-Lutz et al 2008). A study in Italy of 14 wild *Artemisia* species found similar volatile oils but wide variation in concentration, and found that *Artemisia abrotanum* was the only species to contain the monoterpene ascaridole, which is anthelmintic (Mucciarelli et al 1995). Tarragon *Artemisia dracunculus* is milder and used as a culinary herb and contains oxygenated monoterpenes (Kordali et al 2005a).

## A POWERFUL HERB

Wormwood is an intriguing herb, strong, powerful and much valued in the past; a sister herb of *Artemisia vulgaris* 'the mother of herbs', and named after the great goddess Artemis herself. Grieve tells us how Diana/Artemis instructed the centaur Chiron in its use. The victor of the chariot races of the festival of Latinae was given a decoction of wormwood to drink, Pliny records, since he was a person worth keeping alive. Hildegard named it the 'principal remedy for all ailments'. Yet this is no sweet-smelling rose, but a herb of pungency and bitterness, yet with a quality of warmth. 'It is very warm and has much strength' says Hildegard. Fuchs suggests the name 'apsinthion' derives from the Greek meaning 'undrinkable'. With the exception of rue, wormwood is the bitterest herb known 'but it is very wholesome', is Grieve's appraisal. Cook described it bitter and strong to the highest degree, and Pelikan notes that from 'the harshness of its scent' we can appreciate right away that it is a herb with 'forces composing a unique pattern of actions'. Culpeper uses this herb to deliver, in coded terms, and indeed as diatribe in places, his astrological herbal lore arcana: 'he that reads this, and understands what he reads, hath a jewel of more worth than a diamond; he that understands it not, is as little fit to give physick. There lies a key in these words which will unlock (if it be turned by a wise hand) the cabinet of physick; I have delivered it as plain as I durst; it is not only upon wormwood as I wrote, but upon all plants, trees and herbs; he that understands it not, is unfit (in my opinion) to give physic'.

Galen maintains that in every wormwood there is a double power. Some authors speak of a two-fold nature. Mesue, cited by Bauhin, refers to wormwood as 'of dual substance', one hot, bitter, salty, purging, clearing obstructions; the other, earthy, styptic, invigorating by toning the

THE WESTERN HERBAL TRADITION

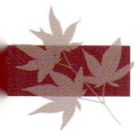

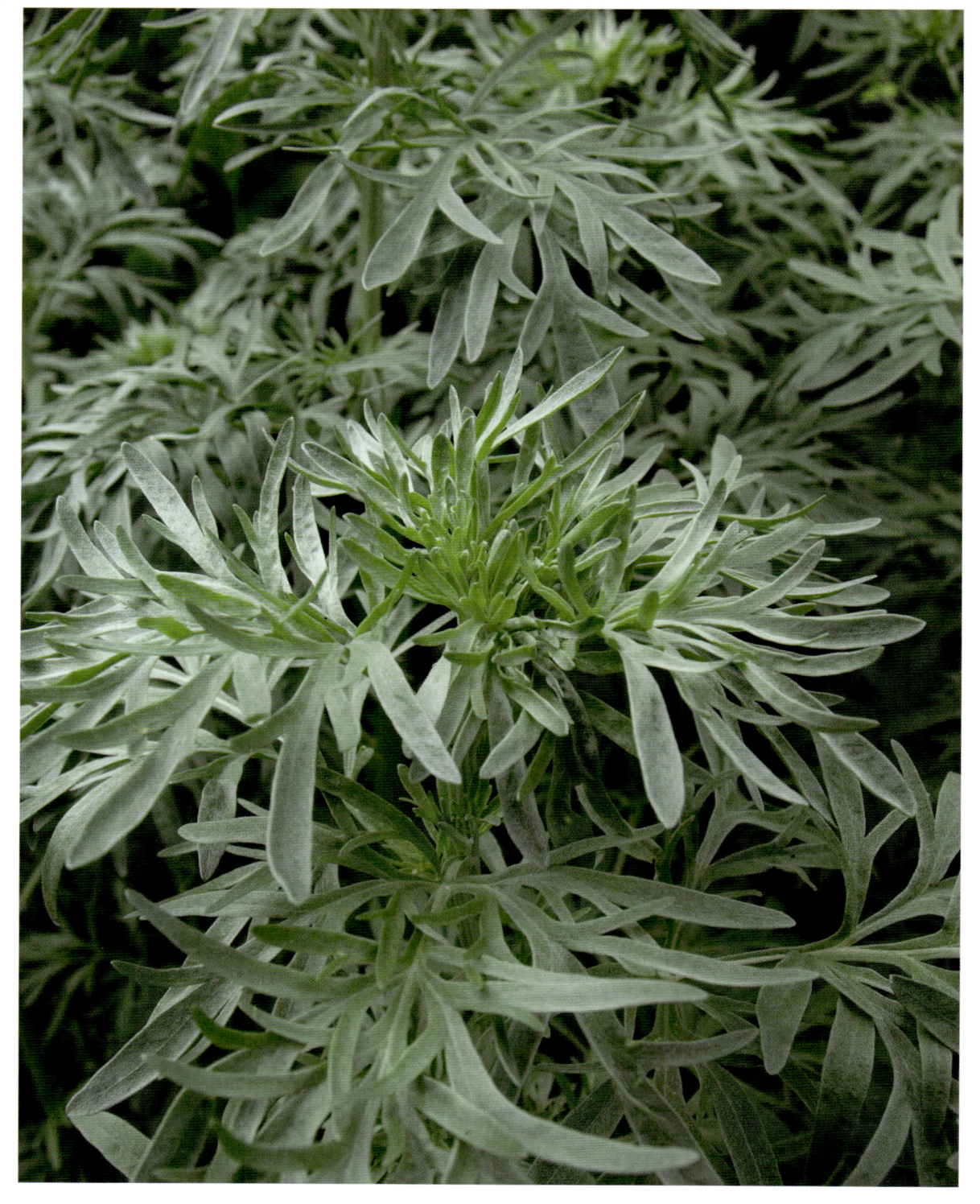

**Figure 11.1** *Artemisia absinthium*, wormwood (a garden in Yorkshire, May).

parts. The bitter action comes first, then the tonic. Ibn Sina writes similarly of an earth element and a volatile. The Salernitan herbal mentions two opposing virtues: it is laxative because of its heat and bitterness, and it is astringent because of its bulk, its substance and its pungency. It is hot in the first degree, dry in the third, according to Galen and many authors after him, although the Salernitan herbal says hot and dry in the second degree. Culpeper judges it hot and dry in the first degree 'viz. just as hot as your blood, and no hotter'. Gerard has it hot in the second degree, dry in the third and Mesue hot in the first degree and dry in the second.

## IDENTITY

There is as usual some debate about the identity of the wormwood of the Ancients and the delineation of its range of actions is not without some contention. Beck at least translates the apsinthion of Dioscorides as *Artemisia absinthium*. Dioscorides (III 23) names three wormwoods: the 'familiar' wormwood of which the best grows in the Pontic region and Cappadocia; Seriphon absinthion thalassion, which is sea wormwood, 'wormseed' according to Beck; and a third kind that grows in Galatia called santonicon, which does the same thing as seriphon. Galen commends Pontic wormwood, with lesser leaves and flowers, above others 'which are excessively bitter and loathesome'. The Arabic writers refer to Roman wormwood. Whether Roman wormwood shared identity with Pontic and whether the common broadleaved wormwood equated to the Pontic wormwood of Dioscorides and Galen were questions which exercised considerable debate among the Renaissance authors. Turner, for example, concludes not; Mattioli thinks it is (although of course his wormwood must be Roman by default). Parkinson, having laid out the different opinions on this as usual, and having identified nine wormwoods of his own day (Dodoens has six, Dalechamps 12) then cites Pena and Lobel's study on the matter which concludes that it is, that Dioscorides was merely specifying where the herb with the best properties grows, and that Galen preferred Pontic as a means of excluding the other two varieties. Both Cook and Grieve, and more recently Schulz et al (1998), refer to Pontic/Roman wormwood as a variety weaker than common absinthium. Culpeper simply uses the opportunity afforded by Roman wormwood to insult the church; 'it may be called so because it is good for a stinking breath, which the Romans cannot be very free from, maintaining so many bad houses by authority of his Holiness'.

Parkinson's discussion on wormwood's identity contains in its detail two interesting considerations. Firstly that the properties of a herb will differ with location: '[Dioscorides and Galen] shew in what place the most vigorous of that kinde doth grow, which property it obtaineth, more by the goodnesse of the place, injoying the commodity of a free and cleare ayre ... then by the nature of the hearbe itselfe. Then of the scent, that it is more aromaticall than others, yet hereby they intimate that others are sweet, although not so much, which is well knowne likewise to be the benefit of the place where it growth, for some hearbes are more or lesse sweet, or more or less stinking, which transplanted doe alter; as Agrimony and divers others are sweet in some place and nothing at all in others'. This rather supports the modern information on the lability of thujone content with location, season, drying conditions and other variations, and might account too for the earlier discrepancies of perceived degree of qualities. And secondly that the apothecaries were not necessarily to be trusted to dispense the appropriate herb, 'but by this is said you see that the vertues of our common Wormewood are so excellent, that we need not seeke for another kinde to performe those that are commended on wormewood; and therefore I the more mervaile at our Apothecaries, that take the sea wormewood, in stead of the Romane or Ponticke, and use it rather than the common, onely because there is lesse bitternesse therein, than is the common and therefore more pleasing to the taste, when as the properties are no way answerable'. Miller, at a later date, makes the same mention, possibly citing Mattioli, implying that the apothecaries gave the less bitter sort in order to sell more and thus increase profit rather than dispensing the best medicinal variety. Culpeper adds his own refinement, that since the sea wormewood is the least bitter and the weakest 'it is fittest for weak bodies, and further for those bodies that dwell near it, than those that dwell far from it; my reason is, the sea ... casts not such a smell as the land doth. The tender mercies of God being over all his works, hath by his eternal Providence, planted Seriphon by the seaside, as a fit medicine for the bodies of those that live near it'. The use of sea wormwood and the confounding of names continued right up to relatively recent times. Grieve records that the drug 'Absinthium' (rarely employed) was directed in the British Pharmacopoeia to be extracted from *Artemisia maritima* 'which possesses the same virtues in a less degree, and is often more used as a stomachic that the common wormwood. Commercially this often goes under the name of Roman wormwood, though that name really belongs to *A. Pontica*'.

## A DIGESTIVE HERB

Wormwood seems to be a herb par excellence for the whole digestive tract. Most authorities prize its actions in this respect. Dioscorides says it has astringent and warming properties; it is diuretic; it can purge the bilious elements through the stomach and bowel; is a preventive for nausea; drunk with hartwort or Celtic nard it is good for flatulence

THE WESTERN HERBAL TRADITION

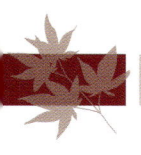

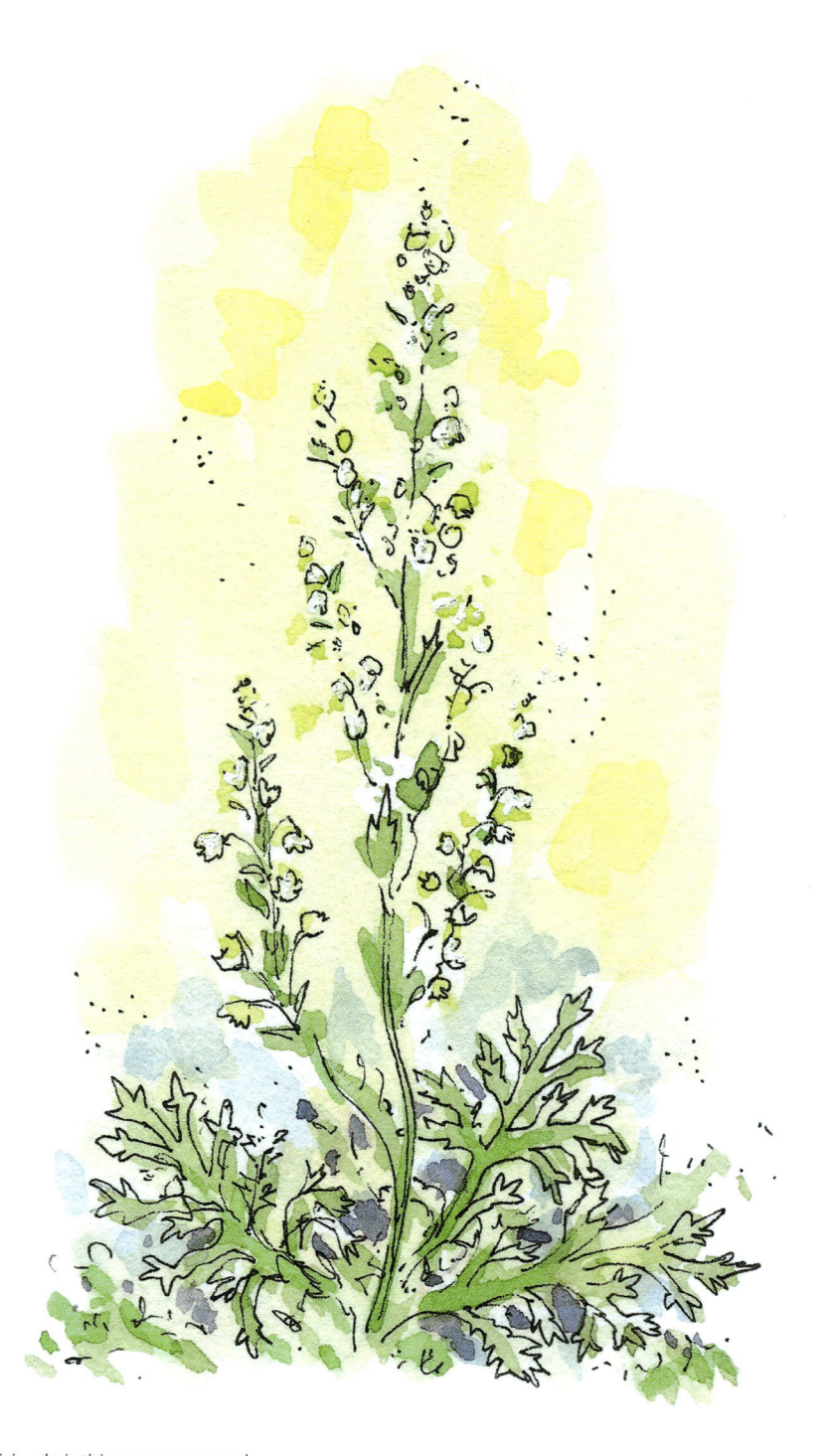

**Figure 11.2** *Artemisia absinthium*, wormwood.

and stomach pains; and a daily infusion or decoction of three cyathi (135 mL) remedies lack of appetite and jaundice. He advocates two external applications for gastrointestinal conditions: plasters made with Cyprian cerate help chronic conditions of hypochondria, liver and stomach, and those with unguent of roses are used for the stomach. For spleen disease or oedemata, it is mixed with figs, soda and darnel meal, although it is unclear whether this is for internal or external use. Dioscorides reports the custom around Propontis and Thrace of making a wine, absinthitis, from wormwood, used for the conditions mentioned, only if the patient has no fever. The same wine is drunk in spring as aperitif to bring good health. The juice, however, should not be taken internally, at least not neat, 'since it is bad for the stomach and gives headaches' he says. In relation to the juice Dioscorides adds 'the juice is adulterated with the watery part that runs out when olives are pressed; it is boiled down and combined with the juice'. Whether this then renders it potable, he does not specify.

A further gastrointestinal use in Dioscorides is against poisons: wormwood as alexipharmic. It is drunk with vinegar to remedy choking from poisonous mushrooms, and with wine against pine thistle, hemlock, bites of the shrew and of the great weever. Inevitably the detail is ambiguous territory: Dodoens says with wine 'it resisteth all venome but chiefly Hemlocke and the bitings and stingings of spiders, and other venomous beasts'; Parkinson reads 'being taken in wine it is a remedy against the poison of Ixia (which as I said before, is the roote of the blacke chameleon, and with Pliny translated viscum, Mistletoe or Birdlime) of Hemlocke, the biting of that small beast or Mouse which we call a shrew, and the biting of that sea fish called Dracomarinus, which is called a Quaviver'.

Galen accounts for the properties of *Artemisia pontica* in that its astringency is greater than its sharpness or bitterness; it is also cleansing, he says, strengthening and drying and the juice is much hotter (Parkinson cites this as 'better', although others repeat 'hotter') than the herb, although he does not berate the juice for all that. As in Dioscorides, Galen says the plant propels biliary humours of the belly downwards. It also evacuates via urine, especially if heat is in the veins, although he cautions that because the astringency overcomes the bitterness, wormwood will not serve for phlegm which is in the stomach nor in the lungs.

Pliny writes in similar vein. It is good and wholesome, he says; it strengthens the stomach aloft (is this perhaps our later appreciation of increase in muscle tone of the lower oesophageal sphincter), evacuates choler downwards, is diuretic, keeps the body soluble and the belly in good temper; it is good for liver infirmities. He repeats Dioscorides' warning about avoiding the juice, or rather syrup of wormwood made from the juice, since it is offensive to the stomach and head. With the ill humours of the stomach cleansed, it will bring appetite and help concoction, i.e. digestion. Pliny's suggestion for helping the spleen is with vinegar or in figs or with gruel, although he is equally unclear on mode of application. His remedy for windiness of the stomach is with seseli, Celtic nard and vinegar; with rue *Ruta graveolens*, pepper and salt it cleanses the stomach of raw humours, occasioned by want of digestion. For jaundice it should be taken raw with parsley (or with raw parsley) or maidenhair; a decoction with cumin seed *Cuminum cyminum* taken warm eases pain of the belly and colic by wind.

The *Old English Herbarium* carries two entries for wormwood: in one *Artemisia absinthium* L., Wermod is described for external use for sores and worms (see below), while an earlier entry for 'Wormwood (*Artemisia pontica* L.), artemisia leptefilos, Mucgwyrt', which 'has the smell of elder', covers external application of the herb simmered in almond oil as a poultice on the stomach for stomach ache, 'within five days the person will be well', and for the juice mixed with oil for trembling of the tendons.

## BROAD CONSENSUS

The Arabic writers mention varieties of absinthium from their own experience. Serapio says the best comes from the Indians, Ibn Sina prefers those from Armenia and the mountains of Turkey and speaks too of one from Jordan 'which smells nicely'. They mainly repeat the commendations of the ancient writers. Serapio includes its use for abscesses of the liver and stomach, repeats Galen's lack of effect on phlegm in the stomach and Dioscorides' warning about the juice as harmful to the stomach. He cites Mabix on opening obstructions, loosening the belly and curing jaundice because of its heat. It is Ibn Sina who talks about the dual properties of the plant and explains this effect; it stops (at least the one from Jordan) diarrhoea thanks to an earth element in it and purges and opens up blockages thanks to the volatile element. Ibn Sina is ambiguous about taking the juice; wormwood, he says, is 'a fantastic and lovely herb to repair appetite when taken as a broth and/or as a squeezed juice during ten days, each day 3 obols (1800 mg). As wine it strengthens the stomach and renders other benefits, or the herb, especially taken as a squeezed juice during ten days, each day 3 dirhams (8.925 g) helps jaundice and dropsy'. Yet after recording the figs, soda and chaff as medicinal bandages for the spleen, familiar from Dioscorides and Pliny, he follows with the, also familiar, expressed juice as not good for the stomach; his citing of medicinal bandages for the liver, stomach and sides, and pains and hardness in the organs, and in wax with henna oil for the liver and sides, and with roses or rose oil for the stomach echoes Dioscorides, yet later we find again a further reference to the juice as helping with old fevers – both juice and fever counter to indication in Dioscorides.

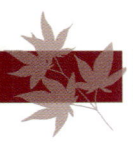

Hildegard in the 12th century says it warms the stomach, purges the intestines and makes good digestion possible.

Our Renaissance authors mainly cite the ancients. Parkinson is very thorough and adds a 'receite' from the *Hortus Medicus* of Camerarius, for yellow jaundice 'take saith hee of the flowers of wormewood, rosemary and blacke thorne of each alike quantity; of saffron halfe that quantity; all which being boyled in Renish-wine, let it be given after the body is prepared by purging etc.'. Parkinson, when citing Pliny, also refers to eating a few leaves of wormwood to defend one from 'surfeiting and drunkennesse'. Dodoens, on this point, says 'if it bee taken fasting in the morning, it preserveth from drunkennes that day'. Culpeper's tract on wormwood is very distinctive and full of imagery 'To give and example here He [Mars] had no sooner parted with the Moon, but he met with Venus, and she was as drunk as a hog; Alas poor Venus, quoth he; What! Thou a fortune and be drunk? I'll give thee antipathetical cure; Take my herb wormwood, and thou shall never get a surfeit by drinking'. Parkinson adds that the opening of obstructions and purging by urine and strengthening of the liver and stomach accounts for its commendation in tertian and other lingering agues; perhaps here supporting Ibn Sina's reference to its virtue in old fevers, i.e. intermittent fevers. Parkinson refers too to a property of sweetening bad breath: 'The vinegar wherein wormewood is boyled, is especiall good for a stinking breath that commeth from the gums or teeth, or from corruption in the stomacke'. Bauhin on this point cites Mesue that the herb is used cooked in vinegar or wine with lemon peel to amend bad breath, gingivitis or 'rotting makemals' in the stomach.

Dodoens similarly follows the ancients, and his language is splendid 'it is good against the windinesse, blastings of the belly, against the paynes and appetite to vomite, and the boyling up or wamblings of the stomacke, if it bee drunken with Annis-seed, or Sesely'. Gerard speaks of 'clensing by urine naughtie humours'. He adds a further observation 'and it often happens that with violent and large vomiting the sick man fainteth or swouneth or when he is revived doth fall into a difficult and almost incureable tymponie [bloating] especially when disease doth often happen; but from these dangers wormwood can deliver him, if when he is refreshed after vomite and his strength anyway recovered, he shall a good while use it in what manner he think good'. He adds too how wormwood withstands all putrefactions, this presumably helping low acid conditions and risk of enteric pathology through lack of sterilization of food. Turner reprises Dioscorides, Galen and Pliny, although he says it is not good taken in an ague. While Dalechamps cites Mesue that it helps putrid fevers, even if continuous, Culpeper is clear and graphic: 'A poor silly countryman hath got an ague and cannot go about his business; he wishes he had it not and so do I; I will tell him a remedy, whereby he shall prevent it. Take the herb of Mars, wormwood, and if infortunes will do good, what will fortunes do?'

Bauhin covers the ancients and the Arabic writers very thoroughly. He cites Mesue, presumably following Galen, that wormwood purges phlegm very little or not at all, but then contrasts Avenzoar's judgment that it does indeed purge phlegm. Dalechamps mentions the same contrast, saying Avenzoar calls wormwood a 'phlegm purger'. Fuchs reads similarly. Culpeper appears to rate the herb highly: 'the sun never shone upon a better herb for the yellow jaundice than this', he says, and repeats Camerarius' recipe, though 'put it not in saffron till it is almost boiled'.

## LATER FLUCTUATIONS

The reputation of wormwood in the 18th century is not so easy to assess. Quincy groups it as Detergent, class 4 of the Balsamics. He describes it as stomachic on account of its bitterness: it is a great detergent, he says, and therefore prescribed in the jaundice and even in dropsies, but then he adds that this use is now laid aside and it is little regarded as stomachic. Miller, on the other hand, indicates no fall from grace. He says it is accounted good and helpful in all disorders of the stomach, as weakness, loss of appetite, vomiting and surfeits, following previous uses quite closely. They strengthen the viscera and are of service in dropsies, jaundice and in tertian and quartan agues, and kill worms (see below), given infused in water, ale or wine. The number of preparations enumerated as available in the shops indicates lively use: a simple water, a greater and lesser compound water, a simple and a compound syrup, an oil by infusion and decoction, an oil by distillation, an extract and a fixed salt. Hill too indicates current use, and still the inevitable debate on species, in his day 'all kinds of wormwood are stomachic, good against obstruction of the viscera. The common kind is the strongest, but insufferably nauseous. The sea wormwood is the kind most used but the Roman is vastly preferable to them all. The sea wormwood is sold in the markets under the name of Roman wormwood, and is almost universally used as such by the apothecaries; but the error is very great; and the other is so common in gardens and lives and increases so freely in them, that a supply is easy'.

Use in America seems to have fluctuated. Ellingwood has no reference to *Artemisia absinthium*, only to *Artemisia pauciflora*, Levant wormseed, santonica (see below). Cook echoes Quincy. He refers to use of the leaves and flowers of wormwood as stimulating and relaxing tonics, bitter and strong to the highest degree and acting upon the stomach and gall-ducts. He relates how it improves appetite and digestion and slightly influences the bowels, for which effect, he says, 'it has been a favourite addition to tonic preparations for low and bilious conditions, intermittent jaundice, hypochondria and similar maladies'. While a small amount is useful in these cases, especially when 'there is present decided languor and sluggishness of action,' he nevertheless indicates infrequent application: 'though its intense bitterness has pretty much driven it from use'.

## BITTERS

By Cullen's time the bitters were acknowledged as a particular group of plants with specific actions. Cullen lectured on their capacities under both bitters and tonics, and he divides the bitters into hot and cold, amara calida and amara frigida, wormwood, of course counting among the calida. Bitters are seldom simple, he says, but combined with other qualities. More recently Schulz et al (1998) differentiate simple, aromatic, astringent and acrid types. 'Proper tonics are bitters' Cullen says. His appraisal both encompasses the applications we have met through the tradition above, other uses from the past to be covered below, and anticipate our modern conception of their bitter actions. On the common qualities he discusses, he offers his own experience, which does not always corroborate the general claim. The 'common qualities' include:

1. action on the stomach; increasing appetite for food and promoting digestion of it, the improvement depending upon an increase in tone of the muscular fibres, hence 'restoring tone to that organ'; correcting acidity and flatulence, checking fermentation, and relieving the stomach from abundant mucus or phlegm. This improved state, communicated to other parts of the system improve the tone of the whole
2. resolving visceral obstructions, hence useful in jaundice and dropsy, although Cullen suggests this is supposed, rather than found
3. diuretic, possibly directly so but there may be other mechanisms, he estimates
4. for intermittent fevers, through their tonic power in the stomach
5. for continued fevers, although their effect is ambiguous
6. sudorific, although only with a sudorific regimen
7. further down the alimentary canal 'pretty certainly laxative', good in spasmodic colics and particularly useful in dysentery
8. emmenagogue, not perceived so by Cullen
9. resolving coagulations produced by falls and contusions, again unestablished by Cullen
10. anthelmintic (discussed later).

This list is followed by two external uses: for cleansing and healing foul ulcers Cullen found bitters useful, and universally employed in fomentations for discussing tumours. Here Cullen is more doubtful of their efficacy. He covers also the use of bitters for gout but has reservations on their long-term use, which may result in apoplexy.

Grieve recommends wormwood as a good remedy for enfeebled digestion and debility. A light infusion of the fresh tops is excellent for all disorders of the stomach and helps promote appetite and digestion, and prevent sickness after meals, but she cautions that if too much is taken it will produce the contrary effect. Grieve includes too a recipe from Dr John Hill of 1772: 1 oz of flowers and buds in an earthen vessel, pints of boiling water poured on and left to stand all night. The following morning the clear liquid is taken with 2 spoonfuls of wine at three draughts hour's distance from each other; 'whoever will do this regularly for a week will have no sickness after meals, will feel none of that fullness so frequent from indigestion, and wind will be no more troublesome; if afterwards, he will take but a 4th part of this each day, the benefit will be lasting'.

In herbal medicine today bitters form a mainstay of practice. The human taste receptor that responds to a variety of bitter compounds has been identified (Behrens et al 2004). Schulz et al (1998) record how the stimuli in the mouth by reflex induce gastric and biliary secretions, arguably only where they are below optimal level, and their reflex action on the cardio-vascular system, decreasing heart rate and cardiac stroke volume. Mills (1991) offers full expression of their use. Unlike Cullen, he designates them 'cold', yet he expresses the paradoxical temperament of wormwood, one of the bitterest plants, but its acrid constituents 'raise its temperature'. Mills records how the broad applications of the bitters stem from their many capacities, as they:

1. increase appetite
2. increase digestive secretions, hence not only improvement of digestion but less likelihood of enteric infections, and not necessarily a contraindication in hyperacidity
3. protect gut tissues since sphincter tone is increased, mucosal regeneration promoted and enhanced recovery from pancreatic disease
4. promote bile flow, hence good liver function
5. enhance pancreatic function, thus possibly useful in late onset diabetes mellitus with a normalizing of pancreatic hormone secretion
6. act as a tonic, promoting good health.

The uses documented by Mills recall a number of familiar applications from tradition and add new ones: he lists their use for biliary disorders, including gall bladder disease and some instances of high cholesterol, liver conditions, loss of appetite, reactive hypoglycaemia, chronic inflammatory diseases of the skin, joints, vascular system, bowels, migraines and fevers. Schulz et al (1998) emphasize the psychological component of appetite, citing a trial in which bitters improved appetite in people with gastric achylia, despite their inability to produce stomach acid. The bitter taste too is necessary. The same range of effects cannot be achieved if this is bypassed by using, for example, coated pills.

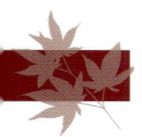

## WORMS AND SAFETY

An action associated with bitters in general and wormwood in particular is that of anthelmintic. Nevertheless, experience is not uniform. Dioscorides, notably, does not document wormwood as anthelmintic. He reserves the designation for seriphon, sea wormwood 'boiled down either by itself or with rice and consumed with honey it destroys intestinal and round worms, gently purging the bowels', although it is bad for the stomach, he adds. It will do the same boiled with lentil gruel, and moreover fattens the sheep (Dodoens extends this to beeves, sheep and cattle) that graze on it, presumably by ridding them of worms. Santonicon acts similarly. I can find no reference from Galen to the use of wormwood for worms, only sea wormwood, as Dioscorides. There is a small debate here about Galen's declaring sea absinthium as of the same sort and taste similar to absinthium, while Dioscorides says seriphon, sea wormwood, more approaches abrotanum than absinthium. Mattioli says it is a case of deciding who is at fault, although Parkinson holds they cannot differ so much in judgment and that the place in Dioscorides or Galen is 'perverted by some writer's fault'.

Pliny, however, does appear to commend wormwood for 'worms of the belly'. He writes too of a 'device' to put the leaves of wormwood in figs for administration to children to avoid their bitterness. This may well also refer to a use against worms. Parkinson's coverage of Pliny carries no such commendation. Neither Turner nor Mattioli appear to commend wormwood for worms. Dodoens carries a small reference to worms under wormwood but this is in the context of oil for 'fleas, flyes, knats and wormes', an extension of Dioscorides' recommendation for repelling mosquitoes (discussed below) and unlikely to refer to worms of the belly, which he covers under the usual sea wormwood: 'boyled by it selfe, or with rice, or with any other food or meat, and eaten with hony, slayeth both long and flat wormes, and all other kinds whatsoever, loosing the belly very gently. It is of like operation being layd to outwardly upon the belly or navel, and for this purpose it is of more strength and virtue than all the other kindes of Wormewood; but it is more hurtfull to the stomacke'. The seed too is good for all kinds of worms, he adds. Gerard does suggest wormwood for worms, an inner and an outer application. Culpeper suggests sea wormwood is to be given to children and the elderly for worms because it is weaker, but he exhorts the use of common wormwood for this purpose for those who are stronger 'for the others will do but little good'. Bauhin, citing Mesue, mentions only dried herb of wormwood applied with cloths to overcome tinea, and that the juice with peach kernels (no longer used due to its cyanide content) kills and draws out worms from the ears and from other parts. Serapio appears to make no mention of worms. Ibn Sina has a reference to worms but it runs 'decoction of wormwood on its own or with rice or chickpeas and drunk with honey kills worms but easily weakens the stomach', almost word for word a repetition of Dioscorides on sea wormwood. Hence the tradition for wormwood for worms from these authors appears variable. Other tradition is firmer but whether based on erroneous interpretation of the ancients is difficult to tell. The Old English Herbarium is very clear on this matter 'if worms are a bother around the anus, take equal amounts of absinthium (wormwood), horehound and lupine. Simmer them in sweetened water or in wine. Put it on the anus 2 or 3 times, and it will kill the worms'. It is notable that this text carries only two uses for this wormwood *Artemisia absinthium*, wermod, and both external (the other for bruises, see below) and reference to the firmer tradition of gastrointestinal tract use only for Pontic wormwood, although again for external use. Hildegard carries a reference only to ear worms. The Salernitan Herbal does refer to gut worms: 'when the worms called lombrics are in the intestines the juice of absinthe with juice of betony or centaury or peach kernels can be given'.

Miller carries a reference to killing worms, as does Quincy, so its reputation as anthelmintic is current in the 18th century. Cook records its popularity in the treatment of worms: it is good for the stomach worm, he says, 'when the stomach is languid and the abdomen tumefied and flaccid'. Ellingwood only has an entry for santonica, Levant wormseed, which rids worms and which he praises from his experience to relieve reflex irritation. Dosage appears to be crucial: two grains (130 mg), he says, caused the death of a feeble child. Cullen seems not too persuaded of sure efficacy against worms, neither of wormwood nor anthelmintic bitters in general. Skelton, however, is convinced otherwise. He says almost any strong vegetable bitter, given at bedtime and fasting with a pretty strong purgative, will expel the round worm. He recommends the powdered herb as more efficient than the infusion, although treating children is more problematic since they dislike bitters in any form. He offers a prescription: wormwood powder 1 oz,    oz senna powder *Senna alexandrina*, 2 oz common salt. Mix and take a tablespoonful in a teacupful of cold water night and morning. Eat nothing 3 hours before taking the medicine at night or 3 hours after taking in the morning. These doses seem excessive. In cases of children the powders alone, he says, can be made into a conserve or mixed with treacle, taken at a dose of a teaspoon or tablespoon night and morning. General health should be attended to. A further recipe for adults is 1 oz wormwood dried herb, 1 drachm ginger powder *Zingiber officinalis*, infuse in     pints boiling water in covered vessel, allow to cool, strain, press, add 6 oz treacle and take a teacupful at bedtime every night. This will remove *Ascaris lumbricoides*, according to Skelton.

Grieve records the flowers dried and powdered as a 'most effectual vermifuge', and the essential oil, as spirituous extract rather than that distilled in water, as a worm expeller. While Weiss acknowledges wormwood's use for threadworms, by a tea taken internally and a retention enema of a strong decoction, he rather supports the ancient advice of Dioscorides, that wormwood is 'not very effective against worms. *Artemisia cina*, Levant wormseed is the real worm remedy used against both threadworms and roundworms'. Wormwood's reputation as anthelmintic continues today, although still with some reservations. The British Herbal Pharmacopoeia records it as an anthelmintic, with indications for nematode infestation and specific indications for infestation with *Enterobius* or *Ascaris*. Bartram suggests internal and topical applications; as a strong tea injected into the rectum by enema, or a single dose of 5–10 mL much diluted and taken on an empty stomach, repeated fortnightly. Wood, more recently, is more reserved, quoting Neil that it is useful, injected (enema) for pin worms, but is less effective for more potent parasites. Chevallier and Mills & Bone record it as an anthelmintic, although none offers a specific dosage. Barker gives a dosage of up to 2 mL for shorter periods as anthelmintic. Hoffman calls it 'a powerful remedy against worm infestations, especially roundworm and pinworm, taken powdered in pill form'. Menzies-Trull recommends taking it on an empty stomach with syrup night and morning, with an enema on days 1 and 3. Mills (1991) records it 'appreciably antiparasitic'. However, he notes the necessity of working with relatively toxic material, although exploiting the differential aspects of metabolism in host and parasite, and hence this should only be done with care by the experienced. We now recognize different families of helminths and use of information from what is in this case a questionable tradition needs more evaluation.

## EMMENAGOGUE? HORMONES?

Cullen notes a claimed, but to him unproven, emmenagogic action to the bitters. Wormwood is recorded with this property. The British Herbal Pharmacopoeia does not record this action for wormwood, despite such a property in both the sister herbs, *Artemisia abrotanum* and *Artemisia vulgaris*. Indeed there is no strong modern tradition for its use in this regard, even when designated emmenagogue, other than cautions against its use in pregnancy, carried by all our modern authors. Mills & Bone expand the caution to association with foetal malformation, and contraindication in breast feeding. Only Bartram recommends its use for abnormal absence of periods and Menzies-Trull for atonic vaginal discharge and leucorrhoea. Mills (1991), together with strong cautions, mentions its use for spasmodic dysmenorrhoea and relief of pain in childbirth. Wood lists it for amenorrhoea, infertility, menstrual cramps and painful parturition but does not discourse further, and Barker (2001) records an anecdotal transient worsening of premenstrual tension symptoms in susceptible individuals, preferring different plants to bring on delayed periods. Beyond this there is little discussion. Past tradition is only a little more fulsome with its recommendations in this regard. Dioscorides is clear – it draws down the menses both when drunk and used topically with honey. Pliny's 'topically' is as a pessary to provoke periods, in honey and wrapped in a lock of wool. Pliny is the only author to express a use in pregnancy to cure pregnant women of their strange longings – hopefully not by any means too drastic. Some Renaissance authors cite Dioscorides on its emmenagogue action but expand no further, while Dodoens and Gerard, despite recording Dioscorides closely, omit this reference altogether, perhaps due to abortifacient sensitivities. Culpeper is circumspect with his 'it helps the evils of Venus and the wanton Boy by antipathy'. Serapio makes no further comment on such a use, nor Mesue, cited by Bauhin and Dalechamps. Ibn Sina reads much like Pliny: wormwood powerfully induces urination and menses, especially as a bougie with honey-water. Emmenagogue action is not mentioned by Miller, nor Quincy, nor later in Grieve. Cook carries only that it is a little stimulating on the uterus, taken advantage of in atonic amenorrhoea. The Salernitan Herbal carries instruction to induce menstrual flow by giving wormwood juice as a pessary and making a suppository of absinthium, Artemisia (vulgaris) and ordinary oil or musk oil 'which is better'. As might be expected *The Trotula* (Green 2001) offers a greater number of recommendations. There is a remedy containing sea wormwood, betony, pennyroyal and mugwort, boiled and the water mixed with fumitory juice, for scant menses emitted with pain. For excessive flux two plasters made from wormwood with animal grease should be tied upon the loins and the belly. For descent of the womb aromatics are mixed with wormwood and the belly anointed with a feather. For a difficult birth, rue, mugwort, opopanax and wormwood are ground with oil and sugar and applied to the pubic area or navel. For exit of the womb after birth a woman should bathe in juniper, camphor, wormwood, mugwort and fleabane. There is also a rare remedy for men, for swelling of the testicles: marshmallow, wormwood, vervain, chamomile, henbane, mugwort and cabbages, these herbs to be ground with honey, boiled and applied with wine two or three times a day. It is notable that all these remedies are for external use. Green (2001) discusses Latin binomials for the herbs in her text.

113

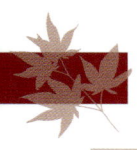

## MENTAL HEALTH

The applications of wormwood continue with its reputation as a herb against melancholy. This action may well be as attributable to the effect of its bitter nature on the liver, as well as the general tonic effect so roundly affirmed from application thus far. There is support of a humoral nature for bitters working through the spleen in hypochondriac melancholy where an overheated spleen causes noxious vapours to rise to the heart and brain. Some modern authors, among them Chevallier, Menzies-Trull and Hoffman, refer to use in depression/melancholy but not a lot of guidance as to source is given. Grieve gives a recipe of 1 oz of herb infused 10–12 minutes in one pint of water taken in glassful doses to relieve melancholia, but again no source is offered. The tradition does not appear in the ancients. Hildegard is an early mention, with a recipe of fresh wormwood pounded and expressed through cloth added to wine cooked with honey, so that the wormwood overcomes the wine and honey flavour, to be drunk every other day, to check not only melancholy, but 'it will ease sickness in the loins and make your eyes clear'. Serapio cites Mabix that an infusion or decoction, especially mixed with epithymum, will cure melancholy. Otherwise there seems to be no specific mention among the Arabic writers, nor our other sources.

There is a little more written on wormwood as a nervine. Grieve calls it a nervine tonic, embracing the idea of vermouth made from wormwood, named from Wermuth, 'preserver of the mind', deriving from its medicinal virtues as nervine and restorative. 'If not taken habitually', she says, 'it soothes spinal irritation and gives tone to persons of highly nervous temperament'. Menzies-Trull also designates it nervine, a stimulant of the central nervous system and heart for 'nervous and physical exhaustion with fatigue'. Wood explores wider fields in this regard. He documents his use of the herb for hopelessness and for people who have suffered severe trauma, physical and mental, 'brutalised by the reverses of life', with depression of life forces in general. He suggests it is indicated in 'thin, scrawny, malnourished individuals', yet he has used it with success, he says, for the 'large, waterlogged and stiff'. Is this the earlier 'dual quality' on another level? Bartram suggests its use for assisting withdrawal from benzodiazepine addiction. From tradition, the closest association in respect of nervine is that of headache. The National Botanic Pharmacopoeia, in the not too distant past, records use of wormwood for some nervous affections, especially headache. Although Dioscorides and others say the juice causes headache, other applications are commended to ease it, including the use recorded in the Salernitan herbal of wormwood juice in hot water and sugar for pains in the head arising from the stomach. The majority of other remedies involve variations on external application. Hildegard says take the juice in warm wine and wet the entire head, including eyes, ears and neck, on going to bed and cover the head with a woollen cap until morning. This will also relieve head pain from gout and the more 'inner pain of the head'. Bauhin and Dalechamps both record a suggestion from Mesue of taking wormwood and the root of field cucumber cooked in wine, water or oil, and binding sponges soaked in this mixture to the head to ease migraine. Parkinson says bathing the temples with distilled water should ease headache from an old cause.

Too much wormwood, as we have seen, will have the opposite effect. Presumably Dioscorides' caution about the juice is founded on experience of reaction that might now be attributed to particular constituents, in particular thujone, which leads to the cerebral dysfunction, epileptiform seizures, delirium and hallucinations that Schulz et al (1998) record. A detrimental effect is not unnoticed in tradition. For example, Cook notes that larger doses or long continued use lead to excitement of the stomach, pulse and brain, although he estimates it is not narcotic but has a slow and persistent stimulating and tonic action upon both the heart and nervous centres. Cullen writes in similar vein, that some authors strongly asserted its narcotic power, although, he says, Linnaeus knew of people taking wormwood daily for 6 months with no narcotic effect. Nevertheless, Cullen estimates the odour as 'temulentans – giving some confusion of the head'. He records the earlier custom of drinking 'purl', a wormwood infused ale which intoxicated more than other ales. He concludes that every bitter 'when largely employed', has 'a power of destroying the sensibility and irritability of the nervous power. The question of safety surrounding absinthe has some relevance here (see the discussion below under safety issues).

Internal dosages need only be small. Bartram records an average dose of 1–2 g of fluid equivalent three times a day, tea of 1 teaspoon to each cup of cold water steeped overnight and drunk in the morning; liquid extract 1:1 in 25% 1–2 mL in water; tincture 1:10 in 45% 1 teaspoon three times a day. This seems rather large, and smaller doses should be effective. Barker suggests 0.1–0.25 mL in combination. Menzies-Trull warns 'always use a small dose – this is a very stimulating remedy'. Cook recommends 5–15 grains (325–975 mg) three times a day, usually given as infusion. Half an ounce in a pint of boiling water is strong enough, he says, and 2–4 drachms (8–16 mL) of this is a dose. 'In combining it with other tonics I seldom use more than    oz of this in each gallon of the preparation' he says, 'for it is too concentrated an article to employ in such large doses as are generally used'. Cullen says tinctures are best by short infusion, anticipating here later findings on thujone extraction. Wood recommends micro doses, one drop per day is often enough, he says. I never use more than 5 mL per week and find this dose effective.

## EXTERNAL USE

It is remarkable how many instances are found through the tradition of external application of herbs, through a variety of inventive means, for more internal conditions; a mode of treating that is far less practised today; and wormwood has been no exception. For the more usual topical applications for skin and joints, for example, wormwood is not normally encountered among the more frequent recommendations. Bartram records an infusion of 1 oz to a pint applied to muscles in rheumatic pain, and Menzies-Trull refers to a number of external applications, but otherwise mention is rare. Given, however, wormwood's strong gastrointestinal reputation, it is interesting to note Wood's appraisal of the herb as having survived in modern American herbalism largely as a medicine for the muscular and skeletal system. He cites Cook's enthusiastic recommendation of it as 'a good fomentation in sprains, rheumatic and other sub-acute difficulties about the joints; and in bruises and local contusions/congestions'. Cullen records the reputation of bitters, especially aromatic bitters, in general as cleansing and healing foul ulcers, including checking of the progress of gangrene, and in fomentations for discussing tumours.

The further external applications that Dioscorides and Pliny record are repeated through many texts and other uses join them. For example, Dioscorides' recommendation of wormwood with honey and soda as an unguent for sore throats, reappearing through the Renaissance authors in various guises, is echoed in Miller 'a cataplasm of the green leaves beat up with hog's lard was commended to Mr Ray by Dr Hulfe as a good external remedy against swelling of the tonsils and quinzy'. This is cited presumably from practical experience, although no other specific external application appears either in Miller or Quincy from that time. A use with honey for 'black eye' in Dioscorides appears similarly in Pliny as applied with honey for bruises and in Mesue, cited by Bauhin, it reads 'parts inflamed by rubbing or bruised are wonderfully helped by the herb heated with honey or wine and a little cumin and applied'. The *Old English Herbarium* refers to absinthium for 'removing bruises and other sores from the body' using cloths soaked in infusion of wormwood, and if the flesh is tender simmer the herb in honey and then apply. For the pontic wormwood, the juice mixed with oil and rubbed on will stop trembling in the tendons and quiet the tremors (and hung over the door it will keep the house from harm). Regarding Dioscorides' treatment for ears, the honey mix helps purulent ears and the vapour of the decoction is good for earaches; Pliny has the smoke of burnt wormwood or the powdered herb mixed with honey and applied. Mesue, cited by Bauhin, expands with the ears fumigated by wine or water in which wormwood is cooked are freed from pain, tinnitus and deafness. Infected ears do buzz and hearing is then often temporarily reduced, so this is not necessarily as inflated a claim as it at first might sound.

Use for the eyes is more contended. Dioscorides says wormwood boiled down with grape syrup can be used as a poultice for very painful eyes. Macer citing Pliny says applied with honey it clears the eyes. Dodoens fills out the recommendation 'the wormewood mingled with honey is goode to be layd to the dimness of the sight and to the eyes that are blood shotten or have blacke spots [Dioscorides' earlier 'black eye?] And with the same boiled in Bastard [wine] or any other sweet wine, they use to rub and strake painefull bleered eyes'. Quincy, much later, however, maintains because the herb is hot and dry it will hurt the sight by drying up or dissipating the animal juices too much 'whereby optic nerves have sometimes also wanted their due supplies', and Cullen likewise says 'wormwood (and other bitters may be) down from the time of the ancients, like sage, affects the eyes with uneasy dryness, weakness, contraction and inflammation attended with headache. Ibn Sina, however, is more positive: wormwood is useful with long standing inflammation of the eyes; especially that of Jordan, applied on a bandage on the eye area helps burning; together with Armenian clay on a bandage it comforts pulsation in the eyes and redness and swelling.

Yet more useful applications from Dioscorides follow, with the facility of wormwood, put in drawers and chests, to preserve clothing from moths; documents written with ink made using an infusion of wormwood instead of just water will not be eaten by mice; Ibn Sina adds too that it helps the ink colour to last, I presume not just because it is not eaten; it will prevent mosquitoes (gnats, flies and more in other versions) from biting, if the body is rubbed with the oil. This latter may have a modern link. Tick-borne diseases such as Lyme disease are significant worldwide, and a study was carried out to identify plant materials which repel the nymph of the main European tick *Ixodes ricinus* L. (Jaenson et al 2005). Oil of *Rhododendron tomentosum* (formerly *Ledum palustre*) 10% in acetone was highly effective (95%) and extract of *Artemisia absinthium* leaves in ethyl acetate was effective (75%) (Jaenson et al 2005). The extract was thujone-free and the main compound was myrtenol acetate (78%).

Ibn Sina adds further uses: it brightens the skin of the face and helps baldness; dough with wormwood helps heal urticaria; for haemorrhoids and anal fissures, although whether internal or external use is not clear. Hildegard recommends wormwood for toothache 'either from rotten blood or from purging of the brain', cook equal amounts of wormwood and vervain in a new pot of good wine, strain, drink with a little sugar and tie warm herb around jaw on going to bed. She also recommends an infused oil for chest pain with cough, and a salve of wormwood, deer tallow and deer marrow, applied in front of a fire, for gout. Pliny says seasickness can be avoided if one gets used to drinking wormwood.

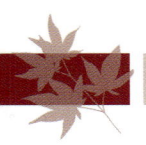

Finally, three more suggestions from Pliny: kibbed heels can be cured by bathing them in a decoction of wormwood; placed under the pillow it procures sleep, but only if the potential sleeper is unaware of its presence; the ash of wormwood mixed with oil of roses colours hair black.

## CURRENT USE

Wormwood continues to be used in traditional medicine in Europe. Guarrera (1999, 2005) sought out elderly people in rural areas of Central Italy and interviewed over 300 people in 175 localities. Use of the leaves as anthelmintic was reported in 26 localities and use for lack of appetite in 10 localities. One respondent referred to use of aerial parts as an effective antiemetic (one spoon infused in a glass for 5 minutes, and drunk morning and evening) (Guarrera 2005).

Pelikan speaks of the wormwoods having a gesture of 'swelling herbage' combining with airy structures radiating outwards', the astral sphere drawn deeply into the etheric forces of the plant. They are plants with many tiny flowerheads and permeated throughout by a bitter taste – 'a strange synthesis', says Pelikan, 'producing volatile oils containing bitters'. Their attraction of the astral bestows a 'stimulant and roborant principle' for the gastrointestinal tract, promoting bile. If too much is taken, the astral that should be active in the metabolism reaches instead the nervous system, resulting in neurological dysfunction. Wormwood, with its deeply divided leaves, has to do with the intervention of the astral and the I (ego) in the digestive system, allowing good appetite and digestion, efficient liver and gall bladder function and resistance to disease. The tonic effect is acknowledged 'with the ability to take hold more firmly of this part of the physical body, there is greater energy and enjoyment of life'. The volatile oil is toxic, Pelikan notes, as in absinthe, where, according to Rudolf Steiner, the air principle prevents the astral from engaging properly with the organs of the body, the reproductive organs being particularly damaged.

This remarkably powerful, warming aromatic bitter still has its place in contemporary use. The British Herbal Pharmacopoeia lists its actions as bitter, stomachic, choleretic and anthelmintic. Further actions of the constituents are added by Mills (1991). He refers to antiinflammatory, antiseptic, astringent and tissue repairing capacities, which address both the gastrointestinal use and wider application. Weiss praises its gastrointestinal qualities roundly: it is 'a very ancient, well proven stomach and gall bladder remedy', for atonic and achylic stomach conditions, to aid food digestion and ease distension from gases; 'one of the best remedies for biliary diskinesia', for a troublesome gallbladder; it 'holds a special place among drugs used to treat dyspepsia', used for atonic states of the stomach and gallbladder, occurring particularly in asthenic patients; 'Wormwood is an excellent aid' for conditions related to a weak stomach such as constitutional arterial hypotension; it is additionally recommended for influenza and weakness following infection. From current literature Wormwood appears to be a herb of choice in anorexia, achlorhydria in the elderly and to serve as a very useful bitter tonic for sluggish liver and associated conditions, following a long history of application. Wormwood seems to have a quite extraordinary association with 'food' that appears in no other plant. I have found it useful not only for patients with anorexia, but for individuals who have some unease in their relationship to food generally – for people who overeat and well as undereat, and it is probably quite unrelated, but so far each one has had a difficult relationship with their mother. There seems, following Wood, to be a possibly related dimension of use of wormwood as a temporary companion for help in aspects of 'bitterness in life'. I have heard too, anecdotally, of its use in a life too cushioned, to introduce a 'bitter' element for strength and toning. Should we here be pondering the twofold nature observed through the history of the herb?

## RECOMMENDATIONS

- Achlorhydria and lack of tone in the digestive organs, particularly in the elderly.
- Atonic dyspepsia and some cases of stomach acidity.
- Anorexia and difficulties with food.
- Bad breath.
- Nausea and vomiting.
- Overindulgence in food and/or alcohol.
- Sluggish liver and bowel activity and associated range of conditions – skin, joints, etc.
- Depression associated with atonic liver/liver congestion.
- Gall bladder problems.
- Colic, flatulence and bloating.
- Tonic after illness to regain strength, and in constitutional arterial hypotension.
- Tonic in nervous exhaustion.
- External application for aching muscles and joints.
- Topical wash with honey for ulcers and other skin erosions.

Dosage: the *British Herbal Pharmacopoeia* recommends 1–2 mL three times a day of dried leaves and flowering tops. It also recommends 1–2 mL of a 1 : 1 liquid extract three times a day, but I prefer 5 mL per week of tincture.

# CONSTITUENTS

Reviews: Bisset & Wichtl (2001), Bradley (2006), Mills & Bone (2005), Williamson (2003).

## Volatile oils

A review of 19 commercial samples from 15 European countries found significant variation:

total 0.1–1.1% (107 components), monoterpenes: myrcene 0.1–39%; ketones: alpha-thujone 1–11% (mean 4%), beta-thujone 0.1–65% (mean 9%); oxygenated monoterpenes: 1,8-cineole 0.1–18% and their acetates: trans-epoxy-ocimene 0.1–59.7%, trans-sabinyl acetate 0–70.5%; oxygenated sesquiterpenes: chamazulene 0–6.6% (Orav et al 2006).

Chemotypes have been identified with thujone and/or cis-epoxycimene as the main components (Boroni et al 2006) but others contain no thujone. In the following examples, the concentrations of ketones and oxygenated monoterpenes, including acetates, are picked out and the list is given in descending order of ketone concentration.

ketones: thujone 0–36.3%; oxygenated monoterpenes: trans-sabinyl acetate 9–36% (dried, 10 samples, 6 sites, Lithuania) (Judžentienė &Mockutė 2004).

ketones: beta-thujone 59.9%, alpha-thujone 2.34%; oxygenated monoterpenes: sabinyl acetate 18.1% (wild, Argentina) (Sacco & Chialva 1988).

ketones: beta-thujone 14–45%; oxygenated monoterpenes: cis-epoxyocimene 11–37% (dried leaf and flowering heads, Croatia) (Juteau 2003).

ketones: beta-thujone 1.3%, camphor 17.1%; oxygenated monoterpenes: cis-epoxy-ocimene 24.8%, trans-chrysanthenyl acetate 21.6% (dried flowering heads with leaves, wild, Italian Alps) (Mucciarelli et al 1995).

ketones: beta-thujone 10.1%, monoterpenes: myrcene 10.8%; oxygenated monoterpenes: trans-sabinyl acetate 26.4% (Lopes-Lutz et al 2008).

ketones: thujone 0.7%, camphor 1.4%; oxygenated monoterpenes: borneol, 1,8-cineole, terpinen-4-ol, traces only of acetates; sesquiterpenes: chamazulene 17.8%, nuciferol butanoate 8.2%, caryophyllene oxide (aerial parts, wild, Turkey) (Kordali et al 2005b).

Total 0.31% (68 components), oxygenated monoterpenes: p-cymene 16.8%; ketones: no thujone; sesquiterpenes; oxygenated sesquiterpenes: caryophyllene oxide 25.3% (dried, flowering heads, Greece) (Basta et al 2007).

oxygenated monoterpenes: cis-epoxy-ocimene 27–39%, chrysanthenyl acetate 29–43% (leaves after flowering period, four extraction methods, Spain) (Ariño et al 1999).

65 components: oxygenated monoterpenes: cis-epoxyocimene 23–50%, chrysanthenyl acetate 11–37% (dried leaf and flowering head, France) (Juteau et al 2003).

The monoterpene ketone thujone is a significant compound. A review of 29 studies found that total thujone varied 0–70.6% (mean 18%), alpha-thujone varied 0–60% and beta-thujone varied 0–70% (Lachenmeier & Kuballa 2007). In nine samples where total thujone was 0–36% (mean 21%), the ratio of isomers also varied significantly so that alpha-thujone was 12–99% (mean 42%) and beta-thujone was 1–88% (mean 58%) of total thujone (Judžentienė & Mockutė 2004).

The concentration of each individual volatile oil varies significantly depending on time of year (Jutea et al 2003) and location (Judžentienė & Mockutė 2004). In plants of the same chemotype grown in five locations at different altitude in Italy, concentration of alpha-thujone was 0.3–1.4% and of beta-thujone was 8.7–37.7% (Bononi et al 2006). A study of dried material found that after 1 year, total concentration fell from 0.29 to 0.08% and the relative concentration of some oils changed but that of thujone remained level (Blagojević et al 2006).

*Artemisia pontica*, total 0.2–0.9%, ketones: alpha-thujone 0–30%, beta-thujone 0–4.2 (Lachenmeier & Kuballa 2007).

## Sesquiterpene lactones

Guanolide dimers: absinthin (and isomer anabsinthin), anabsin, artabsin (Kasymov et al 1979), absintholide (Beauhaire et al 1984).

Absinthin 0.2–0.28%, artabsin 0.04–0.16%, which are bitter (Lachenmeier 2007a).

Germacrene type: artabin (Uzbechistan, wild) (Akhmedov et al 1970).

beta-santonin, ketopepenolid-A (cultivated, Cuba) (Perez-Souto et al 1992).

## Phenypropanoids

### Phenolic acids

Total 2.6%, chlorogenic, syringic, coumaric, salicylic and vanillic acids (Canadanovic-Brunet et al 2005).

## Flavonoids

Total 1.3%, quercetin and glycosides (Canadanovic-Brunet et al 2005).

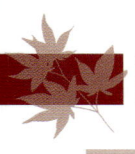

## RECOMMENDATIONS ON SAFETY

1. Do not use in pregnancy.
2. Do not use in porphyria (Bonkovsky et al 1992).
3. The volatile oil should not be taken internally.

A man of 31 drank 10 mL of essential oil of wormwood, thinking it was absinthe. He became agitated and incoherent with tonic and clonic seizures, and developed acute renal failure resulting from rhabdomyolysis (myoglobin release due to muscle injury). He recovered after 8 days of hospital treatment and had normal serum electrolyte, creatine kinase and creatinine concentration after 17 days (Weisbord et al 1997).

The possible association between ingestion of ketones and convulsions has received much attention. Two cases of convulsions have occurred in association with use of volatile oil of sage *Salvia officinalis*, which contains ketones (Burkhard et al 1999). Convulsions have been induced in rats by injected oil of hyssop, which mainly contains pinocamphone (Millet et al 1981). Thujone was first isolated in 1845 and it is argued that thujone is the convulsant constituent in wormwood. Intraperitoneal injection of thujone was convulsant in mice (Höld et al 2000) and the action was blocked by earlier intraperitoneal administration of diazepam or phenobarbital. Höld et al (2000) showed that alpha-thujone acts at the noncompetitive blocker site of the γ-aminobutyric acid (GABA) type A receptor and blocks ion-flow through the channel, which is activated by GABA (Olsen 2000). These receptors are the primary mediators of inhibitory neurotransmission so this is an antiinhibitory action that could lower the threshold for seizures as this action is found with other convulsants (Olsen 2000). Another team (Deiml et al 2004) argue that alpha-thujone inhibits 5-HT3 receptors by channel blockade which enhances the channel-blocking potency of serotonin (5-HT) and thus elevates mood. The animal studies on ketone-containing oils are discussed in the chapter on hyssop (Chapter 19). Their relevance to the internal usage of the herb or tincture is tenuous, but, taken together, the studies discussed here support the advice against internal use of the volatile oil.

4. Use caution with the dose of the tincture which should be used at the lowest effective dose but the cautions based on toxicity associated with the use of absinthe have been exaggerated.

There are two issues of interest: could a tincture or tea be dangerous because of the content of thujone and related ketone components such as camphor and thujyl acetate and, if so, would it be possible to take an excessive dose in a tincture or a tea? This discussion will be on use of the whole plant not the oil. Whilst some wormwood contains no thujone, this ketone could contribute to, for example, the nervine and antibacterial actions of wormwood. This has been suggested by Juteau et al (2003), who found that non-thujone containing samples of volatile oil showed no antibacterial action (three bacteria) and only moderate inhibition of two yeasts. Antibacterial action was also associated with a higher concentration of thujone in the two oils tested (five bacteria, including *Pseudomonas aeruginosa*) but other constituents were also active (Blagojević et al 2006).

A shadow has been cast over wormwood because of the debate on the safety of the alcoholic drink Absinthe, which is distilled using wormwood. Absinthe is distilled from a macerate of *Artemisia pontica* and *Artemisia absinthium* and other herbs, often aniseed and fennel and sometimes hyssop (Lachenmeier et al 2006a). It was developed in Switzerland and commercial production began in 1797 and increased such that the annual production in Pontarlier, France was estimated at 10 million litres in 1905 (Lachenmeier et al 2006a) where the main manufacturer was Pernod Fils (Lachenmeier et al 2008). It was banned in many countries by 1915 but is now available again (Thujone info 2009). There is substantial variation in quality and production methods, and quality assurance of Absinthe has been extensively reviewed by Lachenmeier et al (2006a).

Absinthe was considered to be associated with symptoms of 'absinthism' such as convulsions, hallucinations and sleeplessness (Lachenmeier et al 2006b). However, consumption of alcohol was very high in France (Padosch et al 2006). Strang (1999) argues that the role of ethanol poisoning in alcoholism was underestimated and this was the cause of symptoms thought to be due to Absinthe. The evidence for an association between psychiatric problems and Absinthe was hotly debated in the latter part of the 19th century by French physiologists (Luaute et al 2005). Absinthe was banned after a determined campaign by the temperance movement in France, who sought to decrease consumption of alcohol, and claims that Absinthe exacerbated epilepsy were used to support this campaign. These claims were based on the clinical experience of the main protagonist Dr Valentin Magnan and on his subsequent use of crude animal experiments in public demonstrations (Luaute et al 2005, Padosch et al 2006). Dyes were also claimed to be the cause of symptoms associated with absinthe (Padosch et al 2006) and Lachenmeier (2007a) notes that some samples in his analysis of 23 present-day samples of Absinthe contained dyes not included on the label.

The connection with convulsions has excited added interest as it has been argued that the mental health problems of the artist Vincent Van Gogh (1853–1890) were associated with his excessive consumption of Absinthe, resulting in mood swings linked with exacerbation of temporal lobe epilepsy in the presence of an early limbic lesion (Blumer 2002). It has also been argued that the symptoms of Van Gogh could be explained by attacks of porphyria associated with excessive consumption of Absinthe and thus camphor (Bonkovsky et al 1992). The porphyrogenic action of terpenes, in particular camphor, was shown to be dose dependent in vitro and it was argued that consumption of 500 mL of Absinthe in a day could lead to a dangerous concentration of thujone (Bonkovsky et al 1992). The diagnosis of temporal lobe epilepsy for Van Gogh, on admission to hospital in Arles in 1888, tends to support the first of these two hypotheses (Blumer 2002).

The debate on the safety of Absinthe is controversial and coloured by different views on the reintroduction of the sale of Absinthe in Europe. Since the early 1990s Absinthe has been available again in Europe with a legal maximum of 35 mg thujone/kg of Absinthe (EEC 1988) in bitters and 10 mg/kg in alcoholic beverages with more than 25% volume of alcohol. Research to show whether different products comply with this ruling has revealed great variation in thujone concentration. In a sample of 23 current products, concentration of thujone was 0–70 mg/L (Lachenmeier 2007a). A review of 147 Absinthe products analyzed by four different centres found that 55% of samples contained under 2 mg thujone/kg Absinthe and 5% contained more than the legal limit of 35 mg/kg (Lachenmeier et al 2006b).

The concentration of thujone has been linked with the safety of Absinthe and therefore the concentration has been investigated in a range of samples. Results depend on the recipe, extraction of thujone and concentration of thujone in the source material. A study of 13 samples of vintage Absinthes found 0.5–48 mg thujone/L with a median concentration of 33.3 mg/L (Lachenmeier et al 2008). Interestingly, the highest concentrations were found in four samples of Pernod Fils Absinthe which had been manufactured before the ban in 1915 and were found to still contain 42–48 mg thujone/L. In another study, three different sources of wormwood were used to manufacture Absinthe according to three recipes. In the resulting nine samples of absinthe, the concentration of thujone was 0–4.3 mg/L and it has been argued that the concentration of thujone in pre-ban absinthes may have been low (Lachenmeier et al 2006b). Lachenmeier & Kuballa (2007) argue that some figures given are based on overestimates of thujone concentration due to use of theoretical figures or because of confusion of similar results for thujone and linalool in chromatography (Lachenmeier et al 2006a). Hyssop is also used in the manufacture of Absinthe and pinocamphone was found in 23 out of 32 samples but at concentrations considered safe (Lachenmeier et al 2008).

The sources above show that the oil and absinthe vary significantly in composition and thujone concentration but Lachenmeier et al (2006b) assert that consumption of absinthe does not produce a dangerous thujone intake. Padosch et al (2006) review the literature on safety and question whether the excitatory action of thujone was the cause of absinthism. Lachenmeier (2007b) summarizes the argument and suggests that absinthe should be appreciated for its taste, not for its purported thujone content.

The references given above include detailed discussion of the safety of Absinthe, but how might the concentration of thujone in herbal medicines be estimated? The possible dose of thujone in a prescription of a tincture depends on variables such as the original concentration of volatile oil in the sample, which is likely to be highest in fresh plant material but will vary widely depending on the source. The extraction of thujone depends on the concentration of ethanol in the tincture and the time period of maceration. Gambelunghe & Melai (2002) prepared two tinctures of leaves from the same source: a maceration in 20% ethanol for 1 month yielded 0.2 mg/L beta-thujone, whereas a maceration in 95% ethanol for 6 months yielded 62 mg/L of beta-thujone. The amount and source of the wormwood is not given. A study comparing distillation and percolation found that no thujone was extracted during percolation in 30% ethanol (Tegtmeier & Harnischfeger 1994). We found no studies on extraction from fresh samples, but this could support the recommendation made by Cullen for a short maceration. To estimate the amount of thujone in a 1:5 tincture containing 200 g of herb in 1000 mL tincture, we used the values given in a summary of 29 reports where the mean concentration of volatile oil was found to be 0.5% (maximum 1.6%) and mean thujone was 18% (range 0–70.5%) (Lachenmeier & Kuballa 2007). Taking the mean of 18% thujone in 0.5% volatile oil, and complete extraction of the volatile oil (which is unlikely), a daily dose of 3 mL per day would give a mean daily dose of 0.56 mg of thujone, which Lachenmeier et al (2006b) argue is far below the level where adverse pharmacological effects would occur. The studies on Absinthe and thujone have been summarized very briefly in this discussion, but include substantial experimental data and discussion of the results. The conclusion is that the dose of thujone in a tincture may be low, and use of wormwood tincture can be recommended without concern.

## REFERENCES

Akhmedov IS, Kasymov SZ, Sidyakin GP 1970 Artabin – a new lactone from *Artemisia absinthium*. Chemistry of Natural Compounds 6:634.

Ariño A, Arberas I, Renobales G, et al 1999 Influence of extraction method and storage conditions on the volatile oil of wormwood (*Artemisia absinthium* L.). European Food Research and Technology 209 126–129.

Barker J (2001) The medicinal flora of Britain and Northern Europe. Winter Press, West Wickham, Kent.

Basta A, Tzakou O, Couladis M 2007 Chemical composition of *Artemisia absinthium* L. from Greece. Journal of Essential Oil Research. Online. Available:

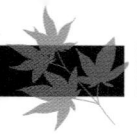

http://findarticles.com/p/articles/mi_qa4091/is_200707/ai_n19434085 28 April 2009.

Beauhaire J, Fourrey JL, Guittet E 1984 Structure of absintholide a new guaianolide dimer of *Artemisia absinthium* L. Tetrahedron Letters 25:2751–2754.

Behrens M, Brockhoff A, Kuhn C 2004 The human taste receptor hTAS2R14 responds to a variety of different bitter compounds. Biochemical and Biophysical Research Communications 319:479–485.

Bisset NG, Wichtl M (eds) 2001 Herbal drugs and phytopharmaceuticals, 2nd edn. Medpharm, Stuttgart.

Blagojević P, Radulović N, Palić R, et al 2006 Chemical composition of the essential oils of Serbian wild-growing *Artemisia absinthium* and *Artemisia vulgaris*. Journal of Agricultural and Food Chemistry 54:4780–4789.

Blumer D 2002 The illness of Vincent van Gogh. American Journal of Psychiatry 159:519–526.

Bonkovsky HL, Cable EE, Cable JW, et al 1992 Porphyrogenic properties of the terpenes camphor, pinene, and thujone: (with a note on historic implications for absinthe and the illness of Vincent van Gogh). Biochemical Pharmacology 43:2359–2368.

Bononi M, Giorgi A, Cocucci M et al 2006 Evaluation of productivity and volatile compound quality of *Artemisia absinthium* L. planted in Valle Camonica (Italy). Journal of the Science of Food and Agriculture 86:2592–2596.

Bown D 1995 Encyclopedia of Herbs. Dorling Kindersley, London.

Bradley PR 2006 British herbal compendium, vol 2. British Herbal Medicine Association, Bournemouth.

Burkhard PR, Burkhardt K, Haenggeli C-E, et al 1999 Plant-induced seizures: reappearance of an old problem. Journal of Neurology 246:667–670.

Canadanovic-Brunet JM, Djilas SM, Cetkovic GS, et al 2005 Free-radical scavenging activity of wormwood (*Artemisia absinthium* L.). Journal of the Science of Food and Agriculture 85:265–272.

Davis PH (ed) 1975 Flora of Turkey, vol 5. Edinburgh University Press, Edinburgh.

EEC 1988 Council Directive of 22 June 1988 on the approximation of the laws of the Member States relating to flavourings for use in foodstuffs and to source materials for their production 8/388/EEC. Online. Available: http://www.fsai.ie/legislation/food/eu_docs/Flavourings/Dir88.388.pdf 6 August 2008.

Deiml T, Haseneder R, Zieglgansberger W, et al 2004 [alpha]-Thujone reduces 5-HT3 receptor activity by an effect on the agonist-induced desensitization. Neuropharmacology 46:192–201.

Gambelunghe C, Melai P 2002 Absinthe: enjoying a new popularity among young people? Forensic Science International 130:183–186.

Green MH (ed) 2001 The Trotula. University of Pennsylvania Press, Philadelphia.

Guarrera PM 1999 Traditional antihelmintic, antiparasitic and repellent uses of plants in Central Italy. Journal of Ethnopharmacology 68:183–192.

Guarrera PM 2005 Traditional phytotherapy in Central Italy (Marche, Abruzzo, and Latium). Fitoterapia 76:1–25.

Höld KM, Sirisoma NS, Ikeda T, et al 2000 Alpha-thujone (the active component of absinthe): gamma-aminobutyric acid type A receptor modulation and metabolic detoxification. Proceedings of the National Academy of Sciences of the United States of America 97:3826–3831.

Jaenson TG, Palsson K, Borg-Karlson AK 2005 Evaluation of extracts and oils of tick-repellent plants from Sweden. Medicinal and Veterinary Entomology 19:345–352.

Judžentienė A, Mockutė D 2004 Chemical composition of essential oils of *Artemisia absinthium* L. (wormwood) growing wild in Vilnius. Chemija 15:64–68.

Juteau F, Jerkovic I, Masotti V, et al 2003 Composition and antimicrobial activity of the essential oil of *Artemisia absinthium* from Croatia and France. Planta Medica 69:158–161.

Kasymov SZ, Abdullaev ND et al 1979 Anabsin a New Di Guaianolide from Artemisia absinthium. Chemistry of Natural Compounds 15:430–435.

Kordali S, Kotan R, Mavi A, et al 2005a Determination of the chemical composition and antioxidant activity of the essential oil of *Artemisia dracunculus* and of the antifungal and antibacterial activities of Turkish *Artemisia absinthium*, *Artemisia dracunculus*, *Artemisia santonicum*, and *Artemisia spicigera* essential oils. Journal of Agricultural and Food Chemistry 53:9452–9458.

Kordali S, Cakir A, Mavi A, et al 2005b Screening of chemical composition and antifungal and antioxidant activities of the essential oils from three Turkish *Artemisia* species. Journal of Agriculture and Food Chemistry 53:1408–1416.

Lachenmeier DW 2007a Assessing the authenticity of absinthe using sensory evaluation and HPTLC analysis of the bitter principle absinthin. Food Research International 40:167–175.

Lachenmeier DW 2007b Estimation of thujone in pre-ban absinthe. Online. Available: http://www.gtfch.org/cms/images/stories/media/tb/tb2007/s430-438.pdf.

Lachenmeier DW, Kuballa T 2007 Behaviour of thujone during distillation and possible concentration ranges in pre-ban absinthe. Journal of the Science of Food and Agriculture 87:2147–2151.

Lachenmeier DW, Walch SG, Padosch SA, et al 2006a Absinthe – a review. Critical Reviews in Food Science and Nutrition 46:365–377.

Lachenmeier DW, Emmert J, Kuballa T, et al 2006b Thujone – cause of absinthism? Forensic Science International 158:1–8.

Lachenmeier DW, Nathan-Maister D, Breaux TA, et al 2008 Chemical composition of vintage preban absinthe with special reference to thujone, fenchone, pinocamphone, methanol, copper, and antimony concentrations. Journal of Agricultural and Food Chemistry 56:3073–3081.

Lopes-Lutz D, Alviano DS, Alviano CS, et al 2008 Screening of chemical composition, antimicrobial and antioxidant activities of *Artemisia* essential oils. Phytochemistry 69:1732–1738.

Luaute, JP, Saladini O, Benyaya J 2005 Toxicite neuropsychiatrique de l'absinthe. Historique, donnees actuelles. Annales Medico-psychologiques, revue psychiatrique 163:497–501.

Millet Y, Jouglard J, Steinmetz MD, et al 1981 Toxicity of some essential plant oils. Clinical and experimental study. Clinical Toxicology 18:1485–1498.

Mills S 1991 Out of the Earth. Viking Arkana, London.

Mills S, Bone K 2005 The essential guide to herbal safety. Churchill Livingstone, St Louis.

Mucciarelli M, Caramiello R, Maffei M, et al 1995 Essential oils from some *Artemisia* species growing spontaneously in North-West Italy. Flavour and Fragrance Journal 10:25–32.

Olsen RW 2000 Absinthe and γ-aminobutyric acid receptors. Proceedings of the National Academy of Science 97:4417–4418.

Orav A, Raal A, Arak E, et al 2006 Composition of the essential oil of *Artemisia* absinthium L. of different geographical origin. Proceedings of the Estonian Academy of Sciences 55:155–165.

Padosch SA, Lachenmeier DW, Kroner LU 2006 Absinthism: a fictitious 19th century syndrome with present impact. Substance Abuse Treatment, Prevention, and Policy 1:14 Online. Available: http://www.substanceabusepolicy.com 15 June 2009.

Perez-Souto N, Lynch RJ. Measures G, et al 1992 Use of high-performance liquid chromatographic peak deconvolution and peak labelling to identify antiparasitic components in plant extracts. Journal of Chromatography 593:209–215.

Sacco T, Chialva F 1988 Chemical characteristics of the oil from *Artemisia absinthium* collected in Patagonia (Argentina). Planta Medica 54:93.

Schulz V, Haensel R, Tyler VE 1998 Rational phytotherapy. Springer-Verlag, Berlin.

Strang J 1999 Absinthe: what's your poison? British Medical Journal 319:1590–1592.

Tegtmeier M, Harnischfeger G 1994 The influence of different extraction-proceedings on the amount of thujone in extracts of absinthii herba and thujae herba. European Journal of Pharmaceutical Sciences 2:127.

Thujone info 2009 Online. Available: http://www.thujone.info/index.html 22 June 2009.

Weisbord SD, Soule JB, Kimmel PL 1997 Poison on line – acute renal failure caused by oil of wormwood purchased through the Internet. New England Journal of Medicine 337:825–827 Erratum: 1997 New England Journal of Medicine 337:1483.

Williamson E 2003 Potter's Herbal Cyclopaedia. CW Daniel, Saffron Walden.

# CHAPTER 12
# *Artemisia vulgaris*, mugwort

## DESCRIPTION

**Family: Asteraceae**  **Part used: leaves, flowering tops**

*Artemisia vulgaris* L. is a vigorous, hardy, woody perennial found throughout Europe, although it is less common in the north. It is a commonplace weed in disturbed ground and waste places, where it forms dense stands. It is an aggressive weed in Canada, where it has spread rapidly as it propagates easily from small fragments of rhizome (Barney & Di Tommaso 2003). The *Flora of Turkey* (Davis 1975) gives 22 *Artemisia* species, including *Artemisia absinthium*, *Artemisia vulgaris*, *Artemisia santonicum* and *Artemisia abrotanum*.

Erect, branched, ribbed reddish stems (50–180 cm high) bear alternate, stalked, pinnately lobed leaves, which are smooth and green on the upper side and white and downy beneath. Upper leaves are unstalked, entire and lanceolate.

Dense, tapering panicles of inconspicuous, oval, rayless, reddish flowerheads (2–3 mm across) occur in July to September. Both leaves and flowerheads are very variable.

**Other species used:** Tarragon *Artemisia dracunculus*, southernwood *Artemisia abrotanum* (Bown 1995). A study in Italy of 14 wild *Artemisia* species found similar volatile oils in all but wide variation in concentration. *Artemisia abrotanum* was the only species to contain enderoperoxide, which is anthelmintic (Mucciarelli et al 1995).

### Quality

Mugwort becomes very woody and flowering tops should be collected as soon as they come into flower but not earlier as the concentration of volatile oil is higher during flowering.

We might rightly think that the English name for *Artemisia vulgaris*, mugwort, suggests some use for the plant in beer-making or as a substitute for tea. Indeed, both were done, according to Grieve: mugwort was a substitute for expensive tea among the working classes in 19th century Cornwall and the dried flowering plant was decocted with malt liquor and added to beer in the days before the introduction of hops into beer-making at the end of the 15th century. Since then, Grieve tells us 'until recent years, it was still used in some parts of the country to flavour the table beer used by cottagers'. Dodoens mentions casting the plant into barrels or hogsheads of beer to stop them going sour. Fernie (1897) has another interpretation, copied by Grieve, that mugwort is the wort or plant for moughte – moths or maggots – recalling the documented use of wormwood laid among clothes to prevent their being eaten by moths.

Pliny offers two origins of mugwort's Latin name artemisia: in honour of the goddess Diana (Artemis in the Greek pantheon), because of its special operation to cure diseases of women, or after Artemisia II, who was the wife of Mausolus (377–353 BC), ruler of Caria, a land in Asia minor now an area of southwest Turkey. The mythology of Artemis includes the story of her birth when, on emerging from the womb, she helped to deliver her twin, Apollo the sun god. In this way she became known as the goddess of childbirth, although she remained chaste ('parthenis' or virgin) and so childless herself. Her name was given to various members of the *Artemisia* genus because of their actions on the female womb and menstrual cycle (O'Dowd 2001). Artemisia II was renowned for her extraordinary grief at the death of her husband, entertaining no new husband but pining away until her death 2 years later. It was said that she mixed some of her husband's ashes into her daily drink. At Halicarnassus she had built a majestic burial tomb to her husband, which was considered one of the seven wonders of the world. The ruins of this mausoleum are to be found in modern Bodrum.

Turner affirms in his entry for mugwort that neither of the two kinds of this herb is the 'artemisia' of Dioscorides and Galen. Dioscorides has an entry for 'absinthion' or wormwood and another for 'artemisia' – the very name that mugwort is called in the Latin herbals of Turner's contemporaries. Dioscorides provides no description of absinthion because it is 'well known', but states that artemisia is similar to it, although with larger, shinier

©2009 Elsevier Ltd, Inc, BV
DOI: 10.1016/B978-0-443-10344-5.00017-3

THE WESTERN HERBAL TRADITION

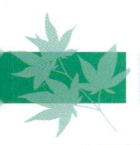

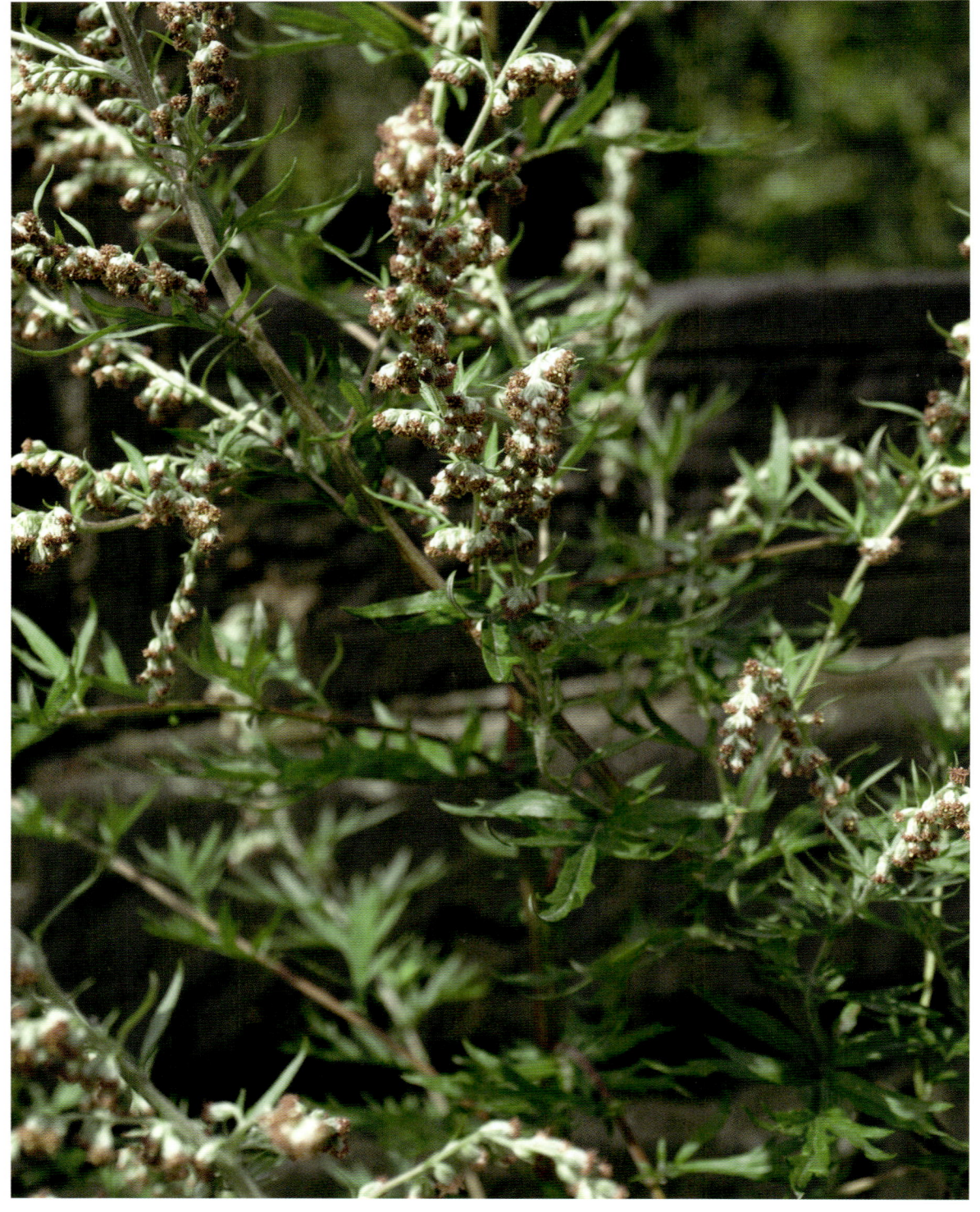

Figure 12.1 *Artemisia vulgaris*, mugwort (Yorkshire, August).

leaves. As to location, he says that artemisia grows, by and large, on coastal lands. It is known today that mugwort flourishes across the whole of the northern temperate region and is common in the southeast Mediterranean. Actually, Dioscorides (III 113) describes two kinds of artemisia: that with relatively broader leaves and a more delicate kind with narrower leaves and small white flowers oppressive in scent. Next there is reference to another herb found inland which some call by the same name, a small plant with a single stalk and slender stems full of yellowish flowers. In the next chapter (III 114) on ambrosia, a small shrub with numerous branches and leaves similar to those of rue surrounding the base of the stem, Dioscorides says that some call this artemisia too. This is clearly not mugwort but Beck identifies none of them as *Artemisia vulgaris*. Instead, the first, larger kind is designated *Artemisia arborescens*, also called wormwood, or mugwort, or sagebrush, a species common to Mediterranean areas; the smaller is *Artemisia campestris*, the field southernwood; and ambrosia is *Artemisia maritima*, a sea wormwood. Thus Beck is in agreement with Turner that Dioscorides does not describe mugwort among the Artemisias.

There are several hundred species of *Artemisia* identified today. The three artemisias listed one after another by Dioscorides, including the inland kind, are worthy of note according to Van Arsdall (2002), since three artemisias are also grouped together in *The Old English Herbarium*, although they do not correspond to the first three of Dioscorides. In the Anglo-Saxon text all three are styled mucgwyrt or mugwort, but they are identified by Van Arsdall, respectively, as *Artemisia vulgaris* or mugwort, *Tanacetum vulgare* or tansy and Artemisia leptofilos, a Greek name for field southernwood *Artemisia campestris*. Van Arsdall suggests that identification of each herb may have altered over the centuries to match where the compiler lived, since in any one area it is possible to find a number of *Artemisia* species, and a practitioner would have to learn which one was meant from one who knew the plants of that area.

It is clear that in attempting to identify the modern *Artemisia vulgaris* in historical texts, there is much opportunity for a confusion of names, not only among the many species of the genus, but also with those of the *Tanacetum* genus, namely tansy and feverfew *Tanacetum parthenium*. Tansy and mugwort both have erect stems and may have both been styled Artemisia monoklonos at one time or another. In the case of feverfew, to which the Greek name 'parthenion' is given in Dioscorides, the confounding of artemis/artemisia and parthenis/parthenion is possible. Moreover, feverfew is called matricaria by Parkinson and Culpeper but this name, meaning 'care of the mother/ womb', is included in Bauhin's alternative names for mugwort, along with parthenis. Mugwort is also designated mater herbarum or 'mother of herbs' by the Salernitan herbal and in Parkinson and Gerard, the latter adding that of the alternative names, 'most of these agree with the right artemisia, and divers of them with other herbes, which now and then are numbred among the mugworts'. Bauhin affirms that many different herbs were called artemisia in his time. Among them was another member of the Asteraceae, the Roman chamomile. For, tansy, feverfew and Roman chamomile share with mugwort heating and drying qualities, a bitter taste and gynaecological uses. It may be, as Van Arsdall indicates, that these plants too may have substituted for mugwort in different places and times.

Our central issue, however, is whether the artemisia of Dioscorides is mugwort. Fuchs in Germany shows no hesitation in accepting that the beyfusz of his country, called armoise by the French and Artemisia latifolia or broadleaved artemisia by the Italians, is the artemisia of Dioscorides, Galen and Pliny, and he quotes them exactly on the plant's medicinal actions. It is to be found in wet, uncultivated, rough places and should be gathered when in full flower. Dalechamps is equally confident of the identification, although the depiction in his herbal of armoise is not convincing. Mattioli, on the other hand, presents a much more lucid analysis of how he concluded the same. He recognizes the two coastal types of artemisia in Dioscorides as being very common in Tuscany: these mugworts are the same in terms of appearance, taste and smell, they share the same properties and only differ in size. Thus he is dumbfounded by the assertions of his fellow countryman and leading physician Antonio Musa Brassavola (1500–1555) that the smaller artemisia, which Dioscorides describes as oppressive in scent, is matricaria or feverfew, and that the artemisias may have a single stem like the inland plant mentioned by Dioscorides as being called artemisia by some. Thus Brassavola is guilty in Mattioli's eyes of expanding the two kinds of coastal artemisia into three separate species. Here lies the confusion between mugwort, the more strongly smelling feverfew *Tanacetum parthenium*, and the single-stemmed tansy *Tanacetum vulgare*, and it is confusion, says Mattioli, since feverfew flowers look nothing like those of mugwort and tansy is not a small plant like the 'third' inland kind of Dioscorides. Mattioli finds that Ruellius (Jean Ruel 1474–1537) is in agreement with him that the two coastal types are mugworts but Ruellius shares Brassavola's opinion that the third kind is tansy. The monks who have translated Mesue, says Mattioli, pass on both errors, that lesser artemisia is feverfew and the third kind is tansy and Fuchs is also found guilty of this mistake. Mattioli instead cites other 'diligent investigators of simples', very probably including specialists in ancient Greek language, who reckon that the third kind of artemisia is a later addition to the original text of Dioscorides and a simple error in Pliny, who confused it with ambrosia. As evidence for this assertion he notes that Galen, Paul of Aegina, Oribasius and Serapio cite Dioscorides but do not mention a third kind of artemisia. Furthermore, Mattioli's own collation of corrections based on the oldest manuscripts of Dioscorides and Oribasius generously made available to him by

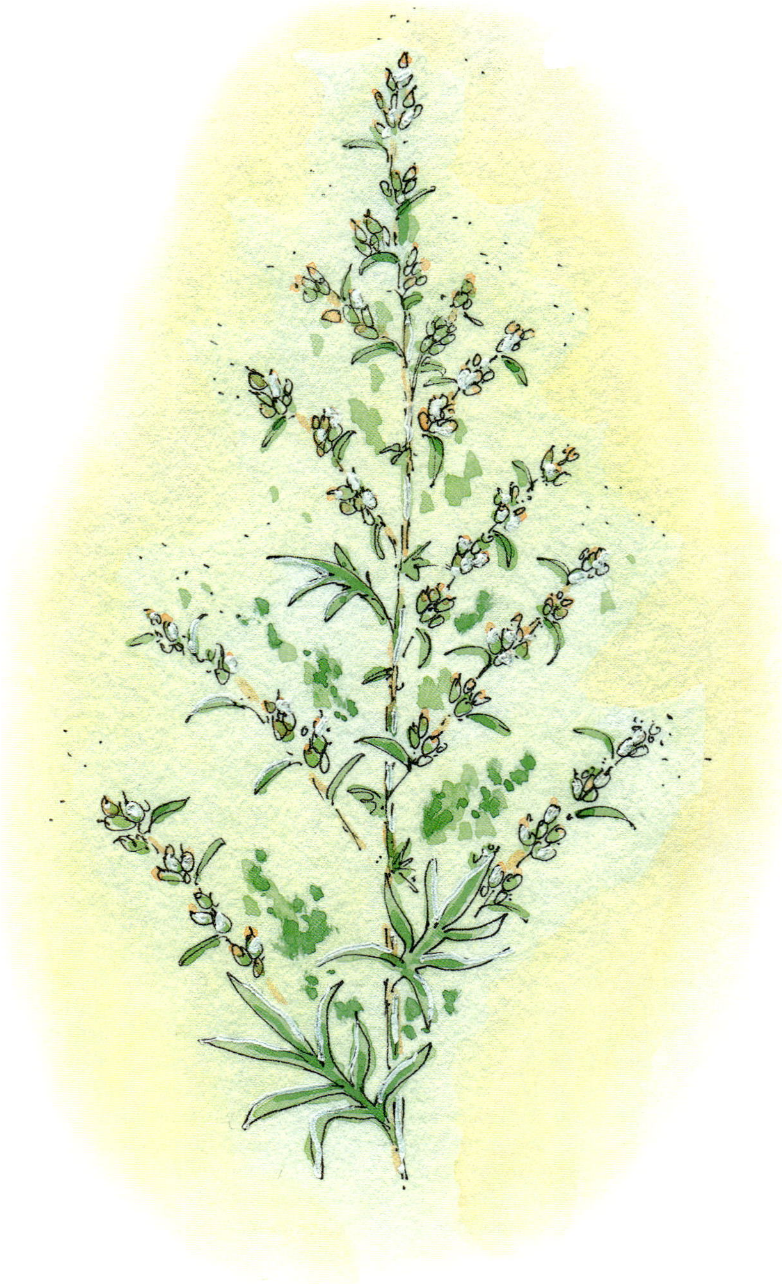

THE WESTERN HERBAL TRADITION

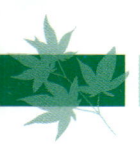

Figure 12.2 *Artemisia vulgaris*, mugwort.

Gabrielle Falloppio (1523–1562), chair of anatomy and surgery at the university of Padua, show that Dioscorides really only discusses two kinds of artemisia. This is apparent in Beck's translation of the standard edition of the Greek text (1906–1914) by Max Wellmann after a full census of extant manuscripts.

We might conclude, therefore, that if feverfew, tansy or Roman chamomile was substituted for mugwort at times, it is likely to be based on these errors of identification that have been passed down through modified versions of Dioscorides and a confusion of names in Apuleius, more than a knowledge of equivalent empirical effects. Mattioli has made the picture clearer but seemingly not to the satisfaction of Dodoens, who links armoise and beyfusz with the English mugwort but equates them with Artemisia leptofilos, the old Greek name for field southernwood mentioned above. Dodoens insists that this is also called Artemisia tenuifolia or narrow-leaved Artemisia in Latin, the fourth kind of artemisia in Dioscorides and the third in Apuleius! Bauhin explicitly rejects this attribution, following Mattioli that it is an insertion into Dodoen's copy of Dioscorides, where originally only the two kinds of Artemisia are described. Mattioli mentions Artemisia tenuifolia separately as a plant of field borders and by water channels that is good topically applied for stomach and joint pains. Dodoens has repeated these locations but more usefully adds that mugwort can appear in two colours: that with reddish stems and flowers, and another with green branches tending to white. In all other respects, they are the same. Gerard follows suit, and more ably describes the latter sort as having a darker green upper surface of the leaves and a hoary or greyish-white colour underneath. He adds his own third kind, which has a pleasant smell similar to that sea southernwood and a whitish appearance all over, and grows by the sea around Rye and Winchelsea castle and at Portsmouth. Parkinson prefers to distinguish between greater and lesser mugworts, both of which may have green stems and leaves that are green on the upper surface and hoary below, or equally with red stems and more deeply coloured flowers. Both kinds are to be found in various places, by waysides and small water courses, but the small mugwort far less often. The common mugwort is called *Artemisia vulgaris*, he says, because it is found in many countries (this has been italicized as it is a current binomial, although Parkinson was writing before Linnaeus). Culpeper simply copies word for word Parkinson's description of mugwort and his presentation of its medicinal virtues, only adding that it is ruled by Venus. Bauhin seems to accept the artemisia with larger shinier leaves from Dioscorides as the mugwort of his day and he exactly cites Dioscorides, Pliny and Galen on the actions and indications of artemisia, its location by the sea, and adding also the recommendation of Hippocrates that if the placenta is not delivered after childbirth, then artemisia is better than all other herbs to effect this. He then rather cautiously concludes 'but even if it [artemisia/mugwort] does not correspond at all to the history of the Greeks concerning artemisia, and this cannot be confirmed by any author, it should nevertheless not be completely rejected, for the power of artemisia [mugwort] is very great in gynaecological matters'.

## A GYNAECOLOGICAL REMEDY

So what do our classical writers say about the uses of artemisia in gynaecology and do those attributed to mugwort differ? Dioscorides recommends a decoction of the herb in a bath to draw down the menstrual blood and to bring out the foetus and the afterbirth. This is achieved by a warming and thinning effect, which could also procure an abortion. A pessary made from the juice of artemisia mixed with myrrh *Commiphora molmol*, or three drachms (12 g, increasing to 15 g in Ibn Sina's entry) of the leaves given in drink will similarly draw out the menstrual blood or contents of the womb. The herb liberally plastered onto the lower abdomen will bring on a period and the decoction added to the bath water will treat uterine closure and inflammation. Pliny mentions only the pessary as cleansing for the uterus, with oil of iris or figs as a substitute for myrrh. Galen records that both artemisias have a heating effect in the second degree or above and are moderately drying in the first or second degree. They are of thin parts and can be used for fomentations of the uterus. Apuleius mentions no gynaecological uses and may be writing of Mattioli's Artemisia tenuifolia instead.

Having cited the classical texts, Bauhin moves to describe the gynaecological uses commonly known in his time for Artemisia rubra or 'ruddy' mugwort, seemingly one of the kinds of mugwort described by Dodoens, Gerard and Parkinson above. He regards the qualities of mugwort to be extremely hot and dry in the fourth degree, and cites the Salernitan Platearius on this matter. Also like the Salernitans, he recommends the leaves above the root and the fresh herb over the dried but the Salernitan text suggests finding mugwort in sandy places, mountains and gardens rather than only by the sea. Bauhin cites Brunfels concerning a decoction of the plant with mace *Myristica fragrans*, an elaboration on Dioscorides, taken two or three times daily for heating the female organs, stimulating suppressed menses and expelling the afterbirth 'and whatever bad things adhere to these parts'. This may include the tumours which Macer mentions. The distilled water taken as regularly will effect the same, and a wine made from mugwort approaches the strength of pennyroyal *Mentha pulegium* in treating these conditions. Bauhin also draws on the Salernitan herbal for a use of mugwort against sterility due to dampness, and warns that if the problem is due to dryness then giving mugwort will worsen the condition. We can understand this by recalling that one of Galen's causes of dryness in the body is the use of heating foods and medicines and mugwort is a heating herb. The Salernitan text explains that it is possible to decide whether to give 'arthemisia' (mugwort) or not from the woman's complexion: if she is fat, then an excess of moisture in the womb is supposed the cause of her sterility, whereas a lean body suggests that an imbalance of dryness is at the root of her problem. The Salernitan text called *Trotula* on the treatment of women (Green 2001) makes a preliminary statement that women may be divided into two groups: those requiring heating medicines and those requiring cooling ones. The two types are to be discerned by use of a piece of lint the size of a little finger, moistened with oil of pennyroyal or laurel or another hot oil, tied round the thighs with string and inserted into the vagina at night. If it is drawn further inside, then it indicates a cold womb; if it is expelled overnight, then it testifies to the heat of the womb. Suitable treatments for a womb that is too hot and dry include marshmallow *Althaea officinalis*, violets *Viola odorata* and roses in water. Heating medicines should be contraindicated for women with a reduced fecundity due to dryness. For sterility due to moisture Bauhin wants an electuary or thick syrup to be made, whose recipe lies in the Salernitan herbal: equal parts of powdered mugwort leaves, astringent bistort root *Polygonum bistorta* and heating nutmeg *Myristica fragrans* are cooked with honey to the right consistency, then added to a decoction of mugwort. The Dioscoridean hot compress of mugwort leaves over the womb, or of an oil made from them, or a decoction in a bath with the addition of bay leaves are also listed in the Salernitan text, with a comment that these are to be preferred to the electuary.

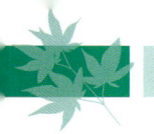

According to the Salernitan herbal, if a woman drinks 'arthemisia' decocted in wine, she will not give birth prematurely. This may imply that she is pregnant when she takes the drink. Macer's herbal warns that arthemisia causes abortion, as does the 17th century translation of Dioscorides by John Goodyer (1934) while the original Greek text is more open to interpretation. However, it is not unreasonable to conclude that if a herb can cause the menses to flow, it can bring on a miscarriage of a foetus, for 'an emmenogogue is an agent that stimulates the menstrual function: thus, if there is a pregnancy, an emmenogogue will also cause an abortion' (Riddle 1991). It may be that the Salernitan writer means such a drink to be taken only by those women whose wombs were sufficiently moist and slippery as to risk miscarriage, in which case 'arthemisia' will dry up the superfluous moisture or, as we might understand it, bring a lax uterus into tone and strengthen its retention of the foetus. Given to a woman without such superfluous moisture or laxity, 'arthemisia' may cause overcontraction of the womb and expulsion of the foetus.

The compress or fomentation of Dioscorides has slight elaborations in other texts: Dalechamps suggests that mugwort can be mixed with barley flour and applied to the belly; in Macer it is mixed with red wine or simply tied onto the belly overnight; Parkinson recommends that it is mixed with other herbs and decocted and that the woman then sits over a bowl of the steaming liquid to promote menstruation, facilitate labour or expel the afterbirth. A remedy for difficult parturition in the *Red Book* of the physicians of Myddfai states that fresh mugwort must be bound to the left thigh of a woman unable to give birth to her child, but it must be removed as soon as she has delivered, lest it cause haemorrhage.

To sum up the gynaecological uses of mugwort, our authors up to the end of the 17th century do not stray from the indications given by Dioscorides: to provoke suppressed menstruation, to facilitate labour and the expulsion of the afterbirth and to cleanse the womb in the treatment of uterine diseases and perhaps, for women of a certain temperament, as a preparation for conception and as protection against miscarriage. The principal use of mugwort is for female complaints, writes Quincy, so that it is held in the highest esteem by midwives and nurses, while later in the 18th century both Miller and Hill only mention its use for promoting menstruation, and for distempers of the female sex such as hysteric fits or the vapours. The leaves are used in infusion or the official syrup of Artemisia is given. Wren reaffirms its employment as an emmenogogue for obstruction of menstruation, usually in combination with pennyroyal *Mentha pulegium* and southernwood *Artemisia abrotanum*, both emmenogogues, in an infusion of 1 oz of herbs to 1 pint of boiling water, taken in wineglassful doses, variously measured as $1\frac{1}{2}$ to 2 fl oz or three to four tablespoons, approximately 45–60 mL. Hool advises mugwort for an adolescent girl whose periods are delayed, although experience tells us that menarche occurs at different ages and the judgment that menstruation is delayed is better not made too quickly. The National Botanic Pharmacopoeia includes painful menstruation as an indication, as does the British Herbal Pharmacopoeia, which also specifies delayed or irregular menstruation and functional amenorrhoea, at a dose of 0.5–2 g of the dried herb three times daily, with large doses to be avoided.

John Stevens, an associate of Coffin and active in political work advancing the cause of herbal medicine in mid-19th century England, notes that cold is very frequently the cause of period pain and that heat will generally remove it (Stevens 1847). He therefore advocates the regular Thomsonian treatment, including a vapour bath, and this he asserts will in most cases be effective when these distressing affections occur. He also recommends that the woman sits over the steam of a strong decoction of mugwort, and foments her abdomen with hot bitter herbs, such as wormwood, tansy and hops. Injections into the vagina of warm mugwort and yarrow tea can also be beneficial. This approach echoes the methods of Dioscorides, Trotula and Parkinson already discussed, but the tea to be drunk in wineglassful doses during the distressing symptoms is formulated along Thomsonian lines: equal amounts of mugwort, pennyroyal *Mentha pulegium* and thyme *Thymus* species in infusion, to which is added guaiacum *Guaiacum officinale* ¼ oz and the same amount of a specific formula ('no.6 rheumatic', composed of 16 oz myrrh *Commiphora molmol* dissolved in one gallon of brandy in a water bath with 1 oz cayenne pepper *Capsicum minimum* added).

A current view recommends emmenogogues such as mugwort not only to stimulate menstrual flow and function but 'in a wider sense to indicate a remedy that normalizes and tones the reproductive system' (Hoffmann).

Artemisia is not limited in use to acting as an emmenogogue. Dioscorides states that it breaks urinary stones and remedies retention of urine. Pliny affirms the same, for which the herb should be given in sweet wine, and adds that it protects him who carries it on his person from witchcraft and sorcery, poison and venomous beasts, particularly toads, and will prevent a traveller from feeling fatigue on his journey. Taken in wine, it will counteract an excessive dose of opium. Of these indications Galen mentions only kidney stones. Apuleius gives the use of Artemisia for travellers and as a protection against all evil, but states its benefits for digestive pains when taken in water and honey, while pounded in fat and rubbed onto the feet, it takes away their pains.

The four uses cited in Apuleius are repeated in the *Old English Herbarium*. Hildegard picks up the use for the digestion: mugwort, she says, is very hot and its juice is of great value, healing ailing intestines and warming a cold stomach. It is particularly useful when a person has eaten rotten food or drink and has abdominal pains. In this case he should eat the pureed plant, or take it with meat or lard, and it will draw to itself and purge the offending substance. Likewise, the expressed juice of mugwort made up with honey can be laid on to discharging wounds, covered with egg white and tied with cloth, and repeated until the corruption is resolved. Macer says that mugwort comforts the stomach. The Salernitan herbal suggests powdered mugwort in mead for abdominal pains due to cold, or else pine resin vapour should be introduced into the lower regions of the body, followed by sitting over a tile on which mugwort is heated.

This use of mugwort for the digestion, passing down through the Middle Ages from the herbal of Apuleius, is mentioned very little among Renaissance writers. Mattioli writes separately of Artemisia tenuifolia, crushed into almond oil and rubbed onto the stomach to ease pains there. This application is repeated by Dodoens, who gives his mugwort the same Latin name, and by Gerard, who does not, suggesting that Gerard may simply have copied Dodoens. Thereafter, no mention is made of mugwort for digestive problems in our authors for nearly 400 years (save for Hool who suggests an infusion drunk and a fomentation applied to the belly in cases of abdominal pain, and Grieve who cites a passage from Culpeper unknown to us). The *British Herbal Pharmacopoeia* gives poor appetite, nervous indigestion and intestinal worms as indications. Pelikan adds heartburn, hyperacidity and colic. Weiss, however, suggests that mugwort is superfluous for such purposes despite its volatile oils and bitter terpenoids when its close relative wormwood is available.

The indications of artemisia in Dioscorides for urinary problems are picked up by Renaissance and early modern writers but are rarely given much attention after Culpeper. The *Old English Herbarium* attributes relief of urinary retention to another mugwort, that is tansy. In the 19th century Fox says the infusion of mugwort promotes perspiration, urine and menstruation, and is good for hysteric fits. Diaphoretic and nervine tonic actions are listed in the National Botanic Pharmacopoeia, while Grieve emphasizes the herb's effect on the nervous system above diuretic and diaphoretic actions. An infusion of 1 oz of mugwort to 1 pint of water, she says, taken warm in half-teaspoonful doses for fevers and the common cold, which Hool says will be dealt with speedily when taken in half-teacup doses, becomes a tonic for them both when taken cold three times daily, owing to its bitterness and aromatic character. In support of its use for palsy and epilepsy, Grieve cites Gerard: 'it cureth the shaking of the joints inclining to the palsie', but the full quotation in Gerard continues 'and helpeth the contraction or drawing together of the nerves and sinewes'. In fact Grieve is only copying Fernie's (1897) partial quotation of Gerard; at least she does not go as far as he in suggesting that mugwort is scentless because it contains no volatile oils.

Gerard's misquoted assertion may be simply a re-interpretation of Dioscorides' use of mugwort for joint problems: he recommends that for blood hardening around joints, the stems of the plant should be boiled with oil of roses and the sick man rubbed all over with this liquid before sleep. In Dodoens this same preparation cures the ache, shaking and drawing together of the sinews. Parkinson repeats Bauhin's proposal of a warm decoction of mugwort, chamomile *Matricaria recutita* and agrimony *Agrimonia eupatoria* to bathe the joints and remove pain in the sinews and cramp, while Apuleius recommends an ointment of mugwort for pains in the feet. Hool also recommends mugwort for rheumatism and gout: to subdue inflammatory swelling, bathe the part for 1 hour in a hot infusion, then apply a poultice of chickweed *Stellaria media* or slippery elm *Ulmus fulva*. Bruises, poisoned hands or wounds, whitlows, abscesses, carbuncles, even tumours are amenable to this topical treatment if, he says, it is persevered with.

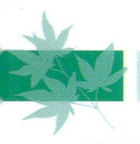

## NERVOUS AFFECTIONS

There are writers other than Grieve who consider mugwort a nervine. Ibn Sina records the benefit of artemisia in headache due to a cold cause and in nasal catarrh while the Salernitan herbal, reflecting Arabic influences, recommends a hot opiate taken with a decoction of artemisia for migraine. Bauhin cites the empiric Wirtemberg, who guarantees relieving within an hour a headache due to cold by washing the head with a decoction of mugwort in wine, then laying on the hot leaves. This is a version of a cure for migraine from Arnold de Villanova, Bauhin points out, mentioning also that mugwort in wine or lavender water can be used in cases of paralysis. Other uses in Bauhin's day include inducing sleep, treating scabs on the head, clearing jaundice and preventing dropsy, and reversing prolapse of the anus. In this last case, the anus is first fumigated with myrrh *Commiphora molmol* and colophonia before a hot poultice of mugwort cooked in red wine is applied.

Quincy classifies uterine medicines under nervous simples, where these 'hysterics' must be differentiated from carminatives and from cephalics and cordials, now under one heading for 'what is cordial must be cephalic as the head hath a principal share in agreeable sensations'. The uterine medicines, notable for their strong scent and distinguishable by smell into odoriferous and foetid plants, are serviceable for menstrual obstructions, which cause a great many symptoms and can bring the whole system of the body into disorder: what were previously termed the 'fits' or 'rising of the mother', or 'suffocation of the womb'. Quincy states that where this has occurred through an irritation of the nerve fibres or 'titillation' of the senses, then those herbs which are offensive and disagreeable in both smell and taste – the very opposite of cordial medicines – are required to calm the excessive stimulation by virtue of a clammy and viscous substance which envelops and entangles the subtle juice of nerve fibres. A second condition he terms 'uneasiness of the womb', which may arise from the obstruction of regular menses or from the lodging of 'some disagreeable matter upon their glands', which can turn into tumours. 'Hysteric' remedies increase the force of circulating blood and render it thinner for easier flow in the required discharges, or by their detersive qualities 'open those glands and by degrees wear away obstructed tumours'. In his entry for mugwort, Quincy simply mentions its use for female complaints, without differentiation into irritation of the nerves or uneasiness of the womb. Certainly mugwort is strongly scented but not pleasant enough to put in a vase in the home. On this basis, it could be considered the opposite of cordial and a remedy to calm over-stimulated senses. Its heat and emmenogogue action fits it for treatment of uneasiness of the womb.

Current herbalists too suggest beneficial effects on the nervous system for uterine remedies such as mugwort: Hoffmann suggests it may ease depression and tension, perhaps due to the volatile oil content. Wood says it reduces tension and corrects a constrictive tissue state and cites LeSassier for its particular suitability for weak, sensitive women or those who have suffered abuse, poverty, obstetric injury, difficult pregnancies and damaging abortions, provoking a 'withdrawal of spiritual aspirations from the womb, from sex'. It is clear that these uses are not based on the same conception of action as that of Quincy's 'hysterics'. For the same reason, there is no mention of mugwort for pre-menstrual syndrome, a state which might have correlations with Quincy's 'titillation of the senses', but for which an imbalance of the female sex hormones is usually cited as the causal factor today.

Let us also consider briefly, for completeness and comparison, the old Hippocratic concept of the wandering womb as recorded by *The Trotula*. 'Suffocation of the womb' occurs when the womb is drawn upwards, causing stomach upset and loss of appetite from overwhelming frigidity of the heart. There is sometimes even syncope, when the pulse vanishes. At other times, the woman may become doubled-up or so contracted that her head is drawn to her knees; she may suffer loss of vision and speech, her nose distorted, the lips contracted, she grits her teeth, and the chest is elevated upwards. It happens because corrupt female seed abounds excessively in her body and is converted into a sort of poison. A cold vapour ascends to organs nearby, such as the heart and lungs, causing the above symptoms. To draw the womb back into place, foul smells are put to the nose to repel the womb, and the woman's vagina is anointed inside and around with pleasantly scented oils to attract the womb back into place. The womb may also descend out of place, causing a weakening of ligaments and an abundance of cold humours. This could arise from cold air entering the body from below, from walking on cold stone, from a cold bath, or from giving birth. Treatment is the opposite, with pleasant scents applied to the nostrils and unpleasant things to the womb. For prolapse, the belly is anointed with aromatics mixed with wormwood, being applied with a feather. Culpeper later recommends the use of burdock leaves *Arctium lappa* to effect these treatments, while Cook, in his *Woman's Herbal Book of Health* of 1920, warns of walking on cold floors in bare feet and identifies many female complaints as due to cold, for which his remedy was pennyroyal *Mentha pulegium* tea freely. Cook could not believe that the womb was able to wander around the body troubling other organs, but the aetiology and 'symptom-picture' could remain, leading to a remedy of which the author of *The Trotula* would have approved.

The mention of mugwort used as moxa is not found in our authors before the 18th century, when Quincy names Sir William Temple in connection with it, and Miller talks about it as a famous cure of gout. This use continues today. Conversely, the antidoting of opium by mugwort disappears with Culpeper, despite the use of laudanum in the 18th and 19th centuries, except as one of a long list of indications in Menzies-Trull and a mention in Wood. Its use against poison in a metaphorical sense, warding off evil, protecting the wearer against harm and the evil eye has been persistent in folklore. Mabey (1996) records a sprig of mugwort being worn to this day as a charm at the annual open-air parliament on Tynwald Hill on the Isle of Man. Among practitioners of plant-spirit medicine, mugwort is a key herb. Brooke (1992) associates mugwort with clairvoyant powers, the ability to see clearly, and with creativity and self-expression. Richter (2002), in an article we have not yet accessed, points out that mugwort is regarded as a magical plant by the Teutonic peoples and the Anglo-Saxons. Its name 'mater herbarum' or mother of herbs speaks not only of its place in the first rank of gynaecological and urological herbal medicines, but also of its protective or apotropaic characteristics valued in Christianity. (Fernie (1897) says that mugwort is mistakenly named mother of herbs by Macer but we have not found the Latin words he cites.) The Salernitan herbal says mugwort combats bad thoughts and devils flee from the plant. Bauhin relates some of the magical practices he has witnessed: garlands of mugwort are worn on St John's eve then cast into the midsummer fire as misfortune is cast off the wearer, thus the plant is called St John's crown, portions of old dead roots called 'coals' and dug up from under the roots of mugwort are worn as a protection against epilepsy and fevers, Jacob Vallich commends mugwort to ward off the devil, and mugwort and sage can be carried on the person to prevent tiredness on a journey. This last of course is an elaboration on Pliny. The Myddfai physicians counsel an egg-shell full of the juice of mugwort and garlic taken in the morning to ensure neither hurt nor tiredness on the journey, whatever distance is walked. The common denominator here is mugwort. The English herbalists Gerard and Parkinson cannot suffer these superstitions. Gerard talks of the 'fantastical devices invented by poets' seen in the ancient writers which tend to witchcraft and sorcery and the great dishonour of God. He refuses to repeat them, whereas Parkinson cites Bauhin's 'idle, superstitious and irreligious relations' although it is 'both unseemly for me and unprofitable for you' to repeat them, before he laments on 'the weake and fraile nature of man!'

To sum up, the main action of mugwort is as an emmenogogue, however, Bradley (2006) cites a single study on mice in which mugwort did not demonstrate a uterine stimulant effect. Mills and Bone suggest that 'probably the most frequent indication for such remedies in earlier times was to bring on delayed menstruation; in other words, many 'emmenagogues' were used for birth control, as abortifacients'. This is particularly so, claims Riddle (1991), when the herb is said to expel the dead foetus, 'a common circumlocution for abortion'. In our sources there is no mention of a dead foetus, save for Wood's citation of Salmon in the late 17th century.

Mugwort as a member of the Artemisia genus has bitter tonic effects and these may be additionally beneficial where the herb is prescribed primarily for gynaecological problems. For primary treatment of the digestive system, however, surely wormwood is a better choice. In broad terms, Wood wants mugwort as a restorative to the injured female nature and he cites Paracelsus: 'What is Venus but the Artemisia that grows in your garden?' Wormwood is given over to Mars by Culpeper.

There are nervine tonic effects attributed to mugwort. Hoffmann states simply that 'of the many plants that stimulate the menstrual process, some also have a tonic effect. Simply triggering menstruation implies nothing more than that'. Numerous claims for a wide range of conditions of the nervous system that mugwort can treat are listed in the negative monograph of the Commission E, but further research is needed to substantiate such claims.

I know of a colleague who has used mugwort to achieve a pregnancy in cases of unexplained infertility, in combination with pennyroyal and *tansy Tanacetum vulgare*. I have effected the same in a case of an overweight, that is, excessively cold and moist, female, at a dose of 10 mL per week of each herb, taken daily in divided doses.

Given the great variability of pharmacological constituents, fresh plant preparations of the flowering plant should be used where possible due to the higher concentrations of volatile oils at flowering. Also, from the point of view of safety, decreases in total terpene concentration with increase in leaf age correlate with decreases in phytotoxicity.

## RECOMMENDATIONS

- Use for delayed menstruation, functional amenorrhoea, dysmenorrhoea and pre-menstrual syndrome.
- In combination with tansy and pennyroyal in cases of unexplained infertility. In all gynaecological uses, mugwort is more appropriate in presentations with signs of cold and dampness.
- Mugwort also provides a bitter tonic action but where digestive problems are the primary indication, wormwood *Artemisia absinthium* should be preferred.

Dosage: The *British Herbal Pharmacopoeia* 500 mg to 2 g three times a day of dried aerial parts and notes that large doses should be avoided.

For unexplained infertility, 0.5 mL of the tincture mixed with 0.5 mL each of tansy and pennyroyal and with other supporting herbs as the prescribing herbalist regards as necessary three times daily for a period of treatment designed to facilitate conception.

The fresh herb gathered while in flower and the specific tincture should be used.

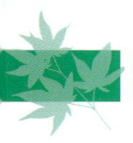

## CONSTITUENTS

Reviews: Bradley (2006), Linley (2002), Williamson (2003).

### Volatile oil

Total 0.2–0.4%, monoterpenes: sabinene 0–8.4%, alpha-pinene 0.1–12.9%; oxygenated monoterpenes: 1,8-cineole 2.6–17.6%, chrysanthenyl acetate 0–23.6%; ketones: alpha-thujone 0–12.9%, beta-thujone 0–20.2%; sesquiterpenes: germacrene D 5.3–15.5%, carophyllene 2.5–12.2% (wild, seven sites, Lithuania) (Judžentienė & Buzelytė 2006).
Monoterpenes; oxygenated monoterpenes: borneol 7–29%, 1,8-cineole 0.8–12.6%; ketones: beta-thujone 0–8.7%, camphor 0.8–55%, chrysanthenone 3–19%; sesquiterpenes: caryophyllene oxide 2–21% (France) (Jutea unpubl. In Jerkovic et al 2003).
Total 0.09–0.61% (81 compounds) monoterpenes: alpha-pinene 1.3–15.5%, alpha-phellandrene 0.4–12.9%; oxygenated monoterpenes: trans-chrysanthenyl acetate 0–24.6%, 1,8-cineole 4.6–16.6%; ketones: beta-thujone 5.3–20.8% (wild, four samples June–Sept, Croatia) (Jerkovic et al 2003).
Total 0.03–0.15%, oxygenated monoterpenes: borneol 5.6–27%, 1,8-cineole 0–15.1%, ketones: beta-thujone 1–9%, artemisia ketone 0–14.9%, camphor 2.3–12.9% (wild, four samples June–Sept, France) (Jerkovic et al 2003).
Monoterpenes: mycene 9–70%; oxygenated monoterpenes: vulgarole 3–25%, 1,8-cineole 0.5–26.8%, borneol 1.5–14.6%; ketones: beta-thujone 1.8–20%, alpha-thujone 0–5.7%, camphor 3.2–18.5% (wild, four sites, Italy) (Nano et al 1976).
Monoterpenes; oxygenated monoterpenes; ketones: alpha-thujone 56.3%, beta-thujone 7.4%, camphor 3% (wild, India) (Misra & Singh 1986).
Monoterpenes: camphene 9%; oxygenated monoterpenes: trans-verbenol 7%; ketones: camphor 47.7%; sesquiterpenes: beta-caryophyllene (wild, Italy) Mucciarelli et al 1995).
Total 0.06%, monoterpenes: sabinene 13.7%; oxygenated monoterpenes; ketones: beta-thujone 13.5%; sesquiterpenes: beta-caryophyllene (wild, Serbia) (Blagojević et al 2006).
Monoterpenes, irregular: artemisia triene, santolina triene; oxygenated monoterpenes: artemisia alcohol, santolina alcohol, santolinyl acetate; ketones: thujone 35%, camphor 30% (Näf-Müller et al 1981). The authors associate the irregular monoterpenes with the fragrance of the oil.
In a study which identified 135 compounds, vulgarole was identified as a characteristic compound that could be used to identify *Artemisia vulgaris* samples for quality assurance (commercial, Germany) (Wőrner & Schreier 1991, Wőrner et al 1991). Linley (2002) argues that vulgarole is not always reported but this may reflect the methods used in different studies.
Studies have shown wide variation in the presence of and concentration of volatile compounds (Blagojević et al 2006, Bradley 2006). For example, in the above studies the concentration of the ketones varies substantially: alpha-thujone 0–56%, beta-thujone 0–21%, camphor 0–55%. Concentration varies with time of year (Jerkovic et al 2003) and some studies found it to be higher during flowering (Nano et al 1976, Thao et al 2004). Leaf and flower oils were found to be similar (Thao et al 2004).

### Sesquiterpenes

Sesquiterpenes: Sesquiterpenes 3–25%; sesquiterpene alcohols 3–10% (wild, four sites, Italy) (Nano et al 1976).
Sesquiterpenes: eudesmane acids (fresh, wild, Germany) (Marco et al 1991).
Sesquiterpene lactones: yomogin, a eudesmenolide (cultivated, Philippines) (Tingo et al 2000).

### Polyphenols

Total 0.1%, flavonoids 0.04% (fresh leaves, cv. Green Boy, cultivated, Mauritius) (Bahorun et al 2004).
Hydroxycinnamic acids 6–9%: chlorogenic acid 0.8–1.3%, dicaffeoylquinic acids (flowering tops, 13 wild samples, 12 commercial, France) (Fraisse et al 2003).
Dicaffeoylquinic acids (flowering tops, wild, France) (Carnat et al 2000).

### Coumarins

Dracunculin (Murray & Stefanović 1986).

### Flavonoids

Quercetin, quercetin dimethyl ethers, quercetin trimethylether in all samples; also chrysosplenetin chemotype (nine samples), artemetin chemotype (11 samples) (wild, 40 populations, Bulgaria) (Nikolova 2006).
Flavonol: quercetin; flavone: apigenin (no luteolin) (cv. Green Boy, cultivated, Mauritius) (Bahorun et al 2004).
Quercetin and glycosides, kaempferol and glycosides, isorhamnetin (wild, Korea) (Lee et al 1998).

Flavones: Luteolin and glycosides, eriodictyol and glycosides, vitexin, apigenin and flavone methylethers (wild, Korea) (Lee et al 1998). The concentrations of luteolin and eriodyctiol were 10 times higher than for any other flavonoid.

## RECOMMENDATIONS ON SAFETY

1. Do not use in pregnancy and lactation.

Bradley (2006) suggests this caution is based on the traditional usage in amenorrhoea rather than on any studies, in which case the use of mugwort to prevent miscarriage in certain women could be a subject of research.

2. Do not use if the patient has an allergy to mugwort or other Asteraceae (see elecampane Chapter 20), birch, celery, hazelnut, kiwi fruit or peach.

Mugwort pollen is a common aeroallergen and mugwort 9-kd protein is homologous to birch (see wild celery). Some food allergens such as hazelnut, kiwi fruit and peach may also interact but this depends on the particular allergen (Pastorello et al 2002).

A study in Tenerife on 24 patients with asthma or rhinitis who were sensitized to mugwort found that 21 also had positive skin-prick test to *Matricaria chamomilla*, and 17 to other Asteraceae pollens. The authors suggest that sensitization to mugwort may be a major risk factor in reactions to teas made from chamomile (de la Torre Morín et al 2001). Allergies are argued to be associated with the western lifestyle but a recent study in four regions of China on 6304 people with asthma and/or rhinitis found that 72% were positive for skin prick tests to 13 common aeroallergens: 58% responded to dust mites and 11% to mugwort (Li et al 2009).

3. No *Artemisia* products should be used for chemoprophylaxis of malaria.

*Artemisia annua* has been shown to be useful in the treatment of malaria (de Ridder et al 2008) but not as a prophylactic. The active compound artemisinin has a short half-life (Balint 2001) and is not therefore suitable in prophylaxis.

A traveller to West Africa who used *Artemisia vulgaris* as prophylaxis developed malaria. An in vitro investigation showed that mugwort had no effect on parasite growth (Kurtzhals 2005).

## REFERENCES

Bahorun T, Luximon-Ramma A, Crozier A, et al 2004 Total phenol, flavonoid, proanthocyanidin and vitamin C levels and antioxidant activities of Mauritian vegetables. Journal of the Science of Food and Agriculture 84:1553–1561.

Balint GA 2001 Artemisinin and its derivatives: an important new class of antimalarial agents. Pharmacology and Therapeutics 90:261–265.

Barney JN, Di Tommaso A 2003. The biology of Canadian weeds. 118. *Artemisia vulgaris* L. Canadian Journal of Plant Science 83:205–215.

Blagojević P, Radulović N, Palić R, et al 2006 Chemical composition of the essential oils of serbian wild-growing *Artemisia absinthium* and *Artemisia vulgaris*. Journal of Agricultural and Food Chemistry 54:4780–4789.

Bown D 1995 Encyclopedia of herbs. Dorling Kindersley, London.

Bradley PR 2006 British herbal compendium, vol 2. British Herbal Medicine Association, Bournemouth.

Brooke E 1992 A woman's book of herbs. The Womens Press, London.

Carnat A, Heitz A, Fraise D, et al 2000 Major dicaffeoylquinic acids from *Artemisia vulgaris*. Fitoterapia 71:587–589.

Davis PH (ed.) 1975 Flora of Turkey vol 5. Edinburgh University Press, Edinburgh.

De Ridder S, van der Kooy F, Verpoorte R 2008 *Artemisia annua* as a self-reliant treatment for malaria in developing countries. Journal of Ethnopharmacology 120:302–314.

De la Torre Morín F, Sánchez Machín I, Garcia Robaina J, et al 2001 Clinical cross-reactivity between *Artemisia vulgaris* and *Matricaria chamomilla* (chamomile). Journal of Investigative Allergology and Clinical Immunology 11:118–122.

Fernie WT 1897 Herbal simples approved for modern uses of cure. Boericke & Tafel, Philadelphia. Online. Available: http://www.gutenberg.org.

Fraisse D, Carnat A, Carnat AP, et al 2003 Hydroxycinnamic acid levels of various batches from mugwort flowering tops. Annales Pharmaceutiques Francaises 61:265–268.

Goodyer J 1934 The Greek herbal of Dioscorides. In: Gunther R T (ed.) The Greek herbal of Dioscorides. Goodyer J (trans). Hafner, London.

Green MH 2001 The Trotula. University of Pennsylvania Press, Philadelphia.

Jerkovic I, Mastelic J, Milos M, et al 2003 Chemical variability of *Artemisia vulgaris* L. essential oils originated from the Mediterranean area of France and Croatia. Flavour and Fragrance Journal 18:436–440.

Judžentienė A, Buzelytė J 2006 Chemical composition of essential oils of *Artemisia vulgaris* L. (mugwort) from North Lithuania. Chemija 17:12–15.

Kurtzhals JA 2005 Ineffective change of antimalaria prophylaxis to *Artemisia vulgaris* in a group travelling to West Africa (Article in Danish). Ugeskrift for Laeger 167:4082–4083.

Lee S-J, Chung H-Y, Maier CG-A, et al 1998 Estrogenic flavonoids from *Artemisia vulgaris* L. Journal of Agricultural and Food Chemistry 46:3325–3329.

Li J, Sun B, Huang Y, et al 2009 A multicentre study assessing the prevalence of sensitizations in patients with asthma and/or rhinitis in China. Allergy 64:1083–1092.

Linley PA 2002 *Artemisia vulgaris*. In: Wright CW (ed.) Artemisia. CRC Press, London, p 39–48.

Mabey R 1996 Flora Britannica. Sinclair-Stevenson, London.

Marco JA, Sanz JF, Del Hierro P 1991 Two eudesmane acids from *Artemisia vulgaris*. Phytochemistry 30:2403–2404.

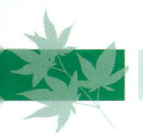

Misra LN, Singh SP 1986 α-Thujone, the major component of the essential oil from *Artemisia vulgaris* growing wild in Nilgiri Hills. Journal of Natural Products 49:941.

Mucciarelli M, Caramiello R, Maffei M, et al 1995 Essential oils from some *Artemisia* species growing spontaneously in North-West Italy. Flavour and Fragrance Journal 10:25–32.

Murray RDH, Stefanović M 1986 6-Methoxy-7,8-methylenedioxycoumarin from *Artemisia dracunculoides* and *Artemisia vulgaris*. Journal of Natural Products 49:550–551.

Näf-Müller R, Pickenhagen W, Willhalm B 1981 New irregular monoterpenes in *Artemisia vulgaris*. Helvetica Chimica Acta 64:1424–1430.

Nano GM, Bicchi C, Frattini C, et al 1976 On the composition of some oils from *Artemisia vulgaris*. Planta Medica 30:209–215.

Nikolova M 2006 Infraspecific variability in the flavonoid composition of *Artemisia vulgaris* L. Acta Botanica Croatica 65:13–18.

O'Dowd MJ 2001 The history of medications for women. Parthenon Publishing Group, London.

Pastorello EA, Pravettoni V, Farioli L, et al 2002 Hypersensitivity to mugwort *(Artemisia vulgaris)* in patients with peach allergy is due to a common lipid transfer protein allergen and is often without clinical expression. Journal of Allergy and Clinical Immunology 110:310–317.

Richter C 2002 Artemisia – Mother of all herbs. Zeitschrift fur Phytotherapie 23:68–80.

Riddle J 1991 Oral contraceptives and early-term abortifacients during classical antiquity and the Middle Ages. Past and Present N132:3–32.

Stevens J 1847 Medical reform, or physiology and botanic practice, for the people Birmingham: John Turner. Whittaker, London.

Thao NTP, Thuy NT, Hoi TM, et al 2004 *Artemisia vulgaris* L. from Vietnam: chemical variability and composition of the oil along the vegetative life of the plant. Journal of Essential Oil Research 16:358–361.

Tingo XT, De Guzman F, Flora AMTV 2000 Phytochemical analysis and hemodynamic actions of *Artemisia vulgaris* L. Clinical Hemorheology and Microcirculation 23:167–175.

Van Arsdall A 2002 Medieval Herbal Remedies: The Old English Herbarium and Anglo-Saxon Medicine. Routledge, London.

Wellmann M 1906–1914 Pedanii Dioscuridis Anazarbei De materia medica, 3 vols. Weidmann, Berlin.

Williamson E 2003 Potter's Herbal Cyclopaedia. CW Daniel, Saffron Walden.

Wörner M, Schreier P 1991 Multidimensional gas chromatography/mass spectrometry (MDGUMS): a powerful tool for the direct chiral evaluation of aroma compounds in plant tissues in mugwort (*Artemisia vulgaris* L.) herb. Phytochemical Analysis 2:260–262.

Wörner M, Pflaum M, Schreier P 1991 Additional volatile constituents of *Artemisia vulgaris* L. herb. Flavour and Fragrance Journal 6:257–260.

# CHAPTER 13
# *Centaurium erythraea*, centaury

## DESCRIPTION

**Family: Gentianaceae**      **Part used: aerial parts**

*Centaurium erythraea* Rafn. is a variable biennial or annual found throughout Europe, mainly on calcareous soils and dry grassy places, including sand dunes and chalky uplands (Gibbons & Brough 1992). There are about 14 species of *Centaurium* in Europe but there is disagreement over their identification and infraspecific hybrids occur which are also interfertile so the identity of local populations can be unclear (Tutin et al 1973). The *Flora of Turkey* (Davis 1978) gives five *Centaurium* species, including *Centaurium erythraea*.

Smooth, erect stems (10–50 cm) arise from a basal rosette of smooth, oval, greyish-green leaves and bear opposite, narrow, smooth stem leaves with three veins. Small, tubular, pink flowers with five petals occur in summer in a branched inflorescence at the top of the stem. Many small seeds form in cylindrical capsules and the anthers coil after dehiscence.

### Quality

Collect when in flower (Bisset & Wichtl 2001). Bradley (2006) states that the greatest bitterness is in two esters of sweroside found in the flower ovary. Wild collection should be avoided as calcareous grassland is a priority habitat listed on the UK Biodiversity Action Plan (2009). This annual plant is a priority for cultivation, especially as Cullen (1775) states that plants are larger and more bitter when grown on fertile soil.

Studies on the taxonomy of the Gentianaceae disagree (Meszáros et al 1996, Mansion & Struwe 2004) and there is debate on the number of species because of variation within species depending on environment. There is some hybridization between *Centaurium erythraea* and other species such as lesser centaury *Centaurium pulchellum*, which is a smaller annual with no basal rosette and fewer flowers often found on moist grassland near the sea, seaside centaury *Centaurium littorale*, which has distinctive narrow oblong leaves (Stace 1991) and is found in sandy turf and dunes, and perennial centaury *Centaurium scilloides*, which is distinguished by its procumbent habit with rounded, stalked leaves on the creeping stems, and is a rare plant found on cliff tops (Sterry 2006).

**Other species used:** *Centaurium uliginosum*, *Centaurium littorale*, *Centaurium pulchellum* (Van der Sluis & Labadie 1981). Culpeper also refers to a yellow variety with larger, darker green leaves and the stem passing through the middle of the leaf. This could be yellow wort *Blackstonia perfoliata*, an annual (Stace 1991) that is locally common on calcareous grassland. Culpeper also refers to a white flowered species, which could be *Centaurium tenuiflorum*, an annual and similar to *Centaurium pulchellum*, which is usually pink but rarely white. *Centaurium tenuiflorum* and *Centaurium scilloides* were both listed as vulnerable in the UK in 1994 (UK Biodiversity Action Plan 2009). *Centaurium erythraea* is listed as vulnerable and *Centaurium uliginosum* is listed as endangered in the Czech Republic, and *Centaurium erythraea* is listed as threatened by wild collection in Hungary (Lange 1998).

## LESSER CENTAURY, GREATER CENTAURY AND CHIRON, THE CENTAUR

Dioscorides (III 7) describes lesser centaury with an angular stem over a span long, resembling St John's wort or oregano, with flowers faintly purple like rose campion, small and longish leaves like rue, fruit like grains of wheat and a small useless bitter root. The use of comparisons is interesting: St John's wort *Hypericum perforatum* also has a smooth stem with small opposite leaves and a branched flowerhead. This description can be taken as common centaury. The only discrepancy is that, as Fuchs comments, according to Dioscorides, it grows in marshy places whereas 'everyone knows that with us it grows commonly in hard, dry, grassy fields and meadows'.

Dioscorides uses the name centaury for two plants: the lesser centaury and the greater centaury (III 6), which is a metre tall with blue flowers, serrated walnut-like leaves and a substantial red root. It is probably a knapweed in

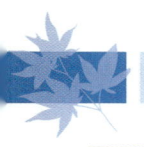

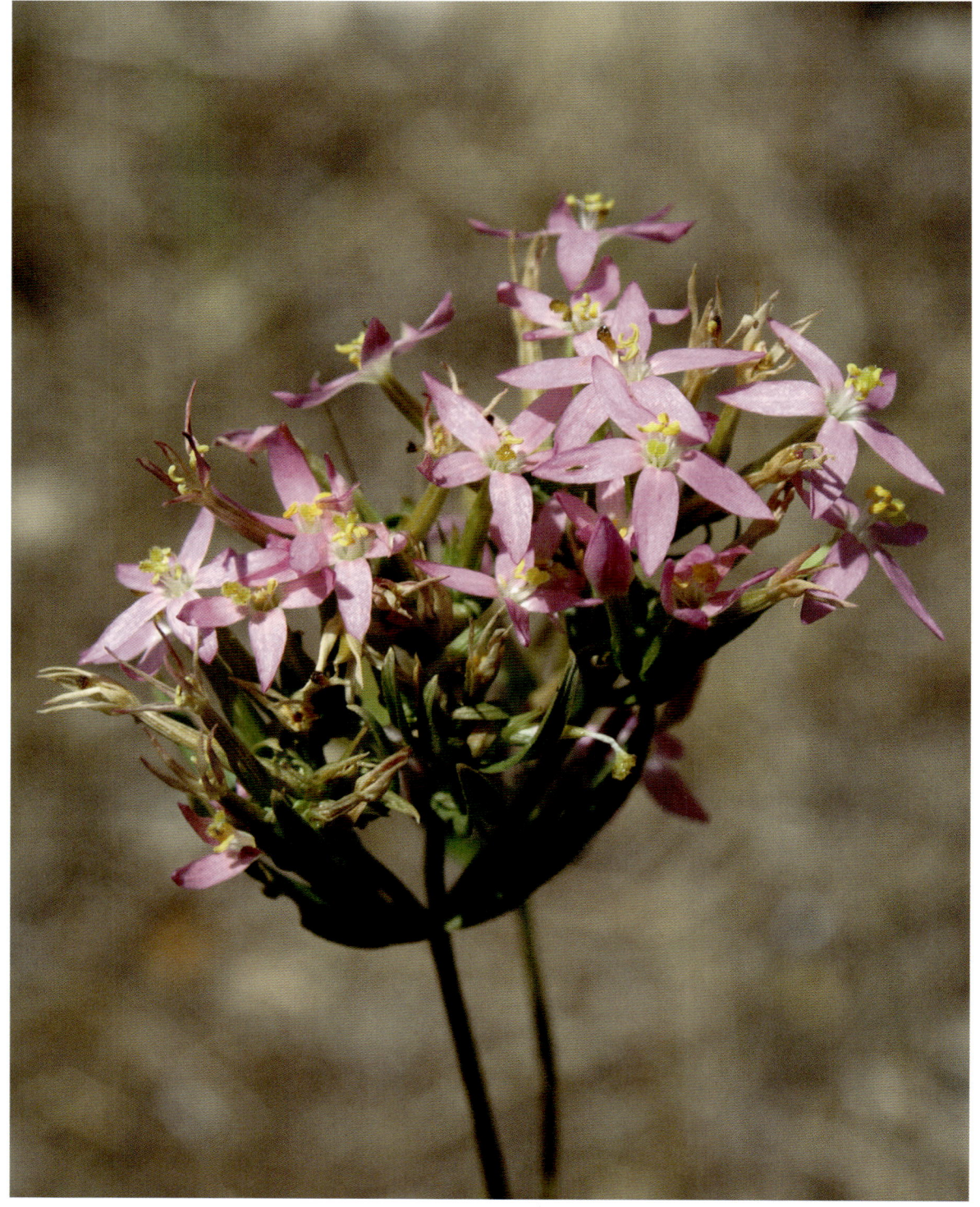

Figure 13.1 *Centaurium erythraea*, centaury (near Fondi, Italy, July).

the genus *Centaurea*. Lesser means the smaller of the two related plants, and this monograph discusses the use of the lesser centaury, which is now called common centaury and remains in use today. The illustration given by Fuchs is of centaury (1980) and later authors such as Culpeper and Miller continue to refer to 'the red ordinary small centaury'.

The two plants are very distinguishable but this introduces the possibility of confusion between the two entries in subsequent herbals. The listing of two unrelated species is significant as centaury is one of the four panaceas ascribed by Pliny to Chiron, the centaur who is the archetype of healers (Bostock 1855). The four panaceas were Asclepion, Heracleon, Chironion and Centaurion, and Dawson (1949) gives Centaurion as *Centaurea centaurium* L. The association with Chiron, the centaur indicates the long usage of these plants and associates both with wound healing. For example, in the Iliad of Homer, which describes the Trojan War, Eurypylos says, 'Cut the arrow out of my thigh … and put kind medicines on it, good ones, which they say you have been told of by Akhilleus, since Kheiron, most righteous of the Kentauroi, told him about them' (Theoi Project 2008).

Old ulcers that refused to heal were called Chironian, as if requiring Chiron himself to heal them (Dawson 1949). The connection is worth investigating as centaury was used by Chiron to treat what was ultimately his fatal wound, as he eventually died because of a wound that could not be healed. Chiron, the centaur 'half like a horse, half a god', was the son of Saturn (Cronos) and the nymph Philyra who was a daughter of Ocean. Chiron lived with his wife Chariclon in a cave on Mount Pelion in Greece and was the tutor of Asclepius, god of medicine, and reared Achilles (Dawson 1949). When Hercules was passing by on his labours in search of the Erymantian boar, Chiron was accidentally wounded by one of Hercules' poisoned arrows. One version states that he was wounded in the knee by an arrow meant for other centaurs and Hercules applied a healing herb, and another version states that Chiron dropped the arrow on his left foot by mistake. The arrow was poisoned with the blood or gall of the Hydra, and this fulfilled the prophecy of Chiron's daughter that he would long for death, although immortal, and his death would be caused by a serpent. Chiron was immortal and could not die, but was released from immortality by Prometheus, who offered himself to Zeus to be immortal in Chiron's stead.

The significance of these events as recounted by Ovid is heightened by the presence of Achilles, who mourns for his mentor, which links this archaic event with the events of the Trojan War (Brookes 1994). Brookes also comments that Ovid uses the word 'foot' rather than 'hoof' and notes the linkage with the eventual death of Achilles from an arrow-shot in the foot. He further notes a linkage with the eventual death of Hercules, who died on a pyre to escape the pain caused by a shirt sent by his wife Deianira. The shirt was smeared with the blood of the centaur Nessus, which was infected by the Hydra.

Returning to the recommendations of the mortals, greater centaury has a large, red astringent root and, comparing the two entries in Dioscorides, the emphasis is more on wound healing for greater centaury than it is for common centaury, and common centaury may not be the wound herb of Chiron. However, it is also strongly recommended for use in wounds. Mattioli argues that the Arabic writers confounded lesser and greater centaury and thus the texts are unclear, but later texts also lack clarity. Some authors consider them together whereas others give two entries.

## WOUND HEALING

The initial advice of Dioscorides on centaury is unclear as he refers to the 'small useless root' of common centaury but then recommends the pounded root as a plaster for injuries, and to cleanse old ulcers to form a scar. Mattioli cites Galen as stating that the root of lesser centaury is ineffective but the aerial parts are most useful. Galen states that the bitter quality permeates them yet there is a little astringency, which makes it an ideal drying medicine without being harsh or stinging: 'Therefore, large wounds are closed up by anointing of this fresh herb; and old ulcers which can hardly be induced to scar over, are scarred over by using it in the same way. Dried, it is put among the herbs with gluing and drying properties, those evidently which are destined by nature to heal sinuses and fistulas and soften old hardnesses, and to heal malignant ulcers'. Fuchs also cites Galen giving the same details, and the advice is repeated by Dodoens and in less detail by Gerard. Serapio writes similarly and advises common centaury for fistulas and indolent or deep ulcers either as the fresh plant or as the dried plant with emollient herbs. Ibn Sina describes the two centauries but does not distinguish in his recommendations. He states that centaury cleans fresh wounds and closes old ulcers, and that dried centaury is used in preparations for plasters for use in fistulas, including 'lacrimal fistulas'. This last recommendation for use in fistulas is also made by Dodoens, who advises the powder of dried aerial parts.

We find that Culpeper recommends the fresh herb bruised and applied to close up fresh wounds and for old ulcers and sores 'perfectly to cure them both although they are hollow and fistulous'. Later recommendations are less specific: Miller suggests external use in fomentations against swellings and inflammations. Quincy refers to the fomentation as discutient, dispersing morbid matter, whereas Coffin refers to use of a strong tea in scrophula (see the discussion under figwort, Chapter 28) and long-standing ulcers without specifying whether it be drunk or applied.

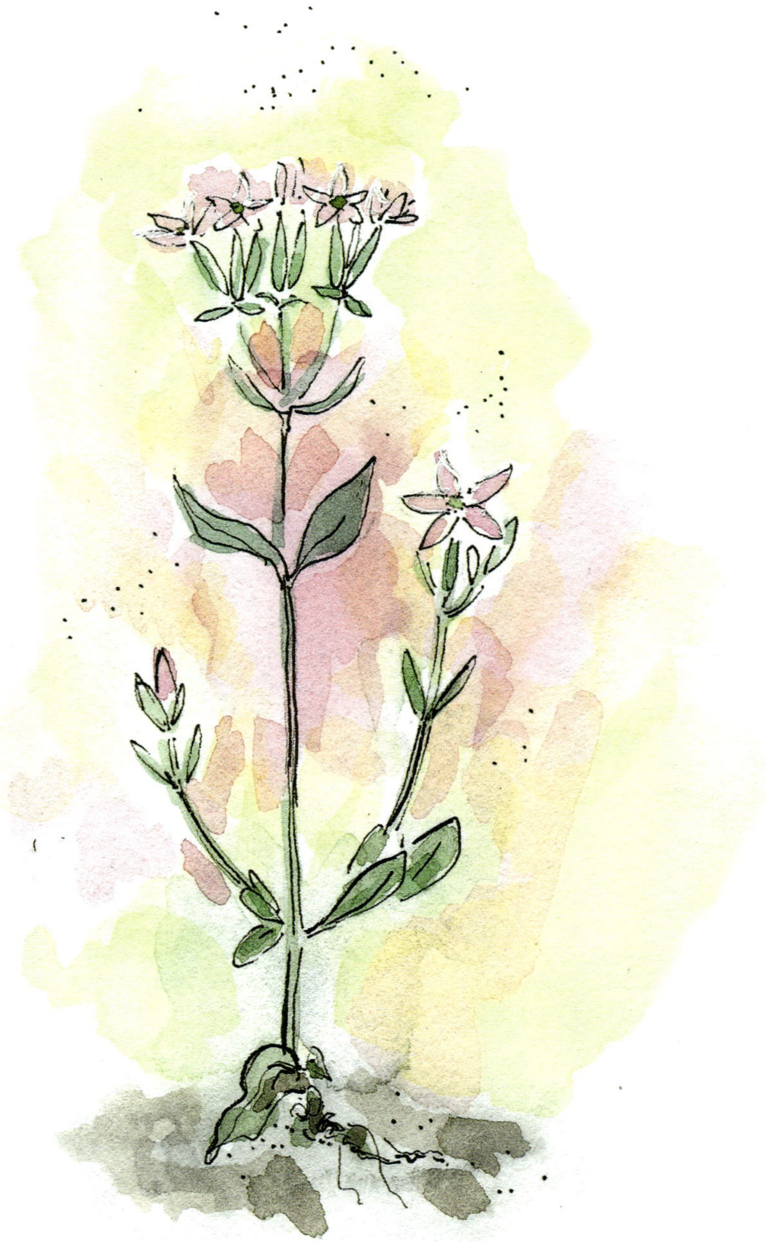

THE WESTERN HERBAL TRADITION

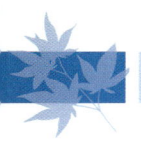

Figure 13.2 *Centaurium erythraea*, centaury.

Further external usages are explained by Dioscorides, who describes the preparation of juices from the aerial parts collected when in seed. The fresh herb is soaked for 5 days, boiled hard, strained and then boiled again until it reaches a honey-like consistency. Given the scarcity of centaury, and the difficulties of producing a sterile preparation, then this preparation would present some challenges. Dioscorides recommends the juice for eye conditions, cleansing with honey 'those elements that cast a shadow over the eyes'. This is repeated by Fuchs, citing Galen, and by Dodoens, Parkinson and Gerard. Another external recommendation that is hard to interpret is made by the Salernitan herbal, which recommends local application of the juice with leek juice for 'worms in the ears'. This could be otitis external or Beck suggests ear wax. This is also repeated by Parkinson, who recommends the decoction dropped into the ears to remove 'worms'. Culpeper repeats Parkinson and both recommend external usage for scabs, freckles and spreading scabs of the head. This is copied by Grieve and thus has been copied onto websites which give herbal information. The transmission of the texts is unclear and recommendations are not possible for this paragraph.

## 'HIP AILMENTS' AND MUSCULOSKELETAL CONDITIONS

The herb is consistently recommended both for external usage and internal usage and it is not always apparent which is being recommended. First I will discuss external and internal usage for muscular pain and arthritis, and then move on to internal use as a bitter, which is the most common usage today.

Dioscorides states that the decoction of the root is a suitable enema for hip ailments delivering blood and relief. Gunther (1933) gives this as 'a fit glister (enema) for the Ischiaticall, draweth out blood and easing the pain'. Serapio writes that the decoction is useful as an enema to treat sciatica as it expels choleric humours. Turner uses the text of Dioscorides and states that 'the broth is good for sciatica as it draweth the blood and easeth the pain'. Descriptions of hip pain sound more like osteoarthritis of the hip or septic arthritis than the use of the term sciatica today to describe pain extending from the hip down the leg. Fuchs, citing Galen, states that some pour the decoction on hip pains. Ibn Sina may shed more light on use in hip ailments as he advises centaury for muscle tears and the appearance of pus there. He advises use of an enema in sciatica, nerve pain and tears and that if blood comes out then this is beneficial. This version is more clear than in some authors and suggests that he means discharge of blood from the wound and thus cleansing of the wound. Gerard comments that although the ancient authors consider that centaury purges by stool, he has never found it so but has found it useful in sciatica. Some authors such as Dodoens suggest that blood in the stool is a useful result of treatment, which cannot be the case.

Dioscorides also advises the juice for 'ailments around the tendons', which is given as diseases of the sinews by Turner and Dodoens. Mattioli, citing Galen, states that it is counted among those which heal rheumatic afflictions, for which those medicines are best which are strongly drying and somewhat astringent but not too sharp. Fuchs gives this slightly differently, specifying that centaury is useful in rheumatic afflictions where vehement drying and astringent qualities are needed without any sharpness. These recommendations are followed by Parkinson and Culpeper with the addition of ague and old joint pains; 'with other things to dry up rheum'. The area around the joints was visualized as being stretched because of the flow of the phlegmatic humour into the area, and thus herbs were needed to dry up or promote the flow of this humour (Culpeper et al 1655). This links with the descriptions of temperament: centaury is described as hot and dry in the third degree by Ibn Sina, and hot and dry in the second degree by Dodoens and Culpeper.

Bauhin states that the pills are useful for those with sciatica, defects of the nerves and gout. Riviere (Culpeper et al 1655) discusses gout and its causes. The word 'gout' was used for gout as we understand it today, and also for pain in other joints, including sciatica or hip gout. Centaury continued to be used for gout and Grieve notes its use in the once famous Portland powder, which was a recipe purchased and published by the Duke of Portland (Thomson 1815). The powder contained equal portions of aerial parts of centaury, germander *Teucrium chamaedrys*, ground pine *Ajuga chaemapitys* and the root of gentian *Gentiana lutea* and birthwort *Aristolochia* species. Two of these ingredients are no longer used: *Aristolochia* species have been banned because of an association with kidney failure (MHRA 2003) and *Teucrium chamaedrys* has been associated with cases of serious hepatotoxicity linked with the use of slimming teas (Larrey et al 1992). The dose of Portland powder was 1 drachm (4 g) to be taken every morning, fasting for 3 months; then ¾ dram (3 g) for a further 3 months and so on for a year; then ½ dram (2 g) on alternate mornings for a further year. Buchanan and Kean (1987), however, cite Heberden as saying that this remedy rose too fast and fell too far.

There is a linkage between external usage in old wounds, in sciatica and disease associated with the tendons and with internal use for gout. Other bitter tonics such as bogbean *Menyanthes trifoliata* continue to be used internally in musculoskeletal pain. Ferrie (1897) refers to use of the hot infusion of centaury for muscular rheumatism.

Quincy suggests that some say it is febrifuge, especially in tertian fevers and Hill states that 'country people cure agues with it'. Again this usage appears to be based on the recommendation of Galen, who described it as evacuating the choleric humour from the body. Galen is cited by Dalechamps as linking use of the decoction for tertian fever with the action of expelling bile via the rectum. The French version of Mattioli adds to the discussion of centaury by proposing that the decoction helps greatly the tertian agues, for it makes bile leave downwards, and thus it is called febrifuge, 'chasse-fièvre'.

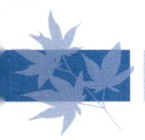

## BEST BITTER AND VISCOUS HUMOURS

Having looked at external application and usage for painful joints, we come to the main current usage of centaury, which is as a bitter. Employment as a bitter tonic with an influence on bile flow appears to have been continuous since the time of Dioscorides. This usage is continued into more modern texts and one gains the impression that authors are writing from experience. For example, Coffin states 'for many years we have used it with great success where the digestive organs have been seriously impaired'. This is repeated in current texts such as Hoffmann who refers to it as indicated primarily in anorexia especially if associated with liver weakness, indigestion and any condition where a sluggish digestion is involved. My personal experience is that it is an excellently well-tolerated herb and useful in poor appetite in the elderly and in small children.

Interestingly, however, we still have Dioscorides to thank for the original recommendation 'the root boiled and drunk, dispels through the bowels matter that is bilious and thick'. Mesue, cited by Serapio, advises 2 drachms (8 g) in decoction to purge thick phlegm. Ibn Sina recommends centaury for obstructions of the liver and as a remedy for a hardened spleen both as a drink and applied topically, which recommendations are repeated by various authors including Culpeper. Ibn Sina advises 6 g as a decoction for colic and states that sometimes the decoction cleanses mucous and unripe humours as well as yellow bile.

Mattioli states that Galen wrote an entire treatise on centaury dedicated to the town of Papia and argues that it removes bile and phlegm, which the greater centaury does not. Fuchs also cites Galen at length and advises centaury to purge bilious and thick humours and resolve obstructions of the liver. Fuchs also cites Pliny as recommending 1 drachm (4 g) in 1 hemina (about 270 mL) of water with a little salt and vinegar to purge the bowels and draw down the bile. Turner states that it drives out choler and gross humours via the belly, and Dodoens advises it boiled in water or wine for this purpose but links this usage with sciatica. Parkinson states that it thins the blood and humours and purges choleric and green humours. Culpeper states that it purges choleric and gross humours, and is especially good for the blood. He recommends a decoction of aerial parts for colic and jaundice; it 'opens obstructions of liver, gall and spleen' as well as being useful for gout and cramps in joints. Quincy claims that it 'discusses and absturges viscous humours' and increases discharge by stool or urine but also helps to thin these humours for evacuation through the skin. Quincy recommends a decoction or infusion in wine.

Macer argues that centaury 'dries up the wild humours of a man's spleen' which has been 'often proved'. Fuchs cites Galen as stating that it is good for those whose nerves are affected. Mattioli says that there are those who recommend it for those affected by nerves, in that it empties out and dries harmlessly those things which are full. Dalechamps gives this as 'those with nervous afflictions or who are full of humours'. Bauhin suggests that advice for use of centaury in nerve disease such as apoplexy, paralysis and epilepsy is based on the action of centaury to 'pull things away from the intestine'. Reading these recommendations, one thinks of the importance that Fuchs gives to pictures as representing the form and thus the nature of the plant. Words can sometimes express so little about the actions and quality of a herb. The advice of Macer makes one think of the pure, clean bitter taste of centaury, as if it would regulate flow and thus purify the spirit.

Modern authors such as Menzies-Trull and Wood recommend centaury in depression associated with digestive disturbance and Wood gives the recommendation of Fernie (1897) for use in 'languid digestion' with heartburn after food. He also discusses the connection between this action and the use of the Bach flower essence of centaury for courage and to help the person to speak out.

Pelikan describes centaury as 'open and friendly yet reticent'. He refers to the medicinal function of bitters as to 'make the ether body inclined to receive the astral body', hence the etheric aspect of the organs serving metabolism will be suffused with astral influence, allowing a vigorous and healthy response to the ingested food. 'The right appetites will then arise, the fluid organism will be toned and conscious awareness strengthened'.

Returning to the physical, usage as an anthelmintic is not mentioned by Dioscorides but it is recommended by Ibn Sina and then the Salernitan herbal for 'worms in the belly.' Apuleius advises the herb crushed in vinegar for worms and this appears in Turner, Dalechamps, Parkinson and Culpeper. Parkinson, copied by Culpeper, states that he has found it useful.

A continuing theme is that centaury is both bitter, thus creating an appetite, and a pleasant stomachic in indigestion. Culpeper claims that 'the herb is so safe you cannot fail in the using of it'. Other writers note its agreeable and pleasant nature including Miller, Quincy, Cullen, Coffin, Robinson, Fox, Fernie, Hool and Grieve. Some authors, such as Gerard and Hill emphasize a powerful action on the liver and use of the powder in jaundice.

Pelikan links this dual action to centaury as it develops more in the direction of stem and stalk than the more usually flower-centred gentians and will therefore work on the 'rhythmic element in metabolism'. It is thus useful, he says, for 'lack of appetite, poor gastric function, gastritis, heartburn, to stimulate hepatic and biliary activity and in cases of jaundice'. According to Zeylstra (1985a), centaury is used for heartburn and hyperacidity and he cites Kniepp as advising it for heartburn and to relieve the stomach of superfluous winds. Zeylstra (1985b) advocates taking bitters at least 30 minutes before meals and sipped in water for maximum effect. The Myddfai also emphasize use as a bitter stomachic, advising centaury for poor appetite, pain in the cardiac area (possibly heartburn) and pain extending to the shoulder, which could be referred pain from the gall bladder.

My experience of using it as a tincture is that it is a bitter tonic that is effective without being too strong. Coffin recommends it alone, with other bitters or with raspberry *Rubus idaeus* in weak and debilitated patients where the digestive organs are seriously impaired. Hool recommends a tonic for the delicate or elderly: centaury ½ oz, raspberry *Rubus idaeus* ½ oz, infuse in 1 pint. Take a wineglassful (60 mL) four times a day.

The *British Herbal Pharmacopoiea* recommends it as a carminative in dyspepsia, in anorexia and in children with gastric or hepatic weakness. Schulz et al (1998) and Hoffmann list it in their discussion of bitters and note its use in anorexia. Menzies-Trull suggests that it is also useful when there is oversecretion of bile.

There are other bitters, and for ecological reasons this herb is not the first choice. However, it is of particular service in people with low energy, including elderly people with poor appetite and my experience is that is very effective and well tolerated. It is also the herb of choice for children, who sometimes combine poor appetite with susceptibility to infections. The authors refer to its use in painful joints and when the nerves have been upset, and this leads to a recommendation for use where the person is debilitated due to illness. An example of this is traditional usage in Scotland of an infusion as a tonic, particularly to improve the appetite in tuberculosis sufferers (Beith 1995). I might include centaury where there are aches and pains associated with chronic fatigue syndrome or fibromyalgia.

## EMMENAGOGUE?

The expulsive action of centaury on humours leads us to another action of the herb. Hoffmann includes centaury in his list of bitters that are also emmenagogue but the evidence for this statement needs some discussion. Both greater centaury and centaury are referred to as 'drawing down the menses' when used as a pessary. Riddle (1991) cites Oribasius, writing in the 4th century AD, as listing the following herbs for an antifertility action: beaten wormwood, pennyroyal, century plant, thyme, rue and others. As discussed in other monographs, the meaning of the word emmenagogue varies and can refer to abortifacients, herbs useful if the menstrual cycle is irregular and herbs traditionally used in the management of labour. Riddle (1992) discusses the many problems in interpreting texts. He argues that the word emmenagogue was used as a code and that herbs were used as contraceptives throughout history, in particular to avoid conception.

The evidence on centaury is particularly difficult to interpret as two dissimilar herbs are discussed by the authors. With regard to greater centaury, Discorides states that 'the root draws down the menses and the embryos/foetuses when whittled, shaped like a pessary and applied to the uterus. The juice accomplishes the same'. With regard to lesser centaury, Dioscorides states that the juice, probably of aerial parts, 'induces menstruation and abortion when used as a pessary'. Ibn Sina affirms that centaury stimulates urine and the menses, and expels the foetus. The Salernitan herbal states that it provokes menstruation as a poultice, or pessary. Turner advises that the juice 'laid in with wool in the natural place, bringeth down womens sickness', and Dodoens suggests use of a pessary for the same purpose and to expel the dead child. Parkinson refers to centaury as emmenagogue, to expel the foetus and ease period pains. Culpeper advises it for the pain associated with a still birth. To conclude, it could be argued that this suggests caution in use of a tea in pregnancy (see Recommendations on safety).

## ALEXIPHARMIC PANACEA

Finally, centaury is recommended as an alexipharmic, for example by Quincy. Alexipharmics are substances considered to protect the heart against poison, in particular after venomous bites. Apuleus proposes the herb crushed in vinegar to dispel the poison after a bite of a viper. Parkinson and Culpeper recommend 1 drachm (4 g) of powder for snakebite in wine, and Culpeper adds that is 'wonderful good against the biting and poisons of an adder'. This links with a use as an antidote to poisons. Pliny refers to the Gauls using it against poisoning.

The healing of inflammation from wounds and protection against wounds or snake bites is an ancient theme in the use of centaury as it was an ingredient in Mithridatum. This remedy is based on a formula sent by Zopyrus, physician to King Ptolemy of Egypt, to Mithridates VI (d. 63 BC), King of Pontus, which is an area west from Trabzon on the southern shore of the Black Sea. The formula contains 20 aromatic plants, including ginger, myrrh and centaury, of which 15 remained in the formula of 36 ingredients proposed by Celsus (Norton 2006) This is advocated for protection against poisons in food or venomous bites, and 'serious conditions' by Celsus (25 BC-50 AD), a Roman doctor who wrote a substantial work on medicine, which was published in 1478 and was thus one of the first printed books (Spivack 1991).

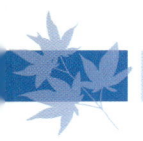

This formula was used as the basis of Theriac by Galen and remained in pharmacopoeias to the 17th century. Discrepancies and substitutions in the Theraic of Mithridates were one of the spurs to the production of the *Pharmacopoeia Londinensis*, published in Latin in 1618 (Griffin 2004). Other compound medicines such as Theriac Londinensis, London treacle, were also used to resist pestilence (Woolley 2004). Pestilence, in the days of infectious disease, plague, contaminated water and badly stored food was a much broader concept than snake bites, so alexipharmic remedies can be seen as preventing disease in a wider sense. Although transmission by bacteria had not been identified, the contagious nature of many diseases was well-known (Nutton 1983).

Jerusalem balsam was another panacea used in Europe that was formulated at the Franciscan monastery of St Saviour in Jerusalem at the beginning of the 17th century (Moussaieffa et al 2005). Centaury was included in one formula of 40 ingredients found in Venice which dates from the early 18th century. Given the earlier discussion of internal and external use of centaury, it is interesting that the same remedy was used both externally on wounds, including gunshot wounds and fistulas, and also daily in small doses in food to resist infectious diseases. This recalls Ibn Sina and Apuleius, who both advise that internal usage will heal wounds. Apuleius advises a decoction in water boiled down to a third part. Centaury continues to be used today in Turkey for chronic inflamed wounds, either as a tea of aerial parts or as a salve made with olive oil (Berkan et al 1991).

Brooke (1992), maybe in a reference back to the story of Chiron, Hercules and Achilles, argues that centaury is useful to face the day with courage, to stand up for yourself, and to drink 'before a long journey where trials of strength are to be attempted'. The alexipharmic action in treating wounds and acute infection could be used again in current herbal medicine in treatment in acute situations, and the concept of an antidote taken regularly in small doses of herbal medicines to protect against infection remains a potent symbol of the power of herbs to preserve health.

## RECOMMENDATIONS

- External usage for chronic wounds is recommended by all the authors and the detailed advice of Galen suggests experience with this herb. Although this usage has not been continued to the present day, the authors do give it prominence and it could be reintroduced as long as the source of the plant material is sustainable.
- Internal usage for arthritis, muscular and joint pain can be recommended, particularly associated with depression, fibromyalgia or where the person is recovering from illness.
- The *British Herbal Pharmacopoiea* recommends it as a bitter, aromatic and stomachic for use in anorexia, dyspepsia and in children with gastric or hepatic weakness. One has to broaden this recommendation to usage wherever there is poor appetite, also in conditions such as irritable bowel syndrome where a mild but effective medicine is required. Given the emphasis by the authors on the action of centaury to drive out choleric humours, phlegm and unripe humours, then it may have a more dynamic action on the bowels as a tea than in the more common modern form of a tincture.
- The authors recommend a decoction of aerial parts in flower. A decoction for use in acute situations such as wounds, bites or stings could include centaury alongside other herbs such as yarrow *Achillea millefolium* and comfrey leaf *Symphytum officinale*.
- A small dose in a medicine to prevent reoccurrence of a chronic condition such as irritable bowel could be seen as harking back to the recommendation as an alexipharmic.

Dosage: the *British Herbal Pharmacopoeia* recommends 2–4 g three times a day of dried flowering aerial parts.

Ibn Sina gives the dose of 6 g for colic and uterine pains, which corresponds, somewhat astonishingly, with the daily dose given by Commission E (Blumenthal 1998). The doses used by herbalists as medicines are often very small, for example 10–15 mL weekly of a 1:5 tincture, which is equivalent to 400 mg daily.

## CONSTITUENTS

Reviews: Barnes et al (2007), Bisset & Wichtl (2001), Bradley (2006), Mills (2003), Williamson (2003).

### Secoiridoid glycosides

Secoiridoid glycosides are bitter compounds that are characteristic of Gentianaceae, and representatives of three types are found: swertiamarin; sweroside and two related compounds, gentiopicroside and gentioflavoside. Secoiridoid glycosides

are the main compounds found in centaury but derivatives of the iridoid glycoside loganic acid and intermediate compounds (secologanol and centauroside) are also found (Jensen & Schripsema 2002). Particularly bitter esters of secoirioid glycosides accumulate in the seeds (Van der Sluis & Labadie 1981).
Total 1.2%: swertiamarin, sweroside (Kumarasamy et al 2003a), gentiopicroside (Kumarasamy et al 2003b).
Swertiamarin 0.5–8.8%, gentiopicroside, no sweroside (wild, five populations, Bulgaria) (Nikolova-Damyanova & Handjieva 1996).
Swertiamarin (predominant), gentioflavoside, dihydrocornin (Do et al 1987).
Monoterpene iridoid alkaloids gentianine, gentianidine, gentioflavine were derived from iridoid glycosides (Handjieva et al 1991) and anaerobic incubation of swertiamarine with intestinal bacteria showed that three main metabolites were produced, including erythrocentaurin and gentianine (El-Sedawy et al 1989).

### Sterols

Beta-sitosterol, stigmasterol, campesterol, brassicasterol, delta 7 stigmastenol (aerial parts) (Aquino et al 1985).

### Phenolic acids

Hydroxycinnamic acids: p-coumaric acid, ferulic acid, sinapic acid (Valentão et al 2001).

### Coumarins

Isocoumarin (wild, Portugal) (Valentão et al 2003).

### Flavonoids

Flavone: kaempferol (Valentão et al 2001).

### Xanthones

Methoxylated xanthones: eustomin, demethyleustomin (wild, Morocco) (Schimmer & Mauthner 1996).
Methoxylated xanthones: six, including eustomin; tetraoxygenated xanthones (12 samples) (Valentão et al 2002).

## RECOMMENDATIONS ON SAFETY

1. Do not use centaury as a tea during pregnancy.
2. The uses of either centaury as a pessary is obviously not advisable. In contrast, the doses used by herbalists as medicines are often very small and the conclusion has to be that centaury *Centaurium erythraea* is safe in pregnancy used thus.

## REFERENCES

Aquino R, Behar I, Garzarella P, et al 1985 Chemical composition and biological properties of *Erythraea centaurium* Rafn. Bollettino della Società Italiana di biologia sperimentale 61:165–169.

Barnes J, Anderson LA, Phillipson JD, 2007 Herbal medicines, 3rd edn. Pharmaceutical Press, London.

Beith M 1995 Healing threads. Polygon, Edinburgh.

Berkan T, Üstünes L, Lermioglu F, et al 1991 Antiinflammatory, analgesic and antipyretic effects of an aqueous extract of *Erythraea centaurium*. Planta Medica 57:34–37.

Bisset NG, Wichtl M (eds) 2001 Herbal drugs and phytopharmaceuticals, 2nd edn. Medpharm, Stuttgart.

Blumenthal M (ed) 1998 The complete German Commission E monographs. American Botanical Council, Texas.

Bostock J 1855 The natural history. Pliny the Elder. Taylor and Francis, London. Online. Available: http://www.perseus.tufts.edu/hopper 26 Mar 09.

Bradley PR 2006 British herbal compendium, vol 2. British Herbal Medicine Association, Bournemouth.

Brooke E 1992 A woman's book of herbs. The Women's Press, London.

Brookes I 1994 The death of Chiron: Ovid, Fasti 5.379–4414. The Classical Quarterly 44:444–450.

Buchanan WW, Kean WF 1987 William Heberden the Elder (1710–1801): the compleat physician and sometime rheumatologist. Clinical Rheumatology 6:251–263.

Cullen W 1775 Lectures on the materia medica, as Delivered in the University of Edinburgh. Philadelphia, Robert Bell Online. Available: http//books.google.co.uk 24 Mar 09.

Culpeper N, Cole A, Rowland W 1655 The practice of physick … being chiefly a translation of the works of … Lazarus Riverius. Peter Cole, London.

Davis PH (ed) 1978 Flora of Turkey, vol 6. Edinburgh University Press, Edinburgh.

Dawson WR 1949 Chiron the Centaur. Journal of the History of Medicine 4:267–275.

Do T, Popov S, Marekov N, et al 1987 Iridoids from Gentianaceae plants growing in Bulgaria. Planta Medica 53:580.

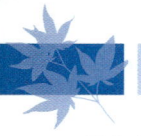

El-Sedawy AI, Shu YZ, Hattori M, et al 1989 Metabolism of swertiamarin from *Swertia japonica* by human intestinal bacteria. Planta Medica 55:147–150.

Fernie WT 1897 Herbal simples approved for modern uses of cure. Boericke & Tafel, Philadelphia. Online. Available: http://www.gutenberg.org.

Fuchs L (1545) 1980 edn. Holzschnitte, die historischen Taschenbücher. Konrad Kölbl, Grünwald bei München.

Gibbons B, Brough P 1992 Wild flowers of Britain & Northern Europe. Chancellor Press, London.

Griffin JP 2004 Venetian treacle and the foundation of medicines regulation. British Journal of Clinical Pharmacology 58:317–325.

Gunther RT (ed.) 1933 The Greek herbal of Dioscorides. Oxford University Press, Oxford.

Handjieva N, Saadi H, Popov S, et al 1991 Separation of iridoids by vacuum liquid chromatography. Phytochemical Analysis 2:130–133.

Jensen SR, Schripsema J 2002 Chemotaxonomy and pharmacology of Gentianaceae. In: Struwe L, Albert VA (eds) 2002 Gentianaceae: systematics and natural history. Cambridge University Press, Cambridge.

Larrey D, Vial T, Pauwels A, et al 1992 Hepatitis after germander *Teucrium chamaedrys* administration: another instance of herbal medicine hepatotoxicity. Annals of Internal Medicine 117:129–132.

Kumarasamy Y, Nahar L, Cox P, et al 2003a Bioactivity of secoiridoid glycosides from *Centaurium erythraea*. Phytomedicine 10:344–347.

Kumarasamy Y, Nahar L, Sarker SD 2003b Bioactivity of gentiopicroside from the aerial parts of *Centaurium erythraea*. Fitoterapia 74:151–154.

Lange D 1998 Europe's medicinal and aromatic plants: their use, trade and conservation. Traffic International, Cambridge.

Mansion G, Struwe L 2004 Generic delimitation and phylogenetic relationships within the subtribe Chironiinae (Chironieae: Gentianaceae), with special reference to *Centaurium*: evidence from nrDNA and cpDNA sequences. Molecular Phylogenetics and Evolution 32:951–977.

Meszáros S, De Laet J, Smets E 1996 Phylogeny of temperate Gentianaceae: a morphological approach. Systematic Botany 21:153–168.

MHRA 2003 Aristolochia. Online. Available: http://www.mhra.gov.uk/Howweregulate/Medicines/Herbalandhomoeopathicmedicines/Herbalmedicines/HerbalSafetyNews/Furthersafetyissues/CON024018.

Mills S 2003 ESCOP Monographs: the scientific foundation for herbal medicinal products, 2nd edn. Thieme Medical Publishers, Stuttgart.

Moussaieffa A, Frideb E, Amarc Z, et al 2005 The Jerusalem balsam: from the Franciscan monastery in the old city of Jerusalem to Martindale 33. Journal of Ethnopharmacology 101:16–26.

Nikolova-Damyanova B, Handjieva N 1996 Quantitative determination of swertiamarin and gentiopicroside in *Centaurium erythrea* and *C. turcicum* by densitometry. Phytochemical Analysis 7:140–142.

Norton S 2006 The pharmacology of Mithridatum: a 2000-year old remedy. Molecular Interventions 6:60–66.

Nutton V 1983 The seeds of disease: an explanation of contagion and infection from the Greeks to the Renaissance. Medical History 27:1–34.

Riddle JM 1991 Oral contraceptives and early-term abortifacients during classical antiquity and the Middle Ages. Past and Present 132:3–32.

Riddle JM 1992 Contraception and abortion from the ancient world to the Renaissance. Harvard University Press, Cambridge, MA.

Schimmer O, Mauthner H 1996 Polymethoxylated xanthones from the herb of *Centaurium erythraea* with strong antimutagenic properties in Salmonella typhimurium. Planta Medica 62:561–564.

Schulz V, Hansel R, Tyler V 1998 Rational phytotherapy. Springer-Verlag, Berlin.

Spivack BS 1991 A C Celsus: Roman Medicus. Journal of the History of Medicine and Allied Sciences 46:143–157.

Stace C 1991 New flora of the British Isles. Cambridge University Press, Cambridge.

Sterry P 2006 Complete British wild flowers. HarperCollins, London.

Theoi Project 2008 Kheiron. Online. Available: http://www.theoi.com/Georgikos/KentaurosKheiron.html.

Thomson AT 1815 The London dispensatory. Longman, Hurst, Rees, Orme, and Brown, London.

Tutin TG, Heywood VH, Burges NA, et al 1973 Flora Europaea, vol 3. Cambridge University Press, Cambridge.

UK biodiversity action plan 2009 Joint Nature Conservation Committee. Online. Available: http://www.ukbap.org.uk.

Valentão P, Fernandas E, Carvalho F, et al 2001 Antioxidant activity of *Centaurium erythraea* infusion evidenced by its superoxide radical scavenging and xanthine oxidase inhibitory activity. Journal of Agricultural and Food Chemistry 49:3476–3479.

Valentão P, Andrade PB, Silva E, et al 2002 Methoxylated xanthones in the quality control of small centaury *Centaurium erythraea* flowering tops. Journal of Agricultural and Food Chemistry 50:460–463.

Valentão P, Andrade PB, Silva AMS, et al 2003 Isolation and structural elucidation of 5-formyl-2,3-dihydroisocoumarin from *Centaurium erythraea* aerial parts. Natural Product Research 17:361–364.

Van der Sluis WG, Labadie RP 1981 Secoiridoids and xanthones in the genus *Centaurium*. Planta Medica 41:150–160.

Williamson E 2003 Potter's Herbal Cyclopaedia. CW Daniel, Saffron Walden.

Woolley B 2004 Heal thyself. HarperCollins, New York.

Zeylstra H 1985a Centaury. New Herbal Practitioner 12:2–6.

Zeylstra H 1985b The pharmacology of bitters. New Herbal Practitioner 12:20–21.

# CHAPTER 14
# *Daucus carota*, wild carrot

## DESCRIPTION

**Family: Apiaceae**      **Part used: seed, aerial parts, root**

Ten *Daucus* species are found in Europe, often near the sea. *Daucus carota* is very variable in morphology and includes several subspecies, which can hybridize with each other (Tutin et al 1968). The culinary carrot *Daucus carota* subsp. *sativus* has a red root. The *Flora of Turkey* (Davis 1972) gives five *Daucus* species, including *Daucus carota*.

*Daucus carota* L. subsp. *carota* is usually biennial and is found throughout Europe in dry meadows, field boundaries, roadsides and coastal areas, and is naturalized in the USA. The other subspecies are mainly found in coastal areas and some are grouped by other authorities as *Daucus gingidium* L. (Tutin et al 1968).

Erect, smooth or bristly stems (10–100 cm) bear pinnate leaves with finely divided leaflets, which smell of carrot when bruised. Solid umbels of white flowers occur in June to August, usually with numerous smooth or shortly hairy, unequal rays (Tutin 1980). The outer flowers are larger and there are some purple flowers in the centre of the umbel. There is a characteristic ruff of conspicuous, linear, pinnatisect bracts. When in seed, the outer flower stems turn in to make characteristic, dense clusters of fruits. Seeds (2–4 mm) are oval, with spines on the ridges.

The root is white but may be red where hybrids occur with cultivated carrots (Hauser & Bjørn 2001).

### Quality

The Apiaceae family includes poisonous plants and presents problems with identification. Subspecies within *Daucus carota* also hybridize, which adds to difficulties in identification of this plant. The dark dot in the centre of the umbel is characteristic in Britain but may not be in Turkey and the Mediterranean. The round cluster of fruits is also characteristic, although this is also found in *Ammi majus* and *Ammi visnaga* (Tutin 1980). According to Akeroyd (2003), it is the only common Apiacea that has a ruff of pinnate, three-lobed bracts surrounding the flowerhead.

Cultivated carrots are also grown for carrot seed oil (Yu et al 2005) and commercial samples of wild carrot seed may be from *Daucus carota* subsp. *sativa*. The white root is considered inedible (Barnes et al 2007).

## CONFUSION OF IDENTITY

Beck's translation of Dioscorides (III 52) on daucus is very clear. It appears as staphylinos agrios in the Greek, translated as *Daucus carota* var. *sylvestris* and *Daucus carota* L., wild carrot and cultivated carrot. There are two kinds, the wild, which is called ceras, and the cultivated. The cultivated, while being more edible, can be used for the same purposes as the wild, but is weaker. Dioscorides describes this wild carrot, identifiable particularly by 'an umbel like that of dill on which there are white flowers, and in the middle there is something small and purplish, as if it were nap on woollen cloth'. However, identifying daucus through further literature is fraught with difficulty.

Dioscorides, confusingly, has another entry under 'Daucos' (III 72) a little later, which Beck introduces as *Athamanta cretensis* L., Daucos. Of this plant Dioscorides says there are three kinds, all described, but not further identified by Beck: the Cretan daucus, which is superior, referred to by some later authors as 'Daucus of Candy/Candie' (Candy was a city in ancient Crete), a second kind similar to wild celery, and a third kind with leaves of coriander, white flowers, head and seeds of dill (or anise according to other translators), with the 'muscarium', the umbel, of carrot (pastinaca following other translations), longish seeds like cumin and pungent.

The four types of pastinaca (the Latin term) referred to by Pliny, according to Andrews (1949) derive from Diodotus. Plutarch, he says, spoke of several kinds, and Oribasius gives stafilinus as a synonym of daucus, called pastinaca by the Romans.

Galen has two separate entries, one in book 6 and one book 8. Book 6 deals with wild daucus 'that some call Staphylinos' (Mattioli suggests this means Galen does not

©2009 Elsevier Ltd, Inc, BV
DOI: 10.1016/B978-0-443-10344-5.00019-7

**145**

THE WESTERN HERBAL TRADITION

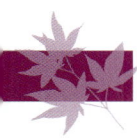

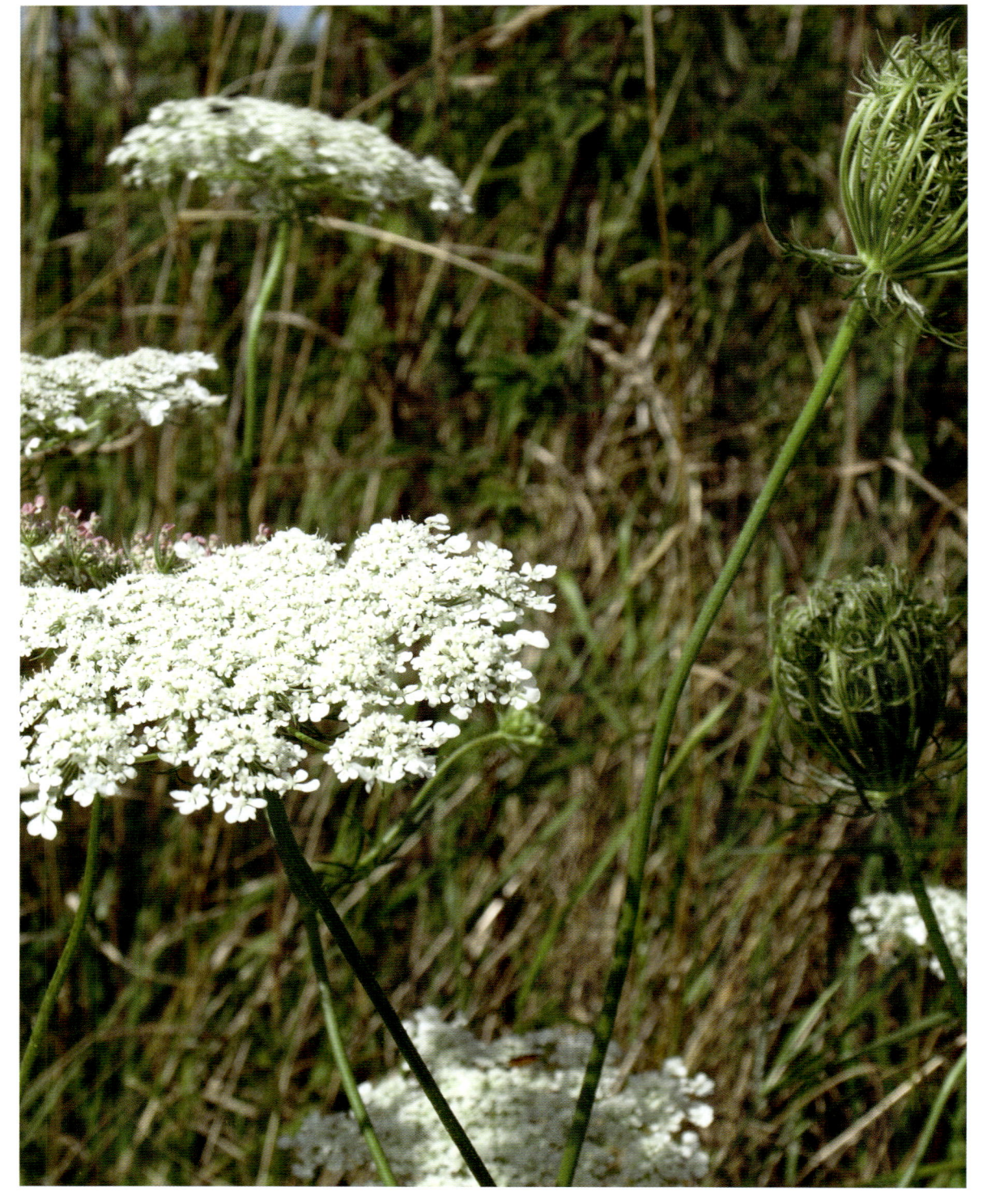

Figure 14.1 *Daucus carota*, wild carrot (Yorkshire, July).

agree the name 'Staphylinos' is appropriate here), and domestic daucus, and book 8 covers domestic pastinaca (sativa) and wild pastinaca (agrestis). If they were plants to be confounded, Mattioli suggests, there would not be two entries. Moreover, if Mattioli's commentary on Dioscorides is to be followed further, the staphylinos of Dioscorides is parsnip and hence does not accord with Beck's classification as carrot. Mattioli is quite insistent that the pastinaca of Dioscorides is not carrot, nor are they the same plant. He maintains there is to be found no author, Greek nor Arabic, who says pastinaca sativa has red roots. He appears to be very familiar with them, for they both grow in Italy, he says, and are eaten in many places, and both have white roots. He tells us of a tradition in Italy that parsnips are eaten (at least in 1554) in lent, roasted with flour in oil (though he advises against this, for they 'incline to Venus'), and often used in place of fish when there is a shortage. (As an aside, I am interested to note that in a vegetarian cookery book I have a recipe for fried parsnips with gherkin butter which the author introduces as 'based very roughly on one I found in an old cookery book called 'Parsnips Fried to look Like Trout'. I tried the recipe on some guests and the blend of flavours, we agreed, does have something of fish about it. I wonder if this stems from this old Italian tradition.) Mattioli affirms, from his considerations, that there are three kinds of daucus, as Dioscorides records, the one growing most frequently in Italy in his time being the one that emulates wild pastinaca. Turner, however, takes Mattioli to task for this error, and argues that staphylinos is carrot. Even Parkinson despaired of identification. There is much debate.

The three-fold grouping of daucus persists through later authors, citing Dioscorides on daucus, of course. Serapio, for example, details the three kinds but makes no comment on their accessibility or accuracy. Dodoens' detail, however, is intriguing. Listing first the daucus of Candie, then the one that resembles wild parsley, he notes that 'both these kinds are yet unknowne'. His third kind he goes to some lengths to identify, recounting Dioscorides' description of leaves like coriander, white flowers, and long seed, yet the 'tufts' (umbels) which the Latin version has as 'like pastinaca', Dodoens records as 'like wild carrot', suggesting that there is at least some tradition of pastinaca as wild carrot. He is then even more specific, and draws in the detail of the purple centre we found in Beck's staphilinos/carrot/daucus: 'For this kind of Daucus, there is now taken the herbe which some do call wilde Carrot, others call it Birds nest; for it hath leaves like Coriander, but greater, and not much unlike the leaves of the yellow Carrot. Its flowers be white, growing upon tuffets or rundels, like to the tuffets of the yellow Carrot; in the middle whereof is found a little small flower or twain of a brown red colour, turning to blacke.'

To confuse matters further, Gerard has a slightly different version, that daucus, described with red roots, is properly called in Greek staphylinos, but in the Latin 'pastinaca sativa' has the addition 'tenuifolia' to differentiate it from garden parsnip with white roots, hence wild carrot is pastinaca sylvestris tenuifolia; and a third kind is daucus of Crete, the true daucus of Dioscorides.

## CLARITY?

Andrews (1949) has written extensively on identification of the carrot in the classical era and it is no uncomplicated matter. The origins and application of the names daukos, staphylinos, pastinaca and carota each offer their own linguistic complexities in the route to establish definition. Daukos, Andrews concludes, was a 'term of generic force', applied to several different plants including wild carrot, species of athamanta and others: 'the common characteristic seems to have been a bitter, pungent root with a cathartic effect …'. In contrast, he continues, staphylinos was a specific term for the cultivated carrot, in use at least as early as the 4th century BC, with the epithet 'agrios', 'wild' to denote wild carrot. The distinction in the classical period between staphylinos and daucos, he says, later broke down and both terms were used for cultivated and wild carrot. Pastinaca was a generic term like daucos and was applied not only to both cultivated and wild carrot, but to other plants too, including parsnip, spawning many common names both for parsnip and carrot across Europe, but usually geographically specific, i.e. referring either to carrot or parsnip, depending on locality. Analysis of carota strays into 'karo' and 'caraway', but he concludes here that 'carota' was a term applied only to the carrot, first met fairly late in the ancient literature, which later became the usual name for the cultivated carrot.

Andrews adds too a further consideration which may throw some light on Mattioli's objection about the colour, at least in terms of the cultivated carrot. Theophrastus referred to yellow- and black-rooted forms of daukon (as wild plants). There is no mention, Andrews says, of colour in Dioscorides, Pliny, Galen and Oribasius – a probably significant omission, since mention might be expected 'by certain of the technical writers of ancient times if these differences existed in the cultivated carrots known to them'. The earliest specific mention is in Simeon Seth in the 11th century speaking of red and yellow types of daukos. Andrews concludes then that the root was probably white. 'This circumstance suggests that the carrot of the classical era was the form with white root surface, developed directly from available wild forms and as yet unaffected by hybridisation with the Afghan anthocyan carrot. In that event, although marked differences in character and quality may have existed, the coloration would have been much the same and therefore would have given no reason for comment'.

## CONSENSUS AND MORE DEBATE

Having laboured these identification problems, the actions of the herbs, staphilinos, daucos and pastinaca, are not at all dissimilar. Mattioli says their properties in Dioscorides and Galen accord so well that in the absence of the one, the other may safely be used. However, some of the detail is again at odds. For Dioscorides says of daucus (three kinds) the seeds all heat, provoke urine, menses and the foetus/birth. It frees from 'torminibus' (colic), sooths old cough; drunk with wine it helps against bites of Phalange (poisonous spider); it breaks/discusses tumours/swellings when applied on them. The use of the seed is stronger in all, but the root of Creticus, when drunk, is very powerful against poisons.

Of staphylinos, Dioscorides (Beck) says 'when drunk or even when applied, its seed sets the menses going, it is suitable for those that pass water painfully and with difficulty, for those with edemata, for pleurisy in potions, and for bites and strokes of wild animals. They say that reptiles do not harm people who have taken it in advance; it also aids conception. As for the root, it, too, is diuretic, aphrodisiac, and expels embryos/foetuses when used as a pessary. The leaves ground and applied with honey, clear cancerous sores completely. The cultivated carrot, which is more edible, is suitable for the same purposes, but it acts more weakly'.

Galen (Book 6), for daucus, says (from Mattioli) it is bitter and has a faculty of heating and therefore extenuat-

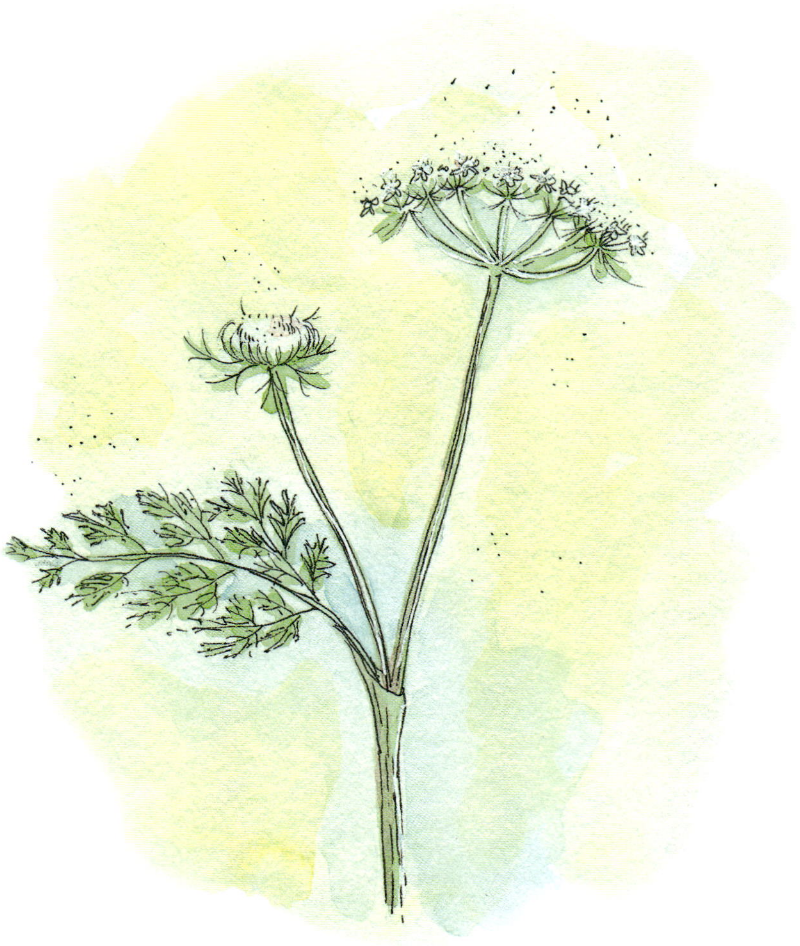

**Figure 14.2** *Daucus carota*, wild carrot.

ing. The root besides has a certain power for stimulating the same to Venus. Agrestis (wild) indeed lacks this wind which is called aphuson, and therefore excites urination and menses.

Galen (Book 8), for pastinaca, says (from Mattioli) all the herb and mainly the seed and the root make urinate and move menstrual flux. It is also somewhat abstersive, and thus some people dress corrosive ulcers with the fresh leaves in purified honey.

So for Dioscorides, daucus has no reference to aphrodisiac nor pro-conception qualities but for Galen this action is present, while for Dioscorides, staphylinos/pastinaca aids conception and is aphrodisiac, but this is absent in Galen's rendering. Perhaps they are both citing an antecedent where identification is obscure or translators have (quite understandably) confounded the plants. Later writers, following Dioscorides and Galen, do not make the situation clearer since a good number of them make claims for 'wild carrot' that appear under either or both pastinaca/daucus, apparently indiscriminately. More recent authors have not solved the problem – even Mrs Grieve is not clear. For example, her Latin/Greek terms for carrot appear under parsnip in Beck, although she does indicate the plants were confused.

## URINARY AGREEMENT

If the aphrodisiac and conception application is ambiguous in ancient writers, other uses are very clear throughout the plant's history, in particular its use for the urinary system. There is surely some link here between effects on the gonads and the urinary system, approaching to some extent the Chinese designation of the kidneys, within which sphere of action the gonads are included, and in Culpeper too Venus rules the womb and kidneys, reflecting somewhat our current reference (albeit more limited) to the genito-urinary system. In practically every entry for daucus through the centuries its reputation as a urinary herb is repeated and is clearly one of the main actions of the plant. For several authors, it is the finest and strongest herb to provoke diuresis. Serapio, for example, says it is the strongest medicine in provoking urine. Cook on the other hand, although speaking of cultivated carrot, which writers agree is weaker than wild, says it is not so strong 'they (the seeds) are too transient to effect a permanent impression, but are a good adjuvant to such diuretics as *Eupatorium purpureum* and peach leaves'. Its reputation as a sound diuretic continues in all our modern herbals. Hoffman, for example, lists it as 'strong' under 'true herbal diuretics', Menzies-Trull defines it as a 'stimulating diuretic'. Linked to diuresis, daucus is celebrated widely for its antilithic properties; Dalechamps records it as official medicine in Italy, France and Germany, and called 'the stonebreaker' in Venice. Culpeper says it will break and expel the stone. Later, Miller reinforces this claim 'the seed infused in ale is accounted an excellent diuretic and good to prevent the stone, and to render its fits less violent; it brings away gravel and provokes urine…' More recently Bartram, for example, lists it as antilithic. With its powerful diuretic and mineral breaking properties (Wood), it follows, in herbal terms, that wider applications are added. Gerard says it remedies dropsy; in more recent herbals it appears for use in gout (Williamson, Hoffman, *British Herbal Pharmacopoeia*) and rheumatism (Hoffman as a diuretic with other remedies).

## REPRODUCTION – MORE DEBATE

Alongside most references to its powerful effect on the urinary system stands fulsome praise for the effects of daucus on the reproductive system through later authors. Firstly we recall Dioscorides' 'aphrodisiac' properties (at least for the plant with the purple bits in the flower centre). Galen made reference to this quality. Turner and Gerard repeat this claim, although Parkinson makes no mention of it (sticking accurately with the straight three-fold version of Dioscorides). Turner has a wonderful turn of phrase here: 'The seed of the garden Daucus hath a certain property also to provoke pleasure … Averroes writeth that the garden carrot is good for them that are slow to the work of increasing the world with children'. As an aid to conception, another claim repeated by some, one is tempted to wonder whether this is simply a consequence of the aphrodisiac properties, or some other more direct influence.

This latter faculty is all the more surprising since its more widely supported action is probably the opposite. For there may be no strong tradition for aiding conception through the herbals but as 'provoking the menses' and 'expelling the foetus/birth' (translation is ambiguous here since 'partus' means both 'foetus' and 'birth') and related female difficulties, the picture is very different. Practically all references carry this theme in some form or other, presumably following Dioscorides in the main. The root according to Gerard 'bringeth forth the birth, and the seed bringeth down the desired sickness', Miller says it provokes the menses and is useful in uterine and hysteric disorders. Bauhin quotes Hippocrates that Daucus moistens the humours of the womb during, or for the benefit of, parturition. Pliny (cited by Fuchs) says the seeds crushed in wine ease suffocations and pains of women sufficient to correct the womb; Culpeper speaks of it 'provoking women's courses' and helping the 'rising of the mother', Apuleius 'for women in labour and not yet purged'. There are obviously pathological conditions that require periods to be provoked. Such a one is offered in *The Trotula* (Green 2001) in that women are moist and cold and need menses (and regular intercourse!) to prevent these properties from overwhelming their constitution, thus any retention of menses carried danger of imbalance and consequent illness. Many women too needed help in childbirth, still birth and miscarriage, and daucus was clearly one of the prime herbs in this regard. Yet Riddle (1997), in *Eve's Herbs*, pushes this argument further and labels daucus 'one of the more potent anti-fertility agents' used orally as a strong contraceptive immediately after coitus. He argues there was a strong oral tradition of means to control conception and birth, and that authors were at more or less liberty to be specific about these practices depending on the social mores of the time and indeed their own personal belief (Pliny, reputedly, was a Stoic and thus anti-abortion), 'emmenagogue' being the 'common circumlocution' for abortifacient/contraceptive capacity in a herb. Riddle seems to make a case for daucus, suggesting some textual record (e.g. Hippocrates, he says, referred to it as abortifacient) citing animal experiments, and interesting anecdotal evidence of very recent use by women in India and the Appalacians – he tells the story of one woman who avoided pregnancy by taking a teaspoon of the crushed seeds of wild carrot after intercourse, until one holiday when she forgot to take the seeds with her and conceived. Four-footed animals, he adds, will not eat wild carrot except after miscarriage. *The Trotula*, however, makes only one mention of daucus, and that for helping to conceive, despite many other remedies for bringing down the menses, including pennyroyal and artemesia. The Salernitan Herbal, from around the same time, also contains no reference to any emmenagogue properties for daucus. This remains a hypothesis. In our modern literature Menzies-Trull and Williamson refer to emmenagogic action, and a number of authors, including Chevallier and Wood, caution against its use in pregnancy. Hoffman, however, is more circumspect. He cites the *Botanical Safety Handbook* 'not to be used in pregnancy unless otherwise directed by an expert qualified in the appropriate use of this substance' but queries whether this conclusion is based on clinical records or extrapolation from in vitro studies on constituents.

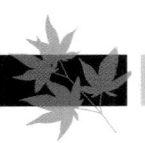

## GASTROINTESTINAL EFFECTS

A third theme in the literature is daucus' use as a gastrointestinal herb. Dioscorides writes of 'gnawings of the belly'. Galen too mentions wind. Culpeper adds his own experience on the matter. He reprises Galen's commendation of garden carrots to break the wind, in complaining of his own difficulties with the vegetable in that regard, 'experience teaches they breed it first' (although Turner says Galen considers the root not easy to digest and has a windy property). Then he follows with the quip 'the seeds of them expel wind indeed and so mend what the root marreth' (it seems the same might be said of the aphrodisiac/conception/abortifacient qualities above).

Other authors comment on this faculty too. Quincy in particular makes a significant departure from the tradition in classing it not as a diuretic or emmenagogue, but under carminatives. He makes no specific notes on this herb, it simply appears between cumin and fennel (interestingly both umbellifers) but its placement is distinctive.

Quincy offers a diverting narration on the origin of the term 'carminative', as many, he says, may not be used to the term. It stems from their fast and effective working 'as if cured by inchantment' since 'carmen' is the Latin for 'song, verse or inchantment'. Quincy complains that these medicines are misused in his day and their efficacy misappropriated, being used by the otherwise unskilled to effect 'miraculous' cures. 'The medicine is used too much by 'Jugglers' who for want of knowledge brought religion into their party and what through ignorance unable to do by rational prescription, and use of proper medicine, they pretend to effect by invocation and interest of heaven'.

The main impetus in consideration of the action of daucus appears to be attributable to its heat in humoral terms, and in some degree to its dryness. It is hot and dry in the third degree, many authors agree, although some say hot in third and dry in second. Andrews (1949) suggests in a note that the word 'daucos' should perhaps be associated with 'daio', meaning 'heat', motivated by the heating property of the seed. Heat, according to Galen, is the element that will attenuate and disperse. Hence for hard conglomerations and heavy, sticky accretions in various parts of the body a hot remedy will break up and release. It has the capacity to make light, make subtle, disperse and rarify through the fine quality of its substance. Daucus, as hot and dry, will 'let down' water from the kidneys, and is emmenagogue through like action on the womb. For the digestive system, Quincy, in a much later time, explains a similar process and despite being professedly 'mechanical' appears to be in deeply humoral territory here. He explains how carminatives are used 'under great disorders from flatus and wind pent up' and speaks of the need for 'what dissipates and dispels such vapours … All these medicines are warm and consist of very light subtle parts … [they] therefore expel substances and invigorate tonic undulation and so obstruction of wind is dislodged.' They can be similarly used topically – 'Also many are discussive topics as they warm, rarify and attenuate obstructed humours'. Daucus' application for old coughs, as commended by Dioscorides and others, can be understood within this capacity too.

## EXTERNAL USE

The herb has been used topically through the traditions. Dioscorides recommends it for ulcers (the leaves powdered into small pieces with honey) – again Galen (cited in Turner) links its action to its heat – it will 'greatly drive forth by evaporation'. Cook gives fuller instructions for the root. While determining it a 'pleasant and diffusive aromatic stimulant, somewhat relaxant, carminative and acting chiefly on the kidneys', Cook reserves his fullest praise for its external effects. 'The boiled roots', he says, 'form an excellent emollient and gently stimulating poultice in irritable ulcers of all grades, but fresh and unboiled roots, finely grated, make a peculiar stimulating application of great value. They are excellent in all low forms of sores such as carbuncles, degenerate abscesses and buboes, and all fetid ulcers of malignant, cachetic and scrofulous grades. They correct the fetor, relieve the aching and quickly promote sound granulation. It is said that they will even abate the suffering of phagedaena (a spreading erosion in an ulcer) and of cancer. They certainly deserve more attention than they have received from the profession, and sores in which it seems impossible to arouse a healing process by ordinary means, will usually improve at once under this application'. Wood, more recently cites this use.

Mrs Grieve bases her recommendations on tradition, as a diuretic stimulant and deobstruent, offering no pharmacological reference. It is an 'active and valuable remedy for dropsy, chronic kidney diseases and affections of the bladder'. Carrot tea, she suggests, from 1 oz herb in a pint of boiling water, used night and morning, can be taken against lithic acid or gouty disposition. The seeds are useful against flatulence, colic, chronic coughs, calculus, jaundice, obstruction of the viscera and as emmenagogue, in accord with tradition. She includes too mention of topical use of the roots for cancerous ulcers, and the leaves with honey for running sores and ulcers.

Weiss says cultivated carrots are particularly valued by paediatricians for thread worms in children. He recommends the child be given nothing but coarsely or finely grated carrots for 1 or 2 days in the active phase of the infection and in the inactive, a drink of fresh carrot juice or one or two fresh carrots for breakfast. Chevallier repeats a similar recommendation for thread worms.

The *British Herbal Pharmacopoeia* mentions the volatile oil daucine, 'which has a nicotine-like odour'. The herb's actions are diuretic, antilithic, carminative, and its indications are for urinary calculus, lithuria, cystitis, gout. Dose 2–4 g or by infusion, liquid extract 1 : 1, 2–4 mL.

## MODERN USES

Modern authors pivot their recommendations largely round the urinary, carminative, antispasmodic and antirheumatic themes, citing mainly the volatile oil and the flavanoids as active constituents in this regard. Some sources also cite the alkaloid daucine, including the *British Herbal Pharmacopoeia*, Hoffman, Bartram and Menzies Trull, but this appears to be a reference to Wren which refers back to a source from the early 1900s and we have found no confirmation of this. A porphyrin content is mentioned by Weiss and Chevallier that stimulates the pituitary gland, releasing increased levels of sex hormones (is this the source of the aphrodisiac tradition?). Wood, in this context too, cites Dr Christopher's opinion of wild carrot as a 'pituitary stimulant', and ponders whether the plant would therefore act on the endocrine cascade, thyroid, kidneys and sex hormones. Menzies-Trull and Bartram both mention the use of daucus for menopause, but there is no other reference to this among our authors.

Chevallier adds a modern commendation of the juice as a 'valuable detoxifier', supporting the liver, stimulating urine flow and removal of waste by the kidneys.

## THE PROPERTIES OF THE CARROT FAMILY

Pelikan's appreciation of Daucus throws a deal of light on the older humoral considerations and offers perhaps an 'inner perception' that approaches an understanding of the nature of the heat and the dryness. He sets it within the carrot family as a whole, a family 'highly sensitive to the interplay' of air and water, light and dark, in which he argues three themes, three 'chords'.

Chord one is reflected by a sort of systole and diastole based on this fine sensitivity. Through the leaves 'light, air, water and earth's minerals' come together and are drawn centripetally into the root where they are held for a time – cosmic forces pulled into the earth. Pelikan refers to this time as the 'year of the root'. The diastole then follows with an exhalation, an opposite movement radiating out into the air, cosmos, in flower and fruit. 'Innumerable flowers float above the green plant like a cloud of stars, loosely combined in an umbrella or domed shape. Individual flowers are insignificant, with little colour, generally a greenish-white. Their scent is faint and not very characteristic. They are open, spread wide; the stamens, too, radiate outwards, so that the radiant principle remains consistent to the very end. We look in vain for flower cups, jugs, crowns, funnels or throats.' There follow inevitably no succulent fruits, but dry hard seeds, yet still continuing the radiant theme with barbs, hairs and such like.

Chord two, Pelikan says, is one of relating strongly to the air, to the extent even of incorporating it. In this family are the multi-divided leaves of many of the characteristic species such as carrot, moving to those of fennel, for example that 'evaporate into the air'. Then there are such examples as the airy leaf sheaths of angelica and the hollow stems of hemlock. The astral body in humans and animals is associated with a process of incorporating air, and enfolding, creating inner organs and allowing independent movement. In plants the domain of the astral remains outside but is expressed in the realm of the flowers in colour, scent, nectar and such, the related warmth revealing itself in volatile oils and other aromatic substances. In the umbelliferae, where air and light and warmth are drawn so powerfully downwards, it becomes clear why the flowers remain insignificant, and with little scent, why the aromas appear in stem and leaf (celery, lovage), and even down to the root where 'fruit-like roots appear' (carrot, parsnip, with colour, smell and sweetness). Yet in the earthy, watery domain such scents remain coarser. Where the astral is incorporated into vital plant processes, in the etheric watery realm, poisons can be expected to manifest, hence water dropwort, water hemlock and hemlock.

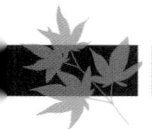

Chord three is that of an enveloping gesture that meets the downward process, producing characteristic gum-resins. The airy volatility of the flower/seed realm and the lignifying mineralizing tendency of the root are mingled. 'Two processes combine: the process of warmth and air coming down from above, condensing in the synthesis of volatile oils and finally becoming fixed as resins are formed closer to the root, and the softening process of latex and mucilage production which takes place between the solid and fluid elements … A volatile fiery principle enters into a sphere of fixedness. A hardening process is softened into plasticity. Latex forms where the two interact'.

Hence, says Pelikan, the medicinal potential can be inferred. In the glandular system, in the digestive and lacteal glands in particular, between the fluid etheric and anabolic and the astral secretory catabolic – 'incretion and excretion' of these glands are promoted. Where the astral intervenes in the fluid etheric, these plants will enhance the astral relationship to the ether body and promote elimination, hence they tend to be diuretic, sudorific and promote fluid elimination in dropsy, coughs and similar. Moreover, remedies in this family are useful where the astral body needs to bring 'stronger formative activity into the aeriform organization where this is inadequate'. Thus they are useful for wind in the digestive tract and as a spasmolytic. 'Spasms in the respiratory and circulatory systems are relieved'. Finally the seasonings in the family again promote strong astral action in digestion.

The carrot specifically, Pelikan says, holds the balance in this family, at its central point, as the rose among the Rosaceae, reaching a harmony of form. The root contains up to 12% sugar (since starches are too solid to form in the carrot), pectin, inositol, lecithin, glutamine, phosphatides and carotene. The latter is a 'light substance' – 'Light activity fills this root with power' – and is found among other places in the visual purple of the eye. The ash contains silica and iron (plus copper, cobalt, nickel and arsenic) and silica is also associated with light (and form). Pelican clearly disagrees with Culpeper in appreciation of the root as a food. It is particularly nourishing for children, he says. He sums up the traditional uses of the root as diuretic and aphrodisiac, the seeds for menstruation and conception, as diuretic and anti-oedematous, 'restoring the rule of the astral body over the fluid organism'.

This appreciation of carrot bears out to an extent the traditional uses and offers some account of their effects.

## RECOMMENDATIONS

- There is no doubt from the tradition that daucus is a strong urinary remedy working through its heat, for use as a diuretic, preventing stone, ridding gravel, against cystitis.
- For related conditions of gout, rheumatic and arthritic complaints, and easing oedema.
- As a gastrointestinal herb as carminative for colic from trapped wind.
- As a topical application, following Cook's hearty recommendations, we have a remedy here that deserves more attention for its capacity to heal old sores of all kinds.
- As a gentle remedy for thread worms.
- As a cough remedy to ease old coughs.
- Through lack of clear evidence it is difficult to conclude daucus' action on the reproductive system: it may be aphrodisiac, it may aid conception, it may be contraceptive (possibly in larger doses) and it most probably provokes menses. It is tempting to designate it a tonic for uterine function but definitive support is lacking, although there is significant traditional usage.

Dosage: The *British Herbal Pharmacopoeia* recommends 2–4 g three times a day of dried aerial parts.

## RECOMMENDATIONS ON SAFETY

1. Do not use during pregnancy

Given the evidence of traditional usage as a contraceptive, daucus should not be used in pregnancy and could be avoided when hoping to become pregnant. Barnes et al (2007) discuss antifertility tests on rats and recommend that daucus should not be used in pregnancy as safety has not been established. An investigation of the antifertility activity of an aqueous extract of a compound product of six herbs, including *Daucus carota* seed, found the product had a 60% antifertility action at 324 mg/kg and the product was found to be safe up to 3240 mg/kg (Gnanasam et al 2002).

## CONSTITUENTS

Reviews: Barnes et al (2007), Bradley (1992), Williamson (2003).

### Volatile oils

A review of carrot seed oils identified four main chemotypes: sabinene 32–60%, geranyl acetate 32–77%, carotol 23–77% and equal parts of all three (Gonny et al 2004).
Total 0.6% (fresh weight) (69 compounds), monoterpenes 38%: alpha-pinene 25%; oxygenated monoterpenes; sesquiterpenes 11%: beta-bisabolene; phenylpropanoids 46%: methylisoeugenol 33%, elemicin 11.4%, beta-asarone 1.2% (aerial parts, end of flowering, commercial);
Total 0.1–0.2%, monoterpenes: beta-pinene 29–39%, sabinene 15–20%, limonene, myrcene (whole plant, before and during flowering, wild, Corsica);
Total 0.6%, monoterpenes: beta-pinene 19%, sabinene 10%, myrcene; sesquiterpenes: carotol 4%, beta-bisabolene; phenylpropanoids: (E)-methylisoeugenol 34%, elemicin 11% (ripe umbel with seeds, wild, Corsica) (Gonny et al 2004). This study found higher concentrations of phenylpropanoids in the ripe umbel with seeds.
Total 0.5–0.7% (103 compounds, 68 identified), monoterpenes 83–95%: sabinene 28–37%, alpha-pinene 16–24%, terpinen-4-ol, limonene; sesquiterpenes 3.7–10.5% mainly caryophyllane-type (seeds, wild, Lithuania) (Mockute & Nivinskiene 2004).
Total 1.06% (31 compounds), monoterpene hydrocarbons 72%: sabinene 40%; oxygenated monoterpenes 25%: geranyl acetate (mature umbel, wild, Poland) (Staniszewska et al 2005). This study in Poland did not find the carotane sesquiterpenes (carotol, daucol and beta-caryophyllene), which have been found in oils from cultivated carrot cultivars, whereas they were found in the previous sample from Lithuania.

### Furanocoumarins

Furanocoumarins were found in cultivated carrot roots but at very substantially lower levels than in other vegetables such as parsnip and celery (Peroutka et al 2007).

### Flavonoids

Flavones: luteolin and glycosides (seeds, wild, Scotland) (Kumarasamy et al 2005).

## REFERENCES

Akeroyd J 2003 The encyclopaedia of wild flowers. Parragon, Bath.

Andrews AC 1949 The carrot as a food in the classical era. Classical Philology 44:182–196.

Barnes J, Anderson LA, Phillipson JD 2007 Herbal medicines, 3rd edn. Pharmaceutical Press, London.

Bradley PR (ed.) 1992 British Herbal Compendium, vol 1. British Herbal Medicine Association, Bournemouth.

Davis PH (ed.) 1972 Flora of Turkey, vol 4. Edinburgh University Press, Edinburgh.

Gnanasam SK, Annamalai T, Narendranath KA, et al 2002 Evaluation of antifertility activity of polyherbal formulation. Indian Drugs 39:330–332.

Gonny M, Bradesi P, Casanova J 2004 Identification of the components of the essential oil from wild corsican *Daucus carota* L. using 13C-NMR spectroscopy. Flavour and Fragrance Journal 19:424–433.

Green MH (ed.) 2001 The Trotula. University of Pennsylvania Press, Philadelphia

Hauser TP, Bjørn GK 2001 Hybrids between wild and cultivated carrots in Danish carrot fields. Genetic Resources and Crop Evolution 48:499–506.

Kumarasamy Y, Nahar L, Byres M, et al 2005 The assessment of biological activities associated with the major constituents of the methanol extract of 'wild carrot' *Daucus carota* L. seeds. Journal of Herbal Pharmacotherapy 5:61–72.

Mockute D, Nivinskiene O 2004 The sabinene chemotype of essential oil of seeds of *Daucus carota* L. ssp. carota growing wild in Lithuania. Journal of Essential Oil Research 16:277–281.

Peroutka R, Schulzova V, Botek P, et al 2007 Analysis of furanocoumarins in vegetables (Apiaceae) and citrus fruits (Rutaceae). Journal of the Science of Food and Agriculture 87:2152–2163.

Riddle JM 1997 Eve's herbs. Harvard University Press, Cambridge.

Staniszewska M, Kula J, Wieczorkiewicz M, et al 2005 Essential oils of wild and cultivated carrots – the chemical composition and antimicrobial activity. Journal of Essential Oil Research 17:579–583.

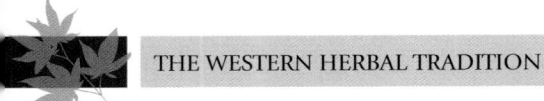

Tutin TG 1980 Umbellifers of the British Isles. Botanical Society of the British Isles, London.

Tutin TG, Heywood VH, Burges NA et al 1968 Flora Europaea, vol 2. Cambridge University Press, Cambridge.

Williamson E 2003 Potter's herbal cyclopaedia. CW Daniel, Saffron Walden.

Yu LL, Zhou KK, Parry J 2005 Antioxidant properties of cold-pressed black caraway, carrot, cranberry, and hemp seed oils. Food Chemistry 91:723–729.

# CHAPTER 15
# *Drimia maritima*, squill

## DESCRIPTION

**Family: Hyacinthaceae**  **Part used: bulb**

*Drimia maritima* (L.) Stearn is a bulbous perennial that grows around the Mediterranean littoral in dry stony and sandy areas. It is found west into Portugal and the Canary Islands, along the North Africa coast, and east into Syria, Israel and southern Iran (Anonymous 2005, Davis 1984). How far it grows inland varies: Davis (1984) states up to 300 m above sea level, but it grows at over 680 m in an inland national park in Apulia, Italy (Perrino et al 2006) and, according to Grieve, at elevations up to 900 m in Sicily.

The basal leaves are flattened (30–100 cm long) and 10 cm wide and appear after flowering and last until the next summer. The scape (leafless stem arising from the bulb) is 100–150 cm tall with a dense raceme of spirally arranged white flowers from September to November. Flowers arise from bulbs over 6 years old (Gentry et al 1987).The black seeds are carried in a three-sectioned capsule.

The large bulbs grow to 15 cm across and form clumps which protrude from the ground. Squill can be grown in warm sunny sites further north, but is unlikely to flower.

The binomial nomenclature of squill has changed over the years and the different opinions lead to its designation in the Hyacinthaceae or in the Scilloideae section of Liliaceae. We have followed Farah (2005), Barnes et al (2007) and the *British Herbal Compendium* (Bradley 1992) in using *Drimia maritima*. Most published work refers to *Urginea maritima* agg. (L.) Baker and this name is commonly used (USDA 2009). The two names can be taken as synonymous.

Linnaeus identified squill as *Scilla maritima* in 1753 and this name can still be found in the literature. The heterogeneity of the genus led to its division and the creation of a new genus *Urginea* Steinheil in 1834 and this genus was recognized as containing squill in 1873 by Baker. In 1977 Jessop reorganized the South African *Urginea* species within the genus *Drimia* and in 1978 the Mediterrranean and Indian species were transferred to *Drimia* by Stearn, which led to the abolition of the genus *Urginea* (Pfosser & Speta 2004). Some authorities maintain the genus *Drimia* with sub-groups, but Speta determined that squill should be a separate genus which he named *Charybdis* and located with *Urginea* and *Bowlea* in Urgineoideae, one of the four subfamilies in Hyacinthaceae (Pfosser & Speta 2004). This determination is supported by Krenn et al (2004) and the debate appears to have some time left to run.

**Other species used:** The *Drimia* genus is centred in South Africa and *Drimia sanguinea* syn. *Urginea sanguinea* and other species are widely used as medicines (Marx et al 2005). *Drimia indica* syn. *Urginea indica* is a similar Indian species (Trease & Evans 1978). *Pancratium maritimum* L. (Amyrillidaceae) is another bulbous plant, with large white flowers, which grows on sandy foreshores around the Mediterranean (Rix & Phillips 1981). It is mentioned as similar in action by the authors, including Dioscorides (II 172) and called sea daffodil by Gerard, but is no longer used in medicine. Gerard refers to *Pancratium maritimum* as great squill and Miller appears to use the term 'red squill' to refer to *Pancratium maritimum*.

### Quality

The bulb is collected in the autumn after flowering and cut into transverse slices after removal of the dry outer membranaceous scales (Trease & Evans 1978). Grieve warns that it should be handled with care as the juice is acrid and burns the skin.

Only white squill should be used. Phylogenetic analysis has found differences between specimens in the eastern and western Mediterranean and *Urginea maritima* agg. includes at least six types, of which red squill, which contains anthocyanins, is cultivated in Egypt as a rodenticide. Ibn Sina calls attention to the poisonous variety and states that pearl coloured bulbs are best. According to Mesue, cited in Turner, the best has shiny peel and grows in a free field in groups. In their detailed entries, Pliny and Bauhin distinguish between red and white squill.

According to Pfosser & Speta (2004), within the species, chromosome number varies and, in this case designated as *Charybdis maritima*, there are diploid, tetraploid, triploid and hexaploid specimens. The specimens look similar and, according to Bradley (1992), squill should be sourced from Spain and the eastern Mediterranean. Pliny (Stannard 1974) describes squill as growing wild in large quantities in the Balearic islands, Ibiza and the Spanish provinces, which suggests this as the source of squill in ancient Rome.

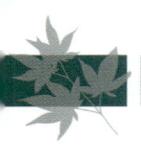

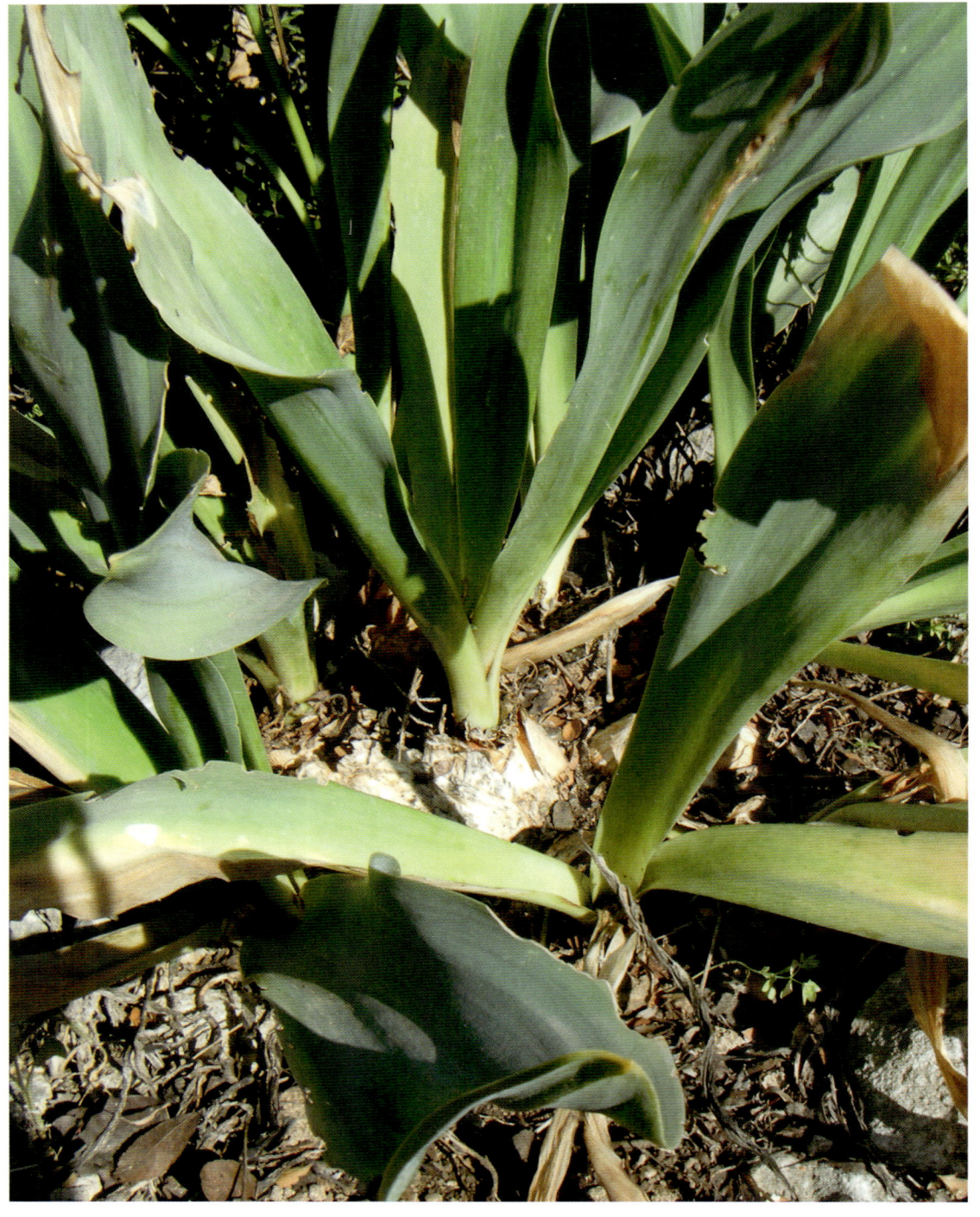

Figure 15.1 *Drimia maritima,* sea onion (near Kizkalesi, Turkey, May).

*Drimia maritima*, squill | Chapter | 15 |

> Propagation and cultivation is discussed in detail by Gentry et al (1987), who ran a large-scale project in southern California. Squill grew successfully without irrigation on dry-farmed grain lands. Squill benefited from coastal mists and yield of scilliroside was higher in mature bulbs which had flowered and in the adventitious roots.
>
> Squill spoils easily in storage because of the high mucilage content and should be stored in a very dry place (Trease & Evans 1978).

## DIURETIC AND EXPECTORANT, BUT MIND YOU COOK IT FIRST

The entry in Dioscorides (II 171) gives an unusual level of detail for the methods of preparation. The relative value of particular preparations such as the vinegar, oxymel and syrup are consistently discussed by the authors. The detail for preparations and dosage is significant as squill contains cardiac glycosides and therefore safe usage depends on careful determination of the dose. Furthermore, an adverse drug reaction was caused by overdosing, and preparation and dosage is a theme in this monograph.

Because of the cardiac glycosides, I will concentrate on the main themes in usage but mention some uses as a general tonic and in external preparations. Dioscorides recommends squill in 'draughts or fragrant prescriptions' for 'those whose micturition we want to set in motion', for oedema, people with chronic coughs, asthmatics and people who bring up blood or phlegm at the dose of 3 obols (1800 mg) in lozenge form with honey. The whole entry for squill in Pliny is very similar with the same dose of cooked squill as a diuretic for dropsy, drunk with honey and vinegar. Ibn Sina gives the same dose in honey for asthma and chronic cough. These symptoms and signs can be the result of congestive heart failure and set the scene for the use of squill down the ages.

Dioscorides recommends three types of preparation: baked squill, cooked and dried squill, which is then macerated in vinegar, wine or oil, and a preparation using a lozenge in honey. These are the basis of preparations given by later authors. Dioscorides states that the bulb is 'sharp and heating' and should only be used after it has been cooked until tender. He recommends wrapping it in dough and baking in an oven or in the embers. He says that the outer parts are stripped off and that it must be returned to the oven if not fully tender. Pliny gives a slightly different method: roast the squill, remove the outer parts, cook in water and take a dose of 3 obols (1800 mg) as a diuretic for dropsy drunk with honey and vinegar. Dioscorides then describes the preparation of the vinegar, wine or oil of squill. The fresh bulb is boiled, cut into pieces, fresh water is added and the water changed until the water is 'neither bitter nor pungent'. Stannard (1974) gives this slightly differently 'The water of the first boiling is poured off, and it is boiled again until the water is neither bitter nor sharp'. Dioscorides then recommends drying the squill in the shade, slicing the bulb and hanging the slices out to dry by threading them on a linen thread so that they do not touch each other. Pliny gives the following preparation for the vinegar: dry the squill as in Dioscorides, plunge straight into vinegar, cover tightly and macerate under a tile in the sunshine for 48 days before the solstice. Mattioli's translation suggests rather maceration during the period of high summer. After maceration, remove the squill and decant the vinegar into another container. The method of Pliny is given by Serapio and Apuleius and, to summarise, all authors state that it must, as Galen says, be cooked to remove its vehemence. Mattioli gives a lengthy consideration of the correct sources of the plant material. He observes that the 'common squill' was used by apothecaries and, on account of the size of the bulb and because it produced bulbils like the squill described by Theophrastus, he had taken this to be correct. However, after comparing the leaves of squill with aloe, to which Dioscorides and Pliny compare squill, he realized that 'common squill' was different as it had leaves more like a lily. He identifies 'common squill' as Pancration, probably *Pancratium maritimum*, which is more lily-like and grows on sandy foreshores in Italy. Mattioli comes to this conclusion based on information from doctors in Spain that on that coast the squills are larger with aloe-like leaves, although not so thick. These squills are considered stronger and more bitter and thus more effective. So, again an author is recommending the use of squill from Spain. Reading this passage, it is easy to see why Mattioli's Commentaries on Dioscorides were so popular. Mattioli is never afraid to comment or disagree with the material from other sources, and extra material is added from his own observations.

## TO SOFTEN AND CUT THE HUMOURS

Dioscorides recommends usage in stomach ailments where the food remains undigested, in jaundice and in colic. He describes squill boiled with honey as assisting digestion very nicely to 'drive the glutinous element down the bowel' but adds the caution that it not be given to people with 'any kind of internal ulceration'. This recommendation for use to purge humours, according to Mesue cited in Turner, or 'bring forth all offensive things from

157

# THE WESTERN HERBAL TRADITION

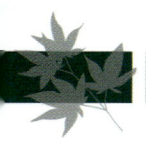

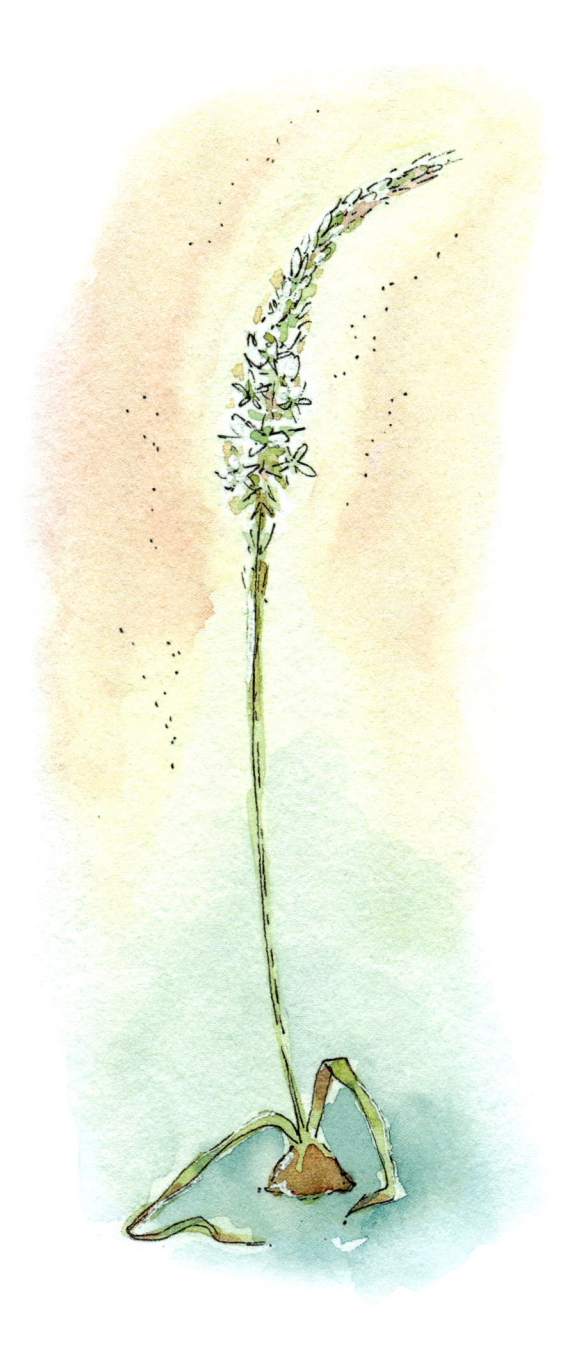

Figure 15.2 *Drimia maritima*, sea onion.

the body' in the words of Culpeper, is repeated by all the Renaissance authors. According to Turner himself, squill 'driveth away slimy matter like shavings of the guts' and he quotes Galen's remarks on its 'marvelous cutting-power'. Mesue describes the process as 'both maketh ripe and ready the matter to be put forth and driveth forth such matters as are made ready'. Ibn Sina followed by Mesue suggests that it 'softens thick and tough humours, cutting them and making them subtle and scouring so that they might more easily come forth'. This recommendation is given in all the later texts.

## THE VINEGAR AS A DAILY TONIC

This action on the digestive tract could be linked with the recommendation for use as a general tonic especially as a daily small dose of a preparation in vinegar. Culpeper suggests a little vinegar of squill taken fasting in the morning before walking for 30 minutes to preserve health, soundness of body and vigour of mind into extreme old age. A daily dose of vinegar is advised in *Sauer's Herbal*, published in America in 1772, for good health, a clear voice, sweet breath, against gum disease and to promote digestive processes (Weaver 2001). Dried squill is described as commonly available in apothecary shops and the recipe given is 16 tablespoons of vinegar poured on 4 tablespoons of dried squill. Keep in a warm place for 14 days, and take a dose of 1 tablespoon every morning. This recipe would need recalculating as a weight of squill to ensure that the dose is safe. Stannard (1974) suggests that squill was commonly known in the ancient world, giving examples including a recipe where it was used to flavour smoked fish in the 3rd century BC in Greece. The recipe ascribed to Dioscorides by Bauhin for use of 65 pints of vinegar suggests usage on a large scale and I wonder whether squill was used as a condiment, since Stannard (1974) mentions Pliny on its use to increase the sourness of vinegar and suggests that the form of reference by Celsus to the vinegar in 1st century AD Rome implies that Celsus expects his readers to be familiar with it. Mesue, cited by Turner, may be giving a clue to this when he writes that squill hinders putrefaction, 'helpeth stopping of the milt and swelling' (enlarged spleen) and thus 'maketh a man's body keep in a young state' and 'maketh a loose body fast and compact'. The heating power of squill is implied by Ibn Sina, who says that it easily damages healthy nerves but heals diseases of nerves and joints, especially paralysis and sciatica (in vinegar or wine), epilepsy and melancholy.

This last recommendation is linked with the temperament of squill. The authors agree that its temperament is fierce. The text of Ibn Sina reflects that of Dioscorides describing squill as caustic, and classifies it as hot in the third degree and dry in the second. Turner discusses whether it is hot in the second degree as claimed by Galen and Averroes, or in the third degree as claimed by Mesue, and concludes from his tasting that it is hot in the second degree. Turner gives the text of Dioscorides, of Mesue and a brief summary of Pliny whereas Fuchs reproduces the whole of Pliny. Turner says that squill grows near the seaside in Spain and Apulia (province of Italy) using different sources from Fuchs who gives it as very cutting and hot in the second, then states, rather confusingly, that it grows everywhere like onions and garlic. The Salernitan herbal gives hot in the second degree but Gerard, who provides a good description and picture, describes it as hot and dry in the fourth degree 'but not so extreme hot as garlic'.

Use as a daily tonic could be implied from its inclusion in Theriacs which were sometimes taken daily in small doses to ward off infection or poison. Although Stannard (1974) reviewed references to dropsy from ancient up to medieval times and found that squill was rarely mentioned or included in the prescriptions, he found consistent mention of use in compound mixtures. This could be because of use in a Theriac given by Galen. Squill was an important ingredient in Galene Ancromachus, the antidote prepared by Andromachus, physician to Nero. According to Griffin (2004) the Galene had 55 ingredients and was the forerunner of Theriacs, which were manufactured until the 18th century. Galen describes Mithridatum and Galene Andromachus in Antidotes I and II. Norton (2006) studied the formula given for Mithridatum by Celsus in the 1st century AD and did not find squill listed. Quincy, writing in the 18th century, argues for use of fresh rather than dried squill.

## EXTERNAL USAGE?

Before returning to cardiac use, there is some external usage to discuss. External usage dates back a long time. Writing in 388 BC, Aristophanes (Stannard 1974) gives a satire on treatment at the Asclepion '...mingled verjuce and squills; and brayed them up together. Then drenched the mass with Sphettian vinegar. And turning up the eyelids of the man, plastered their innersides, to make the smart more painful' – definitely not to be tried. However, there are some consistent recommendations. Dioscorides and Ibn Sina propose use in fissures on the heels, and Dioscorides suggests squill baked and smeared on for thin-necked warts and chilblains. The *Old English Herbarium* says that for chilblains, the adventitious roots of the same plant, pounded with vinegar and bread and laid on the sore 'cure the condition in a wonderful way'. The Salernitan herbal recommends external usage for gout, paralysis and pain in limbs provoked by cold and this is repeated by later authors. The preparation is a maceration in oil and wine for 15 days, cooked and added to wax.

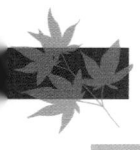

## BACK TO DIURESIS AND DYSPNOEA

Returning to the indication for use in oedema and as a diuretic, Aliotsa et al (2004) portray squill as having been consistently used as a diuretic although Stannard (1974) in his extensive review was less conclusive. The *Old English Herbarium* gives a slightly different preparation for dropsy: dry the squill completely, take the inner part and simmer in water and then mix warm with honey and vinegar. Give three cupfuls and 'quickly the disease will be drawn out through the urine'.

The list of conditions given by Dioscorides suggests an expectorant action as well as the action to support cardiac function, but could mainly refer to support of the heart as we must remember that the role of the heart as pump was not known. Turner's version of Dioscorides' asthma is breathlessness and he renders Beck's 'fragrant prescriptions' as 'spicy compositions'. Miller lists the vinegar, wine, oxymel and troches, and gives a clear summary 'hot, bitterish, opening and alternating, good to cleanse the lungs of tough viscid phlegm, and of great service in asthmas, and difficulty of breathing, and are often used as a vomit to clear the stomach and help the jaundice and dropsy, they likewise provoke urine and the catamenia'. Weiss argues that the action in right heart failure and cor pulmonale in emphysema is not proven and that the main effect is as a diuretic. He gives a prescription: Tincture *Scilla maritima* 5 mL, *Crataegus monogyna* 10 mL, *Valeriana officinalis* 15 mL, with a dose of 15 drops three times a day. The *British Herbal Pharmacopoeia* summarizes the actions as expectorant, cathartic, emetic, cardioactive and diuretic, and recommends squill in asthma with bronchitis and chronic bronchitis with scanty sputum combined with white horehound *Marrubium vulgare* and coltsfoot *Tussilago farfara*. Menzies-Trull gives the same indications, suggesting squill as useful for atonic tissues and effusion of the pleura, pericardium and peritoneum.

## DOSAGE IS CRITICAL

The next consideration is the dose and the type of preparation: the wine, the vinegar and the oxymel, and a maceration in honey. Preparations in vinegar and honey are given throughout the literature. The original dose given by Dioscorides is 1800 mg of cooked squill and this dose is followed by later writers such as Fuchs. How might one interpret the evidence and recommend on type of preparation and dosage?

Practitioners in Britain are likely to purchase dried material, but given the emphasis on cooking the first advice would be to bring the plant material to the boil to tenderize before using in any preparation.

Hill separates the actions by preparation: wine as a diuretic for jaundice and dropsy, vinegar as an emetic and oxymel for asthma and difficulty in breathing. Quincy gives the same actions and suggests that the emetic action of the vinegar can be tempered by giving the infusion with cinnamon water so that the action is 'downward' as a purgative or diuretic. While observing that it was commonly used as a purgative, Cullen argues that its diuretic and pectoral effects often disappoint. He gives the vinegar and pills, and discounts the use of oxymels along with all other honey syrups.

According to Stannard (1974) squill cooked with wine is recommended for dropsy by Scribonius Largus writing in the early 1st century AD. Dioscorides gives a recipe for the wine: chop 1 lb of dried bulb, put in a linen cloth with 20 pints of new must for 3 months. Bauhin offers a recipe for a wine from the Roman writer Columella to be used to restore the body, for the stomach and for an old cough. The squill is chopped as thinly as possible, the slices are hung in the shade to dry and 1 lb is macerated in 48 pints of wine for 30 days. He adds that some use 1¼ lb and some leave for 40 days.

Bauhin recaps the recipes given earlier by Dioscorides and Pliny and gives amounts of 1 mina (Greek unit, 437 g) in 12 pints of vinegar, macerated in the sun for 60 days keeping the vessel open. He then says that some use 65 pints and some use the not yet dried squill, left for 6 months, which is more cutting. Vinegars can spoil and the wine in the earlier recipes would be reduced to a vinegar, so these recipes need consideration in the light of current methods of preparation.

Mattioli, copied by Bauhin, describes the method of preparation of a macerate in honey. The inner part of raw squill is macerated in a vessel that is placed in the sun in the dog days (high summer), and the honey is poured off and used for epilepsy and other illnesses of the brain, proceeding from cold. Mattioli compares this with the method given by Galen, who gives a similar method of preparation but does not use the squill until the heat has 'resolved and softened' the squill. Mattioli argues that in Galen's method the squill is cooked in the honey to form a juice, citing Galen that squill has a strongly cutting virtue, best used roasted or boiled. Turner cites Mesue as recommending the oxymel or honied vinegar or a mixture of the juice with honey.

Culpeper (1669) expresses the recipe slightly differently: take one squill full of juice, cut in bits, put in a stoppered glass vessel in the sun for 20 days before and 20 days after the rising of the dog star, open the vessel, take the juice from the bottom and preserve with honey. As squill is a Mediterranean plant, we do not know whether Culpeper could have obtained fresh squill. According to Pereira (1853), Pliny tells us that the use of oxymel of squill for cough was discovered by Pythagoras in the 6th century BC but Pliny gives no other detail as he promises to return to the subject in a later volume. Culpeper provides a recipe for a simple oxymel: take 4 lb honey, 2 lb of water, 2 lb of white wine vinegar, boil and remove the scum with a 'wooden scummer', until it becomes the consistency of a syrup. 'It cuts phlegm and is a food preparative against a vomit'.

Calculation of the correct dosage is important in making preparations as the dose of the product depends on the final yield of the preparation. The dose given by Dioscorides of 1800 mg of cooked squill is substantially higher than the dose in the *British Herbal Pharmacopoeia*. Bauhin gives doses of 5–12 fluid drachms (17.5–42 mL) for infusion, up to 3 oz (90 mL) for the oxymel and 2–4 drachms (8–16 g) for the troche (lozenge), and again these are higher than the dose now recommended.

Calculation of dosage can inhibit the introduction of herbs into one's practice. In the 1970s when working in a herbal shop, a prescription was periodically made up for cough in babies, which was syrup of violets with oil of almonds. Syrup of squill was added as an expectorant, maybe because squill is recommended for whooping cough in the *British Herbal Pharmacopoeia*. The same formula is recommended for asthma and coughing in *Sauer's Herbal* as follows: 1 tablespoon of squill honey, 1 tablespoon of sweet almond oil and 2–3 tablespoons of violet juice. Take a tablespoonful every 6 hours. The syrup is prepared by boiling 1½ lb honey until it thickens and adding 1 lb of squill vinegar and boiling a little more to thicken the mixture (Weaver 2001). Squill was not part of my training and I did not try it until years later after reading Robinson (1868), who describes squill as a useful expectorant, especially in chronic bronchitis where the phlegm is tough, viscid and difficult to void. He warns that it must not be used when there is active inflammation in the airways as it can irritate and aggravate a cough rather than relieving it. He gives a dose of 1–3 grains (65–195 mg) as a diuretic and 20 drops of tincture of squill in a wineglass of water at night for cough. Preparations given are the vinegar: 2½ oz dried squill macerated in 1 pint of vinegar for 1 week, add 1½ fl oz spirit as a preservative and the syrup made with 3½ lb sugar to 1 pint of squill vinegar at a dose of 1–2 fl drachms (3.5–7 mL). This proved to raise many issues concerning the Avoirdupois and Apothecaries' system and, although I made the vinegar and tried it in a cough mixture for myself, it was never used on patients as the dose remained problematic. It would have been useful to consult two other sources: the dose of dry bulb in the *British Herbal Pharmacopoeia* is 60–200 mg three times a day, which is expressed in the dose of vinegar BPC 1973 1:10 in dilute acetic acid as 0.6–2 mL. The dose of tincture 1:10 60% (BPC 1973) is slightly less at 0.3–2 mL.

Pereira (1853) gives substantial detail on dosage. He states that the bulb loses about 80% of its weight. So, 3 obols (1800 mg) of fresh squill would be equivalent to 360 mg of dried squill. Pereira gives the dose of the dried powder as 6–15 grains (390–975 mg) as an emetic, 10 grains (650 mg) being the average and advises commencing with 1 grain (65 mg) as an expectorant and increasing until there is slight nausea. The starting dose in the *British Herbal Pharmacopoeia* is 60 mg three times a day, so this is equivalent to the starting dose given by Pereira for use as an expectorant.

Using the US pint of 16 fl oz, the recipe for tincture of squill given by Pereira is 1:8. Macerate 4 oz squill in 2 pints of vinegar at a gentle heat in a covered vessel for 3 days, strain, allow the dregs to settle and remove, add 1 fl oz alcohol. He gives a recipe for oxymel, which like the recipe of Robinson would need further analysis of yield to calculate the concentration of squill in the final preparation and thus the dose. The syrup of squill given is 2 lb sugar to 1 pint vinegar of squill as above, an ingredient of cough mixtures 'as a common remedy for children in cases of cough or cold'.

## CARDIAC GLYCOSIDES

The reason for extra care with the dose is the presence of cardiac glycosides and the following is a brief summary of their actions. Steroidal saponins are almost exclusively found in monocotyledons. Sparg et al (2004) review recent in vitro research into triterpene and steroidal saponins and conclude that there is a wide range of activity in the body. Two types of steroidal saponin affect heart function: cardenolides, which are found in *Convallaria majalis* (Liliaceae), and bufadienolides, which are found in squill, and were first isolated from toad venom (Bruneton 1999). The term 'cardiac glycosides' therefore include cardenolides with a five-membered unsaturated lactone ring attached to the steroid nucleus and bufadienolides with a six-membered doubly unsaturated lactone ring. Cardiac glycosides occur in complex mixtures of related aglycones. The aglycones in bufadienolides vary in degree of hydroxylation and the sugars are mainly glucose and rhamnose (Krenn & Kopp 1998). Breakdown by endogenous enzymes changes the complex mixture during drying. For example, the diglycoside scillaridin, the main bufadienolide in squill, is broken down to proscillaridin, which is considered to be the main active aglycone.

Acid hydrolysis of the bond between the aglycone and the sugar occurs in the acid conditions of the stomach and the uptake and pharmacokinetics of the glycosides is thought to depend substantially on the sugar chain (Albrecht 1999) and on the hydroxylation of the aglycone (Bruneton 1999). Products standardized to 0.2% proscillaridin, at a dose of 100–500 mg daily, are recommended by Commission E (Schulz et al 1993). Proscillaridin lowers the pulse less than other glycosides and has a short duration of action (Bruneton 1999). According to Weiss, it is well tolerated and any toxic symptoms such as nausea are short-lived. It has a low uptake and appears to be extensively metabolized (Andersson et al 1975). Schulz et al (1998) give an absorption rate of 20–30% for proscillaridin and an average half-life of 24 hours.

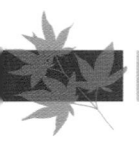

Very briefly, cardiac glycosides inhibit Na+-K+-ATPase and therefore inhibit active transport across cell membranes, which leads to increased intracellular sodium and extracellular potassium. This triggers an increase in intracellular calcium, leading to increased contractility of the myocardium, increased force of contraction and thus increased cardiac output with decreased heart rate. Different modes of action inside the myocyte have been proposed, and the action on other cells may also be useful in chronic heart failure (Schwinger et al 2003). The effects outside the heart are reviewed by Marx et al (2005).

## RECOMMENDATIONS

- Quality and provenance of raw material to be used in herbal preparations need further research for herbal practitioners to feel confident.
- External usage is not necessary.
- The care of patients with chronic heart failure is challenging and the symptoms are not necessarily alleviated by conventional drugs thus squill has a place in the materia medica as an expectorant in noninflammatory conditions of the lungs and as a diuretic in chronic heart failure and cor pulmonale.
- The vinegar and oxymel have a long-standing traditional usage and can be recommended for usage. Calculation of dosage of these products will depend on the method used.

Dosage: the *British Herbal Pharmacopoeia* recommends 60–200 mg three times a day of dried bulb. The minimum dose of 60 mg three times a day is the dose given by Pereira (1853) as the minimum expectorant dose; the maximum dose is half the minimum dose for emesis stated in Pereira.

## CONSTITUENTS

Reviews: Anonymous (2005), Bradley (1992), Barnes et al (2007), Williamson (2003).

### Polysaccharides

Red squill *Urginea maritima*, fructo-oligosaccharides (Spies et al 1992).

### Cardiac glycosides: bufadienolides

Total 0.15–2.4%, scillarenin glycosides: scillaren A, proscillaridin A, glucoscillaren A; glycosides of scilliphaeosidin: scilliphaeoside, glucoscilliphaeoside, 12-*epi*-scilliphaeoside; silliglaucoside, scillicyanoside (Bradley 1992, Kopp et al 1983). *Urginea maritima* sensu stricta, 14 glycosides: proscillaridin A, scillaren A, glucoscillaren A, scilliphaeoside, glucoscilliphaeoside (wild, Pego, Spain, cultivated 1 year, Austria) (Krenn et al 1991).
*Urginea maritima* agg., eight glycosides: proscillaridin A, scilliglaucoside, scilliphaeoside, scilliroside (red coloured bulbs, wild, Tunisia; red coloured bulbs, wild Sardinia). The Tunisian sample had five more glycosides, which were different from the seven extra glycosides in the Sardinian sample (Krenn et al 1994).
*Urginea maritima* agg., total 1%, 41 glycosides (26 new compounds): proscillaridin, glucoscillaren A, scilliphaeoside, scilliroside (wild, Egypt) (Kopp et al 1996).
*Charybdis maritima*, total 1.77%, two new bufadienolides (wild, Spain) (Krenn et al 2000).
*Urginea maritima*, 32 bufadienolides (nine new compounds), one lignan glycoside (cultivated, Japan) (Iizuka et al 2001).
*Urginea fugax*, cardenolides. This is now in a different genus from squill, which is confirmed by the presence of cardenolides (wild, Ibiza) (Krenn et al 2004).

### Flavonoids

Quercetin glycosides, dihydroquercetin glycoside (wild, Spain & Balearic islands) (Fernandez et al 1972).

## RECOMMENDATIONS ON SAFETY

1. Do not use with digitalis and use caution if the patient is taking conventional medicines.

The mainstay of orthodox treatment for heart failure is ACE inhibitors (CKS 2009) but cardiac glycosides are still considered to have a place (Dec 2003). Potential herb-drug interactions involving squill may be extrapolated from contraindications to the use of digoxin and its potential drug–drug interactions. Use caution if the patient is taking a diuretic as potassium depletion is possible (Mills & Bone 2000).

2. Do not use where the patient has hypertension or poor kidney function.

Recently cardenolides such as ouabain and bufadienolides have been shown to be endogenously produced in the adrenal glands (Schoner & Scheiner-Bobis 2007). They are thought to have a role in perpetuating hypertension by increasing contraction in vascular smooth muscle cells and other mechanisms. It is argued that this may be particularly significant where the hypertension is associated with sensitivity to salt or with low plasma renin activity (Haddy 2006).

3. Use caution with the dose.

Side effects are nausea, vomiting, stomach ache, diarrhoea and irregular pulse (Bradley 1992).

Marx et al (2005) review the use of *Urginea sanguinea*, which is commonly used in South Africa for a wide range of diseases. They argue that adverse effects occur because cardiac glycosides affect normal membrane depolarization in all cells, which particularly affects brain function and neurotransmission. Fourteen adverse drug reactions in Pretoria resulting in hospital care are reported by Foukaridis et al (1995). Both authors suggest that traditional healers generally use small doses and that the major cause of adverse effects is patients taking more than the prescribed dose or self-dosing excessively.

A 55-year-old woman died in Turkey 30 hours after cooking and eating squill. She had cooked a bulb for 1 hour and peeled off the outer layers. Bulbs can weigh more than 1 kg so this could have been a large dose. She was hypothyroid and had had a normal ECG the week before as part of her routine care for Hashimoto's thyroiditis. On arrival at hospital her pulse was slow, she was nauseous and became unconscious. She was admitted to the coronary care unit but complete atrioventricular block was followed by ventricular arrythmia and fibrillation which was the cause of death. The authors did not find any other cases in the literature (Tuncok et al 1995).

A 42-year-old woman in Britain who had taken Gee's linctus for many years experienced atrioventricular block as a result of taking a whole bottle daily because of stress in the family. Each 5 mL contains tincture of opium 0.084 mL, squill vinegar 0.5 mL. She made a full recovery after discontinuing the product (Smith et al 1986).

4. Do not use squill in pregnancy, lactation or when the patient could become pregnant during treatment.

*Urginea sanguinea* is used as an abortifacient in South Africa and Marx et al (2005) ascribe this action to the toxic effects of cardiac glycosides. According to Stannard (1974), The Book of Nature of Konrad of Megenberg, which was a translation of a 12th century text, states 'it promotes the menses, and causes abortion in pregnant women, thereby delivering them of their child before their time'.

## REFERENCES

Albrecht HP 1999 Cardiac glycosides. In: Ikan R (ed) Naturally occurring glycosides. John Wiley & Sons, Chichester, 83–122.

Aliotsa GN, De Santo G, Pollio A, et al 2004 The diuretic use of *Scilla* from Dioscorides to the end of the 18th century. Journal of Nephrology 17:342–347.

Andersson K-E, Bertler A, Redfors A 1975 On the pharmacokinetics of proscillaridin A in man. European Journal of Clinical Pharmacology 8:421–425.

Anonymous 2005 A guide to medicinal plants in North Africa. IUCN centre for Mediterranean cooperation, Malaga, Spain.

Barnes J, Anderson LA, Phillipson JD 2007 Herbal medicines, 3rd edn. Pharmaceutical Press, London.

Bradley PR (ed.) 1992 British herbal compendium, vol 1. British Herbal Medicine Association, Bournemouth.

Bruneton J 1999 Pharmacognosy, phytochemistry, medicinal plants, 2nd edn. Intercept, London.

CKS 2009 NHS Clinical knowledge summaries: chronic heart failure. Online. Available: http://www.cks.nhs.uk/heart_failure_chronic.

Culpeper N 1669 Pharmacopoeia Londinensis. London.

Davis PH (ed.) 1984 Flora of Turkey, vol 8. Edinburgh University Press, Edinburgh.

Dec W 2003 Digoxin remains useful in the management of chronic heart failure. Medical Clinics of North America 87:317–337.

Farah MH 2005 Accepted scientific names of therapeutic plants. Uppsala Monitoring Centre, World Health Organization, Uppsala, Sweden.

Fernandez M, Vega FA, Arrupe T, et al 1972 Flavonoids of squill, *Urginea maritima*. Phytochemistry 11:1534.

Foukaridis GN, Osuch E, Mathibe L, et al 1995 The ethnopharmacology and toxicology of *Urginea sanguinea* in the Pretoria area. Journal of Ethnopharmacology 49:77–79.

Gentry HS, Verbiscar AJ, Banigan TF 1987 Red squill (*Urginea maritima*, Liliaceae). Economic Botany 41:267–282.

Griffin JP 2004 Venetian treacle and the foundation of medicines regulation. British Journal of Clinical Pharmacology 58:317–325.

Haddy FJ 2006 Role of dietary salt in hypertension. Life Sciences 79:1585–1592.

Iizuka M, Warashina T, Noro T 2001 Bufadienolides and a new lignan from the bulbs of *Urginea maritima*. Chemical and Pharmaceutical Bulletin 49:282–286.

Kopp B, Jurenitsch J, Czernia B, et al 1983 Separation of cardiac glycosides of *Urginea maritima* by high-performance liquid chromatography; improvement by serial coupling of several polar reversed phase columns. Journal of Chromatography 257:137–139.

Kopp B, Krenn L, Draxler M, et al 1996 Bufadienolides from *Urginea maritima* from Egypt. Phytochemistry 42:513–522.

Krenn L, Kopp B 1998 Bufadienolides from animal and plant sources. Phytochemistry 48:1–29.

Krenn L, Ferth R, Robien W, et al 1991 Bufadienolides from *Urginea maritima* sensu strictu. Planta Medica 57:560–565.

Krenn L, Kopp B, Deim A, et al 1994 About the bufadienolide complex of 'red' squill. Planta Medica 60:63–69.

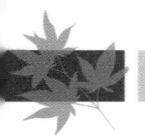

Krenn L, Jelovina M, Kopp B 2000 New bufadienolides from *Urginea maritima* sensu strictu. Fitoterapia 71:126–129.

Krenn L, Hüfner A, Kastenhuber A, et al 2004 Chemotaxonomic relevance of cardenolides in *Urginea fugax*. Phytochemistry 65:2881–2884.

Marx J, Pretorius E, Espag WJ et al 2005 *Urginea sanguinea*: medicinal wonder or death in disguise? Environmental Toxicology and Pharmacology 20:26–34.

Mills S, Bone K 2000 Principles and practice of phytotherapy. Churchill Livingstone, London.

Norton S 2006 The Pharmacology of Mithridatum: a 2000-year old remedy. Molecular Interventions 6:60–66.

Pereira J 1853 The elements of materia medica and therapeutics, vol 2, 3rd edn. Online. Available: http://www.henriettesherbal.com/eclectic/pereira/urginea.html 10 Sept 2009.

Perrino P, Laghetti G, Terzi M 2006 Modern concepts for the sustainable use of plant genetic resources in the Mediterranean natural protected areas: the case study of the Alta Murgia Park (Italy). Genetic Resources and Crop Evolution 53:695–710.

Pfosser MF, Speta F 2004 From Scilla to Charybdis – is our voyage safer now? Plant Systematics and Evolution 246:245–263.

Rix M, Phillips R 1981 The bulb book. Pan books, London.

Schoner W, Scheiner-Bobis G 2007 Endogenous and exogenous cardiac glycosides: their roles in hypertension, salt metabolism, and cell growth. American Journal of Physiology and Cell Physiology 293:C509–C539.

Robinson M 1868 The new family herbal and botanic physician. William Nicholson, London.

Schulz V, Hansel R, Tyler V 1998 Rational phytotherapy. Springer-Verlag, Berlin.

Schwinger RH, Bundgaard H, Müller-Ehmsen J, et al 2003 The Na, K-ATPase in the failing heart. Cardiovascular Research 57:913–920.

Smith W, Gould BA, Marshall AJ 1986 Wenckebach's phenomenon induced by cough linctus. British Medical Journal 292:868.

Sparg SG, Light ME, Van Staden J 2004 Biological activities and distribution of plant saponins. Journal of Ethnopharmacology 94:219–243.

Spies T, Praznik W, Hofinger A, et al 1992 The structure of the fructan sinistrin from *Urginea maritima*. Carbohydrate Research 235:221–230.

Stannard J 1974 Squill in ancient and medieval materia medica, with special reference to its employment for dropsy. Bulletin of the New York Academy of Medicine 50:684–713.

Trease GE, Evans WC 1978 Pharmacognosy, 11th edn. Balliere Tindall, London.

Tuncok Y, Kozan O, Cavdar C, et al 1995 *Urginea maritima* (squill) toxicity. Journal of Toxicology – Clinical Toxicology 33:83–86.

USDA 2009 Plants database. Online. Available: http://plants.usda.gov/index.html.

Weaver WW (ed.) 2001 Sauer's herbal cures: America's first book of botanic healing. Routledge, New York.

Williamson E 2003 Potter's herbal cyclopaedia. CW Daniel, Saffron Walden.

# CHAPTER 16
# *Fumaria officinalis*, fumitory

## DESCRIPTION

### Family: Fumariaceae                                            Part used: aerial parts

*Fumaria officinalis* L. is a scrambling annual found in disturbed and cultivated land throughout Europe. The *Flora of Turkey* (Davis 1965) gives 14 *Fumaria* species, including *Fumaria officinalis*.

Smooth, slender, branched stems of variable height (10–100 cm), bear grey-green, feathery, alternate leaves. Lateral and terminal racemes of purplish pink flowers occur in early summer. Flowers are two-lipped with reddish black tips with two tiny lateral shield-shaped sepals. The seed is a single, round achene and it seeds prolifically.

**Other species used:** There are about 33 closely related annual species in Europe (Tutin et al 1964), and it is likely that others such as *Fumaria muralis* and *Fumaria bastardii* (Sterry 2006) are collected as well as *Fumaria officinalis*. Gerard and Parkinson refer to related species, including yellow corydalis *Pseudofumaria lutea*. This is naturalized in Britain and is quite commonly seen on walls and dry places (Grey-Wilson 1994) but there is no evidence that it can be substituted for *Fumaria officinalis*.

Turner cites Pliny, who refers to a plant listed by Theophrastus as capnos fragmites, fumitory of the hedges. This could be *Fumaria capreolata*, which is a climbing plant with a white body to the flower (Tutin et al 1964) and may be the plant listed by Dioscorides (IV 120) 'the fumitory but some call it phaselion from its resemblance to the bean which has a tendril towards the upper lead. At the top of the stem there are small delicate heads, full of little seeds, tasting very much like black cumin but the leaf tastes like aniseed'.

### Quality

Collection while in flower is recommended by Dodoens and the *British Herbal Pharmacopoeia*, and use of the fresh juice is recommended (see below).

## CLEANSING THE BLOOD

The *British Herbal Pharmacopoeia* gives the merest glimpse of the use of this plant and tersely states that fumitory is used for 'cutaneous eruptions and is specific for chronic eczema'. Barker (2001) amplifies this picture, adding that it can be taken for long periods, thus resolving a chronic condition safely. He links the alterative action to its effects on the digestive organs, which eventually benefit skin conditions. Here, in my experience, is the essential aspect of fumitory: it acts as both a hepatic tonic and an alterative in skin conditions such as eczema without irritating a sensitive constitution.

Culpeper recommends the juice or syrup from the juice 'alongside other more purging or opening herbs' as effective in 'opening up the obstructions of liver and spleen' and 'clarifying the blood from saltish, choleric and burnt humours, which cause leprosy, scabs, tetters, and itches and such like breakings-out of the skin'. Here we see one of the core differences between herbal medicine and conventional medicine: 'cleansing the blood' is a concept that is freely used by patients and reflects vestiges of the humoral tradition.

Eczema can be a complex condition to treat as it occurs in phases, with or without apparent cause (Brown & Reynolds 2006). Possible causes may become clearer through ongoing discussion, but in children atopy is associated with asthma, allergic rhinitis and thus poor sleeping (Brown & Reynolds 2006). Associated problems in eating and sleepless nights raise anxiety levels in the family, who may then try different skin products and dietary regimes in an attempt to follow the often contradictory advice available. The role of the herbal practitioner is to support the patient and to avoid prescribing that is too heavy-handed for the atopic constitution. In my experience, it is possible to exacerbate the itching and soreness, and a gentle prescription in eczema is important as the alterative action must not be severe. Fumitory can act either alone as the hepatic or with another mild hepatic such as dandelion *Taraxacum officinale* or a bitter such as centaury *Centaurium erythraea*. Another alteratives such as cleavers *Galium aparine* (Mills 1991) and an antiinflammatory such as paeony *Paeonia lactiflora* or marigold *Calendula officinalis* could be added. Holistic prescribing depends on evaluation of the

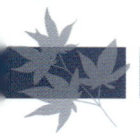

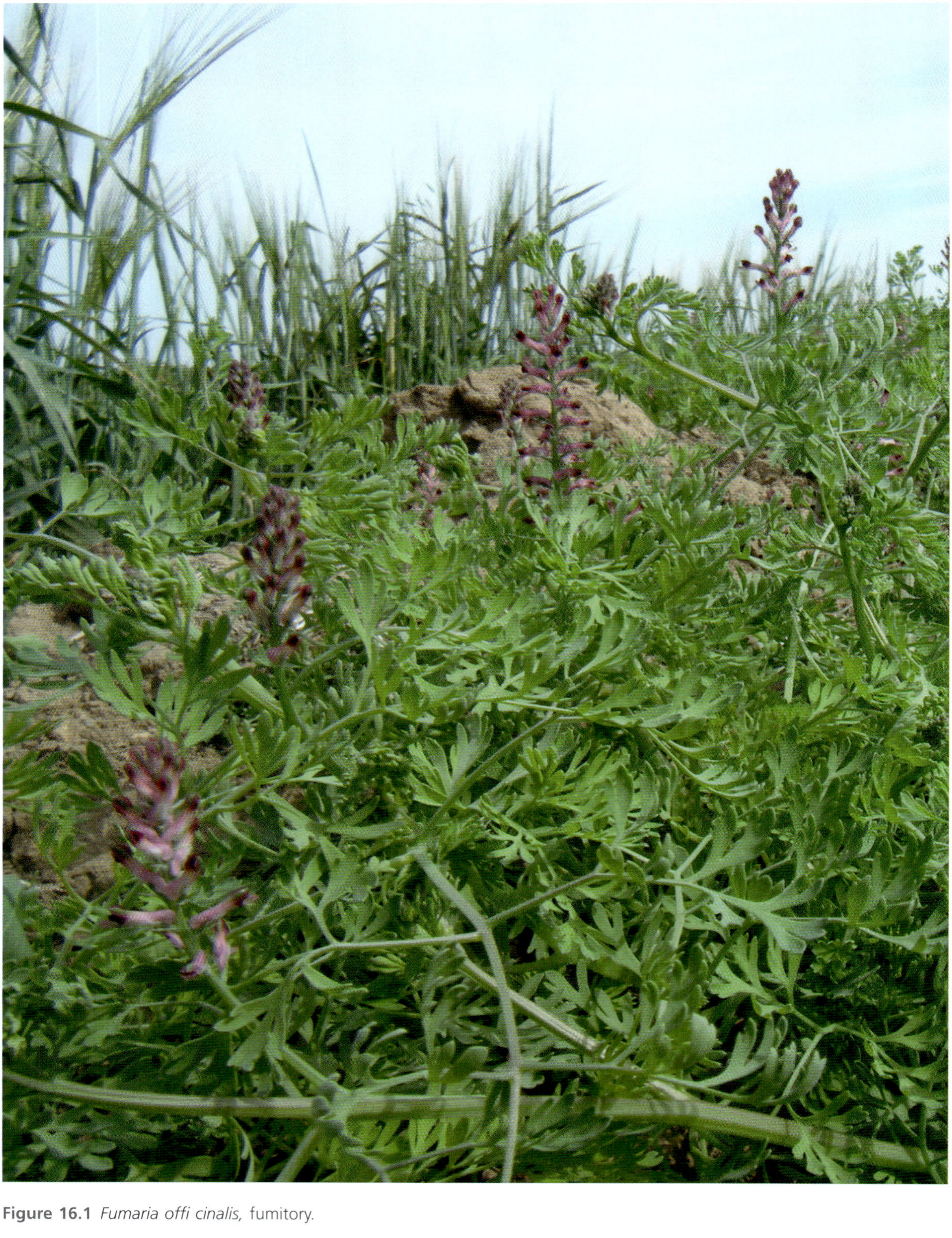

Figure 16.1 *Fumaria offi cinalis,* fumitory.

individual symptoms, tissue function, individual constitution and irritating factors so that the herbs in the prescription supply the necessary actions (Mills 1991).

## DRIVES BILE THROUGH THE URINE

I set out in practice with the clue 'specific for chronic eczema' in the *British Herbal Pharmacopeia*. There seems no doubt that Dioscorides (IV 109) describes a species of fumitory when he writes 'a small shrub-like little herb, resembling coriander, very tender, and abounding in rather pale ash-colored leaves. It has purple flowers'. The herb appears to have been in use for the last 2000 years, so what could our ancestors have told me about fumitory? The first recommendation is for use in liver disease. Dioscorides is brief 'The plant drives bile through the urine when eaten'. Galen agrees as do subsequent authors, including Macer, Fuchs, Dodoens and Bauhin. Culpeper proposes fumitory in 'yellow jaundice' which it 'spendeth by urine, which it procureth in abundance'.

Dalechamps, Bauhin and Parkinson state that Arabic writers attributed many more qualities to this plant. Ibn Sina advises it to cool the blood, to strengthen the stomach and open obstructions in the liver, and the fresh herb as a diuretic, which 'softens the essence'. Dalechamps cites Mesue as saying that fumitory is mainly important as an internal medicine. The references to temperament and humours are developed in Arabic sources but there is disagreement about temperament. According to Bauhin, Mesue describes it as superficially hot but cold in its depths and dry in the second degree, whereas Ibn Sina describes it as cold in the first and dry in the second or third degree. Macer described it as hot and dry and the Salernitan herbal and Fuchs describes it as hot and dry in the second degree. Serapio describes it as bitter and drying, warm, but cold and dry in the second degree. Turner & Dodoens agree that it is hot and dry almost in the second degree and associate its bitterness with its heat. Gerard states that fumitory is not hot 'as some have thought it be' but 'old and something dry'. The authors agree that it is dry but disagree on the temperature. This could be a case of copying older texts but it could reflect on whether the authors used the dried plant as decoction or juice of the fresh plant, with or without seeds.

The Salernitan herbal states that juice of the aerial parts is best and that the dried herb is ineffective, that fumitory should be collected in the evening and always used with a carminative such as fennel *Foeniculum vulgare* to expel wind. The Salernitan herbal recommends for dropsy a syrup made of fumitory and fennel juice, with Esula powder, which is a *Euphorbia* species and not now used. This is repeated by Bauhin. Quincy argues that it gains a detersive quality by taking up minerals from the walls on which it grows, and this makes it good for gravel and obstructions of the urinary passages.

Dosages are given for fresh and dried herb. Mesue, cited by Serapio, gives doses of 5–10 fl drachms (17.5–35 mL) of decoction, 3–7 drachms (12–28 g) of fresh herb and 4–8 fl oz of juice. Ibn Sina gives doses of from 29 to 170 g of fresh herb with sugar, 29 g of dry herb or 9–21 g of powder. The Salenitan herbal recommends 2 fl oz of the fresh juice and this dose is also given by Bauhin & Dalechamps. Dodoens recommends use of the fresh plant, especially when in seed. Cullen gives a dose of 2 oz of decoction. It is noteworthy that 2 fl oz is given by both the Salernitan herbal and Cullen writing much later in the 18th century. The recommendation of the fresh juice by many authors could link with the astringent quality of the phenolic acids (see below). It is also proposed that fumitory exerts a general strengthening action on the digestive system. Dalechamps cites Mesue as stating that it strengthens the stomach, liver and other looser, softer organs by a cold astringency. This is maintained by Culpeper, who states that 'after purging it does strengthen all the inward parts'.

## THE SKIN: PERNICIOUS HUMOURS AND LEPRA

An association is made between internal disease and signs of skin disease. Macer makes this connection through the action of cleansing the blood. Serapio cites Mesue as recommending fumitory to treat the stomach, scabies and the itch, and to remove burnt choler, strengthen the blood and provoke urine. Dalechamps cites Mesue as stating that it purges bile and burnt humours even from the veins, clears and purifies the blood and is therefore useful for disease caused by these humours such as lepra (from the Greek for a scaly skin condition), scabies (which actually refers to eczematous diseases in that erythema and thickening of the skin are combined with pruritis, pustules and ulceration), pruritus, impetigo and serpigo (a contagious, spreading skin condition, possibly ringworm). This use of the same text by two authors illustrates the problem in interpreting the different sources as the citations are similar but offer a different point of emphasis. The list is also used by Parkinson and appears to have been copied by Culpeper. Dodoens, writing in 1551, gives a vivid description: it 'driveth forth by design and siege all hot, cholerish, burnt, and pernicious humours' and is useful in 'foul scurfs, rebellious old sores and the great pocks'.

Hot, cholerish, burnt and pernicious humours certainly sound dangerous but what does this mean? Arabic writers studied the Galenic tradition and the philosophy of Aristotle, who visualized the soul as the set of qualities which define a living being. This can be likened to the set of qualities which defines a skill such as horse-riding or piano-playing, which needs physical, mental and other qualities and cannot in itself be measured (Barnes 1996). Using this concept, the activities of the living person can be visualized as an expression of the original abstract qualities: hot, cold, moist and dry.

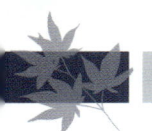

The temperament of a person can be considered as arising from a blend of the four elements: fire, water, air and earth, which are expressions of the original abstract qualities hot, cold, moist and dry. However, the qualities in reality are present in a mixed state not a pure state. Thus fire is hot but tends to dry, water is cold but tends to moist, air is moist but tends to hot and earth is dry but tends to cold (Ullmann 1978). The four fluid humours 'daughters of the elements' nourish the organs which function correctly if properly fed by the flow of humours through the blood vessels. Yellow bile is hot and dry like fire, and blood is hot and wet like air. Black bile is dry and cold like earth, and phlegm is cold and wet like water. Every individual has a temperament, a natural balance of the humours that can be positively or negative affected by lifestyle, which is expressed in the concept of the six non-naturals (see Chapter 6). This brief summary is based on an account by Ullmann (1978) of a work by Al-Majūsi, written in 1294 and subsequently translated into Latin.

Symptoms are clues to assess bodily imbalance and thus suggest possible treatments. The significance here is that if fumitory acts on the flow of bile via the gall bladder, then

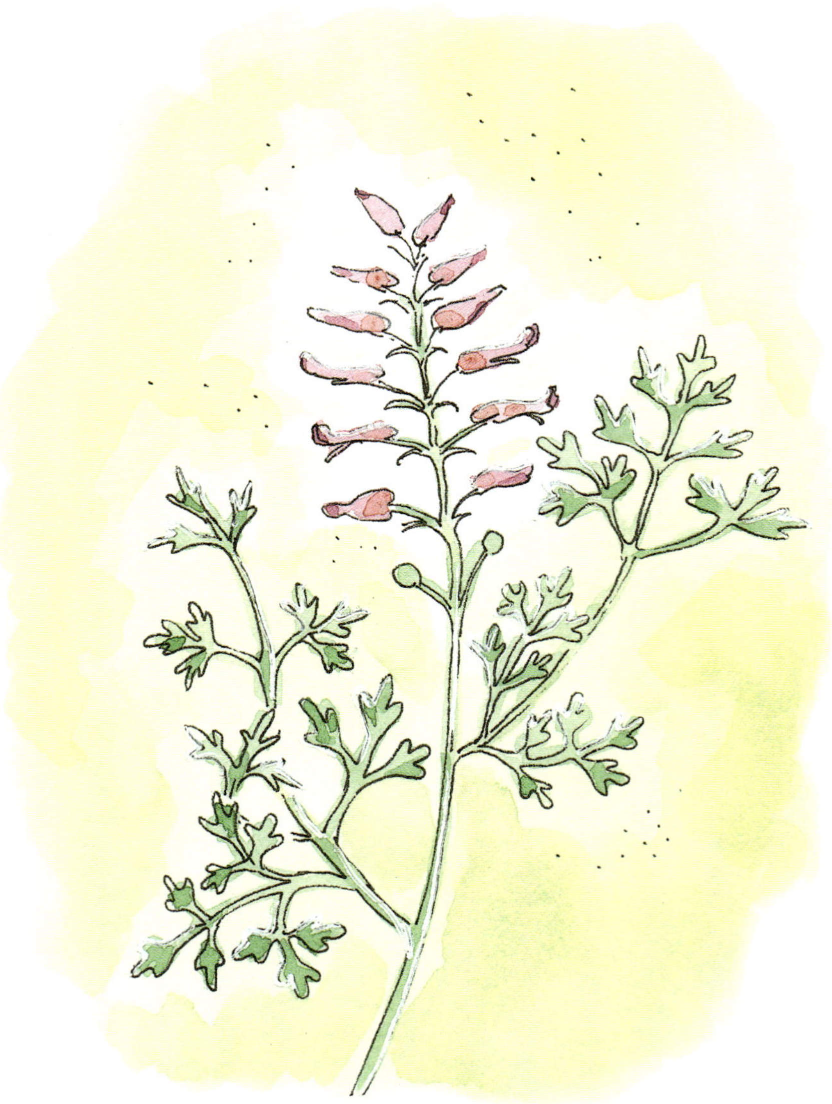

**Figure 16.2** *Fumaria officinalis*, fumitory.

it must improve the digestive processes. However, yellow bile was also considered to flow with the blood, 'thin the blood' and aid blood flow and thus nourishment of the organs. Therefore the action of fumitory is to thin the blood and improve nourishment of the tissues. Yellow bile can become black bile if it is overheated and burned. Black bile can also be overheated and burned and hard, so fumitory is perceived as counteracting these two problems. Excess of burnt humours was considered to lead to malignant disease. Demaitre (1998) portrays the process whereby improperly cooked or burned black bile spreads through the body and leads to hardening, tumours, ulcers, lepra and deep-seated illness. Excess accumulation of black bile also leads to melancholia, that most cold and chronic condition of depression.

The words used for skin disease lead to confusion and need some discussion. Jones (1951) defines lepra as any scaly disease of the skin, scabies, following Celsus, as hardening and reddening of the skin leading to pustules and ulceration, and impetigo as various types of eczema. Norri (1992) reviewed English medical documents 1400–1550 and identified many words associated with skin disease, including lepra (disfiguring skin disease), impetigo (skin eruptions), herpes (yellow, itchy pustules also herpes cingulus meaning shingles), scabies (scabs and itching), serpigo (spreading eruption) and lentigo (freckles, pimples) as well as swellings and growths.

Dalechamps lists lepra, scabies, pruritus, impetigo and serpigo. These terms could include acne, eczema, infected eczema, impetigo and seborrhoeic eczema. It is tempting to argue that fumitory was used in scabies, as we know it today, as well as eczema. Scabies is an intensely itchy infestation caused by mites, transmitted by skin contact. It was common and continues to occur in western societies (Hengge et al 2006) and patients suffering from post-scabies eczema may also consult herbalists.

The reference to lepra and scaliness suggests use in psoriasis. Norri (1992) did not find the word psoriasis, which is derived from the Greek psora, which means itch. Scaliness is more diagnostic of psoriasis than itch, and Glickman (1986) argues that the words lepra and psoriasis were both used for variants of the same condition during the 19th century. The association of lepra with leprosy is disputed by Kaplan (1993), who argues that it refers to skin disease associated with depigmentation. Jopling & Jones (1990) suggest that the word leprosy was used instead of lepra to mean psoriasis in 18th century Manchester. We can conclude that the recommendation of fumitory by Grieve for troublesome eruptive diseases 'even those of the leprous order' is not for use in leprosy, but rather the claim is based on the consistent recommendations of fumitory for skin disease in the 19th century. Robinson (1868) and Knight (1851) repeat the recommendation by Cullen (Clapp 1852) for the use of 2 fl oz of juice or decoction daily in 'skin affections of the worst sort'. Fox refers to it as effective in liver disease and jaundice, but advises it for 'all breakings out of the skin, and find it splendid'. Hool gives a useful 'blood purifying' medicine for eczema and skin disease that contains four herbs included in this book: burdock *Arctium lappa* 1 oz, centaury *Centaurium erythraea* 1 oz, yellow dock *Rumex crispus* ½ oz, fumitory *Fumaria officinalis* ½ oz, teaspoonful of cayenne. Simmer in 3 pints of water for 30 minutes. Cool, strain, take a wineglassful, which is 2 fl oz (60 mL) four times a day.

To conclude our discussion of the connection between liver function and skin disease, we can consider the subtle interplay between bodily functions in a different way. Pelikan offers a potent image of the poppy family, which is very closely connected to the Fumariaceae, as a plant type that demonstrates powerful etheric processes but a strong astral sphere that takes hold of these forces precipitates flowering, and in this consumes them. A play of forces in the type is reflected in a brightly coloured flower that soon loses its petals and then the dramatic, potentially deadly narcotic action of the latex 'the narcotic scent ... tears us away from the world of creative pain which is the world of the physical, earthly, solid and defined objects, and hands us over to a flowing world of images ...'. *Fumaria* species represent a more airy development of the family, the latex has disappeared but the astral incursion still produces alkaloids. Fumitory, despite the air, 'cannot get off the ground', says Pelikan, 'like heavy smoke, fumitory smoulders on the ground with dimly violet flowers'... here is a note of black in the purple' as with poppies. As to its action, it 'promotes all excretory functions, increasing astral activity in metabolism'. Hence we find a 'blood cleansing action' in relation to the skin. 'Skin eruptions and blemishes resulting when metabolism goes in the wrong direction, without restraint, into the sensory skin sphere, will disappear as the ground is taken away from under them.'

## MELANCHOLIA

The airiness of the fumitory as a lightening force links to its usage in melancholy. According to the Salernitan herbal it purges especially the melancholic humour and salted phlegm, which has become hot and dry. Bauhin suggests a conserve of the flowers with sugar for melancholy and bad humours. The melancholic humour is cold and dry and Zerbi (Lind 1988) proposes fresh juice of fumitory for older people as he associates purifying the blood with elevation of the spirits. Quincy calls it 'melancholi fuga' as it prevails against melancholy and he connects the action of purging humours with its use in both jaundice and hypochondriacal cases. According to Hoffmann, some herbalists use bitter tonics alongside nervines when treating depression. Endogenous depression in particular is considered to require tonics to the liver. Wood particularly recommends fumitory when sluggish digestion is accompanied by an underactive thyroid.

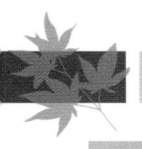

## MORE RECENT USE FOR THE DIGESTIVE TRACT

After the 18th century, there is generally no direct reference to humours but usage remains the same. Miller advises use of the whole plant to cleanse the blood, in scurvy, jaundice, affections of spleen, scabs, itch and leprous disorder. The *Edinburgh New Dispensatory* (1806) states that it strengthens bowel tone, gently loosens the belly and promotes urinary and other natural secretions and is useful in melancholic, scorbutic (resembling scurvy) and cutaneous disorders. Wren lists it as tonic and aperient, useful for deranged stomach, liver and skin affections. Mills (1991) includes fumitory in his list of alteratives to improve elimination in the treatment of chronic disease and Chevallier recommends it in itchy skin disease. Menzies-Trull highlights its antispasmodic qualities in colic and biliary colic and proposes it for hepatic disorders with yawning and excess tiredness. Williamson links the actions with the presence of isoquinoline alkaloids. It is interesting that another plant used as a hepatic tonic and for skin disease is *Mahonia aquifolium*, which also contains isoquinoline alkaloids (Mills & Bone 2000). These alkaloids could support the use of fumitory in digestive conditions as they have been shown in vitro to inhibit *Helicobacter pylori* (Mahady et al 2003), which is associated with gastritis and duodenal ulcers (Kandulski et al 2008).

Usage for the digestive tract continues and Commission E (Blumenthal 1998) approved fumitory for use in 'spastic discomfort in the area of the gallbladder and bile ducts, as well as the gastrointestinal tract', liver and gallbladder complaints and state that it is considered to normalize biliary function. Weiss argues that fumitory has an amphoteric action on bile flow and advises fumitory for 'biliary migraine', relief of pain in the right epigastrium, intolerance of rich food and relief of headache with nausea and vomiting. Weiss cites a study by Giroux et al (1966) as the basis of his proposal that fumitory has an amphoteric action. This study was carried out in France on nine anaesthetized dogs whose bile flow was measured, using a temporary fistula, after intravenous injection of a concentrated aqueous preparation of fumitory (Giroux et al 1966). While the proposal by Weiss is sound, even leaving aside the moral objections to tests on animals, such an experiment cannot be used as evidence to support an equivalent action in oral use by humans.

There has been usage as an antispasmodic, which led to a randomized controlled trial of the use of fumitory in irritable bowel syndrome. The study medication was 500 mg three times a day of aqueous spray-dried extract, standardized to 3.75 mg protopine, and it was taken for 18 weeks by 24 people (71% women, mean age 49) with 58 in the placebo group (Brinkhaus et al 2005). Symptoms improved by over 60% in both groups and there were no significant differences between the groups. Thirty-three per cent (8 patients) in the treatment group reported nine adverse events (constipation, distension, nausea, epigastric pain, nausea, hair loss) and 29% of the placebo group reported adverse events. Irritable bowel syndrome is a multifactorial condition that is difficult to evaluate in clinical trials (Camilleri et al 2007). Use of the Rome criteria for diagnosis of irritable bowel syndrome at recruitment is not mentioned and participants were recruited from a group of patients who had previously been treated without success for some years at the study clinic. Rather unusually for a recent clinical trial, all previous medication was prohibited. Visual analogue scales were used rather than a validated symptom-based outcome measure. One could argue that the trial design did not lead to conclusive results for or against the use of fumitory.

## EXTERNAL USE: MORE QUESTIONS THAN ANSWERS

Recommendations for external usage on the eyes date back to Dioscorides but are difficult to interpret. A general rule is that only fresh teas should be used as eyebaths because of the possibility of bacterial contamination of stored preparations. Users of contact lenses are particularly vulnerable to eye infection caused by contamination of the lenses by bacteria, in particular *Pseudomonas aeruginosa* (Willcox 2007). I have no experience of the *British Herbal Pharmacopoeia* recommendation for external use of fumitory in conjunctivitis. Yet this goes back to Dioscorides, who states that the 'juice is sharp, promotes sharp-sightedness, and produces tears'. Fuchs cites Pliny as stating that the juice 'bites the eyes' like the effect of smoke on the eyes. Bauhin states that the juice or distilled water clears the eyes of heat and Dodoens suggests the juice dropped into the eyes is a singular medicine against the weakness of sight 'especially for such as seem to see small straws'. Dioscorides and subsequent authors also suggest usage with gum to prevent the hair growing back after plucking the eyebrows.

Fumitory provides further examples which illustrate some problems in basing recommendations on historic sources. For example, popular usage in Britain may derive from written rather than oral sources. The infusion, mixed with milk or water, is noted as used in folk remedies for cleansing the skin of blemishes (Allen & Hatfield 2004). However, Grieve quotes Cullen as stating that 'a disorder of the skin ... thought to place the empire of beauty in great jeopardy ... vulgarly known as freckles ... infusion of the leaves ... is said to be an excellent specific for removing these freckles and clearing the skin'. This could link with the recommendation by Gerard for use of fumitory, boiled in whey as a spring tonic for scabs. This recommendation is also made by Turner, Culpeper, Quincy and Miller.

Another problem is in the copying of sources. For example, the Salernitan herbal recommends an ointment for 'mange': walnut oil, very fine furnace soot, fumeterre juice, more juice that the other ingredients, make the ointment and apply when taking a bath. Given in this way three times a week, the preparation 'gets rid of the humour that provokes mange'. Parkinson, followed by Culpeper and Grieve, recommends the same preparation for all sores, scabs, itches, wheals, pimples, pustules that rise in the face, hands or any other part of the skin of the body. The use of similar wording makes it hard to establish whether these authors had actual experience of the recipe. Bauhin gives a similar recipe for an ointment of fumitory and sharp pointed dock with vinegar and honey for all scabies of the skin.

## RECOMMENDATIONS FOR USAGE

- The *British Herbal Pharmacopoeia* lists fumitory as a weak diuretic, laxative and specific for chronic eczema. The recommendations of the authors describe it as a more powerful herb than this, and give substantial support for an effective role in liver disease used as a tea in hepatitis and jaundice which acts to increase loss of bile via the urine.
- The authors also recommend fumitory as an alterative, in combination with other herbs, for all skin disease, in particular psoriasis, and including infections such as scabies and acne.
- Use of the fresh herb or fresh plant juice is consistently recommended throughout the tradition and a syrup of the juice was listed as an official product by Miller.

Dosage: the *British Herbal Pharmacopoeia* recommends 2–4 g three times a day of dried aerial parts.

A dose of 60 mL of fresh juice is given by Dalechamps, Bauhin and Cullen, which is the dose originally given in the Salenitan herbal.

## CONSTITUENTS

Reviews: Barnes et al (2007), Bisset & Wichtl (2001), Bradley (1992), Mills & Bone (2005), Williamson (2003).

### Isoquinoline alkaloids

Review: Bruneton (1999).
Isoquinolines were found in all Fumaria species and protopine was the major constituent (14 species, Turkey) (Şener 2002).
Five categories, protopines 0.13%: protopine, cryptoprotopine; spirobenzylisoquinolines 0.09%: fumarophycine, O-methylfumarophycine, parfumine; phthalide isoquinolines 0.24%: corlumine, adlumine, hydrastine, b cuculline; tetrahydroprotoberberines: sinactine, scoulerine; benzoisoquinilines: reticuline, corydamine (Şener 2002, Seger et al 2004, Sturm et al 2006).
Total 1.3%, mainly protopine and spirobenzylisoquinolines: fumarophycine, O-methylfumarophycine, parfumine, fumaricine, fumaritine, fumariline (wild, France) (Soušek et al 1999).
Subsp. *officinalis*, total 0.54%, mainly protopine and spirobenzylisoquinolines (wild, four samples, Spain) (Suau et al 2002).
Spirobenzylisoquinolines only occur in Fumariaceae (Seger et al 2004).
A study of the industrial extraction of protopine from fumitory found that extraction was greatest using 30 g dried herb/L of 1:1 ethanol/water at 79°C (Rakotondramasy-Rabesiaka et al 2008).

### Phenylpropanoids

Phenolic acids: citric, coumaric, ferulic, fumaric, malic, S-hydroxybenzoic, protocatechuic acid, caffeic acid and its methylester (Soušek et al 1999).
Concentration of hydroxycinnamic esters was 1.3% (freeze-dried and air-dried, cultivated) whereas it was only 0.2% in commercial samples (Hahn & Nahrstedt 1993).

## RECOMMENDATIONS ON SAFETY

1. Do not use externally in eye conditions.
   There are many other herbs to use externally in conjunctivitis and the statement that the herb can also be irritating does not support this recommendation.
2. Mesue, cited in Bauhin, states 'the herb is harmless', and fumitory is interesting in that it is a plant which contains alkaloids but has not been associated with adverse drug reactions or safety concerns.

## REFERENCES

Allen DE, Hatfield G 2004 Medicinal plants in folk tradition. Timber Press, Portland, Oregon.

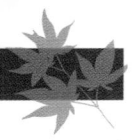

Barker J 2001 The medicinal flora of Britain and Northwestern Europe. Winter Press, West Wickham, Kent.

Barnes J 1996 Aristotle. Oxford University Press, Oxford.

Barnes J, Anderson LA, Phillipson JD 2007 Herbal medicines, 3rd edn. Pharmaceutical Press, London.

Bisset NG, Wichtl M (eds) 2001 Herbal drugs and phytopharmaceuticals, 2nd edn. Medpharm, Stuttgart.

Blumenthal M (ed.) 1998 The Complete German Commission E Monographs. American Botanical Council, Austin, Texas.

Bradley PR (ed.) 1992 British herbal compendium, vol 1. British Herbal Medicine Association, Bournemouth.

Brinkhaus B, Hentschel C, Von Keudell, C et al 2005 Herbal medicine with curcuma and fumitory in the treatment of irritable bowel syndrome: a randomized, placebo-controlled, double-blind clinical trial. Scandinavian Journal of Gastroenterology. 40:936–943.

Brown S, Reynolds NJ 2006 Atopic and non-atopic eczema. British Medical Journal 332:584–588.

Bruneton J 1999 Pharmacognosy, phytochemistry, medicinal plants. Lavoisier Publishing, Paris.

Camilleri M, Mangel AW, Fehnel SE, et al 2007 Primary endpoints for irritable bowel syndrome trials: a review of performance of endpoints. Clinical Gastroenterology and Hepatology 5(5):534–540.

Clapp A 1852 Report on indigenous medical botany and materia medica for 1850–1851. Transactions of the American Medical Association, Philadelphia.

Davis PH (ed.) 1965 Flora of Turkey, vol 1. Edinburgh University Press, Edinburgh.

Demaitre LE 1998 Medieval notions of cancer: malignancy and metaphor. Bulletin of the History of Medicine 72:609–637.

Giroux J, Boucard M, Beaulaton IS 1966 Les modificateurs de la cholérèse: doit-on parler d'amphocholérétique. Thérapie 21:889–902.

Glickman FS 1986 Lepra, psora, psoriasis. Journal of the American Academy of Dermatology 14:863–866.

Grey-Wilson C 1994 Wild flowers of Britain and Northwest Europe. Dorling Kindersley, London.

Hahn R, Nahrstedt A 1993 High content of hydroxycinnamic acids esterified with (+)-D-malic acid in the upper parts of *Fumaria officinalis*. Planta Medica 59:189–190.

Hengge UR, Currie BJ, Jäger G, et al 2006 Scabies: a ubiquitous neglected skin disease. The Lancet Infectious Diseases 6:769–779.

Jones WHS 1951 Pliny, vol 6. William Heinemann, London.

Jopling WH, Jones BEA 1990 Psoriasis and leprosy. Journal of the American Academy of Dermatology 22:321.

Kandulski A, Selgrad M, Malfertheiner P 2008 Helicobacter pylori infection: a clinical overview. Digestive and Liver Disease 40:619–626.

Kaplan DL 1993 Biblical leprosy: an anachronism whose time has come? Journal of the American Academy of Dermatology 28:507–510.

Knight C 1851 Penny cyclopaedia of the Society for the Diffusion of Useful Knowledge. Society for the Diffusion of Useful Knowledge, Great Britain. Online. Available: http://www.books.google.co.uk.

Lind LR 1988 Gabriele Zerbi, Gerontocomia: on the care of the aged; and Maximianus, Elegies on old age and love. Diane Publishing, Pensylvania Online. Available: http://www.books.google.co.uk.

Mahady GB, Pendland SL, Stoia A, et al 2003 In vitro susceptibility of Helicobacter pylori to isoquinoline alkaloids from *Sanguinaria canadensis* and *Hydrastis canadensis*. Phytotherapy Research 17:217–221.

Mills S 1991 Out of the earth. Viking Arkana, London.

Mills S, Bone K 2000 Principles and practice of phytotherapy. Churchill Livingstone, London.

Mills S, Bone K 2005 The essential guide to herbal safety. Churchill Livingstone, St Louis.

Norri J 1992 Names of sicknesses in English, 1400–1550: an exploration of the lexical field. Suomalainen Tiedeakatemia, Helsinki.

Rakotondramasy-Rabesiaka L, Jean-Louis Havet J-L, Porte C, et al 2008 Solid–liquid extraction of protopine from *Fumaria officinalis* L. – experimental study and process optimization. Separation and Purification Technology 59:253–261.

Robinson M 1868 The new family herbal and botanic physician. William Nicholson, London.

Seger C, Sturm S, Strasser EM, et al 2004 $^{1}$H and $^{13}$C NMR signal assignment of benzylisoquinoline alkaloids from *Fumaria officinalis* L. (Papaveraceae). Magnetic Resonance in Chemistry 42:882–886.

Şener B 2002 Molecular diversity in the alkaloids of Turkish *Fumaria* L. species. Acta Pharmaceutica Turcica 44:205–212.

Soušek J, Guédon D, Adam T, et al 1999 Alkaloids and organic acids content of eight *Fumaria* species. Phytochemical Analysis 10:6–11.

Sterry P 2006 Complete British wild flowers. HarperCollins, London.

Sturm S, Strasser EM, Stuppner H 2006 Quantification of *Fumaria officinalis* isoquinoline alkaloids by nonaqueous capillary electrophoresis-electrospray ion trap mass spectrometry. Journal of Chromatography A 1112:331–338.

Suau R, Cabezudo B, Rico R, et al 2002 Direct determination of alkaloid contents in *Fumaria* species by GC-MS. Phytochemical Analysis 13:363–367.

Tutin TG, Heywood VH, Burges NA, et al 1964 Flora Europaea, vol 1. Cambridge University Press, Cambridge.

Ullmann M 1978 Islamic medicine. Edinburgh University Press, Edinburgh.

Willcox MD 2007 Pseudomonas aeruginosa infection and inflammation during contact lens wear: a review. Optometry and Vision Science 84:273–278.

Williamson E 2003 Potter's herbal cyclopaedia. CW Daniel, Saffron Walden.

# CHAPTER 17
# *Galium aparine*, goosegrass

## DESCRIPTION

**Family: Rubiaceae**                                                      **Part used: aerial parts**

*Galium aparine* L. is a vigorous, scrambling annual, found throughout Europe, and was already present as an arable weed in the eastern USA before 1860 (Mack 2003). It is a highly variable species, native to shingle beaches, fenland and alder woodland, and a common weed, often associated with *Urtica dioica* (Taylor 1999). The *Flora of Turkey* (Davis 1982) gives 101 *Galium* species, including *Galium aparine*.

Rough, brittle, square stems (to 300 cm long) with recurved prickles on stem and leaf margins bear whorls of six to eight leaves with bristle-like tips. Tiny white flowers with four petals occur mainly in early summer in clusters which arise from the leaf axils. Different races in Europe germinate at different times depending on local climate and on whether they grow in hedgerows or an open site (Taylor 1999). The abundant, two-lobed, green fruits become reddish and are covered with dense hooked bristles that attach to clothing and passing animals.

*Galium aparine* is distinguished by the length of its stems and its white flowers. *Galium spurium*, which is not used, is a similar naturalized weed, with a slender stem to 1 m, yellowy flowers, and a fruit which becomes black (Gibbons & Brough 1996).

### Quality

According to the *British Herbal Pharmacopoeia*, it should be collected when in flower and forming seeds. Fuchs recommends collection when in seed but, unless the seeds are sought, earlier collection will provide fresher leaf material. The lower part of stem is best cut in situ to avoid collection of dried-out leaves or contamination with soil. It should be dried quickly and turned whilst drying as it blackens and spoils easily. As the physicians of Myddfai observed 'Take care not to leave them out in foggy, muggy weather as the whole virtue of the herb will be destroyed thereby'.

## FRESH PLANT TO RESIST ERUPTIVE POISONS: EAT IT, DRINK IT, MAKE A POULTICE

Dioscorides (III 90) describes goosegrass as having many long quadrangular rough sprays, leaves at a distance lying whorled like madder, white flowers and a hard round seed, somewhat indented in the middle like a navel. His final statement is that, as many children know, the herb clings onto clothing. Here we have a very satisfactory description of *Galium aparine*. This is not the only sticky *Galium* which grows in Turkey but goosegrass and other *Galium* species continue to be used in Turkey today (Baser et al 2004). It is remarkable that a herb which has been in continuous usage has relatively little written about it. There is little research on constituents and this is mainly to determine the sections in the genus. We have used the name goosegrass as the common name rather than the more commonly used cleavers.

Dioscorides states that the juice of the seeds, stalks and leaves in wine can be applied after bites from spiders and snakes. This is one of the places where Dioscorides and Pliny appear to have cited the same source: Pliny, cited in Fuchs, refers to usage in bites from harvest spiders and snakes, and gives a dose of 1 drachm (4 g) of the seeds in wine. The use of the juice against snake bites, by preserving the heart from venom, is repeated by Culpeper.

So, from the beginning there is a reference to the blood purifying action of goosegrass whereas the diuretic action and usage in disorders of the urinary tract are not found until more modern texts. Use of the juice or tea as an alterative alongside external usage is advised by the authors. The physicians of Myddfai in Wales recommend fresh juice of goosegrass in spring and summer, since its healing powers were highly regarded. This text was set down in 1743 but is based on a continuous practice of

©2009 Elsevier Ltd, Inc, BV
DOI: 10.1016/B978-0-443-10344-5.00022-7

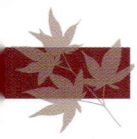

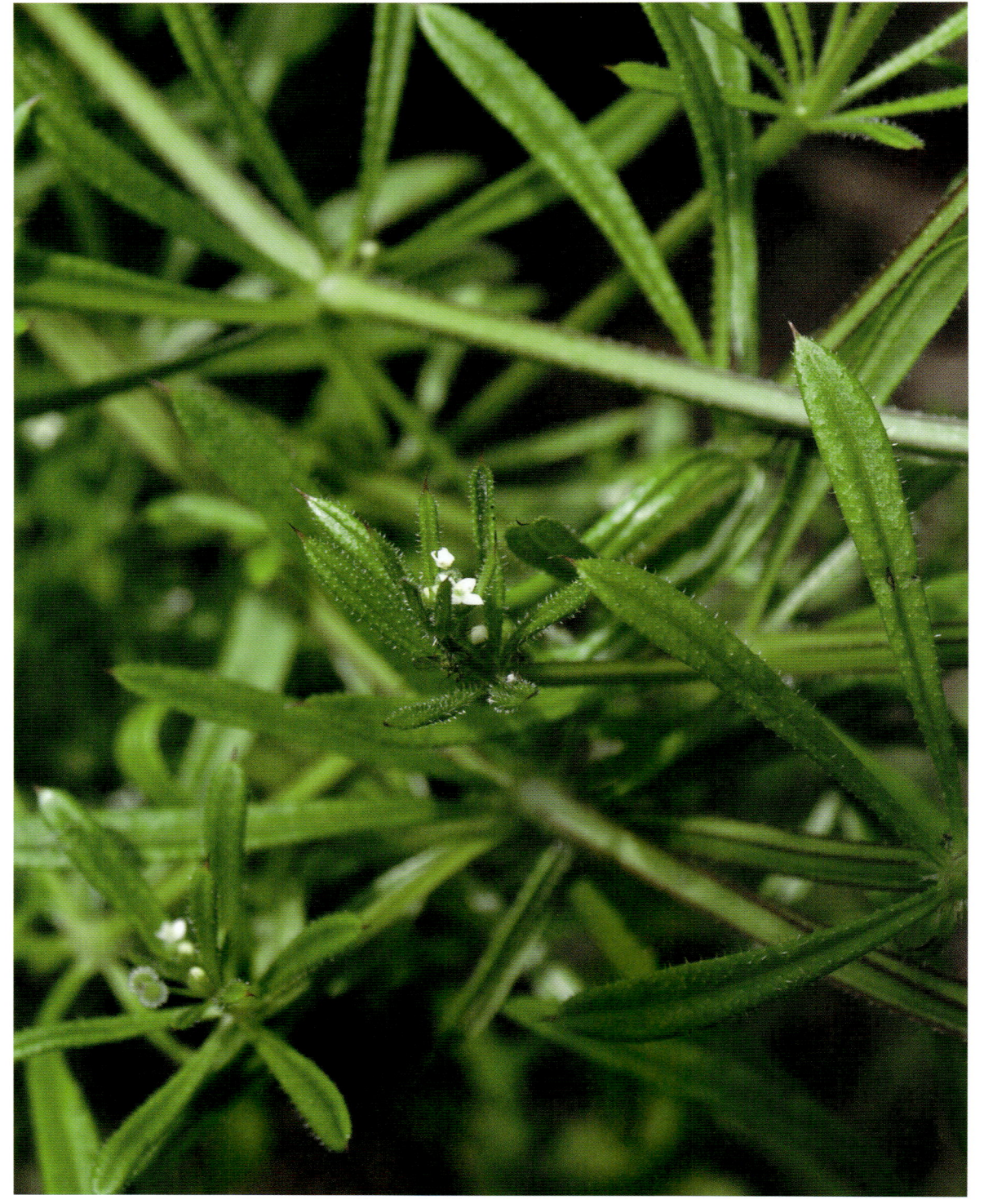

**Figure 17.1** *Galium aparine*, goosegrass (Yorkshire, June).

medicine by one family since the late 14th century. The juice of the plant taken in spring and summer as the patient's only drink 'will completely destroy and expel eruptive poisons in the blood and humours'. The method of preparing and taking the herb is carefully described: the whole herb, leaves, blossoms and seeds should be pounded together well, put in an unglazed earthenware vessel without pressing the plant material down, covered with spring water and left overnight. The infusion is to be taken fresh as the only drink for 9 weeks. The Myddfai text links many diseases with 'an eruptive poison in the blood and humours' associated with 'irregularities in eating and drinking', and thus recommends goosegrass for boils, scrofula and lepra (see the discussion under figwort, Chapter 28), cancer, erysipelas, pneumonia, dropsy, rheumatism and gout, all sorts of fevers, pocks of the skin, all watery diseases of the eyes, head and stomach catarrh, oedematous swellings of the joints, legs, feet and of other parts, inflammations, fevers and oppression of the chest and stomach.

The physicians of Myddfai recommend the use of the juice or decoction of goosegrass externally for eruptions and boils, abscesses, ringworm, dermatitis, ulcers, wounds and burns. In severe cases, the bruised plant itself is applied. Use of the fresh expressed juice, without heat, is also recommended by Coffin and Fox. Coffin advises internal usage in chronic sores (2 fl oz three times a day). Fox recommends 1–4 teaspoons three times a day for eczema, skin disease and 'hard lumps in the glands of the breast or neck' when used alongside an external preparation. The alterative action in skin disease continues to be considered significant (Mills & Bone 2005) and it is recommended for use in eczema and psoriasis. Priest & Priest recommend it for all skin eruptions, including eczema and psoriasis, and as the preferred diuretic in rashes and eruptions. The recommendation for skin rashes in feverish disease reflects that of Felter & Lloyd (1898) who recommend goosegrass in acute erysipelas, scarlatina and 'other exanthematous diseases, in their inflammatory stages'. They advise a tea of equal parts of goosegrass, maidenhair fern *Adiantum capillus-veneris* and elderflowers *Sambucus nigra*, steeped in warm water for 2 or 3 hours, and drunk freely, when cold. They recommend external usage of an infusion made with cold water several times a day for 2–3 months for removing freckles from the face and for 'several cutaneous eruptions'. The link with the use of goosegrass as a diuretic which shortens fevers is also made by Ellingwood (1919). Wood takes the lymphatic action one step further and links this with the nervous system. He states that goosegrass is a 'deer remedy' and so associated with the nervous system. He uses it for inflammation associated with the nervous tract, itchy skin and nodules, in particular as a specific for Dupuytren's contracture and Morton's neuroma.

## EXTERNAL USE ON THE CERVICAL LYMPH NODES

The physicians of Myddfai state that the use of the juice and external application has healed scrofula and cancer, 'when it had destroyed the flesh to the bones'. The use of the term 'cancer' is difficult to interpret, but there are recurring recommendations for use in scrofula. The term 'scrofula', also called the king's evil, refers to large swellings in the cervical glands caused by tuberculosis. However, the meaning of the term is contested (French 1993) and it may include enlarged lymph nodes in general and itchy rashes (see figwort). Dodoens states that 'pounded with hogs grease, it dissolveth and consumeth the disease of the neck called the King's evil, and all hard kernels and wens wherever they be, if it be layed thereto, as Turner writeth'. Culpeper similarly suggests that 'boiled in hog's grease it helpeth all sorts of hard swellings or kernels in the throat, being anointed therewith'. This advice appears to rely on Dioscorides, who states that the herb compounded with lard disperses scrofulous swellings of the glands. Miller gives it as a 'sweetener of the Blood and of service in the King's Evil, for which some give the juices as a great secret'.

Coffin recommends goosegrass in scrofula and indolent ulcers and claims that 'many dangerous cancers have been cured' by taking 2 fl oz of the fresh juice three times daily and the application, where relevant, of a fresh green poultice. This is interesting as it is rare in the 19th century for fresh preparations to be specified. Fox then recommends the use of the fresh herb, made into an ointment with vaseline, for reducing hard lumps in the glands of the neck and breast. The *British Herbal Pharmacopoeia* recommends internal usage for lymphadenitis and use of goosegrass as a specific for enlarged lymph nodes, especially in the neck.

There is an element of chance about the recommendation in books that one chooses to try. I took the recommendation of Fox when first in practice and prepared an oil of fresh goosegrass for use in sore breasts and enlarged cervical glands, and have used it in practice continuously for over 20 years. I make the oil in June before the plant begins to seed. As an example, 2480 g of fresh herb in 4 L of sunflower oil yielded 3100 mL of infused oil. The oil is prepared by roughly chopping and weighing the fresh plant material and filling a large jam pan, and covering it with sunflower oil. It is simmered on the lowest possible heat until the leaves begin to crisp. Then more fresh herb is added and left on the heat until it begins to crisp. Then turn off, cover the pan with clingfilm, steep overnight, strain through a cloth and ensure that the black watery residue is discarded.

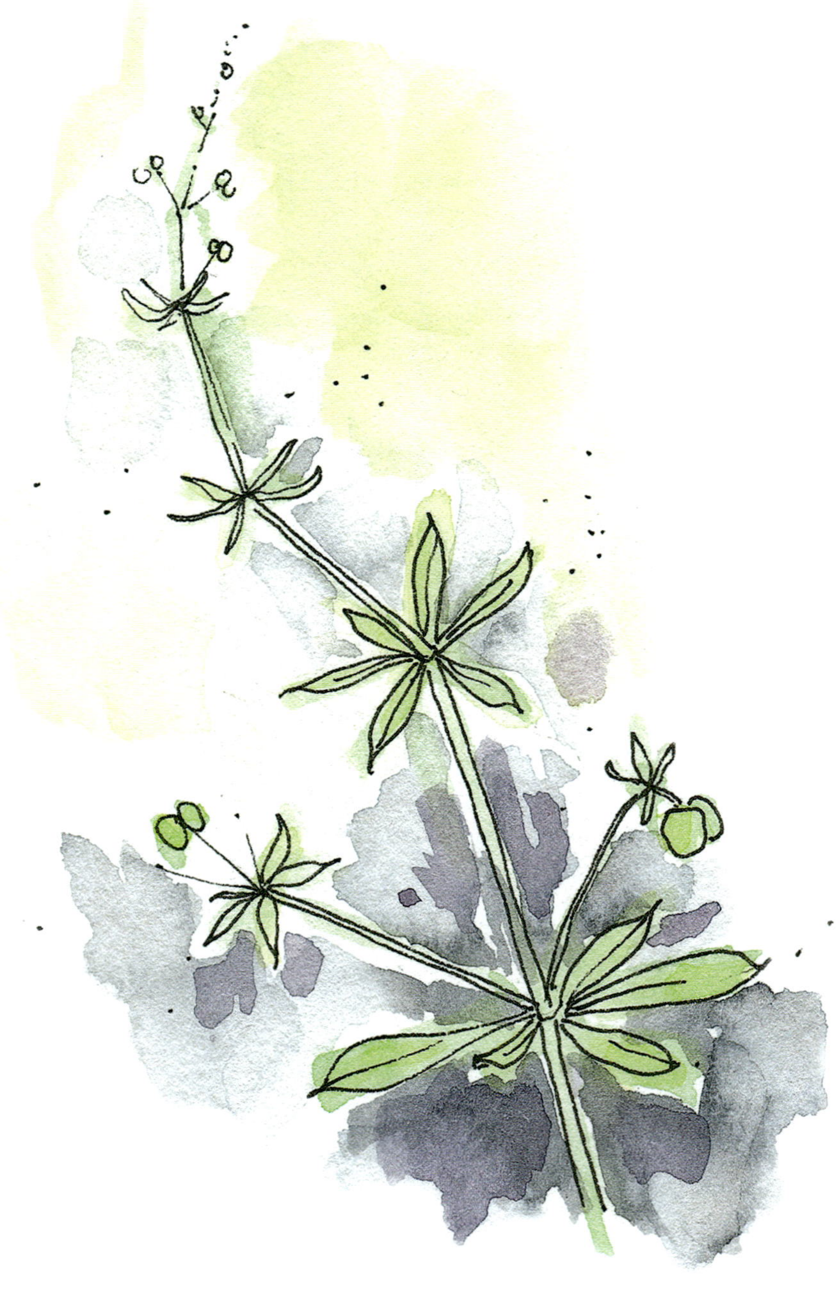

THE WESTERN HERBAL TRADITION

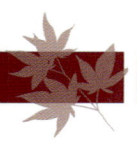

Figure 17.2 *Galium aparine*, goosegrass.

## MORE EXTERNAL USES

The oil can be used alone for premenstrual sore breasts and in the lumpy breasts associated with fibroadenoma. With essential oils and tinctures it is invaluable in external treatment of enlarged cervical glands in throat infections, in sinusitis and in headache associated with sinusitis. I use it as an ingredient in creams for swellings associated with arthritis, and in the treatment of boils with, for example, marshmallow root cream *Althaea officinalis*, tincture of myrrh *Commiphora molmol* and tea tree oil *Melaleuca alternifolia*. My impression is that it is of particular use in decreasing swellings, encouraging lymphatic flow and thus in resolution of infection and inflammation. I had one patient only who appeared to have an allergic reaction to the oil but as it is an oil, I would not use it in eczema as oils can be too heating. A chance decision to follow the advice in Fox is found to have been based on the advice of Dioscorides. I have found this preparation very reliable: what herbalists used to call a 'sheet-anchor'. In writing this book, we have found many external usages which have fallen out of favour, and which could be reintroduced.

The other external use given by Dioscorides is the juice dropped into the ears to treat earache, an application found in Pliny and cited in Fuchs, Dalechamps and subsequent authors. Pliny gives as additional usage: leaves applied to inhibit bleeding from wounds which is also given by Mattioli, Dodoens and Culpeper. This could be a useful first aid measure as *Galium* is used in Turkey to coagulate milk (Deliorman et al 2001). Mattioli and Culpeper also advise the powdered herb to stop bleeding from a wound by closing it up.

## DIURETIC IN THE WIDE SENSE

Use for urinary tract problems is a more recent application. Priest & Priest describe it as a 'soothing, relaxing and diffusive diuretic which increases aqueous excretion, corrects inability to pass normal catabolic wastes, and relieves irritation'. The term 'diuretic' is used in texts on herbal medicine to cover a range of actions and indications associated with urinary function. For goosegrass, these include an increase in flow of urine, use in urinary tract infections, for kidney stones and in strangury. The term 'strangury' is used to mean impeded flow of urine. This indication is given by the physicians of Myddfai, who also recommend use of the fresh juice in dropsy and oedematous swellings of the joints, legs, feet and other parts. Coffin and Fox describe goosegrass as one of the most powerful of all diuretics and so useful in many diseases of the urinary tract, including dropsy. Coffin recommends the juice or decoction for children who start to retain fluid due to inflammation of the kidneys following an attack of scarlet fever. This recommendation links with use in scarlatina and 'other exanthematous diseases, in their inflammatory stages' by Felter & Lloyd (1898). It also suggests a usage in Henoch-Schönlein purpura.

Use in urinary tract infections is a recurring theme. Cook recommends goosegrass in acute conditions, particularly when the urine is too concentrated and scalding, and where urinary flow is impeded by inflammation at the neck of the bladder such as in gonorrhoea, for which he give the dose of ½–1 fl oz (15–30 mL) every 4–6 hours. While the treatment of venereal disease must always be undertaken by a qualified medical practitioner, there is every reason to suppose that the use of an alterative such as goosegrass would support antibiotic treatment. Fox advocates goosegrass in inflammation of the kidneys and bladder, scalding of urine and 'all cases attended with febrile excitement'.

Goosegrass is consistently recommended in the Eclectic texts for its actions on the urinary tract. Scudder (1870) recommends the infusion as one of the best remedies to increase flow of urine and as fast acting in painful urination. Ellingwood (1919) advises use of the infusion, especially where there is dysuria with acute inflammation, and in urinary tract problems associated with enlarged prostate. He particularly values it to resolve fever. Although goosegrass is classified as a renal stimulant, it is a cold remedy and, according to Scudder (1898), should not be used in torpid and debilitated conditions. Wren lists it for 'obstruction of urinary organs, suppression of urine, dropsy, renal obstructions' and use in oedema is also given by the *National Botanic Pharmacopoeia*. Priest & Priest recommend it in scalding micturition, dysuria, irritable bladder and cystitis with marshmallow *Althaea officinalis* and enuresis in children with *Rhus aromatica*. Menzies-Trull also advises it in acute cystitis and in benign prostatic hypertrophy. The *British Herbal Pharmacopoeia* lists it as a diuretic herb noting its use in dysuria and cystitis, although somehow this short entry seems bland and lifeless compared with the earlier sources.

Wood links the usage of goosegrass as an antilithic, describing this as another form of concretion, with its use in fibrous breast tissue. Although the analogy could be farfetched, the alterative action may be affecting both conditions. Goosegrass is recommended for bladder stones and gravelly deposits by the physicians of Myddfai and by Coffin. Wren claims that it is a 'solvent of stone in bladder' as does Grieve. Priest & Priest recommend use in this context with antiseptics such as bearberry *Arctostaphylos uva-ursi*. A combination given by Coffin for stoppage of urine, gravel and 'female weakness (menstrual problems) contains goosegrass, parsley root *Petroselinum crispum*, juniper berries *Juniperus communis*, linseed *Linum usssisitatum* all at 2 oz, 1 oz quassia bark *Picrasma excelsa*, boiled in 1 gallon of water and strained. Then add 1 oz powdered ginger *Zingiber officinalis* and 1 lb honey. The

## THE WESTERN HERBAL TRADITION

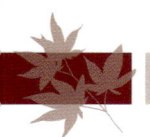

dose is given as 1 tablespoon to half a wineglassful three times daily, which gives a dose of 15–30 mL.

## COOLING OR HEATING ALTERNATIVE?

The temperament of goosegrass is given by Galen, cited by Fuchs and Dalechamps, as slightly heating with subtle parts and a moderately cleansing and drying action. Dalechamps describes it as hot and dry and Culpeper describes it as moderately heating and drying. Yet above, Scudder (1898) argues that it must not be used in cold and torpid conditions as it is cooling. This perception of goosegrass as cooling is also given by Felter & Lloyd (1898), who state that it is contraindicated in diseases of a passive character as it is refrigerant and sedative. This is an important point as it could be the basis of the contra-indication of goosegrass by Coffin in diabetes which is repeated by the *National Botanic Pharmacopoeia*, Grieve and Barnes. It could also be because in untreated diabetes there is already excessive flow of urine, but my impression of goosegrass is that it is predominantly cooling.

There is some support of the mild astringent action given by the *British Herbal Pharmacopoeia*. Mattioli, cited by Dalechamps, and followed by Parkinson then Culpeper, refers to use of the distilled water in dysentery. Culpeper also advises the decoction in jaundice, lasks (diarrhoea) and bloody fluxes. The only reference to tannins is in Bradley (1992) referring to a study published in 1970 which found 2.5–4% condensed tannins. The main constituents identified are iridoid glycosides which are bitter. This could support the advice of Culpeper and Miller, who give a use as a spring tonic. Culpeper advises the herb chopped small, boiled well in watery gruel and eaten to cleanse the blood, strengthen the liver and so keep the body in health and 'fitting it for the change of season that is coming'. The herb taken in broth, with mutton and oatmeal, is said to keep those 'apt to grow fat in a lean and lank state'. Coffin, Cook and Wren state that goosegrass is a mild aperient of the bowels.

It is cooling, but there is also a sense of movement and Menzies-Trull describes it as a vasotonic alterative which cleanses the tissues. Although the *British Herbal Pharmacopoeia* gives only the actions diuretic and mild astringent, it give lymphadenitis as an indication and enlarged lymph modes as a specific indication. Hoffmann emphasizes the action as a lymphatic tonic with alterative and diuretic actions. He particularly recommends it in dry psoriasis.

This herb is an example of a plant where there is no pharmacology to support its usage. The oil is pale green and external usage must rely on a compound which is soluble in oil. The black residue will contain the water soluble iridoid glycosides. Fresh and dried preparations vary substantially as dried preparations are dark whereas fresh tinctures can be a pale straw colour. However, taken as a diuretic, lymphatic tonic and alterative, goosegrass can form a valuable part of a prescription. Used externally, it has a quality which I have not met in any other plant, and which I probably only discovered because the fresh plant was readily available. As Culpeper says 'it growth by the hedge and ditch side in many places of this land, and is so troublesome an inhabitant in gardens, that it rampeth upon, and is ready to choak whatever grows near it'.

## RETURNING TO THE MYDDFAI PHYSICIANS

The commonplace nature of goosegrass allows it to be recommended as a food. The Myddfai text gives a brief account of the four causes of disease: fever caused by excess hot or cold; eruptive poison caused by irregularities in eating and drinking; obstruction in the stomach, veins or hollow vessels which means that the food, drink, blood or humours cannot pass; and boils caused by the entrance of poisons. 'Irregularities in eating and drinking' remain common causes of disease and the recommendation of regular consumption of fresh herbs as food can be overlooked because of the perception of herbs as medicines. The Myddfai text gives a detailed account of the use of goosegrass and offers another recipe for use to make the person strong and healthy. The leaves, flowers and seed should be dried separately in the morning sun, and carefully, for foggy and muggy weather spoils the drying process. An infusion overnight in cold water of either herb, flower or seed, according to what is available is to be taken daily with salt for 1 week. Thereafter, an infusion of the fresh plant material is taken for 9 weeks. During the first 3 weeks of this period the infusion is to be made from the leaves, then the flowers for 3 weeks, finally the seed. Each time the plant material is to be infused for 6 hours. At the end of the day, the infused plant material can be boiled up and the resulting strained decoction taken warm before bed.

In some Renaissance texts it is impossible to know whether the writer is writing from experience or to demonstrate their learning. In contrast, a virtue of the Myddfai text is that it reads as if it is written from practical experience. This will partly be because it is based on a different and more widespread tradition of medical books which listed herbs by indication (Gottfried 1986) and its firm location within a local Welsh context.

## RECOMMENDATIONS

- There is a strong tradition of use as an alterative in 'eruptive poisons' and skin disease.

- As a cooling diuretic in fevers, especially if associated with rashes.
- For urinary tract infections.
- External usage in swollen glands, boils, sore throat, sinusitis and arthritis is consistently recommended throughout the tradition and is recommended from personal experience.

Dosage: the *British Herbal Pharmacopoeia* recommends 2–4 g three times a day of dried aerial parts.

Use of the fresh herb is consistently recommended throughout the tradition. Coffin gives a dose of 60 mL three times a day of fresh juice. The *British Herbal Pharmacopoeia* recommends 3–15 mL three times a day of expressed juice.

External preparations such as an oil in which fresh plant material has been decocted, can be used one to eight times a day depending on whether the conditions is chronic or acute. This makes a useful base oil to which essential oils can be added.

## RECOMMENDATIONS ON SAFETY

- Goosegrass is considered safe in pregnancy and lactation, and no warnings or adverse events were found (Mills & Bone 2005).

## CONSTITUENTS

Reviews: Barnes et al (2007), Bradley (1992), Mills & Bone (2005), Williamson (2003).

### Alkaloids

Three categories, isoquinoline: protopine; beta-carboline: harmine; quinazoline: vascinone, dehydroxdeoxypeganine (wild, Turkey) (Şener & Ergun 1991).

### Volatile oils

Aldehydes and ketones 22%: beta-damascenone 0.2%. Oil mainly composed of non-volatile oils: hexadecanoic acid 22% (wild, Turkey) (Baser et al 2004).
Alkanes: nonacosane, concentrations vary over the summer (Corrigan et al 1978).

### Iridoid glycosides

Asperulosidic acid 0.19%, 10-deacetylasperulosidic acid 0.58% (wild, Turkey) (Deliorman et al 2001).
Asperulosidic acid, monotropein, 10-deacetylasperulosidic acid, scandoside (wild, Bulgaria) (Mitova et al 2002).
Asperuloside, monotropein, deacetylasperulosidic acid (wild, Ireland) (Corrigan et al 1978).

### Polyphenolic acids

The concentration of p-coumaric and ferulic acid was the lowest found amongst 14 plants (Komprda et al 1999). Condensed tannins 2.5–4% (Bradley 1992). These related compounds are listed here as no more recent reference was found.

### Coumarins

Scopoletin (wild, Portugal) (Seabra & Silveira 1993).

### Flavonoids

Flavanone: hesperetin glycosides (Temizer et al 1996).

## REFERENCES

Barnes J, Anderson LA, Phillipson JD 2007 Herbal medicines, 3rd edn. Pharmaceutical Press, London.

Baser KHC, Özek T, Krmer N, et al 2004 Composition of the essential oils of *Galium aparine* L. and *Galium odoratum* (L.) Scop. from Turkey. Journal of Essential Oil Research 16:305–307.

Bradley PR (ed.) 1992 British herbal compendium, vol 1. British Herbal Medicine Association, Bournemouth.

Corrigan D, Timoney RF, Donnelly DMX 1978 Iridoids and alkanes in twelve species of *Galium* and *Asperula*. Phytochemistry 17:1131–1133.

Davis PH (ed.) 1982 Flora of Turkey vol 7. Edinburgh University Press, Edinburgh.

Deliorman D, Çalış I, Ergun F 2001 Iridoids from *Galium aparine*. Pharmaceutical Biology 39:234–235.

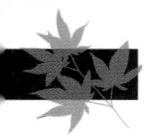

Ellingwood F 1919 The American materia medica, therapeutics and pharmacognosy. Online. Available: http://www.henriettesherbal.com.

Felter HW, Lloyd JU 1898 King's American dispensatory. Online. Available: http://www.henriettesherbal.com/eclectic/index.html 20 April 2009.

French RK 1993 Scrofula (scrophula). In: Kiple KF (ed.) 1993 The Cambridge world history of human disease. Cambridge University Press, Cambridge.

Gibbons B, Brough P 1996 Wild flowers of Britain & Northern Europe. Chancellor Press, London.

Gottfried RS 1986 Doctors and medicine in medieval England. Princeton University Press, Princeton, New Jersey, 1340–1530.

Komprda T, Stohandlová M, Foltýn J, et al 1999 Content of p-coumaric and ferulic acid in forbs with potential grazing utilization. Archiv für Tierernährung 52:95–105.

Mack RN 2003 Plant naturalizations and invasions in the Eastern United States: 1634–1860. Annals of the Missouri Botanical Garden 90:77–90.

Mills S, Bone K 2005 The essential guide to herbal safety. Churchill Livingstone, St Louis.

Mitova MI, Anchev ME, Handjieva NV 2002 Iridoid patterns in *Galium* L. and some phylogenetic considerations. Zeitung für Naturforschung 57c:226–234.

Scudder JM 1870 Specific medication and specific medicines. Online. Available: http://www.henriettesherbal.com.

Scudder JM 1898 The American eclectic materia medica and therapeutics. Online. Available: http://www.henriettesherbal.com.

Seabra RMJ, Silveira A 1993 Phenolic compounds of *Galium aparine* and *Galium broteroanum*. Plantes Medicinales et Phytotherapie 26:49–51.

Şener B, Ergun F 1991 The first isolation of an isoquinoline alkoloid from *Galium aparine* L. Gazi Universitesi Eczacilik Fakultesi Dergisiş 8:13–15.

Taylor K 1999 *Galium aparine* L. Journal of Ecology 87:713–730.

Temizer A, Sayin F, Ergun F, et al 1996 Determination of total flavonoid in various *Galium* species by differential pulse polarography. Gazi Universitesi Eczacilik Fakultesi Dergisi 13:97–103.

Williamson E 2003 Potter's Herbal Cyclopaedia. CW Daniel, Saffron Walden.

# CHAPTER 18
# *Glechoma hederacea*, ground ivy

## DESCRIPTION

### Family: Lamiaceae           Part used: aerial parts

*Glechoma hederacea* L. is a hardy perennial found throughout Europe mainly on damp, heavy soils typically in light shade in woodlands and hedgerows but also on open sites (Hutchings & Price 1998). Pelikan suggests dry and sunny sites that are still shadeless, such as under hedges, walls and fruit trees and by roadsides. The *Flora of Turkey* (Davis 1982) gives one *Glechoma* species, *Glechoma hederacea*.

Creeping square stems bear crenate, dark green leaves with a purplish tinge which are heart-shaped or kidney-shaped. Axillary whorls of two to five purplish-blue flowers occur from March to June on vertical square-stemmed flowering shoots (10–60 cm) between two opposite, stalked leaves. The flower is tubular with a toothed upper lip and a much larger three-lobed lower lip with reddish hairs.

It forms large carpets (ramets) as it spreads rapidly by long stolons which root at the nodes. It is also propagated by seeds which occur in groups of four nutlets in the persistent calyx.

**Other species used**: *Glechoma longituba* (Nakai) Kuprian (syn. *Glechoma hederacea* L. var. *longituba* Nakai) is widely used in China, Korea and the Far East (Zhu 1998).

### Quality

A sample in Germany was found to be *Centella asiatica* (Albert 2005).

---

Ground ivy is one of the first spring plants and the first of the labiates to come into flower and, Pelikan tells us, to transform the cosmic warmth given to the earth in spring into warmth-filled plant nature. After flowering it busies itself in spreading widely through its underground runners. It is thus a plant of the earth, as its English and old Latin names (i.e. hedera terrestris) suggest. Pelikan states that ground ivy has been used as a general metabolic stimulant, especially in spring. It targets the digestive organs, kidneys and lungs, treating calculi and weakness of the bladder, digestive weakness and congestion of the liver and spleen, and tubercular and asthmatic states of the lungs. It has both internal and external uses. However, 'all this is very similar to the action of the other labiates we have been considering'. Indeed, ground ivy has the typical constituents of this family, including volatile oils, triterpenes and phenolic acids, but there is so little published on it compared to other plants in the family. Weiss comments that little is known about the herb and there is no clear reason for its use as a cough remedy. It is not mentioned at all in Mills & Bone, Priest & Priest, Hoffmann and Menzies-Trull. My own experience of the use of ground ivy amongst herbal practitioners is that it is by no means a notable remedy and Wood remarks on how little we herbalists use it today.

What evidence is there that might support the idea that herbalists should be more interested in ground ivy as a medicinal herb? A recent phytotherapeutic monograph (Barnes et al 2007) suggests that the chemistry of ground ivy is well studied and that documented pharmacological activities for its constituents support some herbal uses, although there is a lack of clinical research. On the basis of existing evidence, ground ivy may be considered to possess mild expectorant, anticatarrhal, astringent, vulnerary, diuretic and stomachic properties. Barnes et al consult the *British Herbal Compendium* vol.1, the *British Herbal Pharmacopoeia* and two other herbal textbooks of the 1980s to source the plant's traditional indications: bronchitis and specifically chronic bronchial catarrh, tinnitus, diarrhoea, haemorrhoids, cystitis, gastritis. The dose is 2–4 g three times daily as an infusion or equivalent liquid preparations.

Of particular note is the relative lack of clinical safety and toxicity data for ground ivy. This is by no means unusual for a large number of medicinal plants, but Barnes highlights two facts: that poisoning in cattle and horses

THE WESTERN HERBAL TRADITION

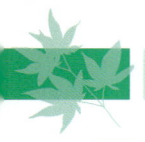

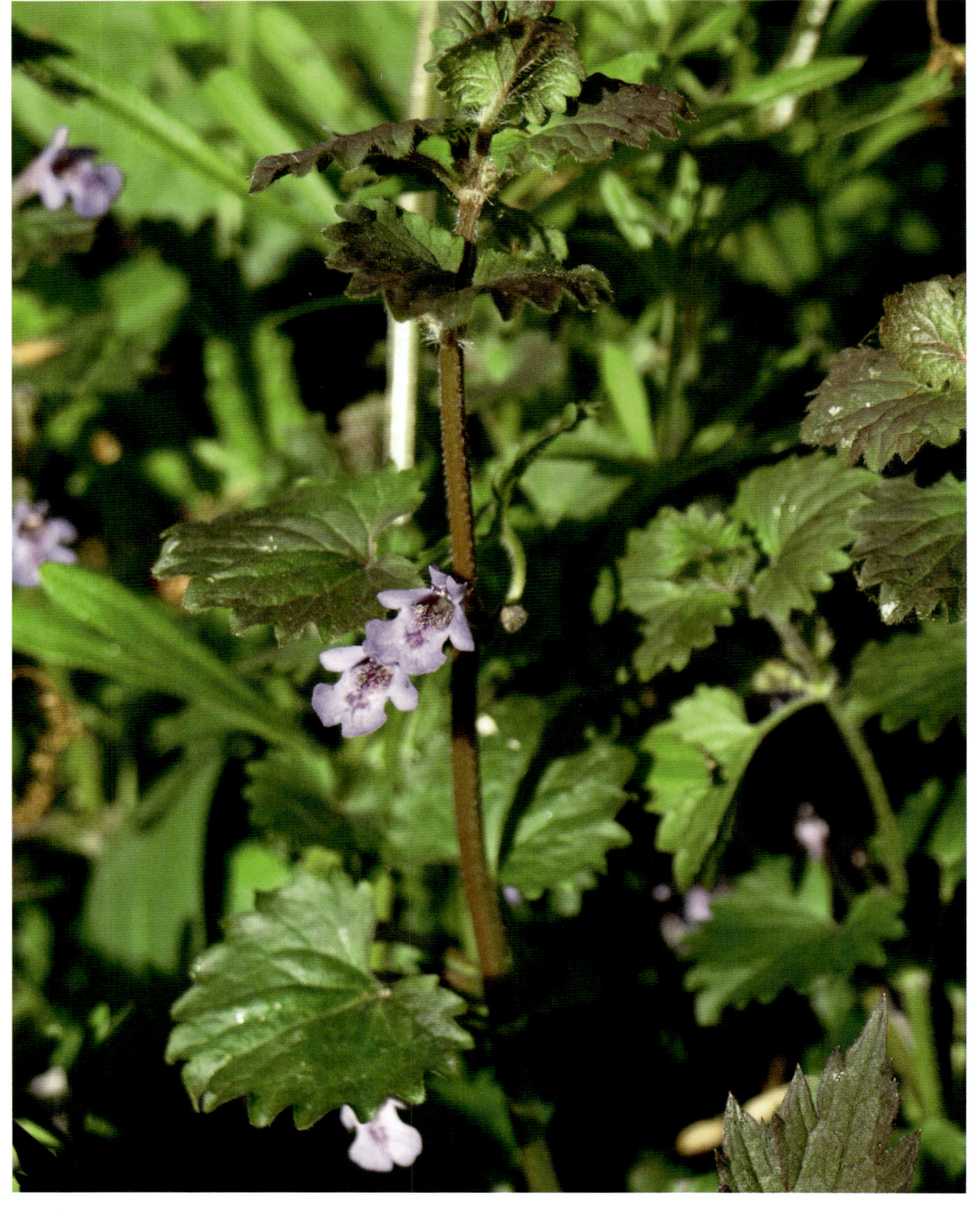

**Figure 18.1** *Glechoma hederacea*, ground ivy (a garden in Yorkshire, May).

has been documented in eastern Europe and that the plant's volatile oil contains many terpenoids, and terpene-rich volatile oils are irritant to the digestive tract and kidneys. A lectin has also been recently identified in ground ivy (Singh et al 2006).

Triterpenes are common constituents of medicinal plants and foods and have been extensively investigated (Ikeda et al 2008) and found to have antiinflammatory activity (Liu 1995). There is growing interest in the elucidation of the biological functions of triterpenoids, some of which are used as anticancer and antiinflammatory agents in Asian countries. Ursolic acid, a natural pentacyclic triterpenoid carboxylic acid, is the major component of some traditional medicine herbs and is well known to possess a wide range of biological functions, such as antioxidative, antiinflammatory and anticancer activities, that are able to counteract endogenous and exogenous biological stimuli. In contrast to these beneficial properties, some laboratory studies have recently revealed that the effects of ursolic acid on normal cells and tissues are occasionally pro-inflammatory. Clinical usefulness is established according to a risk/benefit ratio. This evaluation has not been generally applied to herbal medicines because of a lack of clinical data. Our task here, then, is to review the full tradition of use of ground ivy to appreciate what medical and herbal practitioners of the past have written of the benefits and risks of this herb so that herbal practitioners considering clinical use of ground ivy are in command of the widest knowledge available.

Ground ivy is a plant of central and northern Europe, according to Pelikan, and the neighbouring regions of Asia extending as far as Siberia. Consequently, it is not surprising to find that our Arabic writers do not describe it and the Greek and Roman authors are quite brief in their comments. The leaves of Dioscorides' 'chamaikissos' (IV 125), Greek for the 'ivy of the earth', identified as *Glechoma hederacea* by Beck, are bitter, especially the flowers, according to Galen, and in decoction treat hip problems (Dioscorides and Galen), obstructions of the liver, i.e. jaundice (Dioscorides and Galen), and spleen (Pliny). In the form of an ointment, Pliny adds, it is applied to burns. The editors of Apuleius identify his 'hedera nigra' as *Nepeta glechoma* Benth., but Apuleius is actually describing common ivy instead. This is confirmed in Van Arsdall's edition of the *Old English herbarium*.

Hip problems, one of the indications for ground ivy, are sometimes referred to as sciatica. According to Riviere (Culpeper et al 1655) sciatica and 'ischias' refer to pain in the hip joint. Similar pains in the foot, hand or knee are called podagra, usually meaning gout, chiragra and gonagra, respectively. Pain in other joints is called arthritis. The possible confusion of naming a joint problem sciatica when this word refers to inflammation or irritation of the sciatic nerve today is explained by recourse to the idea that only a nerve could sense and respond with pain to irritation of the joint by the accumulation of a humour there, and, furthermore, that pain is experienced in the thigh rather than in the back in a fair proportion of sciatica sufferers. Dioscorides may have envisaged ground ivy as being able to remove the offending humour and thus free the nerve from irritation.

If the classical writers say little about the plant, we can expect a fuller appreciation from the herbal writers of northern Europe. Fuchs states that 'the strong bitterness and sharpness of the leaves and flowers show that this herb is hot and dry' and he cites Dioscorides, Galen and Pliny as usual – where it is apparent that his edition of Pliny is corrupted because there is no mention of the ointment for burns, instead the dosage of Dioscorides for hip pains is given. He is satisfied that this plant of valleys, steep slopes and cultivated fields near hedges and thickets is the chamaikissos of Dioscorides, also called 'chamaileuce' or 'crown of the earth, because it spreads its stems through the earth and seems to crown it as if with a garland of foliage'. Mattioli, on the other hand, is not convinced that Dioscorides is writing about ground ivy and does not know of any plant fitting his description. Furthermore, Pliny's description, he says, does not match that of Dioscorides. Thus Mattioli does not sanction Fuch's opinion but appends the opinions of Dioscorides and Galen anyway, while doing away with Pliny's reliability on this herb. At least Fuchs provides an appendix of the medical opinions of his day concerning ground ivy and based on Galenic pharmacological theory: the plant's bitterness supports its classical indications, to which he adds its ability to restart suppressed menses, stimulate urine, clear impaired hearing and be effective against the pestilence. He mentions a use among horsemen who have attested to the great success of this plant in treating a plague ('pestis') in horses called 'fibula'.

If we turn to Dodoens, who like Mattioli doubts that this 'hedera terrestris' of the apothecaries, which he says 'is very common in all this country, and groweth in many gardens and shadowie moist places' is the chamaikissos of Dioscorides, we are disappointed to learn from a writer who takes such an interest in his native flora that tinnitus and hard of hearing are the only indications for this plant. Thus Dodoens gives only one of the uses of ground ivy listed in Fuchs.

Tinnitus is also mentioned much earlier by Hildegard as a condition treated by this herb, whose hot and dry qualities and vital energy are somewhat akin to those of the spices. Consequently, if a person who is languishing or whose reason is failing eats it often, soaked in warm water then cooked into a puree or broth and taken with other meats, he will benefit. More specifically, ground ivy targets the head and removes bad humours there, which give rise to tinnitus, poor hearing and other illnesses of that part. In this case, the boiled plant is applied warm directly to the head. Equally it may be applied during a bath to the chest area in cases of pain there 'as if he has internal ulcers'. Macer's herbal does not include ground

THE WESTERN HERBAL TRADITION

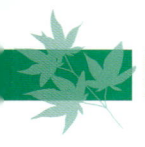

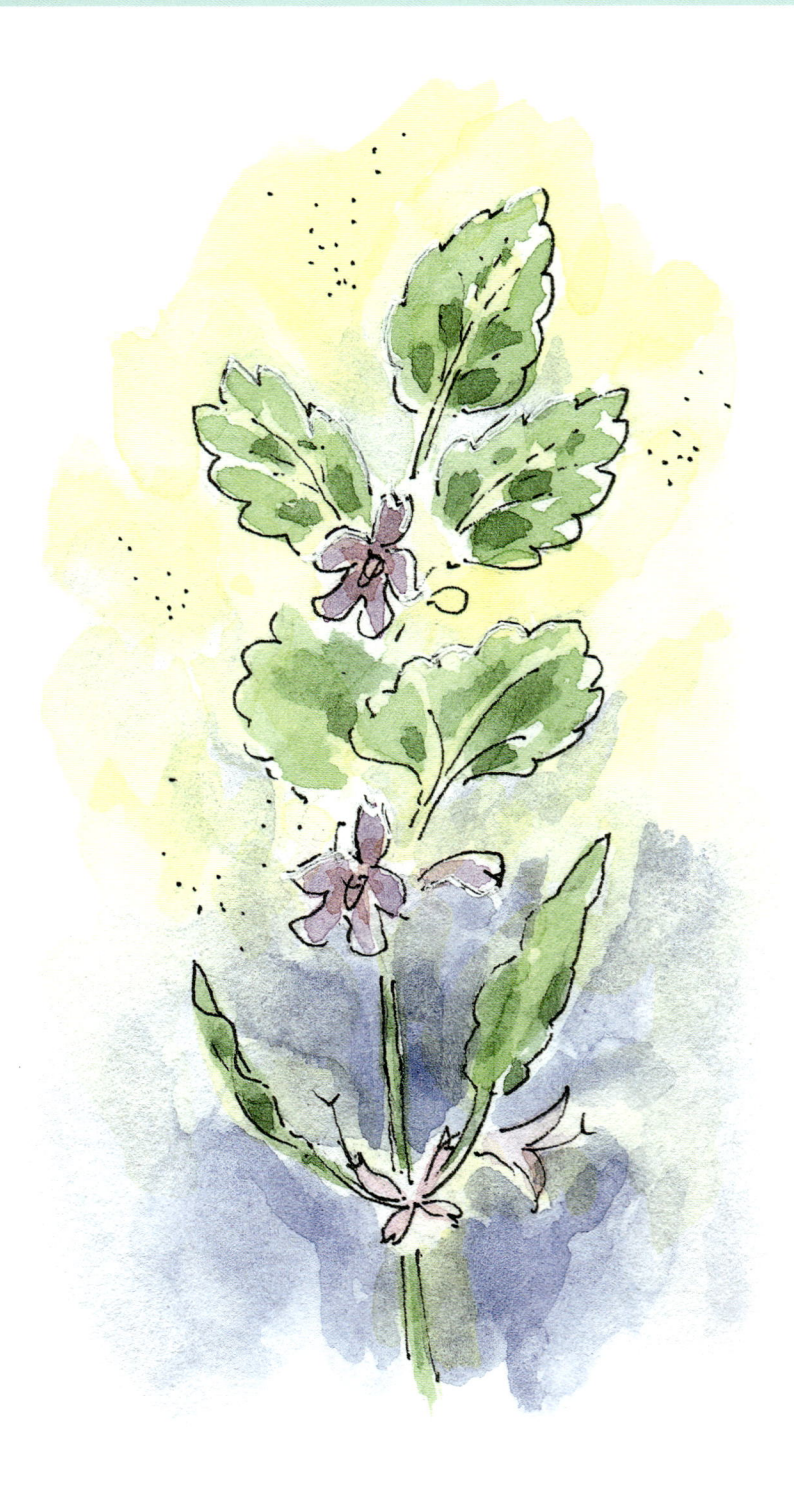

**Figure 18.2** *Glechoma hederacea*, ground ivy.

ivy and it is not clear that the 'sicra' or 'herbe terrestre' of our Salernitan source is definitely *Glechoma hederacea*, but it seems likely. For they accredit it with hot and dry qualities, here in the second degree, and state that it purges bad humours. It is indicated for headache, mange, jaundice and fever. The leaves whiten the teeth when rubbed on and they can be made into an ointment for wounds with plantain *Plantago species* and cinquefoil *Potentilla* species.

The uses of ground ivy in the *Red Book* of the physicians of Myddfai are mainly external. The juice of the plant is dropped into the eye to clear opacity of the lens and specks in the eye. The boiled herb is applied to the head in cases of obstinate ague or intermittent fever while the sufferer is bathing but he must be bled afterwards too. An ointment of ground ivy is used for the bite of a mad dog. Ground ivy is also one of a formula of 19 herbs to be macerated in wheat ale and taken for urinary gravel.

Such medieval uses are not based on pharmacological theory, as we see in Fuchs, not least because there can be no appreciation of the bitterness of the plant when it is applied externally, and the matter of its bitter taste is not mentioned. Equally medical humanists like Fuchs and Mattioli generally omit citing 'corrupted' empirical medieval sources such as Hildegard or the Salernitan herbal.

Returning to the Renaissance authors, we find more information in the Lyons herbal of Dalechamps than that given in the preceding texts. Ground ivy is a plant found almost anywhere in shady and damp places. It is hot and dry in quality and the flowers especially are bitter. These appear in March and last for most of the summer. The leaves are often available all year. It is called hedera terrestris, also mollis hedera or soft ivy and its Greek equivalent malachokissos, and crown of the earth for the same reason as given by Fuchs. Also like Fuchs, Dalechamps is certain this plant is the chamaekissos of Dioscorides and has the virtues cited in the Greek author which have been 'witnessed by the frequent experience of doctors, namely that by its bitterness and by other qualities it is most effective in obstructions and arthritic pains'. He cites the actions of removing obstructions of the liver and spleen, clearing jaundice, remedying hip pains and stimulating the menses and urination. He qualifies the use listed by Fuchs for clearing impaired hearing by explaining that the herb must be rubbed down in the hands and placed into the ears. 'They also say it is effective against the plague' and he gives the example of the treatment of horses. Dalechamps adds to previous entries by citing Hieronymus Bock on additional topical uses: the leaves decocted in a gargle for ulceration and problems of the mouth, throat and neck, and externally applied as a wash for the female genitalia and for itchy skin, while the juice is beneficial for fistulas. Actually, it is Gerard who specifically cites Mattioli on this last use, who requires more exactly a mixing of the juice with verdigris.

Gerard, writing a decade after Dalechamps, does not add to his summary but rather provides an English slant to the text. The woodcut depiction of the plant seems accurate as does Gerard's description. In England, the plant does not flower until April (and Bauhin, for his part, tells us not until May in Basel) but remains so 'till Sommer be far spent' (but only the middle of summer in Basel). Gerard mentions a second kind, found in rocky places in the Provence and Dauphine Departments of southeast France, that is similar to ground ivy in all respect except for longer, larger and lighter-coloured flowers and which is named rock ivy or 'asarina' by de l Obel. The common English names for ground ivy are alehoof, tunhoof – because 'the women of our Northern parts, especially about Wales and Cheshire do tunne the herbe Alehoof into their ale, but the reason thereof I know not' – Gill-go-by-ground and catsfoot. Doubt concerning whether this plant is the chamaekissos of Dioscorides, says Gerard, is dealt with by Dodoens in his *Stirpium Historiae Pemptades Sex* of 1583, where, according to Bauhin, Dodoens writes that he is satisfied with the attribution, in complete contrast to the opinion expressed in his earlier herbal. Gerard cites Dioscorides and Galen, and the use of ground ivy for tinnitus and hardness of hearing, but not those indications rationally derived from the plant's bitterness given in Fuchs and Dalechamps. Indeed, Gerard contradicts the notion that the plant stimulates menstruation by stating that drinking a decoction of the herb in water stops bleeding. Additionally, when boiled in broth and taken it halts diarrhoea. Boiled in mutton broth it helps weak and aching backs, which may suggest a strengthening action on the kidneys. Gerard's other indications are much more reminiscent of the medieval uses already mentioned, namely for purging cold and damp rheumatic humours flowing from the brain into the head, for which the herb is taken in ale, and for problems with the eyes. In this second case, the strained juice of ground ivy, greater celandine *Chelidonium majus* and daisies *Bellis perennis*, mixed with a little sugar and rose-water and dropped into the eyes with a feather, proves itself to be the 'best medicine in the world' for all eye problems, inflammation, spots, webs, itch or smarting, even when the sufferer is virtually blind from the condition. This echoes the treatment for specks and webs in the eyes employed by the Myddfai physicians. The same herbs, but mixed with honey and ale, may be injected into the eyes with a syringe for the same problems in a horse or cow. It seems unlikely that this is the same condition which Fuchs calls 'fibula' in horses. Finally Gerard recommends an ointment of ground ivy for burns by fire and gunpowder.

Gerard's uses of ground ivy for excessive menstruation and for strengthening the kidneys appear in the *London Dispensatory* of the College of Physicians published in 1618 and translated by Culpeper in 1649, but Parkinson's 1640 text explicitly states that the herb is not a treatment for menorrhagia. This is the only substantial difference between his entry and that in Culpeper's herbal, and both are based on Gerard. Additional material in Parkinson, copied by Culpeper, includes the external uses from Bock which Gerard failed to mention, the affirmation of a diuretic and emmenogogue action listed in Fuchs, the use of the juice rather than the rubbed herb topically for tinnitus and deafness, and an extension of the treatment of hip problems from Dioscorides, to include gouty pains in the hands, knees and feet and requiring 3 obols (1800 mg) of herb decocted in 3 cyathi (135 mL) of water drunk daily for 40–50 days. Culpeper wants the decoction made in wine and taken 'for some time'. An apparently new indication, not mentioned before, is for griping pains of the stomach, spleen or belly due to windy and choleric humours. Culpeper identifies this herb as belonging to Venus and especially warming to the bowels. If it opens obstructions of the spleen, he reckons, then it is also beneficial to the melancholic patient. Finally, the herb's use on fresh wounds, such as the bite of a mad dog of the Myddfai text, is extended to cover all inward wounds as well, including ulcerated lungs first speculated upon by Hildegard.

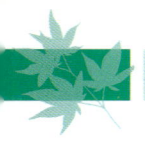

It is generally evident that Parkinson has read a version of Bauhin, although the latter's *Historia Plantarum Universalis* in three volumes was not fully published until 1650. Thus the new indication from Parkinson for abdominal colic may be taken from Bauhin's citation of the full entry from Bock, an entry which Dalechamps only partially listed, for he omitted dysentery. This indication may have become Gerard's diarrhoea in women and Parkinson's colic. Dalechamps seems to be the weak link in the transmission here, while Bauhin is reliably thorough. For instance, Bauhin discusses two diseases of horses: the decoction of ground ivy in wine expels poison through sweat, according to Mattioli, and thus is indicated in pestilence and, applied externally to horses, the infestation called 'feifel'; secondly, an ointment of the herb sold by apothecaries to be applied to plague sores is used by horse riders 'with great effect…when the saddle buckle has torn a horse's flesh'. He cites Mattioli too on the use of ground ivy made by Italian surgeons especially for wounds of the thorax and intestines, who esteem the plant as a trauma potion of certain efficacy. This becomes Parkinson's 'all inward wounds'. Bauhin is his own witness to the application of the herb to the belly for post-partum pains in women and the expulsion of worms in horses, if the herb is chopped up and mixed with oats. For women suffering swelling of the limbs or belly, 3 fl oz of the decoction or distilled water should be applied twice daily. Bauhin states that he has 'used it soundly for 'acipse'(?).

Bauhin also cites three other writers. Camerarius states that in parts of Italy, old ulcers are washed out with the juice of ground ivy, then the powdered herb is sprinkled on to the wound, and for the most part it is an excellent help. Secondly, the famous Dr Ludovic de Leone of Bologna recommends the distilled water taken for 44 days as efficacious for suppuration in the chest. This again may be the source of Parkinson's indication of ulcerated lungs.

Finally, Bauhin draws on a History of America by Lerius for a treatment of diarrhoea amongst a group of colonists: rice gruel was cooked with the juice of ground ivy, then taken from the fire and covered with a cloth, before being transferred to a jar in which egg yolks were mixed, and the whole reheated on a brazier. This soon restored the sufferers to health.

To sum up the actions and indications of ground ivy by the mid-17th century, it is bitter, astringent, diuretic, emmenogogue and vulnerary, being indicated in various conditions of the digestive tract such as dysentery, diarrhoea, haemorrhage and colic; for jaundice and obstructions of the liver and spleen; to strengthen the kidneys and to treat suppurations of the lungs, and various joint pains. Not least, it has many topical uses, for eyes, ears, throat and skin.

## GILL-ALE AND GILL-TEA

When we come to the 18th century, it is not surprising to hear from Quincy that 'this herb is mightily in use both in the shops and common prescription'. Quincy writes at some length about this pungent plant of nitrous and earthy taste called hedera terrestris or chamaekissos. He identifies its actions as abstersive or cleansing, and vulnerary. As well as its beneficial action on liver, spleen, bowels and kidneys, he mentions its prescription in almost all distempers of the lungs and breast, and its reputation to do wonders in tubercles and tartarous indurations of the lungs. Quincy cites Willis' *Pharmacopoeia Rationalis*, written in 1674, in support of the use of the powdered herb in obstinate coughs, especially in young children, and Etmuller concerning a young woman cured of consumption using only a strong decoction of the herb after an initial vomit was prescribed. The remainder of Quincy's entry concerns the correct pharmacological preparations of ground ivy. The infusion is popular in families, but the official syrup available in shops soon spoils, causing it to taste sour and to cause griping. The infusion in malt liquors, known as Gill-Ale and, according to Miller, drunk in great quantities in towns, is highly recommended. The dried plant is better than the fresh, because then the saline parts, where the medicinal virtue lies, are better dissolved into liquids. As a consequence, there is no medicinal benefit in distillations of the plant (so much for the recommendation of Dr Leone of Bologna in cases of suppuration of the lungs cited by Bauhin!) and the suggestion that the spirit of ground-ivy is a great restorative and curer of consumption is simple quackery. Miller adds little to Quincy's words, except to value the syrup and to repeat the commendation of several authors of the herb steeped in brandy, in other words a tincture, as of great service against the colic. Hill does not list the herb at all. Cullen classifies ground ivy as an antispasmodic pectoral 'much talked of, as curing on its own diseases of the breast: and what seems impossible to me but by the surgeon's instrument, an empyema. I can find no foundation for those properties'.

Thus a more negative appraisal of ground ivy takes place at the end of the 18th century and it is removed, as many herbs of the older tradition were at this time, from the official dispensatories of London and Edinburgh, but ground ivy reappears in the writings of Coffin: 'I have long used this herb, and always with satisfaction, although I do not think that it alone possesses so much control over the diseased system as many persons conceive'. He classifies it as an astringent, diuretic and mild tonic which can clear the system of bad humours when used in combination with other herbs. It is best as a tea, infused in a covered vessel, and treats indigestion, the kidneys and all scorbutic diseases. Externally, mixed with chamomile *Matricaria recutita* or fresh yarrow *Achillea millefolium* in a poultice, it is the best such application that can be made for tumours, gatherings or sores. Robinson (1868) restates its use for coughs and other lung complaints, for which an infusion of its leaves with those of elecampane *Inula helenium* and with liquorice root *Glycyrrhiza glabra* in equal quantities may be made. He, like Fernie (1897), draws on Ray's anecdote about a certain Mr Oldacre, who was cured of an inveterate and severe headache by using the expressed juice snuffed up the nose. Fernie (1897) suggests the powdered herb as snuff also. Robinson adds gentle stimulation to the plant's tonic and diuretic actions and quotes Culpeper at some length. Fernie defines ground ivy as diaphoretic, diuretic and somewhat astringent against bleedings. His recipe for an infusion of the herb, the original Gill tea, made with 1 oz of herb to 1 pint of boiling water and sweetened if desired with sugar, honey or liquorice, taken in a wineglassful dose when cool four times daily, is preferable to that of Robinson. Such a tea may be used as a preventative and remedy for lead colic among painters, as reported in the *Organic Materia Medica of Detroit USA 1890*, according to Wood. The National Botanic Pharmacopoeia lists alterative (to treat Coffin's scorbutic diseases), tonic and pectoral actions, and lung and kidney diseases for this herb, the infusion also being serviceable in sore and weak eyes.

Grieve suggests that the entire aerial parts of ground ivy should be gathered in May when the flowers are still fresh, the plant being common and found anywhere in the country on sunny hedge banks and waste ground. Thus there is a string of common names connecting it to hedges like Gill-go-by-the-hedge. She cites Green's *Universal Herbal* of 1832 in reference to ground ivy's power to impoverish pastures by expelling plants which grow near it. Furthermore, cattle, goats and pigs refuse it, and it is positively injurious to horses in quantity, although sheep will eat it. Expanding on Fernie's (1897) comments, Grieve informs us that Gill comes from the French word guiller meaning to ferment beer – ground ivy was one of the main plants used by the Saxons to clarify their beers before hops were introduced, and Culpeper lists it as alehoof rather than ground ivy – but it is also a girl's name, thus the local names haymaids and hedgemaids for those not aware of the reference to brewing. Grieve observes that this aromatic herb with a balsamic odour and bitter taste 'has long been discarded from the materia medica as an official plant in favour of others of greater certainty of action'. She draws her list of actions and uses from Coffin and Robinson, while attributing a diaphoretic action to the juice alone, cites Culpeper and Gerard, remarks on its strong reputation in the past for curing consumption and states that it is especially suited to presentations of pulmonary conditions where the kidneys require toning. The dose of the fluid extract is 0.5–1 fl drachm, which Bartram restates as 2–4 mL.

Few of our modern authors comment on ground ivy. Williamson restates the recent tradition by adding expectorant to astringent, diuretic, tonic and externally antiinflammatory actions, and haemorrhoids to its main indications of respiratory catarrh and bronchitis. These are all reported previously by Bartram, who like Culpeper emphasizes the plants astringent action on the digestive tract. He suggests combining ground ivy in equal parts with agrimony *Agrimonia eupatoria* for irritable bowel, and with a small amount of golden seal *Hydrastis canadensis* for cystitis. Chevallier includes 'glue ear', sinusitis, gastritis and acid indigestion in his list of indications for this 'well-tolerated' herb, based on its anticatarrhal and astringent properties. Wood mentions catarrhal problems troubling the middle ear or commencing in the Eustacian tubes as specific indications of ground ivy and reads the galls formed on it by parasitic wasps mentioned by Grieve as a further indication in cases of cancer where the tongue is dark red in the middle and heat is disorganizing the tissues.

The reputation of ground ivy was made during the Renaissance, peaked in the early 18th century and fell with Cullen. It was sold as a medicinal drink, the widely known Gill tea, on the streets of 18th century English towns when its reputation exceeded its powers. It has kept its place among herbalists until today, but is not in extensive use.

## RECOMMENDATIONS

- As an anticatarrhal, mild expectorant and antiinflammatory in chronic bronchial catarrh, certain presentations of tinnitus, sinusitis and other catarrhal causes of head pain, otitis media and 'glue ear'.
- As an astringent and antiinflammatory in dyspepsia, gastritis, diarrhoea, haemorrhoids, irritable bowel syndrome and abdominal colic.
- As a tonic for the kidneys and in cystitis.

# THE WESTERN HERBAL TRADITION

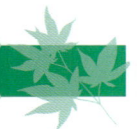

- External use on inflamed skin, for mild burns, sore throats, mouth inflammations, conjunctivitis, blepharitis and irritated eyes.
- Ground ivy no longer has a place in the cure of tuberculosis because chemotherapeutic drugs constitute the appropriate treatment in medicine today. Otherwise, the herb's actions and indications seem to be well represented in modern herbal texts, but further research should be pursued into the benefits of ground ivy in arthritis and gout using Dioscorides' dose of 2 g herb decocted three times daily for 6–8 weeks.

Dosage: the *British Herbal Pharmacopoeia* recommends 2–4 g three times a day of dried aerial parts.

## CONSTITUENTS

Reviews: Barnes et al (2007), Bradley (1992), Williamson (2003).

### Alkaloids
Hederacine A 0.006%, hederacine B 0.005% (Kumarasamy et al 2003).

### Volatile oil
Total 0.03–0.05%, monoterpenes; ketones: pinocamphone, menthone, pulegone (Bradley 1992).

### Diterpenes
Marrubiin (Bradley 1992).

### Triterpenes
Oleanolic acid, ursolic acid (isomers) (Liu 1995).

### Phenolic acids
Caffeic acid, ferulic acid, sinapic acid (wild, Russia) (Vavilova et al 1988).
Phenolic glycosides and phenylpropanoid glycoside: cistanoside E (commercial, Japan) (Yamauchi et al 2007).

### Flavonoids
Flavonol glycosides: apigenin; flavone glycoside: chrysoeriol (Kikuchi et al 2008).
Flavonol glycosides: apigenin, luteolin (commercial, Japan) (Yamauchi et al 2007).

### Lignans
Lariciresinol glycoside, pinoresinol glycoside, syringaresinol glycoside (Kikuchi et al 2008).
Icariol glycoside, coniferyl alcohol glycoside (commercial, Japan) (Yamauchi et al 2007).

### Lectin
Gleheda, structurally similar to a legume lectin with affinity to glycoproteins (leaves) (Singh et al 2006).

## RECOMMENDATIONS ON SAFETY

- Use with caution in pregnancy and lactation. Given the availability of other herbs, such as ribwort *Plantago lanceolata*, for similar indications and the possible poisoning of animals (Barnes et al 2007), it would be prudent to avoid use in pregnancy and lactation.

## REFERENCES

Albert K 2005 Counterfeiting of *Glechoma hederacea*. Pharmazeutische Zeitung 150:31–32. Online. Available: http://www.pharmazeutische-zeitung.de/index.php?id=249&no_cache=1&sword_list[0]=glechoma&sword_list[1]=hederaceae 17 April 2009.

Barnes J, Anderson LA, Phillipson JD 2007 Herbal medicines, 3rd edn. Pharmaceutical Press, London.

Bradley PR (ed.) 1992 British herbal compendium, vol 1. British Herbal Medicine Association, Bournemouth.

Culpeper N, Cole A, Rowland W 1655 The practice of physick ... being chiefly a translation of the works of ... Lazarus Riverius. London, Peter Cole.

Davis PH (ed.) 1982 Flora of Turkey, vol 7. Edinburgh University Press, Edinburgh.

Fernie WT 1897 Herbal simples approved for modern uses of cure. Boericke & Tafel, Philadelphia. Also online. Available: http://www.gutenberg.org.

Hutchings MJ, Price EAC 1998 *Glechoma hederacea* L. (*Nepeta glechoma* Benth., *N. hederacea* (L.) Trev.). Journal of Ecology 87:347–364.

Ikeda Y, Murakami A, Ohigashi H 2008 Ursolic acid: an anti- and pro-inflammatory triterpenoid. Molecular Nutrition and Food Research 52:26–42.

Kikuchi M, Goto J, Noguchi S, et al 2008 Glycosides from whole plants of *Glechoma hederacea* L. Natural Medicines (Tokyo) 62:479–480.

Kumarasamy Y, Cox PJ, Jaspars M, et al 2003 Isolation, structure elucidation and biological activity of hederacine A and B, two unique alkaloids from *Glechoma hederacea*. Tetrahedron 59:6403–6407.

Liu J 1995 Pharmacology of oleanolic acid and ursolic acid. Journal of Ethnopharmacology 49:57–68.

Robinson M 1868 The new family herbal and botanic physician. William Nicholson, London.

Singh T, Wu JH, Peumans WJ, et al 2006 Carbohydrate specificity of an insecticidal lectin isolated from the leaves of Glechoma hederacea (ground ivy) towards mammalian glycoconjugates. Biochemistry Journal 393:331–341.

Vavilova NK, Fursa IS, Oshmarina VI 1988 Hydroxylcinnamic acids of *Glechoma hederaceae*. Chemistry of Natural Compounds 24:251.

Williamson E 2003 Potter's Herbal Cyclopaedia. CW Daniel, Saffron Walden.

Yamauchi H, Kakuda R, Yaoita Y, et al 2007 Two new glycosides from the whole plants of *Glechoma hederacea* L. Chemical and Pharmaceutical Bulletin (Tokyo) 55:346–347.

Zhu Y-P 1998 Chinese materia medica. Harwood Academic Publishers, Amsterdam.

# CHAPTER 19
# *Hyssopus officinalis*, hyssop

## DESCRIPTION

**Family: Lamiaceae**  **Part used: leaves and flowering tops**

*Hyssopus officinalis* L. is a semi-evergreen sub-shrub, native to the Mediterranean region Southern Europe but introduced elsewhere and naturalized on walls in Dorset (Stace 1991) and in parts of Central Europe (Podlech 2001). It can be hardy but may not survive winter weather. It is the only representative of the genus in Europe and four subspecies are identified, although their status is not definite (Tutin et al 1973). The *Flora of Turkey* (Davis 1982) gives one *Hyssopus* species, *Hyssopus officinalis* subsp. *angustifolius*.

Branched, square stems (to 60 cm) bear entire, opposite, narrowly lanceolate leaves with glands on each side. Bright blue flowers, with a characteristic smell, occur from August to October in spikes of dense, whorled clusters of three to seven flowers. The flowers are tubular with a short upper lobe and longer three-lobed lower lip. The tubular calyx is toothed.

**Other varieties**: White forms and pink forms of hyssop are sometimes found, and *Hyssopus officinalis* subsp. *aristatis* is a compact variety with smaller spikes of flowers (Bown 1995).

### Quality

The variability of the volatile oils in hyssop is discussed in an extensive review by Jankovsky & Landa (2002) that also refers to sources in Eastern Europe and Russia. The characteristic odour of hyssop is associated with ketones, in particular pinocamphone and isopinocamphone, but their concentrations vary substantially. A study in Hungary on seed-grown hyssop from nine different sources, found that concentration of pinocamphone varied from 3 to 50%, concentration of isopinocamphone varied from 5 to 50% and limonene varied from 1 to 60% (Veres et al 1996). A study by Fraternale et al (2004) shows variation associated with site of cultivation. A study by Özer at al (2005) found that subsp. *angustifolia* had similar constituents to the main species whereas the studies on var. *decumbens* and subsp. *aristatis* found different constituents (Mazzanti et al 1998, Piccaglia et al 1999).

The colour of the flowers is variable. A study on three wild types of *Hyssopus officinalis* L. with blue, red and white flowers yielded similar total oil concentrations with similar proportions of pinocamphone, isopinocamphone and pinocarvone (Chalchat et al 2001), whereas a similar study found the same main constituents but could distinguish the phenotypes by the relative proportions of each constituent (Kerrola et al 1994).

A study in a semi-arid area of northern Iran found that hyssop was tolerant of dry conditions and yield of volatile oil was no higher with irrigation every 7 days than every 21 days (Khazaie et al 2008). Mean total oil concentration was 1.1% in one year and 0.9% in the next, which is similar to that found in other studies.

## IDENTITY QUESTIONS

Dioscorides (III 25) names his plant hyssopos, but does not describe it since it is 'a well known herb', he says, of which there are two main sorts, the mountain and the garden. It is a pity he did not describe it since we thus inherit the odd circumstance that the hyssop he refers to may not be the *Hyssopus officinalis* used for centuries, which is not an unusual circumstance in itself, but in this case, even where authors dispute legitimacy (and the Renaissance authors could not agree upon this at all), Dioscorides' applications are cited regardless, as those of hyssop. The problem stems from references made by Dioscorides describing other herbs in reference to hyssop. It is details of oregano and a plant named 'chrysocome' (probably *Helichrysum orientale* Gaertn., according to Andrews 1961) in Dioscorides that confuse the picture somewhat; the leaf of oregano, he says, is similar to that of hyssop, and further particulars of the flowers or flower heads of the two plants offer more opportunities for debate.

Of the Renaissance authors, Parkinson seems to have a lot to say about it, contending it is the true hyssop of the Arabians but not that of Dioscorides or other Greek

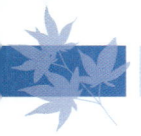

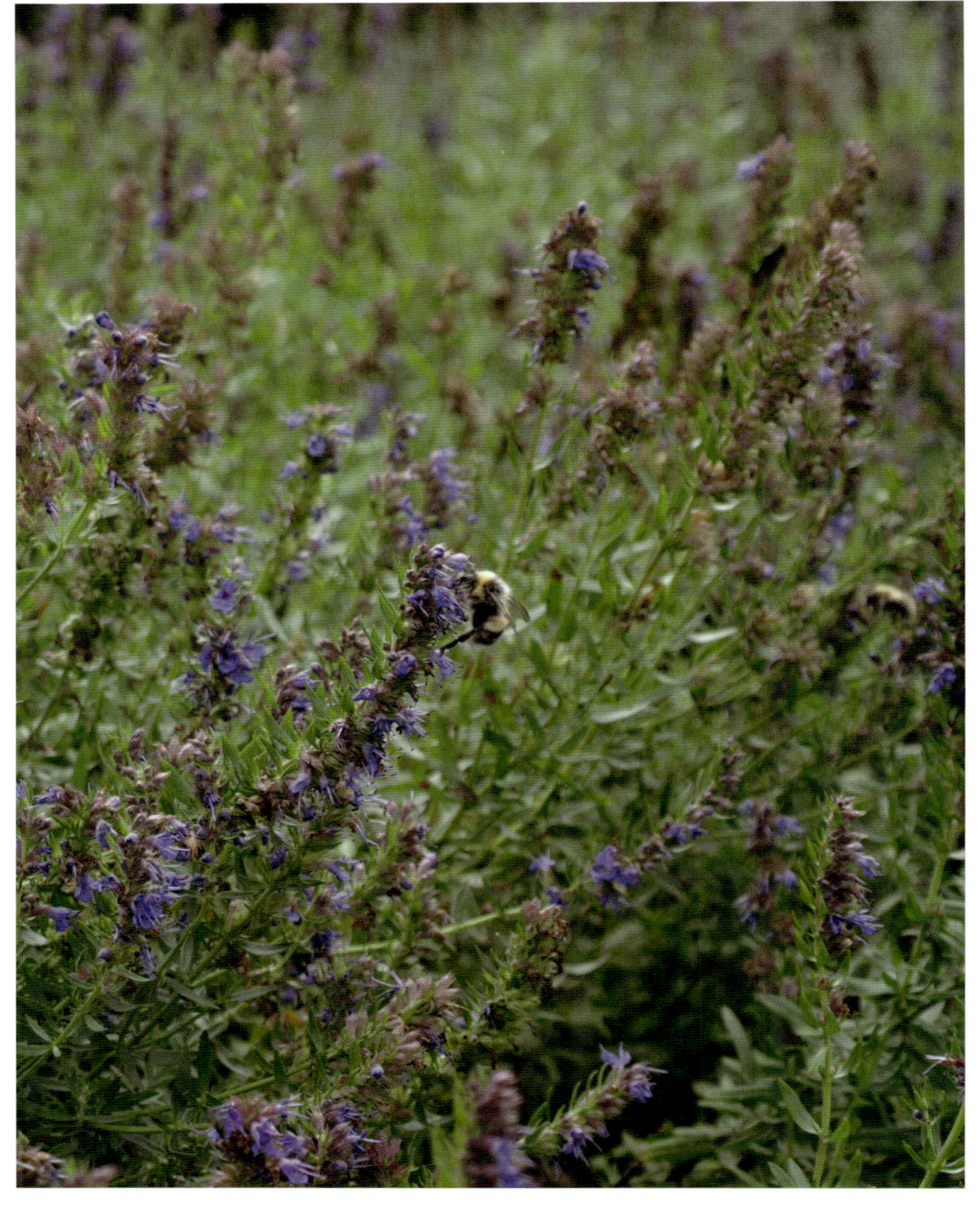

Figure 19.1 *Hyssopus officinalis*, hyssop (Hardwick Hall, Derbyshire, August).

authors 'as all doe acknowledge except Matthiolus'; he continues with alternative suggestions and justifications from various authors but eventually rejects them all. Gerard appends a note to his description of hyssopus parva angustis foliis, dwarf narrow-leaved hyssop, the fifth and last of the hyssops he describes, 'this is by most writers judged to be the hyssop used by the Arabian physicians, but not that of the Greeks which is nearer to Origanum and Marjerome, as this is to Satureia or Savorie'. Dodoens relies on the testimony of other authors, that it is not the right hyssop of the Ancients 'as is sufficiently declared by certaine of the best learned writers of these daies'. Dalechamps restricts himself to a simple 'it is not clear what plant the hyssop of Dioscorides was'. Mattioli puts up a long and stout defence, arguing wrong translations, misassumptions about exact meanings, the leaves of a further plant, 'onitis' *Onitis heracleoticum*, likened by Dioscorides to oregano that correspond clearly to hyssop, the context of hyssop in Dioscorides' collation, and most convincingly of all, that the familiar hyssop plants possess all the strengths and virtues Dioscorides claims for his, 'as I have tested'. Fuch's stance supports Mattioli's although he is far more concise 'Those who think that this is not the true hyssop of Dioscorides are in error. For it clearly has leaves like those of oregano, but slightly narrower. Nothing more than this was noted by Dioscorides.' And from Dioscorides' text this is a reasonable conclusion to reach. Among the several types of hyssop described by Parkinson is one called 'round leaved hyssop', in Latin hyssopus foliis origani, i.e. hyssop with leaves of oregano. His claim of hyssop being that of the Arabians but not the Greeks is difficult to follow since Serapio's narrative (as Parkinson says) likens ysopus to marjoram and then includes Dioscorides' recommendations exactly. Then, despite all, Parkinson concludes his debate quite surprisingly with 'Now although the true Hysope of Dioscorides, and the other Greeks, is not yet certainly knowne, yet assuredly this which is knowne, and generally received, may safely be used in the stead thereof, untill the true Hysope may be knowne', and proceeds with consideration of the 'vertues' according to Dioscorides. Other dissenters follow suit.

Barker (2001) and Grieve both draw attention to references to hyssop in the Bible. Clearly hyssop was a revered and well-used plant in Jewish ritual, but there is much inconclusive debate on hyssop's identity in that context.

The identity matter is still not concluded since Beck's 2004 translation of Dioscorides specifies hyssopos not as *Hyssopus officinalis* but as *Satureia graeca* L. (syn. *Micromeria graeca* Benth.), a kind of savory. Intriguingly, Parkinson's satureia vulgaris, winter savorie, is a '…herbe, very like unto Hysope'. So the debate continues… if pressed, I think I would stand with Mattioli.

Andrews (1961) presents a very detailed study on hyssop in the classical era, tracing first the biblical references (this plant is unlikely to be hyssop, he says) through to Greek and Roman uses and later references to these, considering clues from many perspectives – historical, geographical, linguistic, economic and further. He journeys through ezob and its Semantic origins, oregano, sampsuchum, onitis, micromeria and satureia, among others. His conclusion is that modern hyssop *is* the hyssop of Dioscorides.

## ANCIENT USES AND THE EPILEPSY DEBATE

As in many herbs, Dioscorides and Pliny read very similarly on hyssop, although Dioscorides seems more trim and precise. Galen is very succinct, saying only it is hot and dry in the third degree and 'of thin parts'. Dioscorides says it has a warming property. He recommends it for inflammations of the lungs, asthmatics, a chronic cough, catarrh and orthopnoea (serious asthma, when the patient cannot breathe unless upright (Jones 1956)), boiled with figs, water, honey and rue. The same will kill intestinal worms and can also be used as 'lozenge with honey'. The decoction with vinegar and honey 'expels thick masses down the abdomen'. It will purge the bowel eaten with 'brayed green figs' and will act more strongly as a cathartic mixed with 'garden cress or iris or hedge mustard' (Beck). 'It achieves even fresh and healthy looks'. As a plaster with fig and soda (other authors have nitre/saltpetre here) it is useful for the spleen and for oedemata, for inflammations with wine. Beck's translation continues, 'it also disperses black eye when plastered on with hot water. It is an excellent gargle for sore throat with a decoction of figs and it assuages toothaches when cooked with vinegar and employed as a mouthwash. Its vapour stops inflations ('gaseous' swellings?) around the ears'

Pliny says if the best comes from the Taurus mountains in Cilicia, the second best is from Pamphylia and Smyrna. He maintains it is not friendly to the stomach: it will purge downwards with figs and by vomit with honey; it can be used for serpent stings as a plaster with honey, salt and cumin; as an ointment for head lice and an itchy head. Bauhin quotes Pliny further, reading in places very much like Dioscorides, using hyssop as a gargle for angina (of the throat), as decoction in wine: the purge by vomit with hyssop and honey is better if nasturtium is added; the decoction with salt will drive away phlegm, and with oxymel will remove worms from the belly. Then he adds its use decocted with figs for the spleen and if taken for 16 days treats epilepsy. This is one of a number of references to epilepsy but the trail is somewhat difficult to follow. It could simply be a question of interpretation from yet older texts – Dioscorides has its use with figs for the spleen and *oedemata*, not epilepsy – but there are wider references and complications. Culpepper speaks of

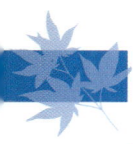

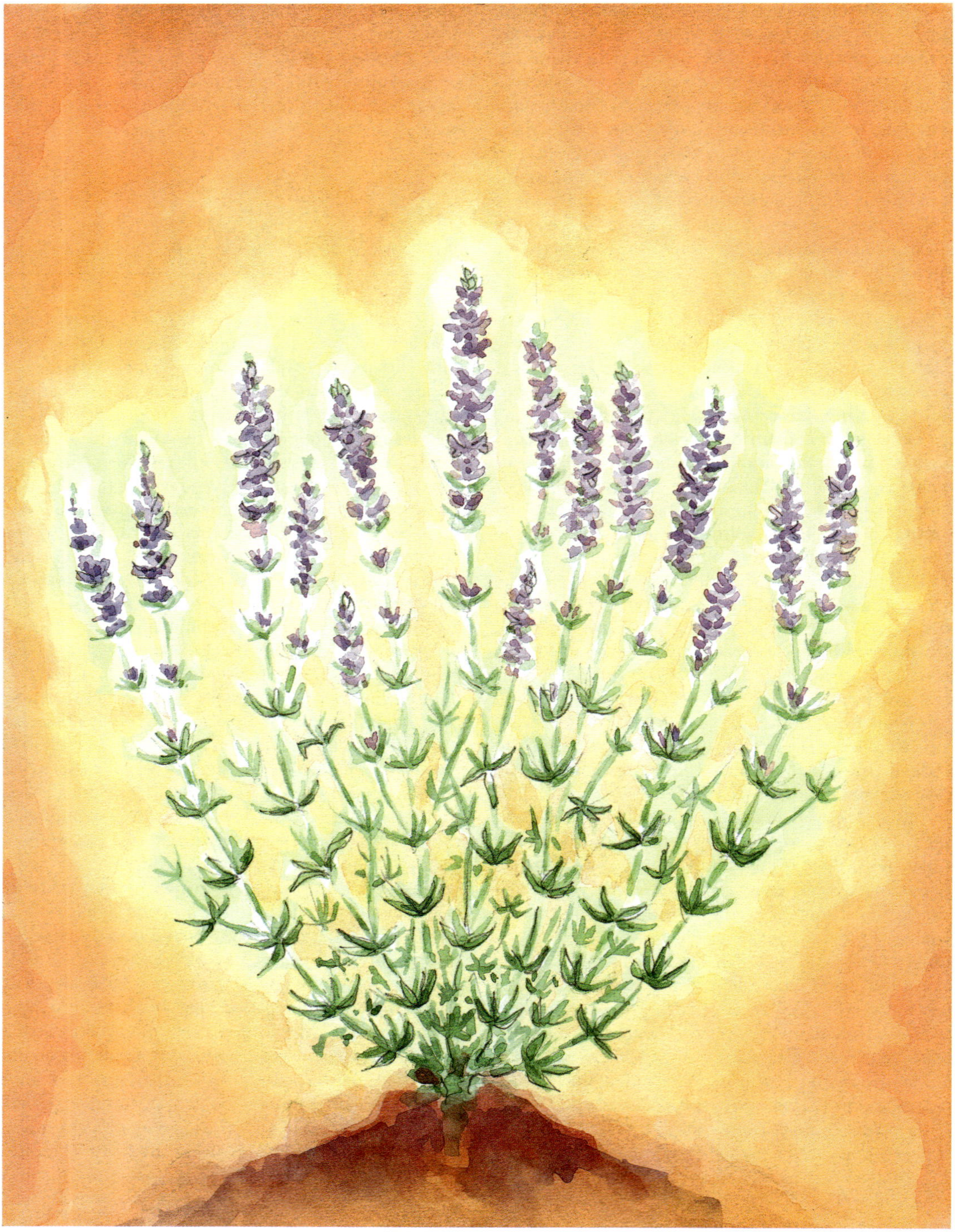

**Figure 19.2** *Hyssopus officinalis*, hyssop.

epilepsy but unattributed to any source. Gerard and Dodoens stick safely with Dioscorides and hence have no reference. Ibn Sina too carries no reference to epilepsy. Parkinson on Pliny has no such reference to epilepsy. Parkinson's epilepsy claim lies under Mattioli – that the oil kills lice, takes away itching of the head and 'helpeth those that have the falling sicknesse', following this with a recipe for such. Bauhin makes a very similar reference to Mattioli's recommendations, including its use for snake bites with salt and cumin, as Pliny above. Dalechamps too cites Mattioli on snake bites, oil, lice, itching and gives the same recipe as Parkinson for an epilepsy preparation. In the 1554 Latin version of Mattioli, there is no such reference, nor in the later 17th century French translation we referred to. This must be an addition to a later Mattioli text. However, the reference reappears in Dalechamps, not under Mattioli (although the snake bites and cumin, lice, itching, thins and purges is there) this time, but attributed to Mesue 'for epilepsy due to phlegm', and, alongside the familiar chest, thinning, gives florid colour to skin, etc., for 'other problems of phlegm in the head'.

The Salernitan herbal refers to epilepsy under hyssop, but has too an intriguing addition, which may open the debate a little, again after the usual reference to decoction in wine and dry fig for cough and cold catarrh, 'for fall of the uvula' – the powder or whole plant placed hot on the head; decoction in vinegar as a gargle without swallowing; the powdered flower sprinkled onto the uvula raised by the finger. Now Bauhin has an entry under peony explained as good for epilepsy because it 'lifts the uvula' – a reference to the humoral view of epilepsy as too much phlegm in the brain, (already a moist organ) (the Latin for 'pituitary gland' translates as 'phlegm'), which phlegm, as distillation from the brain where it fills the ventricles, descends through the cribriform plate and into the nose and hence causes what we would understand as swollen uvula here. Through a herb hot and dry in the third degree, as hyssop, a ridding of phlegm would theoretically ease such problems. Certainly Mattioli speaks of hyssop as helping those affected by phlegm in the brain and nerves, and the applied oil heals nerves (or sinews or tendons) afflicted by cold and strengthens them. Others speak similarly of this capacity in hyssop. Though the link with epilepsy may be tenuous, it is perhaps a way of looking at hyssop's adjuvant action as calming to the nervous system.

## A WARMING RESPIRATORY HERB AND FURTHER APPLICATIONS

From Dioscorides and Galen we have a picture of a warming herb, dispelling cold by heating and thinning. Hyssop's prime reputation lies in its use for the respiratory system: it clears the build up of cold mucus and eases its effects, extending even to the ears. All authors to the present day refer in some way to this virtue. Dodoens specifically recommends the preparation of a lohoch or loch – a 'licking medicine', of middle consistency, between a soft electuary and a syrup – for relief of obstruction, shortness of breath and an old, hard cough. Parkinson offers a recipe for old coughs and voiding tough phlegm; a handful of hyssop, 2 oz figs, 1 oz sugar candy; boil in a quart of Muscadine until half a pint be consumed; strain and take morning and evening. In the more local tradition too this application appears in the Myddfai texts, with hyssop and centaury *Centaurium erythraea* pounded and strained and mixed with white of egg and drunk for 3 days for tightness of the chest; and red fennel and the tops of hyssop, bruised with mallows and boiled to strengthen the lungs, throat and chest.

Its warming influence reaches the bowels too, moving cold, heavy deposits there. The warmth generated inside is presumably responsible for the good colour claimed by Dioscorides and many of those repeating his recommendations. Applied externally it counters inflammation and dissolves bruises. This latter action is perhaps a little more obscure today but can be accounted for in Galenic medicine through the dispersing properties of the herb. As a herb hot and dry in the third degree, additional applications might be expected, such as a general heating in chills, a diuretic and emmenagogic action. For example, Serapio mentions that it softens hardening of the body and is strong against hardness and cold in the womb, kidneys and bladder, 'it helps void crude humours', he says. The Salernitan herbal says it disperses and dissipates humours and is diuretic by its powers to free the urinary ducts. It purges phlegm of the stomach and nutritive organs (little here of Pliny's 'not friendly to the stomach') and is good for diseases of the lungs with heavy phlegm.

Parkinson refers to causing women's courses. The Trotula (Green 2001) of the late 12th century refers to its use as an emmenagogue in 'deficient menses' if the womb is 'so indurated that the menses are not able to be drawn out', in which case carded wool should be dipped in the gall of a bull or another gall, or powder of natron, mixed with the juice of wild celery *Apium graveolens* or hyssop, the wool to be pressed to make it hard and rigid and then to be inserted into the vagina. As we have come across before, a paradoxical use for fertility is also cited for the same herb; thus later in *The Trotula* text hyssop's heating nature is deployed with other herbs to aid conception. Some women are too fat, others to thin to conceive, the author claims. If a woman is phlegmatic and fat, she should 'sit in a bath of sea water with rainwater and add juniper, catmint, pennyroyal, spurge, laurel, wormwood, mugwort, hyssop and hot herbs of this kind' – a potent mix indeed!

Hildegard in the 12th century speaks of hyssop's hot, dry and powerful nature; 'it is of such strength that even a stone is not able to withstand it, and it grows wherever it is sown'.

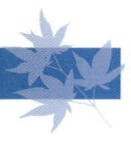

Her applications extend only to lungs and liver 'when it is eaten the liver becomes lively and it cleanses the lungs somewhat. He who coughs and has a pain in the liver, or who suffers from congestion in the lungs, or who suffers both conditions should eat hyssop with meats or with lard and he will be better'. She recommends taking it with liquorice, cinnamon and fennel, fennel in the greater proportion, then decreasing portions of hyssop, cinnamon and liquorice. If the liver is sick 'because of a person's sadness,' she adds, 'he should cook and eat young chicks with hyssop' and drink wine with hyssop soaked in it.

Among the Renaissance writers Culpeper attributes to hyssop the rulership of Jupiter and Cancer, hence useful for liver, stomach and lungs. He gives a succinct yet comprehensive (and by now very familiar from Dioscorides and Pliny) summary of recommendations so far, with rue and honey for coughs, shortness of breath etc.; as oxymel to expel gross humours by stool; with honey to kill worms; with figs for looseness of belly especially with fleur de luce and cresses (these two are contended ground of course); for colour of the body spoiled by jaundice; with nitre for dropsy and spleen; with wine for bruises; with figs for quinsy as a gargle; with vinegar for toothache; its vapours for the ears; with salt, honey and cumin for serpent stings; the oil kills lice and soothes itching of the head; for the falling sickness, tough phlegm all cold griefs of the chest, as a syrup or licking medicine; the ground herb for green wounds with sugar. This latter use, while not in the ancient texts we consulted, appears in a number of the Renaissance and later authors, for example, Parkinson and Robinson (1868).

Hyssop appears to have been used widely in Bauhin's day in a variety of forms: juice, distilled water, syrup, conserve, wine and oil. He quotes Brunfels recommending its use in fomentations, epithemes and baths, in clysters for colic pains and decoction for 'all psoras and skin lesions'.

## LIMITATION

By the 18th century the variety of preparations appears to have been reduced. According to Miller the only official preparation was the simple water. The use to which hyssop was put appears a little slimmed down but enthusiasm for its virtues continued. Miller has it as 'healing, opening and attenuating, good to cleanse the lungs of tartarous humours and helpful against coughs, asthmas, difficulty of breathing and cold distempers of the lungs; likewise reckoned a cephalic and good for diseases of the head and nerves. The bruised herb applied outwardly is famous for taking away black and blue marks out of the skin'. An amount of Dioscorides' applications have gone; the respiratory uses remain, plus a reputation as a general cephalic and good for the nerves, presumably from Pliny.

Quincy praises the use of hyssop but the indications are further shrunken to just the chest 'it is good in many kinds of coughs and disorders of the lungs and breasts which arise from phlegm and viscid humours. It is good in asthmas, promotes expectoration and gives relief in difficulty of breathing. It is almost a constant ingredient in pectoral apozems'. Quincy rates the distilled water of the shops highly: 'This is one of those few simples of which there is a distilled water in the shops that is good for anything. For there comes over with it so much of a warm essential oil, as not only preserves it from *Mother* and stinking (which most simple waters are subject to) but also makes it a good pectoral and efficacious to all those purposes which this herb is given for in any other forms'. For Quincy the herb is warm and detergent and thus belongs to Class 4 of the balsamics, the detergents. The balsamics generally comprise remedies that are 'softening, restoring, healing and cleansing', while the detergents are of even more subtle parts and 'therefore fitter to mix with, attenuate and wear away the contents of abscesses and ulcerations, and those mucous and viscid collections of humours which are apt to adhere to and obstruct the vessels.'

Cullen, in the 18th century, was far more dismissive of the herb, suggesting it is 'properly now neglected in favour of Pulegium'. Moreover, in his experience, the claim to rid bruises from the skin was quite unfounded: 'In ecchymoses, Riolan goes so far as to say, it sucks the blood out of the part, which was seen on the cloth. You see how difficult it is to trust materia medica writers. I have tried Hyssop in such cases and found no other effect than from the application of any other aromatic'.

The herb was used in America. Cook refers to it as a diffusive aromatic, stimulant and relaxing and a mild tonic; for sustaining capillary circulation gently and the nervous periphery; as an expectorant it relieves coughs, for cold with soreness of the chest and as a gargle for quinsy. Again it is apparently valued for its warming and thinning qualities, as a stimulant of sorts, although the capillary circulation is a rare mention, presumably a physiomedical appellation. Its tradition of nervous support continues and Dioscorides comes through again. The herb does not appear in Ellingwood.

Back in England, Fox tells us it is a favourite herb with the working classes and one much grown: 'there is scarcely a garden without this plant'. He adds to the usual asthmas, coughs and colds its use as a drink is slow typhus fevers.

## LATER USES

Late 19th and early 20th century authors are still following Dioscorides, Robinson (1868) almost exactly (via

Parkinson). Hool in the 20th century records a breadth of properties: aromatic, diaphoretic, anthelmintic, aperient, febrifuge, expectorant, diuretic. He says it is a herb highly esteemed in infancy. For bronchitis, hoarseness and cough he gives a recipe: hyssop ½ oz, symphytum ½ oz, pour on 2½ pints of water, boil gently for 10 minutes, strain, sweeten with sugar or molasses, take a wineglassful every 2–3 hours or oftener.

Mrs Grieve attributes the virtues to the volatile oil which, she says, is stimulating, carminative and sudorific; particularly promoting expectoration, and the diaphoretic and stimulant properties too being useful in chronic catarrh. She says it is frequently mixed with horehound *Marrubium vulgare*. Although in her day it was 'seldom employed (as it once was)' as a carminative and for hysterical complaints, she attests to the use of the fresh green tops as tea as an old-fashioned country remedy for rheumatism 'that is still employed'. Is this perhaps an echo of Dioscorides' use for inflammation?

The *British Herbal Pharmacopoeia* records the presence of volatile oil and flavonoid glycosides, including diosmin. Its action is expectorant, diaphoretic, sedative and carminative, with indications for bronchitis and chronic nasal catarrh. It has been used in hysteria, anxiety states and petit mal. Dose 2–4 g; liquid extract 1:1 2–4 mL; tincture 1:5 2–4 mL.

So its old reputation gets fixed in a more modern context and we find reference to epilepsy reappearing with use for petit mal and a recommendation for hysteria and anxiety despite the 'seldom used' of Mrs Grieve. Is this, then, a reflection of its use by herbalists in the 1950s and later?

Among modern authors hyssop's effect is attributed mainly to its volatile oils. It is valued mainly for its upper and lower respiratory applications ridding thick phlegm, with an aromatic tonic, calming and carminative undertow, valuable particularly in children's remedies. Barker (2001), Hoffman, Chevallier and Wood carry this sort of emphasis, although Weiss, a little earlier and over in Germany, suggests it is more carminative than expectorant. Barker and Wood both refer to its capacity to stop sweating, although in some herbals, including the *British Herbal Pharmacopoeia*, it is classed as diaphoretic. Menzies Trull covers a much wider range of therapeutic activities, very inclusive of applications through the tradition, and adds to the above actions; antiviral, antibacterial, anthelmintic, antirheumatic, emmenagogue, dermatological agent, vulnerary and external antiseptic; it is, he says, aromatic and stimulating to mucous membranes from the bitter in the volatile oil; it sustains the capillary circulation and peripheral nerves by diffusive activity; an absorbent remedy which relieves the lungs of excess mucus; he thus recommends it for a wide range of conditions from chronic catarrh and bronchitis, to genital herpes, petit mal, tinnitus (steam treatment), bruises, wounds and body lice. With these recommendations and Hoffman's citing of King's Dispensatory on hyssop as 'used in quinsy and sore throats…in infusion sweetened with honey….leaves applied to bruises… disperse every spot or mark from affected parts…' it is interesting to note we are still working with Dioscorides.

The epilepsy tradition still persists. Menzies Trull lists it above; Hoffman has a confident 'it may be taken for anxiety states and petit mal seizures' and Barker (2001) has a more reserved 'the herb has been used in petit mal'. In modern literature, however, research has indicated the oil of hyssop may provoke epileptic seizures. Chevallier warns of this. Is this a case of Paracelsus' 'dosis facit venenum', the idea that nothing is without poison and only the dose makes a thing not a poison – a dose–response relationship, and that there is some sort of link here? Nevertheless the use of the herb seems quite safe. Hoffman reports no side-effect or drug interaction reported, and Barker (2001) reassures about the use of the whole plant 'Cadeac and Meunier report that the use of the essential oil itself is capable of giving rise to epileptic crises. This should come as no surprise for those who work with essential oils; the toxic dose is very close to the therapeutic dose and does not mirror the therapeutic application of the whole plant extract.'

In Pelikan hyssop is covered within the labiate family, which has, of course, its own defining characteristics. Pelikan entitles the labiates 'plants of warmth', through which they have a special relationship with human beings, all 3000 species in the family having some medicinal properties. The activity of the warmth expresses itself particularly in the production of volatile oils. Pelikan has a vivid description of these 'fiery aromatic compounds', 'In them, warmth has transformed matter to the point where it comes as close as possible to warmth nature'. The warmth nature can be gathered from a variety of indications that Pelikan rehearses. One example is seen in the needle shaped leaf found in many plants of this family. In a good number of plants from various families a change in shape of the leaves can be determined (see Goethe and introduction) from the base upwards as the plant grows, beginning with a longer stemmed more amorphous shape, then spreading outward, gradually indenting further up the stem while pulling closer to it, until the leaf immediately before the flower has only a simple pointed shape. If an elemental sequence is applied to this metamorphosis, the first lowest leaf as earth, the spreading as water, the indenting as air, the pointing as fire (see Bockemuehl & Suchantke (1995), and Hoffmann (2007) for elaboration of these ideas) the leaves of many labiates, rosemary, lavender, thyme, hyssop, savoury and oregano speak clearly of a 'fire' plant. Pelikan here simply refers to the typical labiate as moving thus rapidly to the flowering process and even anticipating it, 'the leaves, even the stems are fragrant, anticipating the flowering aspect; they are filled with warmth and show the inflammatory tendencies of the flower'. To the stimulating and warming actions anticipated through a flowering process that reaches into the leaf region is added, Pelikan says, an influence through the I organization that is associated with warmth. Pelikan hence refers to firing of the metabolism 'anywhere in the metabolic and rhythmic systems'; with 'I activities involved in metabolism, blood production and respiration' influenced by medicinal plants in this family. Since astral activities are not abnormally strong and any 'wayward' astral activity is nevertheless under the control of I warmth, there are no poisonous or narcotic plants in this family. Pelikan summarizes, 'Depending on the particular form of a species the action will be addressed to the blood, gastric region, heart, lungs or uterus'. Hyssop Pelikan describes as camphor-like in the scent of its leaves, which is warming and a bit animal-like, as a badger (Wood, from the other side of the Atlantic, likens the smell to skunk 'which tips us off that it will be deeply penetrating, opening pores and passageways deep inside the body, as well as in the skin…'). The leaf region is abundant, he says. The plant is warming, relaxing and antispasmodic with a medicinal action mainly in the rhythmic system, of use for chronic bronchial catarrh, asthma and regulation of perspiration. The oil, he says, will relieve severe pain.

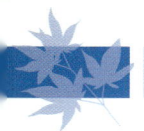

## RECOMMENDATIONS

- Hyssop is a warming plant with application to the lungs and upper respiratory system, ridding cold, hard phlegm, useful for inflammation of the lungs, asthma, old hard cough, catarrh and ear problems. Its recommended use with figs and honey for such indications seems quite apt.
- The decoction as a gargle for sore throats, with or without the addition of honey.
- Its use for the digestive system too seems in little doubt, for a cold stomach and nutritive organs, as a carminative, gentle purgative, with some influence on the liver. If Pliny's observations are applied, then it is good as an oxymel here, or with figs again following Dioscorides.
- Where the above problems are combined, particularly with nervous conditions, hyssop's effects on the nervous system may prove extrabeneficial.
- Externally the infusion may be tried for bruises, likewise an infusion or decoction mixed with honey for wounds, but the tradition is less definitive here.

Dosage: The *British Herbal Pharmacopoeia* recommends 2–4 g three times a day of dried aerial parts.

## CONSTITUENTS

Reviews: Bradley (2006), Williamson (2003).

### Volatile oil

Monoterpenes: beta-pinene 4–9%; oxygenated monoterpenes: bornyl acetate 3–4%, borneol 4%; ketones: isopinocamphone 47–58%, pinocamphone 11–22% (cultivated, Scotland) (Letessier et al 2001).
Total 0.5%, ketones: pinocamphone 14.1%, isopinocamphone 44.7%; sesquiterpenes: elemol 5.6%, germacrene-D-11-ol 5.7% (flowering tops, cultivated, Serbia) (Mitić & Đorđević 2000).
Total 1.2%, 21 compounds, monoterpenes 32.3%: pinene 18.4%, limonene 5.5%; oxygenated monoterpenes (including ketones) 60.5%: pinocamphone 49.1%, isopinocamphone 9.7%; sesquiterpenes 0.35% (grown as annual, India) (Garg et al 1999).
subsp. *officinalis*, monoterpenes: beta-pinene 10.5%, 10.8%; oxygenated monoterpenes: linalool 0.2%, 7.9%; ketones: pinocamphone 34%, 18.5%, isopinocamphone 3.2%, 29%, camphor 0.3%, 5.3% (Fraternale et al 2004). The two figures given for each concentration show that the yield and proportions of each oil was different when plants from the same source were cultivated and then transplanted to two locations at different altitudes in Italy.
subsp. *angustifolius*, monoterpenes: beta-pinene 10.6; oxygenated monoterpenes: 1,8-cineole 7.2%; ketones: pinocarvone 36.3%, pinocamphone 19.6%, isopinocamphone 5.3% (wild, Turkey) (Őzer et al 2005).
var. *decumbens*, monoterpenes: limonene 5.1%; oxygenated monoterpenes: linalool 51.7%, 1,8-cineole 12.3%, (wild, France) (Mazzanti et al 1998).
subsp. *aristatus*, three chemotypes: myrtenol 33% and beta-pinene 19%; 1,8-cineole 23% and beta-pinene 25%; methyl eugenol 44% and limonene 16% (wild, Italy) (Piccaglia et al 1999).

### Phenolic acids

Phenolic acids: rosmarinic acid, caffeic acids (Varga et al 1998).

### Flavonoids

Flowers, total 11.7% (233 plants) (Tsitsina, cited in Jankovsky & Landa 2002).
Flavone: diosmin, maximum in leaves, sepals (Marin et al 1998).

## RECOMMENDATIONS ON SAFETY

- Do not use the volatile oil internally.

Avoid use of the volatile oil externally for adults and do not use in infants.

The epileptogenic action associated with the oil is very unlikely in use of the dried herb as the concentration of volatile oils is low.

Use of oil of hyssop is not recommended because of the potential for high levels of ketones. Millet et al (1981) refer to three cases of convulsions: in a 26-year-old woman after a dose of 10 drops a day for 2 days; in an 18-year-old girl after a dose of 30 drops; and in a 6-year-old girl after a dose of half a teaspoonful of oil. There has been one study showing that oil of hyssop is convulsant in rats, by injection over 130 mg/kg but had no effect at 80 mg/kg (Millet et al 1981). The safety of ketones in oils is reviewed in Chapter 11 on *Artemisia absinthium*. Tisserand & Balacs (1995) advise that hyssop oil should not be used as an inhalation or in massage. This advice is cautious and would not apply to samples of oils characterized as low in ketones.

## REFERENCES

Andrews 1961 Hyssop in the classical era. Classical Philology 56:230–248.

Barker J 2001 The medicinal flora of Britain and Northwestern Europe. Winter Press, West Wickham, Kent.

Bockemuehl J, Suchantke A 1995 The metamorphosis of plants. Novalis Press, Capetown.

Bown D 1995 Encyclopedia of herbs. Dorling Kindersley, London.

Bradley PR 2006 British herbal compendium, vol 2. British Herbal Medicine Association, Bournemouth.

Chalchat JC, Adamovic D, Gorunovic MS 2001 Composition of oils of three cultivated forms of *Hyssopus officinalis* endemic in Yugoslavia: f. albus Alef., f. cyaneus Alef. and f. ruber Mill. Journal of Essential Oil Research 13:419–421.

Davis PH (ed.) 1982 Flora of Turkey, vol 7. Edinburgh University Press, Edinburgh.

Fraternale D, Ricci D, Epifano F, et al 2004 Composition and antifungal activity of two essential oils of hyssop (*Hyssopus officinalis* L.). Journal of Essential Oil Research 16:617–622.

Garg SN, Naqvi AA, Singh A, et al 1999 Composition of essential oil from an annual crop of *Hyssopus officinalis* grown in Indian plains. Flavour and Fragrance Journal 14:170–172.

Green MH (ed.) 2001 The Trotula. University of Pennsylvania Press, Philadelphia.

Hoffman N 2007 Goethe's science of living form: the artistic stages. Adonis Press, New York.

Jankovsky M, Landa T 2002 Genus *Hyssopus* L. – recent knowledge. Horticultural Science (Prague) 29:119–123.

Jones WHS 1956 Pliny Natural History, vol VII. William Heinemann, London.

Khazaie HR, Nadjafi F, Bannayan M 2008 Effect of irrigation frequency and planting density on herbage biomass and oil production of thyme *(Thymus vulgaris)* and hyssop *(Hyssopus officinalis)*. Industrial Crops and Products 27:315–321.

Kerrola K, Galambosi B, Kallio H 1994 Volatile components and odour intensity of four phenotypes of hyssop (*Hyssopus officinalis* L). Journal of Agricultural and Food Chemistry 42:776–781.

Letessier MP, Svoboda KP, Walters DR 2001 Antifungal activity of the essential oil of hyssop *(Hyssopus officinalis)*. Journal of Phytopathology 149:673–678.

Marin FR, Ortuño A, Benavente G, et al 1998 Distribution of flavone glycoside diosmin in *Hyssopus officinalis* plants: changes during growth. Planta Medica 64:181–182.

Mazzanti G, Battinelli L, Salvatore G 1998 Antimicrobial properties of the linalol-rich essential oil of *Hyssopus officinalis* L. var *decumbens* (Lamiaceae). Flavour and Fragrance Journal 13:289–294.

Millet Y, Jouglard J, Steinmetz MD et al 1981 Toxicity of some essential plant oils. Clinical and experimental study. Clinical Toxicology 18:1485–1498.

Mitić V, Đorđevi S 2000 Essential oil composition of *Hyssopus officinalis* L. cultivated in Serbia. Facta Universitatis 2:105–108.

Özer H, Şahin F, Kiliç H, et al 2005 Essential oil composition of *Hyssopus officinalis* L. subsp. angustifolius (Bieb.) Arcangeli from Turkey. Flavour and Fragrance Journal 20:42–44.

Piccaglia R, Pace L, Tammaro F 1999 Characterization of essential oils from three Italian ecotypes of hyssop [*Hyssopus officinalis* L. subsp. aristatus (Godron) Briq.]. Journal of Essential Oil Research 11:693–699.

Podlech D 2001 Herbs and healing plants of Britain and Europe. Diamond Books, London.

Robinson M 1868 The new family herbal and botanic physician. William Nicholson, London.

Stace C 1991 New flora of the British Isles. Cambridge University Press, Cambridge.

Tisserand R, Balacs T 1995 Essential oil safety. Churchill Livingstone, Edinburgh.

Tutin TG, Heywood VH, Burges NA, et al 1973 Flora Europaea, vol 3. Cambridge University Press, Cambridge.

Varga E, Hajdu Z, Veres K et al 1998 Investigation of variation of the production of biological and chemical compounds of *Hyssopus officinalis* L. Acta Pharmaceutica Hungarica 68:183–188.

Veres K, Varga E, Dobos A, et al 1996 Investigation of the composition of essential oils of *Hyssopus officinalis* L. populations. Proceedings of the 27th International Symposium on Essential Oils, Vienna.

Williamson E 2003 Potter's Herbal Cyclopaedia. CW Daniel, Saffron Walden.

# CHAPTER 20
# *Inula helenium*, elecampane

## DESCRIPTION

### Family: Asteraceae (Compositae) — Part used: root

The genus *Inula* includes 90 species which are hardy Eurasian perennials (Bown 1995) and 19 species found in Europe (Tutin et al 1976). *Inula helenium* L. is a robust, hardy perennial, native to Western and Central Asia, but naturalized throughout Europe and in Britain since the Bronze Age (Preston et al 2004). The *Flora of Turkey* (Davis 1975) gives 26 *Inula* species, including *Inula helenium*.

Stiff, erect, hairy stems (to 2.5 m) bear ovate, unstalked leaves and the stalked basal leaves can be very large with prominent midribs. Large, yellow flowerheads (6–9 cm across) with prominent yellow rays occur in loose clusters in June to October.

**Other species used**: *Inula helenium* is also used in Asia as are *Inula japonica* and *Inula britannica* (flowers) (Reid 1987), *Inula racemosa* and *Inula royleana* (Ketai et al 2000, Zhao et al 2006). The essential oils of the annual stinking fleabane *Dittrichia graveolens* syn. *Inula graveolens* (Stace 1991) and *Dittrichia viscosa* syn. *Inula viscosa*, which is native to southeast Europe (Nikolakakis & Christodoulakis 2004), are used as mucolytics for dry cough and asthma.

The genus includes fleabane *Inula conyza* and this can cause confusion. This was recommended in ancient Egypt (Ebers 841) as a strewing herb to repel fleas (Manniche 2006). This could be *Conyza magna*, which Dioscorides (III 136) (Osbaldeston 2000) refers to as a fumigant having tawny yellow, foul smelling flowers. Dioscorides also states that aerial parts of this plant, taken in wine, act as an emmenagogue and to procure an abortion. The name fleabane is also attributed to a number of species, including *Conyza canadense* syn. *Erigeron canadense*, which is native to North America but, according to Grieve, was not found in Europe until the later 1600s.

## HELENIUM

The authors focus on the usage of elecampane in lung disease but also emphasize its use as a warming, tonic herb, especially for the stomach and as a general tonic which influences urinary and menstrual flow. Dioscorides (I 28) gives a reasonable description: rough, stemless leaves, like those of narrow-leaved mullein, large and somewhat pungent, orange-tawny root, propagated with offshoots as the top surface of the root has lumps that can be divided into sections that propagate easily. As Bauhin states, propagation by root is easy and propagation by seed is unnecessary.

Dioscorides (I 29) states that Crataeus refers to another helenium, which grows in Egypt. The description 'spreading like serpyllum', 'leaves like lentils', suggests a thyme. Mattioli refers to this helenium and states that Avicenna made no difference between this and *Inula helenium*. Mattioli also cites Pliny, who gives a similar description and appears to link this plant with the 'tears of Helen of Troy' rather than the supposed link between Helen of Troy and *Inula helenium*.

The preparations given by Dioscorides and Pliny are repeated for the most part by all later authors. Dioscorides recommends a decoction of the dried root to set urination and menstruation in motion, then the 'root itself' as a lozenge made with honey both for cough and orthopnoea (see under hyssop, Chapter 19) and for ruptures, spasms and flatulence. Pliny recommends the powder of dried root for similar indications or the dried powder made into a lozenge. Pliny recommends the root in an aromatic wine to help coughs while Dioscorides speaks of Oinos nektarites, a wine in which elecampane is macerated. Dioscorides finally recommends a confection in grape syrup for the stomach.

## RESPIRATORY USE

I will discuss its use in lung disease and as a tonic for the digestion and nervous system, with a consideration of the

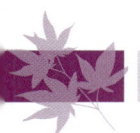

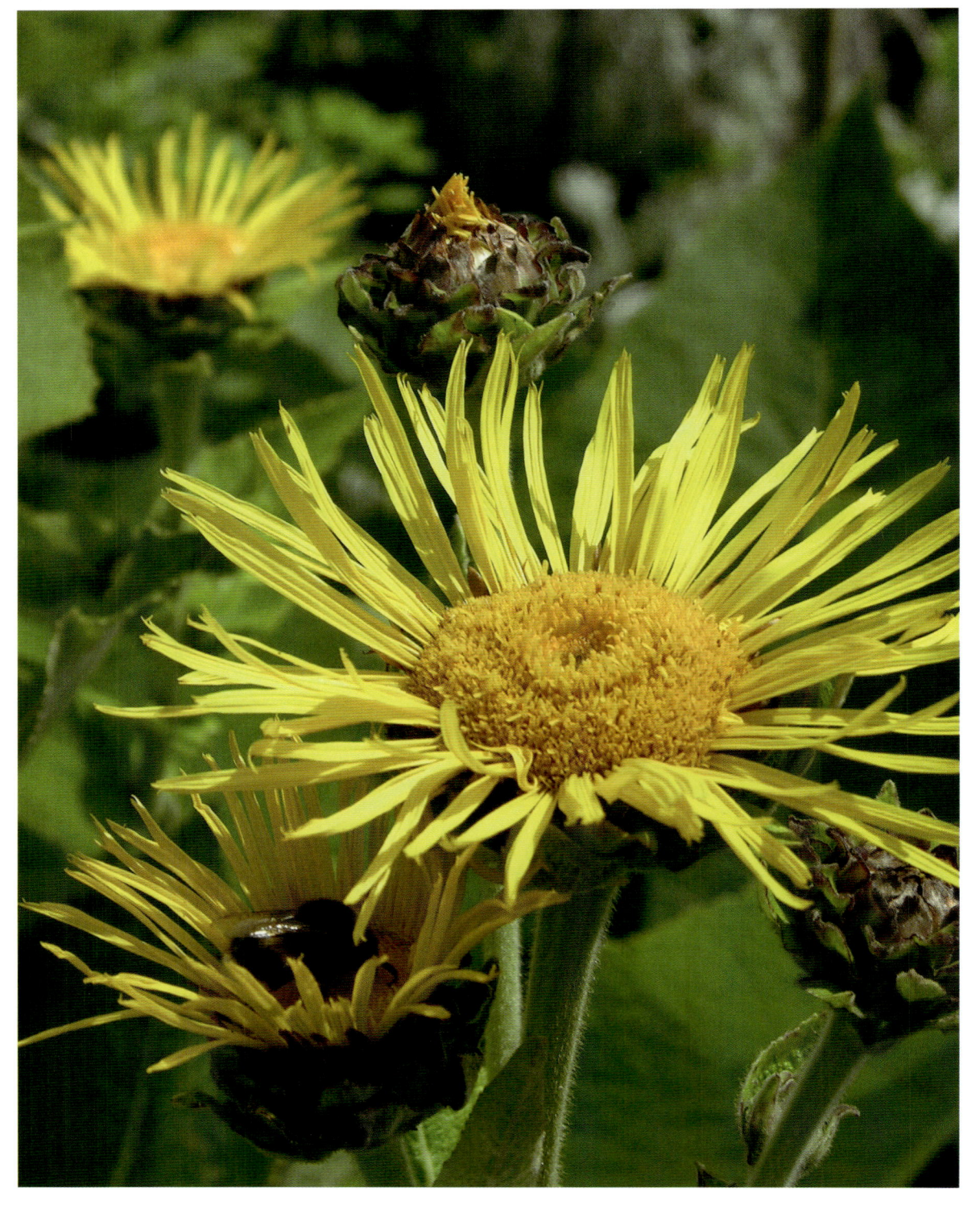

Figure 20.1 *Inula helenium*, elecampane (an allotment in Horsforth, Yorkshire, July).

different preparations. Both authors recommend external use of leaves in wine for hip disease in the case of Dioscorides and pain in the loins and genitals in the case of Pliny, but I will limit recommendations for external usage because of the risk of allergic contact dermatitis.

The recommendations of Dioscorides and Pliny for use in cough and breathlessness are repeated by Serapio, Fuchs, Bock, Bauhin, Turner, Dodoens, Dalechamps, Culpeper, Miller and Quincy. Renaissance authors such as Fuchs, Bauhin and Mattioli refer to widespread cultivation and usage of elecampane. Cough is consistently mentioned whereas recommendations in breathlessness vary as to whether the recommendation is for orthopnea or more specifically for asthma and wheeze. Pliny refers to the windpipe which could be interpreted as referring to wheeze. Ibn Sina recommends the syrup to promote expectoration but also recommends it to invigorate and strengthen the heart.

Galen, cited by Mattioli, notes that while not exactly hot and dry like pepper, it is heating with a superfluous humidity. Ibn Sina gives it as hot and dry in the third degree but observes that, as it has some surplus moisture, it does not heat the body as soon as it comes into contact with it. Ibn Sina, Gerard and Culpeper also describe it as hot and dry in the third degree and Gerard sees the superfluous moisture of the fresh root as abating the hot and dry quality. Equally, it is recommended with heating herbs by Hildegard, who recommends a 'clear drink' with elecampane and galangal as useful, although she advises this mixture only for lung disease where the person is not weakened by other disease.

Pliny, cited by Bauhin, states that elecampane is harmful to the stomach but healthy when mixed with sweet things, and this proposition continues throughout the authors. Mattioli recommends an electuary, a thick preparation of the powder in a syrup made with honey, to remove thick and sticky humours. This recommendation is repeated in the most vivid of terms by later authors. For example, Gerard recommends a lozenge to 'void out thick, tough, and clammie humours, which stick in the chest and lungs. The root taken with honey or sugar as an electuary, cleanseth the breast, ripeneth tough phlegm, making it easy to be spit forth, and prevaileth mightily against the cough and breathlessness, an old cough and such that cannot breathe unless they hold their necks upright'. Turner adds a recommendation for use of the flowers as an electuary with honey for cough, and Turner and Bauhin both advise the decoction of root in cases of spitting of blood and breathlessness.

Syrups are not the only preparation given. Ibn Sina suggests that a preparation in vinegar will reduce its heat and the Myddfai herbalists recommend a preparation using vinegar: for dyspnoea, boil scraped roots of elecampane in white wine vinegar, dry the roots, reduce to a powder, boil the powder with honey and add powdered pepper, take a spoonful night and morning. A similar confection with the addition of roots of mallow *Althaea officinalis* is recommended for cough, taking 'as much as a pigeon's egg' night and morning.

Quincy describes the 'superflous humidity' of Galen as 'somewhat glutinous, tenacious or adhesive' and thus useful in 'wastings and confirmed consumptions' as it 'gives fresh substance and vigour to the solids'. This action links with the use of elecampane as a tonic in chronic disease, which is discussed later. There is some consideration of its use in tuberculosis by an Eclectic practitioner writing in New York (Von Unruh 1915). He discusses his usage of *Echinacea angustifolia* and *Inula helenium* together by injection in 98 cases of tuberculosis. He notes the action of elecampane in controlling night sweats when taken as 20 drops of specific tincture, four to six times per day and also notes an action of increasing and then decreasing expectoration. Recent studies suggest that elecampane may inhibit tuberculosis. An in vitro study using root material isolated 11 natural and semisynthetic eudesmanolides and found that alantolactone and isoalantolactone inhibited *Mycobacterium tuberculosis* (Cantrell et al 1999). An in vitro study found that *Inula helenium* L. subsp. *turcoracemosa*, collected in Turkey, was one of 5 out of 107 plants which showed over 90% inhibition of growth of *Mycobacterium tuberculosis* H37Rv (Tosun et al 2005). Tuberculosis can remain latent for many years until activated (Locht et al 2007) and it is tempting to speculate whether it could be useful to follow the advice of Priest & Priest that it is beneficial where a predispostion to tuberculosis is suspected as so many people worldwide have latent tuberculosis (Frothingham et al 2005).

Later authors recommend the use of elecampane in lung disease but without the same vigour of language as the Renaissance authors. Hill proposes candied elecampane sucked slowly for coughs. Cook recommends it as a warming, stimulating and relaxing tonic to the lungs that leaves a mild astringent effect through the discharge of viscid mucus. He recommends it in coughs where there is a relaxed state with chronic expectoration that is viscid or profuse but not where the lungs are constricted and the cough is dry. He recommends it in lozenges with lobelia *Lobelia inflata*, black cohosh *Cimicifuga racemosa*, and liquorice *Glycyrrhiza glabra*.

Fox advises it in chronic pulmonary complaints and recommends simmering 4 oz for 10 minutes in 2 pints of water, taken in doses of one wineglassful (45–60 mL) every 3 hours, sweetened with honey. The expectorant action is noted in Wren (1988) for cough, consumption and pulmonary disorders. The *National Botanic Pharmacopoeia* notes its use in asthma, bronchitis and lung disease, and as a warm decoction in acute catarrhal affections. Priest & Priest are more specific and describe it as a gently stimulating tonic expectorant for chronic catarrhal conditions that is warming, strengthening and cleansing to pulmonary mucous membranes. They advise it in chronic pectoral states with excessive catarrhal

# THE WESTERN HERBAL TRADITION

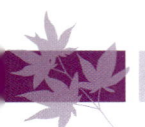

expectoration and where a predispostion to tuberculosis is suspected. They suggest a combination with leaf of comfrey *Symphytum officinale* in chronic bronchitis and tuberculosis, with demulcents in pneumoconiosis and silicosis and with red clover *Trifolium pratense* in whooping cough.

The *British Herbal Pharmacopeia* notes its antitussive action, in particular in the cough of pulmonary tuberculosis and use in the wasting associated with tuberculosis. It is also recommended for irritating cough in children. Hoffmann emphasizes use of a decoction in irritating coughs, especially in children, and use where there is copious catarrh. Chevallier advises it not only in coughs but for all chesty conditions, especially where the person is weakened by illness, as he highlights the tonic action. Bone (2003) cites Felter, writing in 1905, as the source of

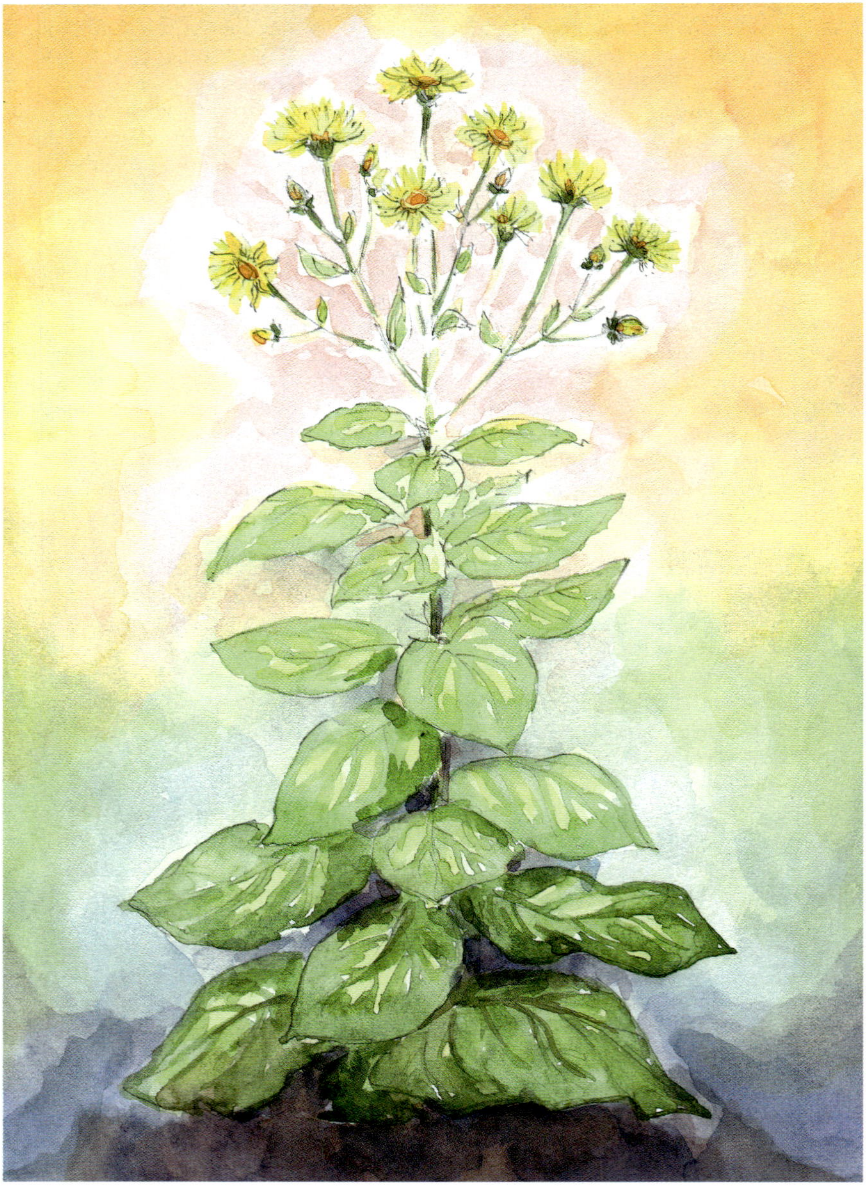

**Figure 20.2** *Inula helenium*, elecampane.

the advice for use in chronic lung disease, especially where there is irritation of the trachea and bronchi, abundant expectoration, in 'teasing' cough and substernal pain and also in acute conditions such as colds and influenza. Menzies-Trull refers to its usage in persistent coughs with substernal pain and to restore the capillary circulation after getting chilled, and suggests a mix for acute bronchitis with mullein *Verbascum thapsus* and yarrow *Achillea millefolium*.

Weiss gives the combination of 2 teaspoons of a mixture of elecampane, root of cowslip *Primula veris* and leaf of coltsfoot *Tussilago farfara* decocted for 5 minutes, left to stand for 15 minutes and taken at a dose of 1 cup three times a day. Bartram highlights its use on old coughs and to remove mucus in advanced lung disease. He suggests a mix of elecampane, root of marshmallow *Althaea officinalis* and yarrow *Achillea millefolium* decocted. Wood recommends it for conditions, including chronic sinusitis and post-nasal drip, where there is yellow or green mucus, particularly where the cough is insufficient to create full expectoration. He makes a useful linkage between the respiratory and digestive aspects of elecampane and recommends it where swallowing of excess mucus has caused indigestion.

## CORDIAL AND CARMINATIVE PREPARATIONS

As well as the emphasis on the value of elecampane in lung disease, it is recommended by the authors as a carminative and as a general tonic. Long-term use is advised by the use of various preparations. The use of cordials and wines recurs. Dioscorides refers to Oinos nektarites: 5 oz of dried root in 6 gallons of must, removed after 3 months. He advises the wine as good for stomach and chest and to expel urine. Hildegard proposes a wine, in which the dried or fresh root is soaked, for 'pain in the lungs', in moderation daily before and after food. Turner suggests the leaves, seasoned and laid up in malmsey, a sweet wine such as Madeira, as good for the stomach. Culpeper recommends an ale or beer made using the roots, drunk daily for clearing and strengthening. Grieve suggests a cordial made from the roots infused in white port with sugar and currants. This last could refer back to Dioscorides, who proposes the root preserved in raisin wine as very good for the stomach. In his introduction Dioscorides expresses his intention to make his instructions for usage clear. If we compare him with later authors, then he was successful in this.

Dioscorides recommends a confection in grape syrup for the stomach and states that confectioners dry the root a little, boil it and then steep it in cold water, place it in a concentrated must and keep it in jars for use. A very similar syrup prepared by boiling down fresh grapes continues to be used today in Greece (Gaifyllia 2008). Turner's version runs 'take the root, dry it a little first, seethe it, afterward steep it in cold water and lay it up in sodden wine for divers uses'. This is an example of the difficulty in interpreting later authors. So similar is the statement of Turner that it may merely be a translation and not a description of usage in the 16th century. Gerard recommends the crystallized root as wholesome for the stomach, taken after supper to help the digestion and Culpeper refers to a syrup or conserve made from the fresh root for cough but also to 'warm a cold, windy stomach'. Fernie (1897) states that elecampane candy was common in 19th century London, sold as flat, round cakes, mainly composed of sugar and eaten daily for asthma.

The demulcent action of these sweet aqueous preparations is supported by the inulin content. Inulin is a storage polysaccharide mainly composed of fructose (maximum 30–40 units) which is also found in other plants such as the tubers of Jerusalem artichoke *Helianthus tuberosus* (Azisa et al 1999, Niness 1999). Inulin has been shown to increase viscosity and is used in low-fat products to improve creaminess (Villegas et al 2007). It is used in specialist foods for diabetes, as it is mainly composed of fructose which does not stimulate insulin release. However, fructose does not suppress appetite, and it is argued that the widespread use of products containing fructose, such as corn syrup, is associated with obesity (Elliott et al 2002). The recommendation of regular usage is as a medicine rather than as a food so would be in smaller quantities.

It is certainly a herb associated both with usage for acute conditions and as a preventative. The recommendation of the lozenge by Dioscorides for 'bites of wild animals', given by Turner as 'bites of serpents', suggests a possible use in acute fevers whereas Miller describes elecampane as alexipharmic, protecting against poisons, and useful in infections and contagious distempers. Fernie (1897) states that 'it was customary when travelling by a river to suck a bit of the root against poisonous exhalations and bad air'.

The recommendations for regular use as a general tonic, not just for use in lung disease, could hark back to Galen's recommendation for use in 'parts troubled by cold and continuous diseases'. The Salernitan herbal recommends it where the 'nerves are afflicted by cold' as does Serapio, who associates use in cold conditions with chronic conditions such as a 'cold cough' and recommends the root cooked with barley for asthma from just such a cold cause. The advice for use as a carminative for wind is repeated and, in the words of Dodoens, 'it promotes concoction and defecation'. The Salernitan herbal proposes the powdered root or decoction in wine for pain associated with wind, and powdered root with double the quantity of cinnamon for 'those who are delicate'; an expensive remedy at the time. Turner recommends it in windiness and Gerard claims that the juice of the root, boiled, 'comforteth the stomach and helpeth', while Culpeper states that it is 'very effective to warm a cold, windy stomach, or the pricking therin or the stitches caused by the spleen'. Culpeper recommends too the decoction of root in wine or the juice as an anthelmintic. Fox lists it as an aromatic, stimulant tonic useful in dyspepsia and hepatic disorders. Grieve particularly recommends it in small doses for atonic dyspepsia with weakness and in the spasmodic pain of dysentery. It is used today with other herbs in Tibet and Mongolia for abdominal pain, enteritis and dysentery (Wenhua et al 2004).

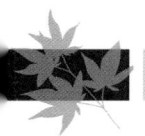

The usage as a general tonic is taken further by Dioscorides, who recommends the decoction of the dried root to promote urination and menstruation. Ibn Sina states that the decoction, and especially the syrup, stimulates urine and the menses. He adds that the initial diuretic effect will decrease and 'those who become accustomed to the use of elecampane will not have to urinate hourly'. Apuleius give a recipe for 'bladder pain' for use of the leaves with celery seed, asparagus root and fennel, bruised in wine and taken warm. Turner, Gerard, Culpeper and Miller repeat the recommendation in anuria and for kidney and bladder stones. Hill states that hardly any plant has more virtues and that it operates by urine and sweat, and Priest & Priest list it as diuretic, alterative and diaphoretic. Ibn Sina, Culpeper, Miller, Cook and Fox repeat the advice of Dioscorides for use to promote menstruation, and Culpeper and Fox add use in period pains.

At this point, the breadth of action of elecampane discussed so far is substantial, and it is useful to look at the way in which Pelikan links the actions on the respiratory system with an overall action on metabolism. He notes in elecampane the movement of the daisy family into production of unusually large leaves and their rise in rhythmic sequence up the stem, gradually gathering more closely to it. He observes the aromatic scent and acrid taste of the root and that the production of aromatic compounds through the volatile oils demonstrates the flowering process pervading the whole plant, right down to the root. Medicinally it will thus stimulate digestion, alleviating inflammation and promoting the flow of bile. The lungs as an organ of the rhythmic system are inevitably served by this plant, since, he says, 'with a plant given so much to the production of a rhythmic sequence of leaves, the metabolism-regulating action extends to the rhythmic system, specifically to the sphere of the lung'.

As if this breadth of action were not enough, elecampane is also recommended to improve the mood. Serapio cites the actions previously given by Dioscorides but adds that, because of its heat, it is useful for weakened nerves and conditions arising from cold such as sciatica and migraine. He cites Hippocrates as saying that elecampane takes away anger and sadness. This link remains in herbal practice to day in that the tonic action of bitters is used to support other herbs in a prescription for depression (Mills 1991).

Ibn Sina states that elecampane provokes headache but disperses it 'especially if it is poured over in cases of mucous migraine'. Hildegard recommends it for migraine and Fernie (1897) for 'congestive headache coming on through costiveness of the lowest bowel'. Hildegard states that it 'clears the eyes' and Bauhin states that the wine is prepared 'everywhere in Germany' and, taken frequently, wonderfully sharpens the sight. Irritation of the eyes from smoke from use of wood fires will have been a substantial problem at that time although there may be entirely no connection between this problem and the recommendation given here.

Mattioli, Parkinson and Fernie ascribe to Pliny the statement that his contemporary Julia Augusta, the daughter of the Emperor Augustus, 'let no day pass without eating some of the roots of Enula condired, to help digestion, and cause mirth'.

## POSSIBLE EXTERNAL USE

Alongside internal use in cold conditions, and thus pain, are recommendations for external use. Dioscorides advises external use of the leaves boiled in wine for 'hip disease.' Galen recommends elecampane for pain in the hip, and chronic pain in the joints. This is repeated by Turner and by Mattioli, who states that it has a rubefacient action. Gerard and Culpeper repeat the recommendation for internal and external use of the root in gout, sciatica and painful joints. Grieve extends the use of an embrocation in sciatica to facial and other neuralgias and Fernie (1897) recommends elecampane specifically for sharp pain in the right elbow joint which recurs daily. The Salernitan herbal recommends the whole plant cooked with wine and oil and placed on the belly for colic or on the kidneys and bladder to promote urination.

Elecampane is also recommended for itchy skin diseases. Hildegard gives an ointment for 'various ulcers and scabies' (the latter referring to eczematous diseases in that erythema and thickening of the skin are combined with pruritis, pustules and ulceration) which includes elecampane. Drury (1985) states that one of the common names of elecampane was horseheal, which referred to its use in the treatment of cutaneous disorders. The Salernitan herbal recommends elecampane macerated in oil for mange, a general term for infectious skin disease in animals. For psoriasis and itch, the Myddfai herbalists propose drinking a decoction three times a day for 9 days, and application of softened, pounded roots mixed with cream every third night for 9 days.

Gerard proposes the decoction or powder, with honey, as an ointment to cleanse and heal up old ulcers. Culpeper also recommends the decoction as a wash for old, putrid ulcers and this is repeated by Grieve. Gerard gives a very similar recipe to the Myddfai herbalists. It is for an ointment for itch, scabs and manginess and the root is boiled very soft and mixed in a mortar with fresh butter and powder of ginger. Culpeper recommends an ointment, for scabies and itch, of the root boiled in vinegar and added to oil of pigs' trotters.

Dodoens, cited in Bauhin, states that there are those who affirm that the decoction, reduced and mixed into an ointment in the thickness of honey, is useful to cleanse old ulcers and promote scar formation. Wood quotes an American herbalist as making a linkage back to the former name of scabwort and using elecampane for proud flesh where a scab is not forming. As he states, this does link with the action in resolving old infections.

Where there is an indication for its usage, elecampane should not be used externally in people with eczema or people with any history of allergic contact dermatitis, and patients should be informed of this possibility. Given the possibility of allergic contact dermatitis (see below), one cannot now support the recommendation of Culpeper for use of the distilled water to cleanse skin from spots, blemishes and morphews (possibly a type of psoriasis). There are many other herbs which can be used externally for pain. However, it is possible that the local antiseptic action of elecampane would make use of external preparations appropriate in some skin conditions.

## RECOMMENDATIONS

- The *British Herbal Pharmacopoeia* lists only the actions of expectorant, antitussive, diaphoretic and bactericidal. The expectorant action and value of elecampane in cough, asthma and both acute and chronic lung disease is supported by many authors. That it is repeated so consistently gives strong support to this recommendation.
- Elecampane is not widely recommended now for self-prescribing because of the risk of allergic contact dermatitis (Bisset & Wichtl 2001). However, for practitioner usage, it is an effective and important herb. It is fortunate that research on this important herb is continuing in the Far East (Huo et al 2008a).
- Use as an effective carminative and general tonic with a diuretic action is consistently recommended with the suggestion that it is also useful to lift the mood. Use of the plant in this way is consistently advised and I have made more use of this herb as a general tonic to good effect since preparing the material for this section.

Dosage: the *British Herbal Pharmacopoeia* recommends 1–2 g three times a day of dried roots and rhizomes. A low dose could be useful in long-term usage, for example 2 mL daily of tincture of the fresh root.

## CONSTITUENTS

Reviews: Barnes et al (2007), Bisset & Wichtl (2001), Bradley (1992), Williamson (2003).

### Polysaccharides

Inulin 44% in autumn, 20% in spring (Bradley 1992).

### Volatile oils

Cyclic sesquiterpenes are the main constituents in the genus (Zhao et al 2006).
Monoterpenes: thymol derivatives 0.19% (Stojakowska et al 2006).
Sesquiterpene lactones, eudesmanolides 3.5%: alantolactone and isoalantolactone which are structural isomers (cultivated, Poland) (Stojakowska et al 2006).
Alantolactone 1%, isoalantolactone 1.3% (collected, Gansu, China) (Ketai et al 2000); alantolactone 1.2%, isoalantolactone 1.2% (commercial, China) (Wenhua et al 2004).
Ten eudesmanolides (Ma et al 2008); other eudesmanolides (commercial, Tibet) (Konishi et al 2002).
Other sesquiterpene lactones: an elemanolide, a germacranolide (Konishi et al 2002), a germacranolde (Huo et al 2008b).

## RECOMMENDATIONS ON SAFETY

1. Pregnancy and lactation.
   Category B2 (Mills & Bone 2005): there is no evidence from studies on women or on animals which supports the safety of elecampane or is evidence of risk.
   Use of elecampane is strongly discouraged in lactation because of the allergenic risk.
2. Allergic contact dermatitis.
   Do not use externally if the patient has eczema or a history of allergic contact dermatitis such as nickel allergy. Use caution on other patients and advise the patient of the risk so that they can discontinue usage if there is any reaction.

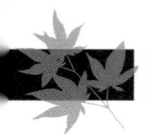

Use caution in internal usage if the patient has a history of allergic contact dermatitis.

Sesquiterpene lactones are widespread in the Asteraceae family (Bruneton 1999) and are lipophilic so dissolve in skin oils. They have been identified as an important cause of allergic contact dermatitis and, in an assessment of 956 compounds, alantolactone was among the 98 substances with significant allergenic effects (Schlede et al 2003).

Allergic contact dermatitis is a red, eczematous pruritus that occurs in response to an allergen but can become lichenified and chronic. It is a type IV delayed-type hypersensitivity cell-mediated reaction with antigen specific T-cell activation that initiates an inflammatory cascade. Many sesquiterpene lactones found in the Asteraceae may act as haptens, which are low molecular weight compounds that bind to polypeptides or glycoproteins and so induce a conformational change. The resulting complex is recognized as an antigen and binds to antigen-presenting Langerhan's cells in the epidermis (Akhavan & Cohen 2003). Subsequent repeat challenge leads to release of phagocytes, which release lysosomal enzymes, monocytes and granulocytes. Nickel is considered to be the most common cause of allergic contact dermatitis (Krob et al 2004).

Sensitization usually depends on dose and requires prolonged local contact, for example 2 weeks (Barile 2004). Asteraceae-related allergic contact dermatitis is associated with occupational risk in florists, horticulturists, farmers and gardeners as sesquiterpene concentration is highest in leaves and flowers (Gordon 1999). Where it results from air-borne irritation, for example by leaf hairs (trichomes), there is a characteristic pattern on exposed areas such as the face, neck and arms but it is also strongly associated with touching Asteraceae, as exemplified by resolution of symptoms when people move house or cease touching the relevant plant (Gordon 1999).

Diagnosis is by patch test either with extracts of Asteraceae (Compositae) or with a sesquiterpene lactone mix which contains alantolactone, dehydrocostus lactone and costunolide (Frosch et al 2006). A 6-year study of patch testing in 2248 patients in Spain found that 16% of the positive patch tests were for a sesquiterpene lactone mix and this represented 0.5% of the patients (Cabanillas et al 2006). A 7-year study in Germany of 285 children, aged 6–12, found that 4% reacted to a Compositae mix and 10% reacted to nickel (Heine et al 2004). In a study of routine patch testing in Denmark, further testing of 129 patients who reacted to a Compositae mix was carried out and positive reactions were found to feverfew 81%, tansy 77%, chamomile *Matricaria recutita* 64%, yarrow 41% and arnica 23% (Paulsen et al 2001). Paulsen (2002) argues that the most common initial cause is probably cultivated or pot plants but that cross-sensitization to other Astereaceae is common. Cross-sensitization is a risk in contact dermatitis (Mitchell 1975) and this is significant because of the increasing use of plants in the Asteraceae family in natural healthcare and toilet products. Aberer & Hausen (1990) also argue that the use of patch testing has increased the incidence of reactions to elecampane.

There are different points of view on the connection between allergic contact dermatitis and eczema. In the study referred to above, Heine et al (2004) found that 37% of the children with positive patch tests also had atopic eczema. Akhavan & Cohen (2003) review the immunological processes in atopic eczema and allergic contact dermatitis and propose that allergic contact dermatitis is not more common in people with atopy than in the rest of the population. However, they also review studies which show a high rate of sensitization to preservatives in populations with atopic eczema, probably associated with high use of skincare preparations.

Paulsen (2002) reviews Asteraceae-associated allergic contact dermatitis and highlights the risk of erythema multiforme-like eruption associated with the use of elecampane externally, and suggests that the incidence of adverse reactions is high given that it is used much less frequently in skin-care and external products than other Asteraceae such as chamomile. A 31-year-old woman in Spain, with a history of nickel and chromate dermatitis, developed an acute rash on the chest 2 weeks after applying a herbal bag whose contents included elecampane. The rash healed after application of a topical corticosteroid but, another 2 weeks later red confluent papules appeared, which spread over the anterior trunk (Mateo et al 1995). There are four other relevant adverse event reports. A 32-year-old woman in Italy presented with diffuse dermatitis after use of a massage liniment for 1 month which began to resolve after stopping the product. The liniment contained *Inula helenium*, *Achillea millefolium*, *Arctium lappa* and *Laurus nobilis*. The woman was shown to react to alantolactone in a patch test. A year earlier, the woman had taken a medicine of *Inula helenium* and had experienced facial eczema at the time. The authors (Pazzaglia et al 1995) suggest that this event acted as a previous sensitizer although Paulsen (2002) comments that other herbs in the mix may also have been sensitizing. A 66-year-old man in Korea, who was a heavy smoker, developed painful oral mucosal lesions after taking a mouthwash product including *Inula helenium* for 3 months (Kim et al 1988). The lesions cleared after stopping the product and recurred when it was started again. Patch tests were positive for elecampane, at a high concentration, and liquorice *Glycyrrhiza uralensis* but reactions to liquorice are extremely rare. A 28-year-old woman in Spain developed an itchy papular rash with blisters a day after preparing an infusion of *Inula viscosa* root to treat haemorrhoids. The rash resolved after oral treatment with steroids, and the authors discuss which sesquiterpene lactone may have been implicated (Pinedo et al 1987). Reactions can also occur to *Dittrichia graveolens* (Thong et al 2008).

This is a contact dermatitis and is not associated with oral use of associated plants. But the question then arises about the internal use of elecampane in people who have allergic contact dermatitis. Lundh et al (2006) argue that people who have allergic contact dermatitis will also be allergic to sesquiterpene lactones in teas. Wintzen et al (2003) describe a woman with recalcitrant eczema and a positive patch test to a Compositae mix. It was found that her diet was very high in Compositae and the condition improved on changing her diet. However, White et al (2007) discuss oral tolerance to nickel associated with ingestion of nickel in the diet, and take the opposite view, which is that the much lower incidence of positive reactions to chrysanthemum in Singapore compared to London is related to the widespread drinking of chrysanthemum tea.

# REFERENCES

Aberer W, Hausen BM 1990 Active sensitization to elecampane by patch testing with a crude plant extract. Contact Dermatitis 22:53–55.

Akhavan A, Cohen SR 2003 The relationship between atopic dermatitis and contact dermatitis. Clinics in Dermatology 21:158–162.

Azisa BH, China B, Deacona MP, et al 1999 Size and shape of inulin in dimethyl sulphoxide solution. Carbohydrate Polymers 38:231–234.

Barile FA 2004 Clinical toxicology: principles and mechanisms. CRC Press, Florida.

Barnes J, Anderson LA, Phillipson JD 2007 Herbal medicines, 3rd edn. Pharmaceutical Press, London.

Bisset NG, Wichtl M (eds) 2001 Herbal drugs and phytopharmaceuticals, 2nd edn. Medpharm, Stuttgart.

Bone K 2003 A clinical guide to blending liquid herbs: herbal formulations for the individual patient. Churchill Livingstone, Edinburgh.

Bown D 1995 Encyclopedia of herbs. Dorling Kindersley, London.

Bradley PR (ed.) 1992 British Herbal Compendium, vol 1. British Herbal Medicine Association, Bournemouth.

Bruneton J 1999 Pharmacognosy, phytochemistry, medicinal plants, 2nd edn. Intercept, London.

Cabanillas M, Fernández-Redondo V, Toribio J 2006 Allergic contact dermatitis to plants in a Spanish dermatology department: a 7-year review. Contact Dermatitis 55:84–91.

Cantrell CL, Abate L, Fronczek FR, et al 1999 Antimycobacterial eudesmanolides from Inula helenium and Rudbeckia subtomentosa. Planta Medica 65:351–355.

Davis PH (ed.) 1975 Flora of Turkey, vol 5. Edinburgh University Press, Edinburgh.

Drury S 1985 Herbal remedies for livestock in seventeenth and eighteenth century England: some examples. Folklore 96:243–247.

Elliott SS, Keim NL, Stern JS, et al 2002 Fructose, weight gain, and the insulin resistance syndrome. American Journal of Clinical Nutrition 76:911–922.

Fernie WT 1897 Herbal simples approved for modern uses of cure. Boericke & Tafel, Philadelphia. Online. Available: http://www.gutenberg.org.

Frosch PJ, Menné T, Lepoittevin J-P 2006 Contact dermatitis. Birkhäuser. Online. Available: http://www.springerlink.com/home/main.mpx 30 Mar 2009.

Frothingham R, Stout JE, Hamilton CD 2005 Current issues in global tuberculosis control. International Journal of Infectious Diseases 9:297–311.

Gaifyllia N 2008 Petimezi: grape syrup (grape molasses). Online. Available: http://greekfood.about.com/od/syrupssauces/r/petimezisyrup.htm 5 Nov 2008.

Gordon LA 1999 Compositae dermatitis. Australasian Journal of Dermatology 40:123–128.

Grieve M 1931 (1984) A Modern Herbal. Penguin Books, Harmandsworth.

Heine G, Schnuch A, Uter W, et al 2004 Frequency of contact allergy in German children and adolescents patch tested between 1995 and 2002: results from the Information Network of Departments of Dermatology and the German Contact Dermatitis Research Group. Contact Dermatitis 51:111–117.

Huo Y, Shi HM, Wang MY, et al 2008a Chemical constituents and pharmacological properties of Radix Inulae. Pharmazie 63 699–703.

Huo Y, Shi HM, Wang MY, et al 2008b Complete assignments of 1H and 13C NMR spectral data for three sesquiterpenoids from Inula helenium. Magnetic Resonance Chemistry 46:1208–1211.

Ketai W, Huitao L, Yunkun Z, et al 2000 Separation and determination of alantolactone and isoalantolactone in traditional Chinese herbs by capillary electrophoresis. Talanta 52:1001–1005.

Kim SC, Hong KT, Kim DH 1988 Contact stomatitis from a breath freshener. Contact Dermatitis 19:309.

Konishi T, Shimada Y, Nagao T, et al 2002 Antiproliferative sesquiterpene lactones from the roots of Inula helenium. Biological and Pharmaceutical Bulletin 25:1370–1372.

Krob HA, Fleischer AB Jr, D'Agostino R Jr, et al 2004 Prevalence and relevance of contact dermatitis allergens: a meta-analysis of 15 years of published T.R.U.E. test data. Journal of the American Academy of Dermatology 51:349–353.

Locht C, Rouanet C, Hougardy JM, et al 2007 How a different look at latency can help to develop novel diagnostics and vaccines against tuberculosis. Expert Opinion on Biological Therapy 7:1665–1677.

Lundh K, Hindsén M, Gruvberger B, et al 2006 Contact allergy to herbal teas derived from Asteraceae plants. Contact Dermatitis 54:196–201.

Ma X-C, Liu K-X, Zhang B-J, et al 2008 Structural determination of three new eudesmanolides from Inula helenium. Magnetic Resonance in Chemistry 46:1084–1088.

Manniche L 2006 An ancient Egyptian herbal. British Museum Press, London.

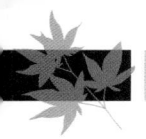

Mateo MP, Velasco M, Miquel FJ, et al 1995 Erythema-multiforme-like eruption following allergic contact dermatitis from sesquiterpene lactones in herbal medicine. Contact Dermatitis 33:449–450.

Mills S 1991 Out of the earth. Viking Arkana, London.

Mills S, Bone K 2005 The essential guide to herbal safety. Churchill Livingstone, St Louis.

Mitchell JC 1975 Contact allergy from plants. In: Runeckles VC (ed.) Recent advances in phytochemistry, vol 9. Plenum Press, London.

Nikolakakis A, Christodoulakis NS 2004 Leaf structure and cytochemical investigation of secretory tissues in *Inula viscosa*. Botanical Journal of the Linnean Society 144:437–448.

Niness KR 1999 Inulin and oligofructose: what are they? Journal of Nutrition 129:1402S–1406S.

Osbaldeston T 2000 Dioscorides de materia medica. IBIDIS Press, Johannesburg. Online. Available: http://www.cancerlynx.com/dioscorides.

Paulsen E 2002 Contact sensitization from Compositae-containing herbal remedies and cosmetics. Contact Dermatitis 47:189–198.

Paulsen E, Andersen KE, Hausen BM 2001 Sensitization and cross-reaction patterns in Danish Compositae-allergic patients. Contact Dermatitis 45:197–204.

Pazzaglia M, Venturo N, Borda G, et al 1995 Contact dermatitis due to a massage liniment containing *Inula helenium* extract. Contact Dermatitis 33:267.

Pinedo JM, Gonzalez de Canales F, Hinojosa JL, et al 1987 Contact dermatitis to sesquiterpene lactones in *Inula viscosa* Aiton. Contact Dermatitis 17:322–323.

Preston CD, Pearman DA, Hall AR 2004 Archaeophytes in Britain. Botanical Journal of the Linnaean Society 145:257–294.

Reid DP 1987 Chinese herbal medicine. Shambhala, Boston.

Schlede E, Aberer W, Fuchs T, et al 2003 Chemical substances and contact allergy–244 substances ranked according to allergenic potency. Toxicology 193:219–259.

Stace C 1991 New flora of the British Isles. Cambridge University Press, Cambridge.

Stojakowska A, Michalska K, Malarz J 2006 Simultaneous quantification of eudesmanolides and thymol derivatives from tissues of *Inula helenium* and *I. royleana* by reversed-phase high-performance liquid chromatography. Phytochemical Analysis 17:157–161.

Thong H-Y, Yokota M, Kardassakis D, et al 2008 Allergic contact dermatitis from *Dittrichia graveolens* (L.) Greuter (stinkwort). Contact Dermatitis 58:51–53.

Tosun F, Kizilay C, Sener B 2005 The evaluation of plants from Turkey for in vitro antimycobacterial activity. Pharmaceutical Biology 43:58–63.

Tutin TG, Heywood VH, Burges NA, et al 1976 Flora Europaea, vol 4. Cambridge University Press, Cambridge.

Villegas B, Carbonell I, Costell E 2007 Inulin milk beverages: sensory differences in thickness and creaminess using r-index analysis of the ranking data. Journal of Sensory Studies 22:377–393.

Von Unruh V 1915 *Echinacea angustifolia* and *Inula helenium* in the treatment of tuberculosis. National Eclectic Medical Association Quarterly 7. Online. Available: http://www.henriettesherbal.com/eclectic/journals/nemaq1915/01-ech-inula-tbc.html.

Wenhua G, Yaowen C, Yin Y, et al 2004 Separation and determination of two sesquiterpene lactones in Radix *inulae* and *Liuwei Anxian* San by microemulsion electrokinetic chromatography. Biomedical Chromatography 18:826–832.

White JM, Goon AT, Jowsey IR, et al 2007 Oral tolerance to contact allergens: a common occurrence? A review. Contact Dermatitis 56:247–254.

Williamson E 2003 Potter's Herbal Cyclopaedia. CW Daniel, Saffron Walden.

Wintzen M, Donker AS, van Zuuren EJ 2003 Recalcitrant atopic dermatitis due to allergy to Compositae. Contact Dermatitis 48:87–88.

Wren RC 1988 Potter's new cyclopaedia of botanical drugs and preparations. CW Daniel, Saffron Walden.

Zhao YM, Zhang ML, Shi QW, et al 2006 Chemical constituents of plants from the genus Inula. Chemistry and Biodiversity 3:371–384.

# CHAPTER 21
# *Lamium album*, white deadnettle

## DESCRIPTION

**Family: Lamiaceae** — **Part used: aerial parts**

*Lamium album* L. is a spreading perennial, common in Britain, found by roadsides and on rough ground in sunny and shady sites. The *Flora of Turkey* (Davis 1982) gives 27 *Lamium* species, including *Lamium album* and *Lamium purpureum*.

Erect, pubescent, square stems (to 25 cm) bear opposite, fresh-green, dentate, stalked leaves. White flowers occur in whorls. The tubed corolla (2 cm) has a curved upper lip, the lower lip has two to three teeth on each side and the calyx is five-toothed. The flowers are creamy-yellow in bud. It flowers for long periods from early spring.

**Other species used**: Culpeper lists white, yellow and red deadnettles. Yellow deadnettle *Lamium galeobdolon*, syn. *Lamiastrum galeobdolon* or *Galeobdolon luteum* (Alipieva 2003) is a perennial plant of woodlands (Stace 1991). It has yellow flowers and taller stems than the white deadnettle. Culpeper describes red deadnettle as an annual with pale, reddish flowers. This is probably *Lamium purpureum* L., which is a common weed.

The *Galeopsis* genus is closely related and some descriptions could be of common hemp-nettle, *Galeopsis tetrahit* L., which is native to Europe and Western Asia and grows on disturbed sites or roadsides. It is a herbaceous annual with hairy stems to 1 m tall with swollen nodes that bear coarsely serrate leaves. The tiny flowers are purple. Bisset & Wichtl (2001) include an entry for Galeopsidis herba, hemp-nettle *Galeopsis segetum*, which has yellow flowers. It is used in lung complaints and as a diuretic and is available under its synonym, *Galeopsis ochroleuca* for the indications of asthma and enuresis.

### Quality

Weiss suggests that the flowers have to be pulled from their calyces one by one but the recommendation of Grieve for the whole herb when coming into flower in May and June is more practical. As *Lamium album* is a robust and common herb, there does not seem to be any need to use the other species.

## ENIGMA

White deadnettle is an enigmatic herb. Its key functions are hard to grasp through the literature and its effects appear more subtle than obvious. Bisset & Wichtl (2001) cite the Commission E monograph where the list of traditional uses is very long and wide ranging. It begins with use for the gastrointestinal tract, for irritation of the gastric mucosa, bloating, flatulence and strengthening the intestine. The cited combination preparations of the herb are exhaustive: for 'nervousness, restlessness, irritation, for sleep disorders, for invigoration, relaxation and stimulation, during the menopause, for female ailments of all kinds, menstrual disorders, 'blood purifying', metabolic stimulation in support of gallbladder and liver function, proneness to biliary gravel, to stimulate the appetite, for neutralisation of gastric hyperacidity, to promote digestion, in flatulence, for stimulation of pancreatic function, regulation of the blood lipid level, irrigation of the urinary tract in inflammatory and spasmodic bladder ailments, functioning of the prostate gland, stimulation of the heart and blood circulation, in dizziness, flickering of the eyes, tinnitus, for increased blood supply to the heart, increased heart capacity, improvement of lymph flow and stimulation of lymph formation, strengthening of the respiratory tract, dissolving mucus, and improvement of vitality and general weakness, especially after illness or surgery'. Use of the flowers alone is for 'catarrh of the upper respiratory tract, local treatment of mild inflammation of mouth and throat mucosa, and for non-specific fluor albus (leucorrhoea)'; externally for mild, superficial inflammations of the skin. However, Commission E suggests efficacy of use for the herb is not substantiated and therefore does not recommend therapeutic use. There is no evaluation on the use of the flowers. It is surprising to find quite so many claims with so little outcome, but it is difficult to trace many of these uses through our texts.

©2009 Elsevier Ltd, Inc, BV
DOI: 10.1016/B978-0-443-10344-5.00026-4

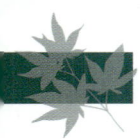

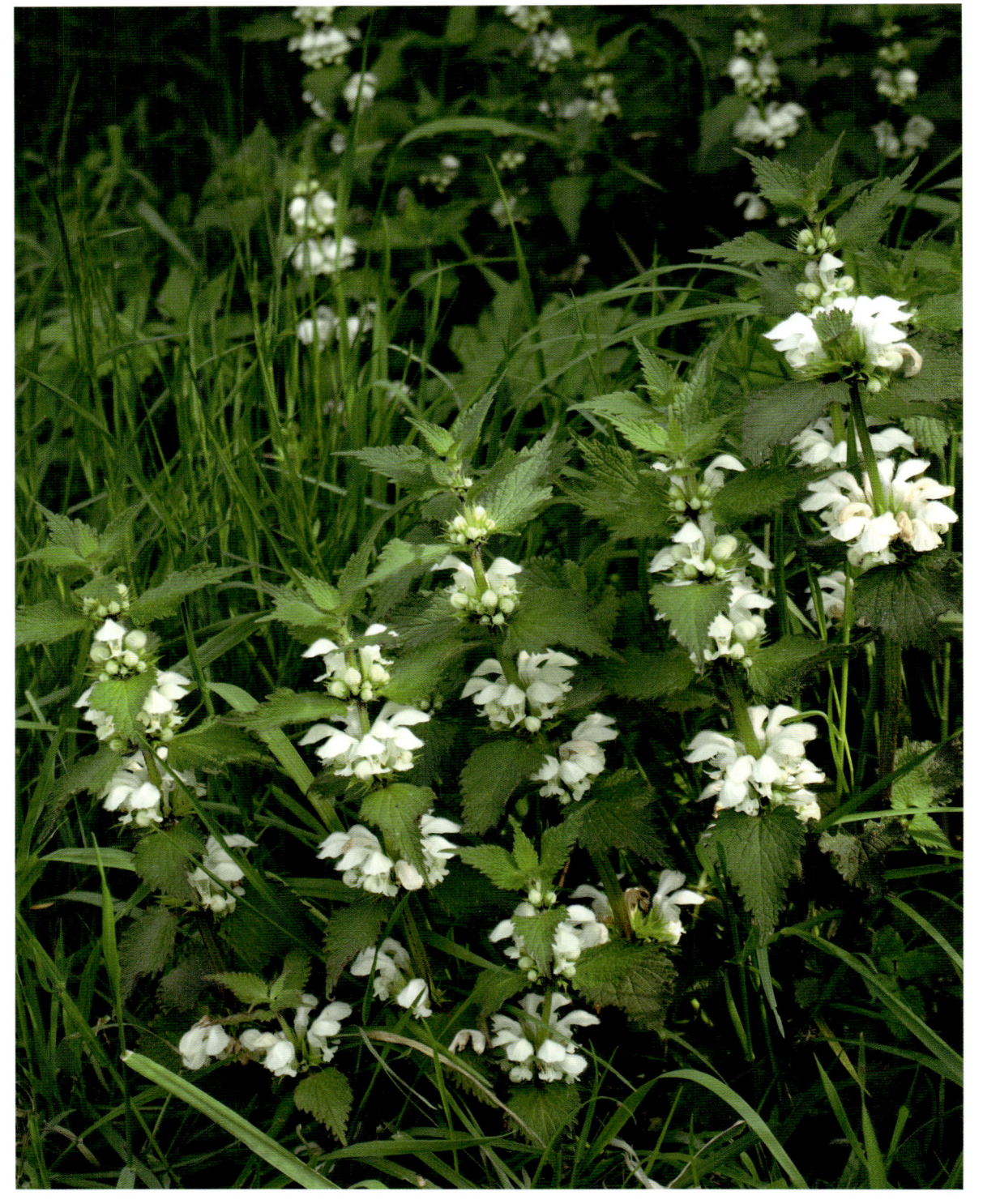

Figure 21.1 *Lamium album*, white deadnettle (Yorkshire, May).

## ELUSIVE IDENTITY

The first difficulty is the usual one of which plant is Dioscorides' lamium and does it correspond to Pliny or anyone else. There is an amount of dispute. Beck identifies Dioscorides' 'leukas' (III 99) as deadnettle, but this is tentative, and comes with a question mark in the index against the Latin binomial. There is little description in Dioscorides' text beyond that the one growing in mountains has wider leaves than the cultivated, is more potent and its fruit is more pungent, bitter and less tasty. Its actions are only against venoms of animals, topically or drunk. Mattioli suggests this text is obviously corrupt and several things are missing. Pliny speaks of 'lamium' and, according to Dodoens of 'anonium' or 'aononium', which with salt will heal contusions and blows, burns and swollen glands, swellings, gout and wounds; and the white it has in its leaves will heal the sacred fires (St Anthony's fire). The trouble is Dioscorides (IV 94) also has an entry called 'galeopsis', otherwise 'galepsis' or 'galeobdolon'. Even the origin of the word is disputed. Mattioli criticises Fuchs' suggestion that the name comes from galea, a helmet, saying that galea is a Latin word, not a Greek one, and the Greeks, 'having no want of words', would not compose names of plants from the Latin. (Grieve suggests galeopsis comes from gale meaning weasel and opsis, countenance, inspired from the flower). Galeopsis resembles the nettle, says Dioscorides, but it has smoother leaves which smell rather foul when ground, and its flowers are delicate and purple. It grows on fences, road edges and building lots. This galeopsis will dissolve indurations, tumours, scrofulous and other swellings of the glands and parotid tumours, applied twice daily with vinegar as a plaster, or the decoction as a rinse. It is applied with salt as a plaster for spreading ulcers, gangrenes and putrid humours. This could be interpreted as Pliny's lamium, or at least a purple variety of it, broadly used for wounds and swollen glands, but may be an entirely different herb. Beck designates this plant brownwort *Scrophularia peregrina*. Most of our Renaissance authors include it among the deadnettles or call it stinking deadnettle, although some authors, according to Parkinson, do think it is a scrophularia. It is impossible to conclude the definitive identity of the plant, and confusion is inevitable. The plant does not appear in Galen.

## RENAISSANCE DEBATE AND USE

The question of identification becomes critical in the Renaissance texts, yet remains elusive. Fuchs distinguishes three types of deadnettle: white deadnettle, lamium proper; spotted deadnettle with purple flowers, *Lamium maculatum*; and yellow archangel, *Lamium galeobdolon*. Turner writes only of *Lamium album*, dede nettle urtica iners/mortua/alba, archangelica. Dodoens has a title archangel or deadnettle, of which there are two kinds: the first, which does not smell, of which there are three sorts, with white, yellow and reddish flowers; the second has a strong and stinking savour, of which there are two sorts which differ only in flower colour, one being pale, the other of a brown red colour, smaller than the flowers of the first deadnettle. This does sound rather like a figwort. Dalechamps distinguishes between lamium, which has white flowers growing by walls and footpaths or yellow flowers growing in shady wooded places, and galiopsis, the foetid deadnettle with purple flowers. He says of galiopsis 'the Ancients and those after them were familiar with the notable qualities of this deadnettle, which was easily distinguished from lamium and the like… yet the images of the species here do not differentiate to my untrained eye'. Bauhin, strangely, since he is usually the differentiator and taker to task, partly confounds the two plants, introducing them as galeopsis or inert nettle, yet specifying different species: white nettle, archangel, Pliny's lamium, which likes damp shady places, ditches and courtyards; spotted deadnettle; yellow deadnettle; the purple flowered with oblong leaves differs by scent in that it is more foetid.

Parkinson sets out his own list of eight: (1) red deadnettle or red archangel, (2) Spanish archangel with flowers of purplish colour, (3) white archangel, (4) long-leafed red archangel, (5) archangel with spotted leaves, (6) archangel with white lines in the leaves, (7) yellow archangel and (8) strange archangel. He details which may be called which and by whom, yet none of these is Dioscorides' galeopsis, for he has a following chapter entitled galeopsis, stinking deadnettle, which he names the true stinking deadnettle of Dioscorides. There follow in Parkinson the yellow stinking deadnettle, the hoary stinking deadnettle, pale stinking deadnettle and the dragon flower. Gerard distinguishes six plants under the heading of archangel or deadnettle: white, yellow, red, Hungary, hedge and 'Hungary nettle with variegated floure'. The hedge nettle, he says, Tragus and Clusius judge to be the true galeopsis of Dioscorides. Matthioli thinks the galeopsis of Dioscorides is not a scrophularia. He speculates whether it could be the lamium with white patches on the leaves, the name galeopsis possibly relating to gala milk in Greek, and whether Pliny was familiar with galeopsis, but eventually does not commit himself to a firm opinion. Culpeper has a red, white and yellow archangel, but, shunning idolatry, is distinctly uncomfortable with the name: 'to put a gloss upon their practice, the physicians call an herb (which country people vulgarly know by the name of Deadnettle) Archangel; whether they favour more of superstition or folly, I leave to the judicious reader.

It is clear these authors recognized and probably worked with the deadnettles; the problem lies in the unreliability of citing Dioscorides' uses of galeopsis for these plants.

THE WESTERN HERBAL TRADITION

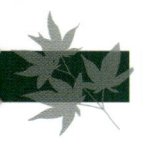

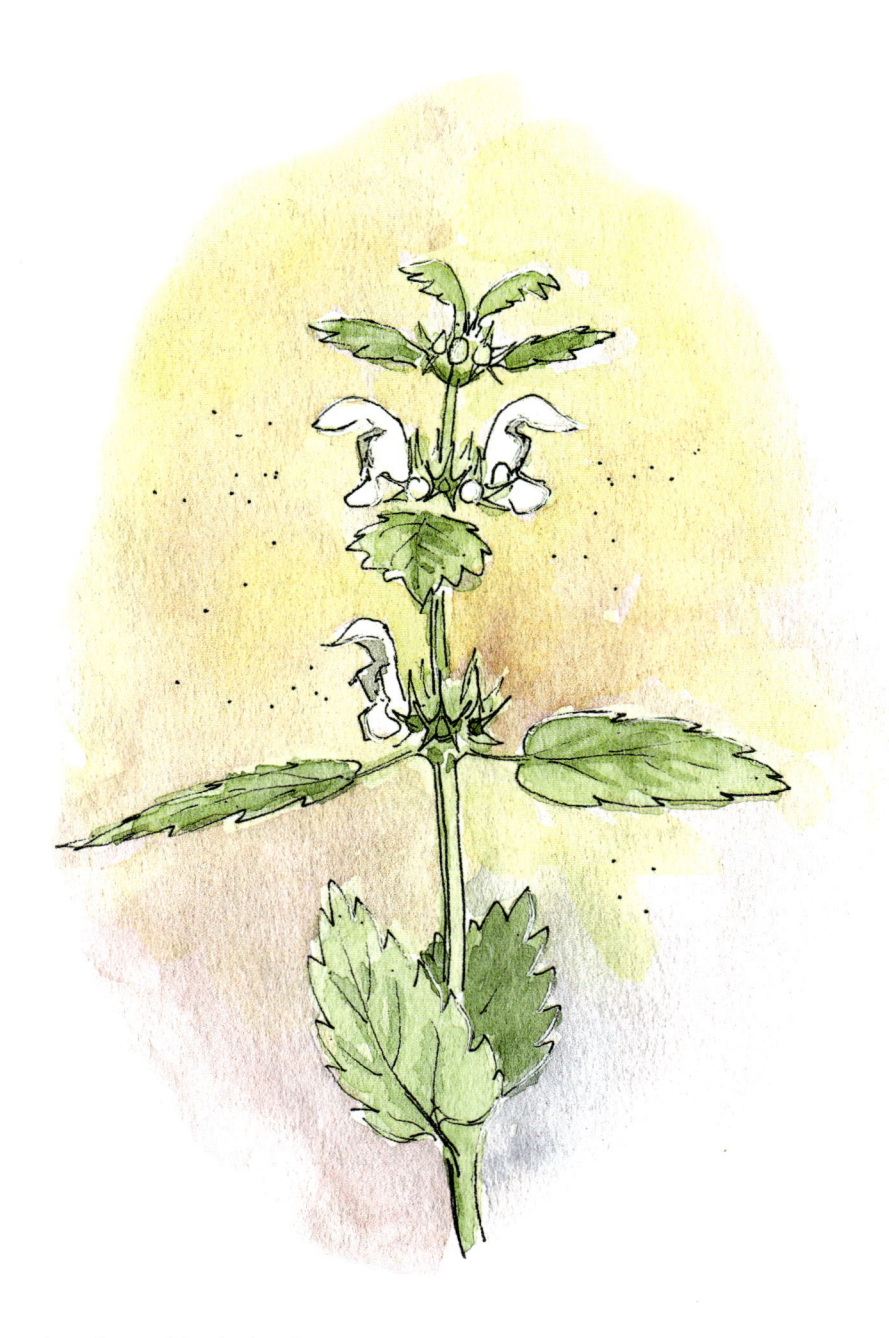

**Figure 21.2** *Lamium album*, white deadnettle.

The questionable similarity of Pliny's lamium compounds the difficulties. Turner sticks with Pliny, although Pliny himself is no reliable source. Turner writes how with a corn of salt it heals places that are bruised, beaten or burnt, and wens and swellings, gouts and wounds. He repeats Pliny's white sections of the leaf for St Anthony's fire. Then he adds a reference carried in most of these Renaissance authors to 'the later writers' who hold that the herb is good for nose bleeds when laid to the back of the neck or shoulder blades. Furthermore, it is a good remedy against 'foul sores, fistulas or false wounds'. Dodoens too stays with Pliny, with no reference to later writers, only that the virtue is like other nettles. Fuchs cites Pliny too, but then adds, singularly, a sort of magical use, how 'certain people among us distinguish the types by the season; the root of the autumnal urtica is bound to the body in tertian agues such that the sick are formally called when that root is dug up and told which root will be lifted out and for whom and by whose son, thus the healing of illness has been handed down'. Quartan agues are treated similarly, with salt added to the root of urtica.

Dalechamps is clear in keeping Pliny and Dioscorides separate. He distinguishes lamium with Pliny's recommendations, adding the usual 'recent practitioners' reference, together with how the yellow archangel is much more effective for wounds, ulcers, swellings, while galiopsis, the leaves, flowers, juice and seed, dissipates hardenings, carcinomas, scrophulous swellings and parotids applied in vinegar as warm cataplasm twice daily, and the decoction applied with salt on gangrenous and putrid sores. Yet we still do not know what plant this is. Bauhin tells us all deadnettles generally are good for ulcers and swellings, and in baths and vapour baths to soften. He then offers different uses for four types: the purple with oblong leaves disperses scrofulous tumours (Dioscorides' galeopsis) and can be smeared on with salt for putrid ulcers, cancerous eating ulcers and corroding sores; the spotted deadnettle should be used as powdered leaves in an egg, sucked, or taken in wine, for obstructions of the spleen; the white deadnettle or white archangel is taken in wine for obstructions of the liver or spleen, and for 'the whites' (leucorrhoea) in women as a conserve in sugar taken daily. This is an early reference to this use. Then follow uses for nosebleed and wounds/ulcers. The yellow deadnettle or yellow archangel has similar uses to the white but is much more effective for wounds, ulcers and swellings. It might be called lamium, he suggests, because the flowers look like hooded ghosts.

Parkinson introduces the deadnettles as hotter and drier than stinging nettles and used with greater success for hardness of the spleen taken both internally and applied hot externally as cataplasm or fomentation. The use for women appears again, but Parkinson recommends the white flowers to stay the whites, and those of the red to stay the reds, i.e. menorrhagia. He adds a number of further uses 'it is thought good to make the heart merry, to drive away melancholy and to quicken the spirits'. Quartan agues, nose bleeds, bruises, burns and such appear too, and for the king's evil, gout, sciatica and aches of joints and sinews, after Pliny. He expands on the wound uses: for inflammations, as a repercussive to drive away humours, to heal all green wounds, for old ulcers, to stop them corroding and spreading and it draws splinters etc. too. The yellow archangel, he says, is best for filthy and corrupt sores and ulcers, fistulae and to dissolve tumours. The stinking deadnettles, including Dioscorides' galeopsis, are boiled in wine and drunk for inward hurts and for the spleen; the warm juice with vinegar is applied for haemorrhoids, warts and 'other such like hard gimes or knots that grow in or about the fundament', for other swellings etc. that grow in the neck or throat and for fistulous ulcers and gangrenes, again mainly following Dioscorides appropriately, assuming the herb is accurately identified. Culpeper follows Parkinson exactly, covering all three of his red, white and yellow archangels, adding only that it is a herb of Venus and its chief use is for women.

Gerard for 'Archangel (or rather the hedge Nettle)' covers Pliny, but seems to broaden more specifically into galeopsis: 'Archangel…stamped with vinegar, and applied in manner of a pultis taketh away wens and hard swellings, the king's evil, inflammation of the kernels under the ears and jawes and also hot fierie inflammations of the kernels of the necke, armeholes and flanks. It is good to bathe those parts with the decoction of it, as Dioscorides and Pliny say'. Later physicians, he says, use a conserve of the flowers to stay the whites, and the flowers baked with sugar are use to 'make the heart merry; to make a good colour in the face, and to make the vitall spirits more fresh and lively'.

So a very unclear picture emerges from the Ancients themselves – are Dioscorides and Pliny speaking of the same plant and if so is it lamium or a scrophularia? The Renaissance authors broaden the debate considerably but do not necessarily help us to a conclusion. Perhaps we can rely a little more firmly on their references to 'later writers', with their recommendations for nose bleeds and gangrenous ulcers and fistulae, since that plant at least is more likely to be identifiable as a deadnettle.

## INTERIM OPINION

Other sources between the Ancients and the Renaissance throw no more light on the matter. The *Old English Herbarium* carries no entry for this plant. Hildegard has a 'blind nettle' but she does not describe the plant. It is hot, she writes, and a person will smile with pleasure on eating it since it touches his spleen so his heart is made happy. The plant will help 'leucoma' in the eye if it is picked and put in spring water for a night, 'then having taken it from the water, heat it in a small dish (plant or water?) and place it warm, over the affected eye'. This is done for three nights and the leucoma will disappear.

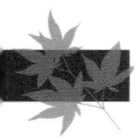

The Myddfai text, again with no description, urges use of deadnettle for two conditions: scabies (which actually refers to eczematous diseases in that erythema and thickening of the skin are combined with pruritis, pustules and ulceration) and menorrhagia. For menorrhagia 'take archangel, pound well with strong red wine, strain carefully, give to drink night and morning freely'. Its use is of great benefit, the text records. It should also be kept dry for winter, taken as a powder, a spoonful in warmed wine, drunk as warm as possible. The pounded root in wine is good to the same purpose. The text then adds if growing the herb in the garden it should be grown apart from other plants, but offers no reason for the isolation. Its use for scabies is external application of the decoction as a wash for the whole body every morning. There is also a recipe for ointment for the same purpose 'boil the residue of archangel and garlic in unsalted butter, make into an ointment and anoint the whole body with this for nine mornings.' The Salernitan herbal is clearly following Dioscorides on leukas for it only records use of the plant, crushed in wine and drunk, for bites of serpents or vipers.

## 18TH AND 19TH CENTURY

Miller and Quincy in the 18th century appear to consider the red deadnettle as Dioscorides' galeopsis. Quincy has an entry under lamium, deadnettle, galeopsis, archangel, but he qualifies the name saying the plant is distinguished Lamium non foetens, folio oblongo (non-foetid lamium with oblong leaf) by Caspar, and Urtica iners floribus albis (deadnettle with white flowers) by Bauhin; there is also a lamium rubrum (red lamium), he says, which is the galeopsis of Dioscorides, and a lamium luteum (yellow lamium). Quincy does not rate the herb highly, commenting, 'The plant itself is of no great esteem'. He accounts its application as soft, lubricating and strengthening, hence given in some female weaknesses as the whites and in heat and difficulty of urine. He confirms its meagre reputation with the discouraging, but practical, remark 'a conserve is made of them in shops, but it is not often prescribed and on that account seldom to be met with fresh and good'. Miller writes about two deadnettles, the white, which is counted specific against the fluor albus and frequently (no agreement with Quincy on this) made use of in a conserve or decoction which is to be continued for some time. Some commend it, he says, against the king's evil and all scrofulous swellings, so Pliny is echoed here. The only official preparation is conserve of the flowers. Then Miller covers lamium rubrum, red archangel, the purpureum foetidum folio subrotundo sive Galeopsis Dioscoridis (the purple foetid lamium with roundish leaf or galeopsis of Dioscorides), which has a strong, earthy, unsavoury smell,

he says. In application of this plant he appears to echo Parkinson (white to stay the whites, red to stay the reds) saying as the former archangel (white) is accounted specific for fluor albus, so this is helpful for 'the excess of the 'catamenia' (menses) and all other haemorrhages'. Furthermore, it is serviceable externally for wounds and inflammations.

Hill writes of *Lamium album* for the whites and all other weaknesses. The flowers only are used, gathered in May, 1 lb beat up with 2½ lb sugar as conserve. I can find no coverage in Cullen. The herb was not used in the USA by Cook nor Ellingwood.

## LATER CONFUSION

Grieve is no less confusing. There is an entry for white deadnettle with no medicinal uses appended, followed by purple deadnettle with medicinal actions and uses – decoction of herb and flowers for haemorrhage, leaves to staunch wounds, dried herb as tea with honey to promote perspiration and act on kidneys, useful in cases of chill. Then, under a subheading 'other species', henbit, spotted deadnettle and hempnettle are described. This is followed by a quote from Gerard on *white* archangel after which the next heading, 'parts used medicinally', begins 'the whole herb collected…', but which herb is meant here is far from clear. Then a further 'medicinal actions and uses' confuses the picture even more. Whichever plant (or plants) is meant, it is astringent in nature, Grieve tells us, and used for stopping haemorrhage, spitting of blood and dysentery. The decoction of the flowers is a blood purifier for rashes, eczema etc., but no source is cited. Reputations from the tradition then follow – healing green wounds, bruises and burns. Culpeper and others follow, on lifting spirits, against quartan agues, and bleeding of nose and mouth applied to nape of neck. She rehearses use in the past for hardness of spleen, the seat of melancholy, the herb applied as a hot plaster. Finally, a further familiar use appears, bruised and mixed with salt, vinegar and lard (sounds like chips!) for reduction of swellings and ease in gout, sciatica and other pains in joints and muscles. Yellow deadnettle has its own entry, *Lamium galeobdolon*. The galeobdolon, Grieve tells us, comes from two Greek words gale meaning weasel and bdolos a disagreeable odour, a reference to the strong odour of the crushed plant. It is used for the same purposes as white archangel, she says.

There is no entry in the *National Botanic Pharmacopoeia*, Wren, Priest & Priest, nor the *British Herbal Pharmacopoeia*.

Weiss is clearer. He writes only of *Lamium album*. The flowers are used, which need pulling from the calyces individually. He stresses its heavy popular use and how women in particular 'keep asking for the drug and using it', although he says he finds little information on its efficacy. He suggests use for leucorrhoea of asthenic young girls, taken internally and used as a genital wash. The flowers make a good family tea too, he says. Treben reinforces a wider folk use, at least in central Europe, in recommending a range of applications. The entry is for yellow deadnettle *Lamiastrum galeobdolon*, but she includes white deadnettle, saying both are 'valuable medicinal herbs'. The leaves and especially the flowers are used. White deadnettle, three cups a day, is good for abdominal and menstrual complaints, cleansing the blood, for sleeplessness and 'diverse female troubles'. Yellow deadnettle is used similarly, but apparently with more emphasis on the urinary system. It is especially used, says Treben, for scanty and burning urine, bladder troubles, serious kidney disorders and fluid retention in the heart, for bladder malfunction in older people and chill in the bladder and nephritis. In renal dialysis she recommends a mix of yellow deadnettle, bedstraw *Galium* species and golden rod *Solidago virgaurea* in equal proportions. The flowers are taken for digestive troubles, scrofula and skin rashes, one cup each morning; externally used for ulcers and varicose veins. So here is filled out a little the traditional uses cited in the Commission E monograph that the chapter began with.

## RESEARCH APPLICATION

White deadnettle has been used in two randomized controlled trials; but yet again the results do not help in formulating recommendations. In a randomized, placebo-controlled trial in Israel, 49 patients with atopic dermatitis (age and sex not given) were treated for 2 weeks with a proprietary product containing *Lamium album*, *Achillea millefolium* and *Eleutherococcus senticosus* (dried herb, ethanolic extracts). Patients were monitored for 8 weeks and assessed using the SCORAD scale and 44 people completed the trial. Improvement was similar for the treatment and placebo groups and was maintained after the active treatment period (Shapira et al 2005). The trial is interesting because there was a significant response to both the treatment and the placebo. Details of the placebo were not reported. Two weeks is a very short treatment period in atopic dermatitis and this is not a formulation which would necessarily be widely chosen in Britain, although the formulation was based on the experience of herbalists.

In the second randomized controlled trial, white deadnettle was used as the placebo in a trial of urtication in arthritis (Randall et al 2000) and proved not as inert as the designers had hoped, illustrating some of the problems of determining a placebo in trials of herbal medicines.

A study of six Lamiaceae, including *Lamium album*, *Lamium purpureum* and *Galeopsis speciosa* (commercial dried herb, methanolic extracts), used three in vitro antioxidant assays. Results for each plant varied between the tests, but *Lamium album* came out well in all three (Matkowski & Piotrowska 2006). A study of four *Lamium* species in Turkey found that the results varied between the species in the different antioxidant assays. The authors suggest that the phenylpropanoids may be the relevant constituents, but also argue that the range of constituents is such that this may not be the case (Funda et al 2007). An in vitro study on the proliferation and viability of human skin fibroblasts using extract of dried flowers (commercial, Poland) was performed to assess whether there was support for the traditional usage of *Lamium* in wound healing (Paduch et al 2007) Only the heptane extract was associated with increased cell proliferation and the authors associate this with the triterpenes found only in the heptane extract. The relevance of this study is unclear as traditional usage is a decoction as a compress.

## MODERN USE

Modern texts, if the herb appears in them at all, mainly limit themselves to white deadnettle, but vary quite widely in their range of applications. Chevallier cites Gerard on lifting the spirits but restricts his internal uses mainly to women's complaints. It is, he says, astringent and demulcent, used as a uterine tonic, to stop intermenstrual bleeding and menorrhagia; traditionally for vaginal discharge; sometimes taken to relieve painful periods. It can be taken against diarrhoea and externally used for varicose veins and haemorrhages. Wood cites Hill. Weiss and a 19th century UK herbalist who records the familiar traditional uses of helping the spleen, whites, flooding, nose bleeds, spitting blood, haemorrhages, green wounds, bruises and burns. The source of some of his specific indications – cough, bronchitis, pleurisy, inflamed prostate, anaemia – is unclear, given his text. Menzies-Trull covers a broad range of uses, although there is no specific discussion of them. Bartram too gives a broad sweep, designating the flowering tops haemostatic, astringent, diuretic, expectorant, anti-inflammatory, vulnerary, antispasmodic and menstrual regulator, with uses including heavy and painful menstrual bleeding, cystitis, diarrhoea, prostatitis, catarrh, and piles, as douche for vaginal discharge, and as an eye douche. He gives a dose of 1–2 teaspoons to a cup of boiling water, taken three times a day; for vaginal douche 2 oz in 2 pints boiling water, cooled

We should perhaps not be too surprised at a more subtle herb here. From Pelikan we learn how deadnettle differs from the more strongly active members of the labiate family, imbued as they normally are with warmth nature, suffused right into the leaves with volatile oils. We might anticipate a gentle action from the shape of the leaves, since, says Pelikan, the leaf shape gives clear indication of the extent of cosmic warmth perfusion. He compares the broad leaves of melissa to the 'needles' of rosemary. So we find 'only traces of labiate warmth' in white deadnettle, 'a faint echo of the fiery labiate theme in a cool, damp, earthy medium'. The flowers however play a key role (as we have seen). They appear to take full part in the labiates' movement towards the animal world, spoken of by Pelikan. The move of the flowers to the horizontal axis, the axis of animals; formation of 'lips, throats and gullets', and the space within the flowers forming the shape of insects' heads. Wax casts, Pelikan tells us, resemble bees' heads with proboscis. One name for lamium is bee nettle; the word lamium, Grieve says, comes from the Greek word laimos meaning throat; and we find from modern research that white deadnettle produces a constituent, phytoecdysteroid, an insect steroid hormone analogue.

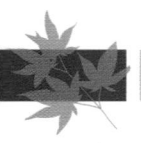

recommendations for this herb that it might deserve after its reputation in central Europe. We can say there is a fairly consistent tradition of use in leucorrhoea, menorrhagia and metrorrhagia internally as tea, tincture or decoction and externally as a douche. It may have broader genitor-urinary applications. For these indications, Barker (2001) recommends an infusion of 10–20 g in 500 mL of water three times a day, and double this strength for douches and compresses.
- Externally as a wash for wounds and ulcers.
- Other uses need more research and confirmation.

Dosage: Barker (2001) recommends 2–5 mL three times a day of 1 : 5 tincture of dried flowering tops, aerial parts.

## RECOMMENDATIONS

- The confusion and lack of clarity in the tradition does not allow us to make the broader

## RECOMMENDATIONS ON SAFETY

No safety concerns are documented.

## CONSTITUENTS

Reviews: Bisset & Wichtl (2001), Bradley (2006), Williamson (2003), Yalçın & Kaya (2006).

### Volatile oil

Total 0.01–0.31% mainly alkanes: squalene; sesquiterpene: germacrene (Yalçın & Kaya 2006).

### Triterpenes

Ursolic acid, amyrin (Paduch et al 2007).

### Iridoid glycosides

C10 type: lamalbid, caryoptoside; C9 type: alboside A, alboside B and isomers (Damtoft 1992).
C10 type: lamalbid, caryoptoside (wild, Bulgaria) (Alipieva et al 2006).
*Lamium maculatum*, C10 type: lamalbid, penstemoside (wild, Bulgaria) (Alipieva et al 2006).
Similar iridoid glycosides in *Lamium album, Lamium garganicum, Lamium amplexicaule, Lamium maculatum, Lamium purpureum* (wild, Bulgaria) (Alipieva et al 2007).
*Lamium galeobdolon*, C9 type and benzoxazinoids (Alipieva et al 2003), which are commonly found in grasses (Frey et al 2009).
*Lamium purpureum* var. *purpureum*, C10 type: lamalbide (Yalçın et al 2008).
Hemiterpene glycoside: hemialboside (Damtoft & Jensen 1995).

### Phenylpropanoids

Total polyphenols 23 mg/g (flowers, commercial, Poland) (Matkowski & Piotrowska 2006).

### Phenolic acids

Chlorogenic acid, 5-caffeoylquinic acid (flowers, wild, Poland) (Budzianowski & Skrzypczak 1995).
Protocatechuic acid, chlorogenic acid, vanillic acid, caffeic acid, *p*-coumaric acid, ferulic acid (flowers, commercial, Poland) (Paduch et al 2007).

### Phenylpropanoid glycosides

Acteoside (verbascoside), lamalboside (Budzianowski & Skrzypczak 1995).
*Lamium maculatum*, acteoside (higher in flowers) (wild, China) (Shuya et al 2003).
*Lamium purpureum*, phenylethanoid glycosides: lamiusides A, B, C, D (wild, Japan) (Ito et al 2006).

### Flavonoids

Tiliroside, rutoside, quercetin and kaempferol 3-*O*-glucosides (Budzianowski & Skrzypczak 1995).
Tiliroside, quercetin glycosides: rutin, isoquercitrin (Paduch et al 2007).
*Lamium maculatum*, 3,7-dimethoxy-quercetin, rutin (wild, China) (Shuya et al 2003).

### Tannins

6–7% condensed and hydrolyzable (Bradley 2006).

### Phytoecdysteroids

These insect steroid hormone analogues are thought to inhibit the activities of some plant-eating insects. *Lamium album* and *Lamium purpureum* are hosts for some moths and butterflies. Highest levels were in young leaves and side-shoots. Abutasterone, inokosterone, polypodine B and pterosterone (aerial parts) (Savchenko et al 2001).
*Lamium maculatum*: 20-hydroxy ecdysone (flower) (Shuya et al 2003).

## REFERENCES

Alipieva KI, Taskova RM, Evstatieva LN, et al 2003 Benzoxazinoids and iridoid glucosides from four *Lamium* species. Phytochemistry 64:1413–1417.

Alipieva KI, Taskova RM, Jensen SR, et al 2006 Iridoid glucosides from *Lamium album* and *Lamium maculatum* (Lamiaceae). Biochemical Systematics and Ecology 34:88–91.

Alipieva K, Kokubun T, Taskova R 2007 LC-ESI-MS analysis of iridoid glycosides in *Lamium* species. Biochemical Systematics and Ecology 35:17–22.

Barker J 2001 The Medicinal flora of Britain and northwestern Europe. Wionter Press, West Wickham, Kent.

Bisset NG, Wichtl M (eds) 2001 Herbal drugs and phytopharmaceuticals, 2nd edn. Medpharm, Stuttgart.

Bradley PR 2006 British herbal compendium, vol 2. British Herbal Medicine Association, Bournemouth.

Budzianowski J, Skrzypczak L 1995 Phenylpropanoid esters from *Lamium album* flowers. Phytochemistry 38:997–1001.

Damtoft S 1992 Iridoid glucosides from *Lamium album*. Phytochemistry 31:175–178.

Damtoft S, Jensen SR 1995 Hemialboside, a hemiterpene glucoside from *Lamium album*. Phytochemistry 39:923–924.

Davis PH (ed.) 1982 Flora of Turkey, vol 7. Edinburgh University Press, Edinburgh.

Frey M, Schullehner K, Dick R, et al 2009 Benzoxazinoid biosynthesis, a model for evolution of secondary metabolic pathways in plants Phytochemistry 70:1645–1651.

Funda N, Yalçın FN, Kaya D, et al 2007 Antimicrobial and free radical scavenging activities of some *Lamium* species from Turkey. Hacettepe University Journal of the Faculty of Pharmacy 27:11–22. Online. Available: http://www.eczfakder.hacettepe.edu.tr/Arsiv/EskiDergiler/01.../ecz-02.pdf.

Ito N, Nihei T, Kakuda R, et al 2006 Five new phenylethanoid glycosides from the whole plants of *Lamium purpureum* L. Chemical and Pharmaceutical Bulletin 54:1705–1708.

Matkowski A, Piotrowska M 2006 Antioxidant and free radical scavenging activities of some medicinal plants from the Lamiaceae. Fitoterapia 77:346–353.

Paduch R, Wojciak-Kosior M, Matysik G 2007 Investigation of biological activity of *Lamii albi* flos extracts. Journal of Ethnopharmacology 110:69–75.

Randall C, Randall H, Dobbs F, et al 2000 Randomized controlled trial of nettle sting for treatment of base-of-thumb pain. Journal of the Royal Society of Medicine 93:305–309.

Savchenko T, Blackford M, Sarker SD, et al 2001 Phytoecdysteroids from *Lamium* species: identification and distribution within plants. Biochemical Systematics and Ecology 29:891–900.

Shapira MY, Raphaelovich Y, Gilad L, et al 2005 Treatment of atopic dermatitis with herbal combination of *Eleutherococcus, Achillea millefolium*, and *Lamium album* has no advantage over placebo: a double blind, placebo-controlled, randomized trial. Journal of the American Academy of Dermatology 52:691–693.

Shuya C, Xingguo C, Zhide H 2003 Identification and determination of ecdysone and phenylpropanoid glucoside and flavonoids in *Lamium maculatum* by capillary zone electrophoresis. Biomedical Chromatography 17:477–482.

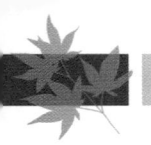

Stace C 1991 New flora of the British Isles. Cambridge University Press, Cambridge.

Williamson E 2003 Potter's Herbal Cyclopaedia. CW Daniel, Saffron Walden.

Yalçın FN, Kaya D 2006 Ethnobotany, pharmacology and phytochemistry of the Genus *Lamium* (Lamiaceae). FABAD Journal of Pharmacological Science 31:43–52. Online. Available: http://www.fabad.org.tr/fabad.org/pdf/volum31/issue1/43–52.pdf.

Yalçın FN, Kaya D, Çalış I, et al 2008 Determination of iridoid glycosides from four Turkish *Lamium* species by HPLC-ESI/MS. Turkish Journal of Chemistry 32:457–467. Online. Available: http://journals.tubitak.gov.tr/chem/issues/kim.../kim-32-4-6-0706-16.pdf.

# CHAPTER 22
# *Ocimum basilicum*, basil

## DESCRIPTION

**Family: Lamiaceae**                                              **Part used: aerial parts**

*Ocimum basilicum* L. is a half-hardy annual or short-lived perennial, which is native to India and Asia and cultivated worldwide (Bisset & Wichtl 2001) It is very variable in morphology (Labra et al 2004). Erect, branching, green stems (to 60 cm) support opposite, soft, bright-green oval leaves, which are slightly crumpled-looking. Whorls (usually six flowers) of small, white, lipped, tubular flowers are borne in terminal racemes (Podlech 2001). The fruit contains four small smooth black seeds. It is propagated from seed.

### Quality

Many cultivars and varieties are used and some are cultivated, especially for the manufacture of pesto (Bown 1995, Vieira & Simon 2006). Simon et al (1999) compare the growth habit and constituents of 42 forms cultivated in the USA, and note that the cultivars of var. *purpurescens* contain a substantial concentration of anthocyanins.

Crosses can occur between any *Ocimum basilicum* varieties, cultivars and related species such as *Ocimum minimum* L. There is substantial variation in composition of the volatile oil and little correlation has been found between phenotype and chemotype (Marotti et al 1996, Grayer et al 2004, Sifola & Barbieri 2006) or genotype and chemotype (Labra et al 2004). Schnaubelt (1999) uses basil as an example of the broad range of healing qualities in aromatic oils, and associates this with the adaptability and vigour of the plant kingdom.

Volatile oil accumulates in trichomes so yield depends on leaf number and size (Sifola & Barbieri 2006). Concentration of volatile oil in basil cv. Sweet Genovese was higher after cultivation at 25°C than at 15°C (Chang et al 2007).

Drying and freezing resulted in loss of concentration and changes in the proportion of each component (Klimánková et al 2008). A substantial reduction from 0.3 to 0.1% was found in the concentration of volatile oil in dried basil after 6 months of storage at 4°C in aluminium polyethylene polyamide bags (Baritaux et al 1993). This was originally a high methylchavicol sample, but the reduction in concentration of methylchavicol from 0.15 to 0.01% after storage, associated with relative increases in monoterpenes, oxygenated monoterpenes and sesquiterpenes, led to important changes in the volatile oil. Similar results are discussed by Grayer et al (1996).

A study of drying methods found that, compared to oven drying at 45°C, air-drying resulted in lower loss of volatile oil and greater retention of the more floral odour of fresh basil (Diaz-Maroto et al 2004). However, the authors argue that oven-drying produced a better product as deterioration could occur over the time-span of air-drying.

---

Most people know basil today. It is used in cuisines across the world, from Thai to Italian, and particularly the famous pesto sauce from Genoa. We may mention it in the same breath as oregano and bay, or imagine how we make use of the fresh and not the dried plant, as we do with coriander or parsley. It must be one of the most frequent pot herbs, sitting in sunny kitchen windowsills across many lands and in many times, as Fuchs records in 16th century Germany and Bauhin in the 17th regarding the reports of scorpions commonly making their homes under pots in Venice.

Yet look in any modern English-language herbal and the chances are that basil will not appear in it. Go back 70 odd years to Maud Grieve's A Modern Herbal, and you will find an entry for basil, with an etymological link to the Greek 'basileus' meaning 'king' and descriptions of several varieties of this 'regal' herb, but no indications or uses! We must agree with Quincy that basil is found in few herbal prescriptions, the only one in his day being the College of Physicians' compound briony water used for hysterical conditions, and with Miller that although the herb has a fragrant scent – fit for the palace was Fuch's assessment of the smell of the 'basilikon', as it was known by the German apothecaries – it is little used in medicine. Apparently, the internal use of basil was condemned by the Ancients.

Culpeper gives us a reasonably accurate description and more information on this sweet or garden basil. This herb

# THE WESTERN HERBAL TRADITION

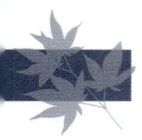

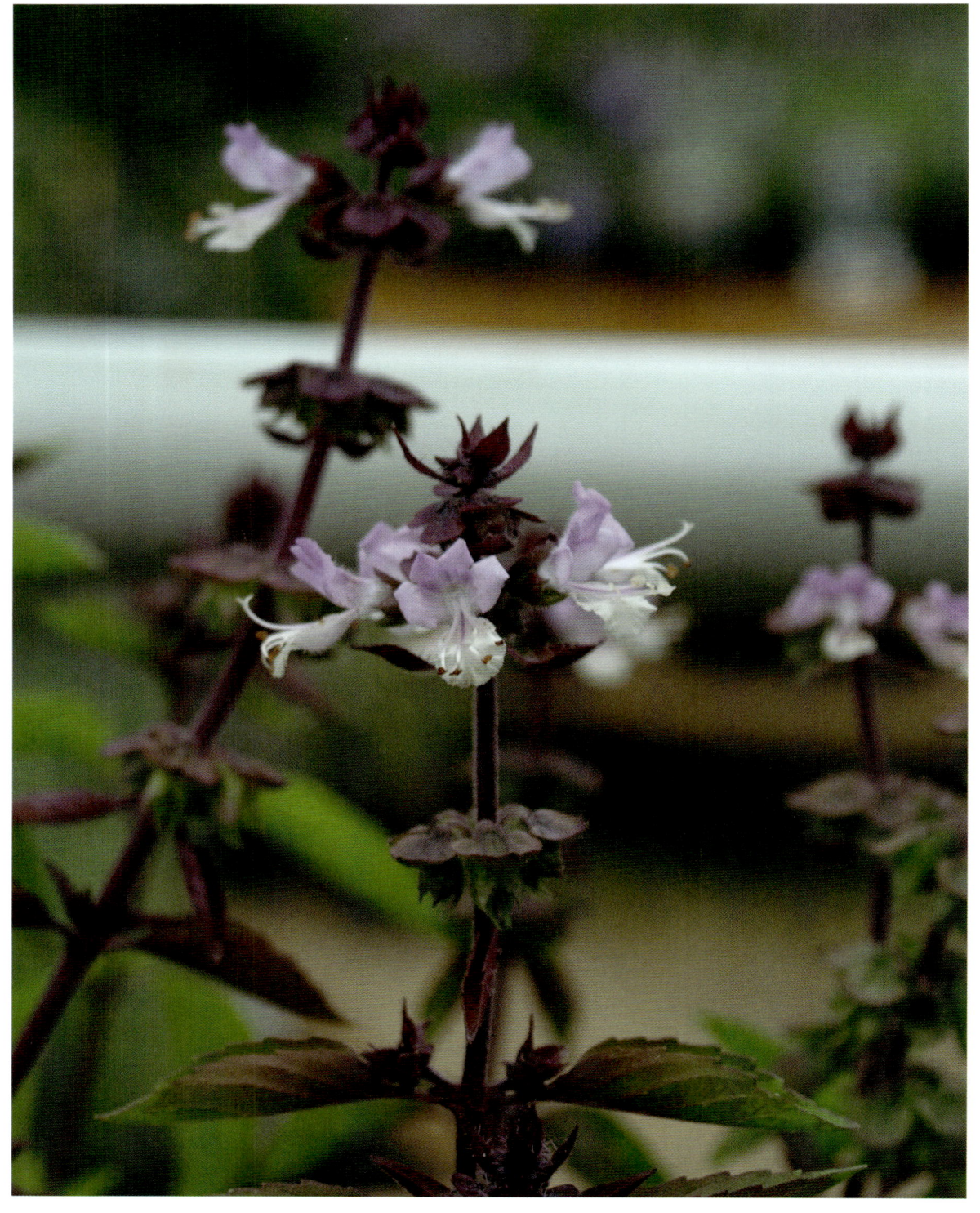

**Figure 22.1** *Ocimum basilicum*, basil (Hidcote, Gloucestershire, August).

of virulent qualities has stirred up argument among the authorities: 'Galen and Dioscorides hold it not fitting to be taken inwardly... Pliny and the Arabian physicians defend it'. Pliny actually gives us both sides of the argument, taking Chrysippus' many criticisms and countering them one by one on the testimony of later writers and physicians. It is not true, Pliny writes, that goats, who eat most things, avoid it. Nor does it make a man witless and bring on lethargy, for a perfume of basil and vinegar is used to bring someone round from a faint or to rouse a person from indolence. Basil vinegar is also good for the stomach, and to break wind upwards, to treat jaundice and dropsy and applied to the belly, to stop (bloody) diarrhoea. It has a diuretic effect, also, and other actions agreed on since the death of Chrysippus three centuries earlier: in the head region a liniment of basil corrects cold in the head, clears catarrh, and with vinegar and oil of roses or myrtle helps headache; the powdered seed is taken as snuff to provoke sneezing to clear the head, or the juice made up with goose grease and dropped into children's ears for problems there. It can be applied to eyes watering with irritation or inflammation. Externally, mixed with a copper compound, it removes warts. Eaten at table with vinegar, the herb strengthens the female womb and can be used to repress breast milk when it is time to wean the child.

Pliny relates without comment the superstitions he has read in Chrysippus concerning basil: that the bruised herb placed under a stone will breed a serpent; or the herb chewed and put in the sun will breed worms and maggots; that basil pounded with crabs or crayfish will attract all the scorpions of the area to gather around the bait; or finally, that if you are stung by a scorpion on a day when you have eaten basil, you will surely die! Pliny has made it clear that basil possesses medicinal qualities, including that of treating scorpion stings (despite Beck's translation of Dioscorides (II 141) which supports Chryssipus' assertion and is credited to the Libyans), when applied externally with wine and vinegar, but how we make sense of some of them is another matter. Can the herb warm and comfort a cold head but also cool and refresh someone in a burning fever? If the herb has some aphrodisiac effect, how does it also repress the rage of choler, the yellow bile humour whose dominance can induce lust?

Culpeper considers the herb to be hot and moist in the first degree. This is a category of Galenic pharmaceutical activity that allows the plant to be used in heating and in cooling prescriptions. Its effect is therefore implicitly balancing or tonic, reducing heat to the body's normal level or cherishing heat where it is lacking. Culpeper, however, limits its actions to a strengthener of the womb, perhaps as an aid to conception, but certainly of help in delivery of the foetus and expulsion of the placenta in labour, and thus not to be taken during pregnancy, for fear of abortion. He thus characterizes the herb more by its sympathy and antipathy to this organ by making it a herb of Mars in Scorpio, which 'as it helps the deficiencies of Venus in one kind, so it spoils all her actions in another'. This designation also reflects the association of the plant with scorpions but obscures its reputed cordial effect of heating the heart (which he listed in his *Catalogues of simples in the new dispensatory*, in the second edition of the *Pharmacopoeia Londinensis* (1669)). He adds instead that it can be applied to poisonous bites and wasp and hornet stings for it will quickly draw the venom to it and 'all poisons draw their like'. Finally, it is observed not to survive alongside rue in the garden, and rue 'is as great an enemy to poison as any grows'. He advises a dosage not above half a drachm (2 g) and ends saying he dare not write any more about it.

Culpeper is hardly promoting basil as a medicinal herb but he exceeds Parkinson, who opines from the first that basil has little application in medicine and is employed rather as a sweet-smelling herb, especially since Dioscorides and Galen think it should not be given internally. Here in Parkinson is the conventional warning about dimness of sight, from too much consumption of basil, and of the plant containing superfluous moisture (hot and moist in the second degree, according to Galen), which would prove harmful to the body over time, if consumed. Topical applications are acceptable: for worms in the belly and for reducing a swollen spleen; snake bites and scorpion stings; the juice with goose grease for earache in children; Pliny's combination with oil of roses and vinegar for lethargy, jaundice and dropsy; the sternutatory action mentioned by Dioscorides and the smell of basil vinegar to repress the tendency to faint; finally, the moistening quality of the plant to help ripen abscesses and pustules, as Galen suggested. Bock, cited by Bauhin, also adds others: that the seed dissolved in rose water and gum overnight is useful for mouth ulcers and other inflammations, chapping of the lips and warts on the breasts. Parkinson knows basil only as a garden plant, reckoning its natural habitat unknown, but he does mention the cordial uses noted by the Arabic writers, in a trembling of the heart or palpitations and for melancholy or sadness, and he explains an aphrodisiac quality with reference to the herb being given to horses to help them breed. He must have read Bauhin's reference to comments by Simeon Seth that basil helps the heart, changing the grief of the soul caused by black bile into cheerfulness and joy, and the head, procuring sleep when steeped in water and drunk.

## CONTRARY OPINIONS IN THE TRADITION

What actually is the opinion of Dioscorides? His recommendations of the commonly known plant are mainly external: the juice for dimness of sight and rheums of the eyes; the plant or its seed as an agent to provoke sneezing (the eyes must be kept shut! Dalechamps thinks they have to be pressed); as an oil, warming and sharp, applied to the vulva as an emmenogogue and abortifacient and to treat constriction; finally for bites of the sea dragon and for scorpion stings. He relates how Africans, presumably living or travelling in areas populated by many scorpions, eat the herb to remain without pain if they get stung. The indication that, applied with barley, oil of roses and vinegar, it helps inflammations may seemingly be taken to refer to conditions of the lungs – Bock, for instance, recommends it for breathing difficulties and old coughs, by clearing thick and viscid humours.

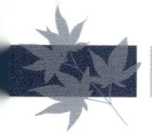

There are, however, internal uses recorded too in Dioscorides' work: the seed taken in drink corrects an excess of black bile, difficulty in urination through a diuretic action and flatulence. Basil will encourage the production of breast milk and helps to soften the stools for easier passing, an effect perhaps linked with the idea that it is a hard food to digest. Fuchs provides other classical sources – Philistio and Plistonicus – for the treatment of constipation, colic and dysentery, and adds that it helps to reduce the intensity of symptoms.

Serapio quotes Hunayn on the view of ancient physicians that basil evinces two contrary virtues: as a laxative for expulsion from the belly and, by the testimony of Hippocrates, as an astringent to retard the bowel motions. Andreas Vesalius, cited by Bauhin, reports that some regard the herb as astringent but the juice as laxative. Ibn Sina reckons the internal consumption of basil generates turbid and melancholic blood from its superfluous humidity, whereas Dioscorides considers it a treatment for black bile. Serapio relates the views of Rufus and Hunayn that basil has a drying effect, is converted quickly to yellow bile according to the former, and useful to dry up moisture after the consumption of unripe fruits in the latter's testimony. The Renaissance writers thus found the record on basil to be highly contrary. Fuch's recommendation, quoted verbatim in the following century by Bauhin, was

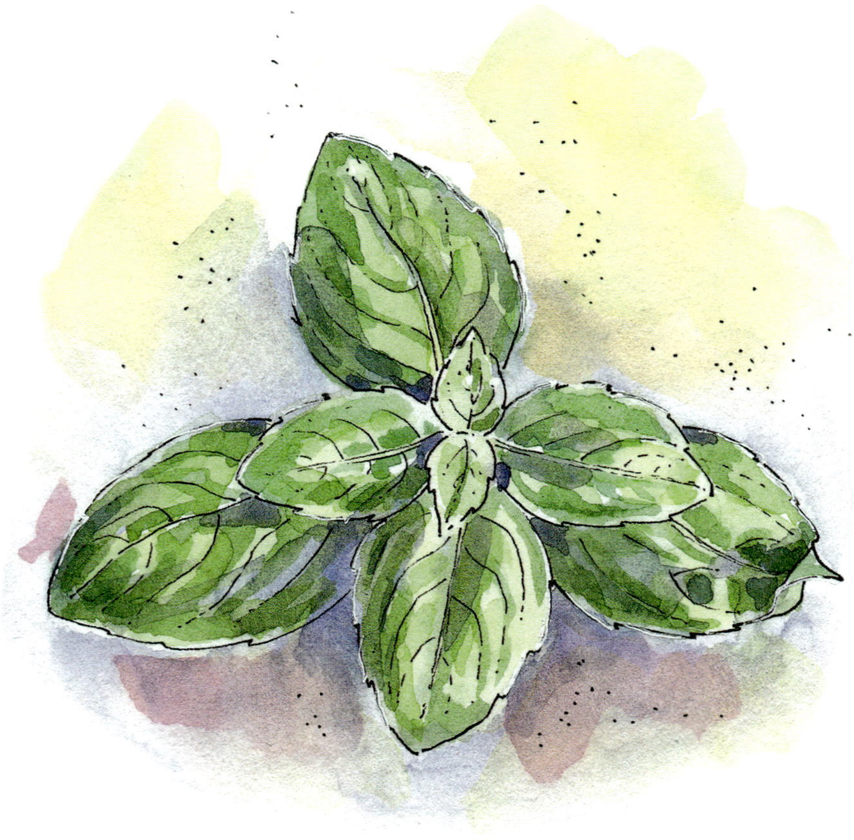

**Figure 22.2** *Ocimum basilicum*, basil.

to solve the contradictions between Pliny and Dioscorides by adhering to Galen's view that basil should be used externally only.

The herbal of Apuleius Platonicus lists two different basils: ozimum, which Fuchs derives from the Greek for 'fragrant', also called basilica and used for head pains, rheums in the eyes and for the kidneys; and herba basilica of three kinds, which treat poisonous bites. Further, the Salernitan herbal differentiates between ozimum, whose seeds are used, and two sorts of basilicum which have a warming and drying quality. Mattioli considers the name ocymum, from the Greek 'ocys' meaning 'swift growing' to relate to the first animal fodder to appear in spring such as green corn and vetch, and nothing to do with ocimum, the true basil. Of this he lists three kinds: those with large long, wide and thick leaves of a lemon apple scent, a smaller version named 'non garyophyllatum', which he matches to Dioscorides' description, to distinguish it from the third kind with the tiniest, narrowest leaves and the strongest scent, the 'clove' basil, the most cordial of all, called the 'native basil' (basilicum gentile) by the Italians. Bock also lays claim to this last kind as that used by the German apothecaries, a medicinally useful herb in contrast to 'Cato's basil', an inferior species and the one thought useless or harmful by classical writers. Mattioli's differentiation according to leaf size is supported by modern botany.

Dodoens also differentiates three kinds, two being large and small garden varieties of a hot and moist temperament, the third a wild basil of a hotter and drier quality. Bauhin notes the contrariness of basil also in relation to how it grows. He states that it likes being watered in the middle of the day under the heat of the sun; that it sprouts sooner if hot water is poured onto newly sown seed. However, quoting Costaeus, who speculates on the feebleness of the plant, which withers if not regularly watered, Bauhin affirms that heat normally relaxes bodies and increases feebleness. If basil requires heat due to a deficiency in its essence, this is countered by its pronounced scent, which is proof that heat flourishes there. Costaeus concludes that basil instead has a laxity of substance, causing its innate heat to be easily disrupted and requiring heat to support its constant need for nourishment.

Thus the story of basil, wild or garden, large or small, until the Age of Enlightenment. With such disagreement reigning, is it any surprise, then, that basil would have easily disappeared from the herbal pharmacopoeia?

Hill in the mid-18th century mentions the Ocymum vulgare majus as better than two or three other varieties but still little used, although it deserves to be much more: the fresh tea he holds as excellent against all obstructions, 'no simple is more effectual for gently promoting the menses and for removing complaints which naturally attend their stoppage'. This entry is copied by Robinson over a century later, although he does add uses for nausea and vomiting. It is absent in Cullen's review of the materia medica and many texts since. Wren renames basil Clinopodium hortus, a carminative occasionally used for mild nervous disorders.

## CURRENT VIEWS

Looking for references to basil in more current texts, the herbals which do not mention it are far greater in number than those which do. Bairacli Levy (1966) is fascinated by the herb and recommends it for culinary use, as an insecticide and as a powerful tonic stimulant and nerve remedy. It is advised for nausea, severe vomiting and indigestion, as well as topically for snake and spider bites and scorpion stings. Schauenberg & Paris (1977) list the infusion of the entire dried plant as a gastric antispasmodic, carminative and galactogogue.

Ody (1993) has a more extensive monograph, listing the actions of basil as antidepressant, antiseptic and tonic, stimulating the adrenal cortex and preventing vomiting, while acting as a carminative, febrifuge and expectorant. She proposes several combinations: as a tincture with wood betony and skullcap for nervous conditions, or with elecampane *Inula helenium* and hyssop *Hyssopus officinalis* for coughs and bronchitis; as a juice mixed with honey in a syrup for coughs, or the juice in a decoction of cinnamon *Cinnamomum zeylanicum* and cloves *Syzygium aromaticum* for chills. Topically, it can be mixed with honey for ringworm and itching skin or the fresh herb can be rubbed on to insect bites to stop itching and reduce inflammation. In combination with motherwort *Leonurus cardiaca* as an infusion it may be given after childbirth to prevent retention of the placenta. The essential oil of basil is also recommended as an inhalant for nervous exhaustion, mental fatigue, melancholy or fear, or, diluted with a carrier oil, it can be massaged in for nervous weakness, or rubbed onto the chest for asthma and bronchitis. The essential oil must not be used in pregnancy.

In the Unani Tibb tradition, basil is still used to raise the vital spirits in depression and grief, and acts as a stimulant nervine for mental clarity (Chishti 1988). Called Shahfaram in Arabic, it is classed as hot and dry in first degree, with cordial, cephalic, diuretic and nervine actions for use in flatulence, bad eyesight, melancholy, rheumatism and influenza. The physiomedicalist Menzies-Trull categorizes basil's primary action as an adaptogenic tonic to the autonomic nervous and cardiovascular systems. He gives a large list of actions and indications, including most from the tradition, whilst adding anti-inflammatory, antispasmodic, stimulant, hypotensive, diaphoretic, antifungal and immunomodulatory actions. Additional indications include sexual dysfunction and fertility problems (by increasing sperm count), exhaustion, motion sickness, withdrawal from cannabis and fungal infections of the skin. The herb influences tissue conditions by relaxing smooth muscle spasm and relieving irritable intestinal conditions. The dried herb can be given in doses of 3 g, or as 30 mL of the infusion or 4 mL of the tincture.

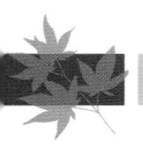

Pelikan emphasizes the warming, stimulating qualities of the mint family, but basil comes from the hotter and damper Hindustan, rather than from the Mediterranean. Nevertheless its stimulation of metabolism in various organs and systems are shared with other members of the family. In the case of basil, its warmth works on the digestive system, relieving spasms and generally calming, while also cleansing the womb to promote sexuality, fertility and lactation, and treating inflammations of the genitourinary system.

Among the phytotherapeutic texts, Schulz et al (1998) limit basil to digestive disorders such as bloating, presumably owing to the volatile oil which exerts a carminative action on the gut wall. Williamson references its actions as aromatic and carminative, with vermicidal activity substantiated in research, antibacterial in human trials on acne sufferers in India, in vitro evidence as an antiviral, and possibly a role in chemoprevention by increasing levels of enzymes responsible for detoxifying carcinogens. She also mentions an analgesic action and a use for diseases of the kidneys but no source is given.

There is newer evidence for an antibacterial action too. A sample of volatile oil (methyl chavicol 86%) was amongst volatile oils which showed antibacterial activity against 25 bacteria in vitro (Baratta et al 1998). A sample of volatile oil (linalool 32%, methyl chavicol 34%, 1,8-cineole 8.7%) showed antibacterial activity and the authors argue that this reflects the proportions of linalool and methyl chavicol rather than the 1,8-cineole as the other volatile oils in the experiment were less active yet had substantially higher concentrations of 1,8-cineole (Bouzouita et al 2003). A sample of volatile oil (linalool 55%, methyl chavicol 12%, methyl cinnamate 7.2%) was found to have a significant in vitro antibacterial action against three multidrug resistant isolates of *Staphylococcus aureus* and against *Staphylococcus epidermidis*, *Pseudomonas aeruginosa* and *Enterococcus faecalis* (Opalchenova & Obreshkova 2003). Significant antioxidant activity was shown in six test systems and the authors argue that this may underlie the antibacterial action (Gülçin et al 2007). In a study of the separate components of the oil, eugenol was found to have the highest antioxidant activity (Lee et al 2005b) whereas antioxidant activity was found to significantly correlate with total phenols (Javanmardi et al 2003). A high linalool sample of the oil showed an action in vitro against *Giardia lamblia*, which is a common parasite associated with diarrhoeal infections (de Almeida et al 2007). These experiments are in vitro and their clinical relevance is therefore limited, but they do support the use of basil as an antibacterial in the digestive tract. It may be that the apparently contradictory laxative and astringent actions on the bowel that basil was evidenced as having among the ancient Greek and Arabic writers can be explained by an antibacterial as well as a carminative action on the gut, which would correct the cause of diarrhoea or remedy the underlying condition supporting constipation.

To sum up, the aromatic basil clearly possesses a carminative action and is a remedy for the digestion. It may correct flatulence and colic, nausea and vomiting, soften stools for easier passing in costiveness but also have a role in treating diarrhoea. There is some evidence that it is a vermifuge, according to Williamson. Furthermore, there is a history of topical use, from the pustules of acne and the irritation and inflammation of insect bites to eye-washes and mouthwashes for oral ulceration. As a diuretic, basil may be useful to disinfect and flush through the urinary tract in conditions giving rise to difficult or painful micturition.

In the Arab tradition basil is valued among the cordial remedies. No mean store is placed on the aroma of a plant and its ability to 'cheer the heart and mind' troubled by worry, grief or painful life circumstances, although Parkinson saw no medical uses in this sweet-smelling herb. This may reflect its foreign origin, the reaction against Arabic medicine of the century preceding Parkinson and the polarized views from the classical tradition. Basil can be regarded as a nerve tonic to calm the system, lift the mood, help sleep and treat functional symptoms such as palpitations. It may have a place in chronic fatigue syndrome and similar deficiency states, especially where gastrointestinal symptoms or a depressed mood are evident, or where chronic pain is experienced, recalling Fuch's comment on the plant's ability to reduce the intensity of symptoms.

As a gynaecological remedy, basil is a gentle cleanser and strengthener of the womb, and may have a role in both facilitating conception and in managing labour. It may encourage breast milk in the nursing mother. It is also a herb to be used with caution, if at all, in pregnancy. Usefulness will depend on achievement of effects through oral doses, which will be more acceptable today than some of the topical applications of the past.

Basil should be considered for catarrh of the respiratory tract, to be used in combination with other herbs in conditions such as sinus congestion and head catarrh, earache, asthma and bronchitis and simple cough.

## RECOMMENDATIONS

- A calming nervine agent to reduce the pain of headaches and neuralgias, and counter depression, anxiety and irritability with tonic effects suitable for chronic fatigue syndromes.
- A topical remedy for pustules, insect bites, ulcers and as an insecticide.
- Flatulence, colic, nausea, vomiting, constipation and diarrhoea, irritable bowel syndrome, intestinal worms.

- A cleanser and strengthener of the womb, encouraging conception but to be used with caution in pregnancy. A reputed galactogogue action.
- An anticatarrhal and expectorant for the respiratory system, including sinus congestion and head catarrh, earache, asthma and bronchitis and simple cough.

Dosage: Culpeper does not go beyond a dose of 2 g of herb, although it is not clear whether fresh or dry is meant. Ibn Sina has a dose of 106 g of the juice, which seems excessive given the safety concerns voiced below. Other historical authors do not specify dosage. Miele et al (2001) estimate that a portion of pesto might contain as much as 10 g of fresh basil with a volatile oil content of 0.5%, therefore a fresh tincture 1:3 of basil taken in a dose of up to 5 mL three times daily delivers half this quantity of fresh herb and should remain within the bounds of safety as far as the ingested levels of methyl eugenol are concerned. We propose this dose, which is 1 mL larger than Menzies-Trull's dose of a tincture of unspecified strength and type, as the upper limit of dosage range for specific tincture of basil. Bartram suggests 2 teaspoons of fresh basil or 1 teaspoon of dried as an infusion, with not more than 3 cups taken daily. We advise that herbalists monitor carefully the responses to basil administered within these dosage ranges in order to better establish dose-related benefits, possible side-effects such as diarrhoea and with the purpose of better clarification of an effective and safe dosage range.

## CONSTITUENTS

Reviews: Bisset & Wichtl (2001), Williamson (2003), *Ocimum sanctum* (WHO 2002).

### Volatile oil

Total 0.4–1.1%, terpenes; oxygenated terpenes: linalool 15.6–32.2%; sesquiterpenes: bergamotene 1–20.2%; phenylpropanoids: methyl chavicol 0–4.2%, eugenol 0–22.2% (fresh, five cultivars, cultivated, Czech Republic) (Klimánková et al 2008).
Terpenes; oxygenated terpenes: linalool 0–85.4%, 1,8-cineole 0.4–13.8%; sesquiterpenes; phenylpropanoids: methyl chavicol 0–88.3%, eugenol 0–38.5% (16 samples, three varieties, one cultivar, cultivated, UK) (Grayer et al 1996).
Total 0.3–0.9%, terpenes: myrcene 0–0.9%, oxygenated terpenes: linalool 41.2–76.2% sesquiterpenes: bergamotene 0–3.4%, cadinol 1.8–7.5%; phenylpropanoids: methyl chavicol 0–41.4% (10 cultivars, Italy) (Marott et al 1996).
Total 0.4–1.5%, terpenes; oxygenated terpenes: linalool 2.7–60.2%, citral 0–65.6%; sesquiterpenes: phenylpropanoids: methyl chavicol 0–74.3%, methyl eugenol 0–34.2%, methyl cinnamate 0–63.1% (18 samples, cultivated, Turkey) (Telci et al 2006).
Oxygenated monoterpenes: linalool 19–37.6%, 1,8-cineole, 7.1–14.2%; phenylpropanoids: methyl chavicol 8.5% (one sample only), eugenol 3.3–24.4% (fresh, nine cultivars, including five used for pesto, cultivated, Italy) (Labra et al 2004).
Linalool 0–50%, 1,8-cineole 0–8.2%, geraniol 0–14.2%, methyl chavicol 0–93.4%, methyl eugenol 41.8% (two samples) (18 samples, cultivated, Spain) (Pascual-Villalobos & Ballesta-Acosta 2003).
Linalool 0–3.2%, methyl chavicol 83.8–88.6% (five samples, cultivated, Togo) (Sanda et al 1998).
Some volatile constituents are also found as aglycones (Politeo et al 2007).
The volatile oil combines both terpenoids such as linalool and phenylpropanoids such as methyl chavicol (estragole). The composition varies with geographical origin (Baritaux et al 1998, Kéita et al 2000) and time of harvest (Nacar & Tansi 2000). Five chemotypes are identified by Grayer et al (1996): high linalool, high methyl chavicol, linalool/methyl chavicol, linalool/eugenol, methyl chavicol/methyl eugenol. These categories were supported with the addition of linalool/methyl eugenol by Pascual-Villalobos & Ballesta-Acosta (2003). Methyl cinnamate is an important component is some samples (Lee et al 2005b), and a study in Turkey identified somewhat different categories: high linalool (mean 48%), high methyl chavicol (mean 68%), linalool 23%/methyl cinnamate 30%, high methyl cinnamate (mean 61%), methyl eugenol, high citral (mean 61%), methyl chavicol 42%/citral 34% (Telci et al 2006). In addition, a study of *O. basilicum*, *O. minimum*, *O. americanum* and *O. x citriodora* identified five categories – high linalool, high methyl chavicol, linalool/methylchavicol, high methyl cinnamate, citral/spathulenol – and showed that the categories did not correspond with the species (26 samples, cultivated, USA) (Vieira & Simon 2006).
The linalool 0.3–67.7% was found to be pure (*R*)(-)-linalool in 11/12 samples, and in 10/11 purchased oils whereas, in *Ocimum sanctum* the main enantiomer was (*S*)(+)-linalool (12 samples, cultivated, 11 purchased oils, Israel) (Ravid et al 1997).

### Triterpenes

Ursolic acid, oleanolic acid (Nicholas 1958).

### Phenolic acids

Total 2.3–6.5% (measured as gallic acid equivalents): rosmarinic acid (23 samples, Iran) (Javanmardi et al 2003).

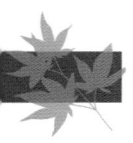

## RECOMMENDATIONS ON SAFETY

1. Use caution with oil of basil and do not use during pregnancy and lactation.
   Culpeper claims that basil is emmenagogue. Price & Price (1995) review different opinions and advise avoiding use of the aromatherapy oil in pregnancy and lactation.
2. Although basil contains constituents whose safety is under review as they have been found to be carcinogenic in animal studies, there is no evidence that this poses a risk in humans.

The phenylpropanoid volatile oils in basil are methyl chavicol (estragole), methyl eugenol and eugenol which are phenyl methyl ethers, also referred to as alkenylbenzenes (Bowles 2003). Another phenyl methyl ether, safrole, has been shown to be carcinogenic in animal tests which are reviewed by Tisserand & Balacs (1995). Safrole has been found to form DNA adducts in rats (Daimon et al 1998) and to be present in the tissues of smokers with oesophageal carcinoma who also chewed betel *Areca catechu*, which contains safrole (Lee et al 2005a).

Methyl eugenol has also been found to form DNA adducts (Burkey et al 2000). However, there are different viewpoints on the safety of methyl eugenol and estragole in foods, which depend on differing interpretation of the animal studies. The opinion of the Scientific Committee on Food (2001a, 2001b) of the European Commission is that the use of foods and spices containing methyleugenol and estragole should be reduced as no lower threshold of safety can be determined. However, other experts argue that the effects are dose dependent and that the low levels in diet are not a significant risk (Smith et al 2002). Rietjens et al (2008) present a model for risk assessment which attempts to calculate a margin of exposure and concludes that methyl eugenol is a low priority for risk management. In any risk assessment, there may be groups who are at particular risk, and Miele et al (2001) discuss this possibility in people who eat substantial quantities of pesto. The main cultivar used for pesto cv. Genovese Gigante can contain high levels of methyl eugenol. Twenty-two pots of young plants from one batch of seeds, all in the same soil, were distributed to 11 sites in Northern Italy. After 4 weeks, the concentration of methyl eugenol in the oils showed marked variation, from 10.6 to 100%, and eugenol was the other main constituent. The conclusion was that it would be safer to use plants higher than 16 cm, which are higher in eugenol as concentration of methyleugenol is higher in young plants below 6.5 cm (Miele et al 2001).

## REFERENCES

De Bairacli Levy J 1966 A herbal handbook for everyone. Faber & Faber, London.

Baratta MT, Dorman HJD, Deans SG 1998 Antimicrobial and antioxidant properties of some commercial essential oils. Flavour and Fragrance Journal 13:235–244.

Baritaux O, Richard H, Touche J, et al 1998 Effects of drying and storage of herbs and spices on the essential oil. Part I. Basil, *Ocimum basilicum* L. Flavour and Fragrance Journal 7:267–271.

Bisset NG, Wichtl M (eds) 2001 Herbal drugs and phytopharmaceuticals, 2nd edn. Medpharm, Stuttgart.

Bouzouita N, Kachouri F, Hamdi M, et al 2003 Antimicrobial activity of essential oils from Tunisian aromatic plants. Flavour and Fragrance Journal 18:380–383.

Bowles EJ 2003 The chemistry of aromatherapeutic oils. Allen & Unwin, Crows Nest, New South Wales.

Bown D 1995 Encyclopedia of herbs. Dorling Kindersley, London.

Burkey JL, Sauer JM, McQueen CA, et al 2000 Cytotoxicity and genotoxicity of methyleugenol and related congeners – a mechanism of activation for methyleugenol. Mutation Research 453:25–33.

Chang X, Alderson PG, Hollowood TA, et al 2007 Flavour and aroma of fresh basil are affected by temperature. Journal of the Science of Food and Agriculture 87:1381–1385.

Chishti GM 1988 The traditional healer. Thorsons, Wellingborough.

Culpeper N 1669 Pharmacopoeia Londinensis. London.

Daimon H, Sawada S, Asakura S, et al 1998 In vivo genotoxicity and DNA adduct levels in the liver of rats treated with safrole. Carcinogenesis 19:141–146.

De Almeida I, Alviano DS, Vieira DP, et al 2007 Antigiardial activity of Ocimum basilicum essential oil. Parasitology Research 101:443–452.

Diaz-Maroto MC, Palomo ES, Castro L, et al 2004 Changes produced in the aroma compounds and structural integrity of basil (*Ocimum basilicum* L) during drying. Journal of the Science of Food and Agriculture 84:2070–2076.

Grayer R, Kite GC, Goldstone FJ, et al 1996 Infraspecific taxonomy and essential oil chemotypes in sweet basil, *Ocimum basilicum*. Phytochemistry 43:1033–1039.

Grayer R, Vieira RJ, Price AM, et al 2004 Characterization of cultivars within species of *Ocimum* by exudate flavonoid profiles. Biochemical Systematics and Ecology 32:901–913.

Gülçin I, Elmastat M, Aboul-Enein HY 2007 Determination of antioxidant and radical scavenging activity of basil (*Ocimum basilicum* L. Family Lamiaceae) assayed by different methodologies. Phytotherapy Research 21:354–361.

Javanmardi J, Stushnoff C, Locke E, et al 2003 Antioxidant activity and total phenolic content of Iranian *Ocimum* accessions. Food Chemistry 83:547–550.

Kéita SM, Vincent C, Schmit J-P, et al 2000 Essential oil composition of *Ocimum basilicum* L., *O. gratissimum* L. and *O. suave* L. in the Republic of Guinea. Flavour and Fragrance Journal 15:339–341.

Klimánková E, Holadová K, Hajšlová J, et al 2008 Aroma profiles of five basil (*Ocimum basilicum* L.) cultivars grown under conventional and organic conditions. Food Chemistry 107:464–472.

Labra M, Miele M, Ledda B, et al 2004 Morphological characterization, essential oil composition and DNA genotyping of *Ocimum basilicum* L. cultivars. Plant Science 167:725–731.

Lee J-M, Liu T-Y, Wu D-C, et al 2005a Safrole–DNA adducts in tissues from esophageal cancer patients: clues to areca-related esophageal carcinogenesis. Mutation Research 565:121–128.

Lee S-J, Umano K, Shibamoto T, et al 2005b Identification of volatile components in basil (*Ocimum basilicum* L.) and thyme leaves (*Thymus vulgaris* L.) and their antioxidant properties. Food Chemistry 91:131–137.

Marotti M, Piccaglia R, Giovanelli E 1996 Differences in essential oil composition of basil (*Ocimum basilicum* L.) Italian cultivars related to morphological characteristics. Journal of Agricultural and Food Chemistry 44:3926–3929.

Miele M, Dondero R, Ciarallo G, et al 2001 Methyleugenol in *Ocimum basilicum* L. Cv. genovese gigante. Journal of Agricultural and Food Chemistry 49:517–521.

Nacar S, Tansi S 2000 Chemical components of different basil (*Ocimum basilicum* L.) cultivars grown in Mediterranean regions in Turkey. Israel Journal of Plant Sciences 48:109–112.

Nicholas HJ 1958 The sterol and triterpene content of the Labiatae family. Journal of the American Pharmaceutical Association 47:731–733.

Ody P 1993 The complete medicinal herbal. Dorling Kindersley, London.

Opalchenova G, Obreshkova D 2003 Comparative studies on the activity of basil – an essential oil from *Ocimum basilicum* L. – against multidrug resistant clinical isolates of the genera *Staphylococcus, Enterococcus* and *Pseudomonas* by using different test methods. Journal of Microbiological Methods 54:105–110.

Pascual-Villalobos MJ, Ballesta-Acosta MC 2003 Chemical variation in an *Ocimum basilicum* germplasm collection and activity of the essential oils on Callosobruchus maculatus. Biochemical Systematics and Ecology 31:673–679.

Podlech D 2001 Herbs and healing plants of Britain and Europe. Diamond Books, London.

Politeo O, Jukic M, Milos M 2007 Chemical composition and antioxidant capacity of free volatile aglycones from basil (*Ocimum basilicum* L.) compared with its essential oil. Food Chemistry 101:379–385

Price S, Price L 1995 Aromatherapy for health professionals. Churchill Livingstone, Edinburgh.

Ravid U, Putievsky E, Katzir I, et al 1997 Enantiomeric composition of linalol in the essential oils of Ocimum species and in commercial basil oils Flavour and Fragrance Journal 12:293–296.

Rietjens IMCM, Slob W, Galli C, et al 2008 Risk assessment of botanicals and botanical preparations intended for use in food and food supplements: emerging issues. Toxicology Letters 180:131–136

Sanda K, Koba K, Nambo P, et al 1998 Chemical investigation of *Ocimum* species growing in Togo. Flavour and Fragrance Journal 13:226–232.

Schauenberg P, Paris F 1977 Guide to medicinal plants. Lutterworth Press, Guildford.

Schnaubelt K 1999 Medical aromatherapy. Frog, Berkeley, CA.

Schulz V, Haensel R, Tyler VE 1998 Rational phytotherapy. Springer-Verlag, Berlin.

Scientific Committee on Food 2001a Opinion of the scientific committee on food on methyleugenol. Online. Available: http://europa.eu.int/comm/food/fs/sc/scf/out102 en.pdf.

Scientific Committee on Food 2001b Opinion of the scientific committee on food on estragole. Online. Available: http://europa.eu.int/comm/food/fs/sc/scf/out104 en.pdf.

Sifola MI, Barbieri G 2006 Growth, yield and essential oil content of three cultivars of basil grown under different levels of nitrogen in the field. Scientia Horticulturae 108:408–413.

Simon JE, Morales MR, Phippen WB, et al 1999 Basil: a source of aroma compounds and a popular culinary and ornamental herb. Purdue Agricultural Research Programs, Purdue University, Indiana. Online. Available: http://www.hort.purdue.edu/newcrop/proceedings1999/pdf/v4-499.pdf 24 March 2009.

Smith RL, Adams TB, Doull J, et al 2002 Safety assessment of allylalkoxybenzene derivatives used as flavouring substances – methyl eugenol and estragole. Food and Chemical Toxicology 40:851–870.

Telci I, Bayram E, Yılmaz G, et al 2006 Variability in essential oil composition of Turkish basils (*Ocimum basilicum* L.). Biochemical Systematics and Ecology 34:489–497.

Tisserand R, Balacs T 1995 Essential oil safety. Churchill Livingstone, Edinburgh.

Vieira RF, Simon JE 2006 Chemical characterization of basil (Ocimum spp.) based on volatile oils. Flavour and Fragrance Journal 21:214–221.

Williamson E 2003 Potter's herbal cyclopaedia. CW Daniel, Saffron Walden.

WHO 2002 WHO monographs on selected medicinal plants, vol 2. World Health Organization, Geneva.

# CHAPTER 23
# *Paeonia officinalis*, paeony

## DESCRIPTION

**Family: Paeoniaceae**                                          **Part used: root**

*Paeonia* are long-lived, hardy, robust herbaceous perennials. The two main European species are *Paeonia officinalis* L. subsp. *officinalis*, 'female paeony', which is found from France across to the Balkans and *Paeonia mascula* (L.) Mill., 'male paeony', which is found around the Mediterranean and in Greece, Turkey, Azerbaijan, Iraq and Iran (Halda 2004). A remnant population of introduced *Paeonia mascula* persists on Steep Holm, an island in the Bristol Channel (Stace 1991). Both species contain several subspecies, which are described and illustrated by Halda (2004) and Page (2005). The two species hybridize if grown together. Both species are considered to be close relatives to *Paeonia lactiflora* (Page 2005). The *Flora of Turkey* (Davis 1965) gives six *Paeonia* species, including *Paeonia mascula* but not including *Paeonia officinalis*.

*Paeonia mascula* has stiff stems (to 75 cm) which bear large compound leaves and the plant forms large clumps. Solitary, large, single, red terminal flowers with up to 10 petals and numerous yellow stamens occur in April. Three to five smooth, curved seed pods split to reveal bright pink unfertilized ovules and shiny, blue-black fertilized seeds.

*Paeonia officinalis* is similar with deeply cut divided leaves. The single red flowers occur slightly later and black seeds are formed.

The tuberous roots of each species are different. *Paeonia mascula* has long thick spreading roots. *Paeonia officinalis* has round tubers joined by root strings.

**Other species used**: *Paeonia lactiflora* Pallas syn. *Paeonia albiflora*, Chi shao yao, Radix Paeonia rubra is an important herb in traditional Chinese medicine (Dharmananda 2002) and Kanpo, Japanese herbal medicine (Kuwacki 1990). It is a very hardy, herbaceous perennial with stems up to 80 cm high, which bear large, white aromatic flowers in May (Halda 2004). It is native to Siberia, Tibet, Mongolia and northern China but has been sourced from cultivation in China for many years. It was introduced into Europe in 1800 and is the ancestor of most garden paeonies currently grown. There are numerous cultivars and natural hybrids which range from white through to deepest red. Other related Chinese species are used such as *Paeonia veitchii* Lynch (Yamamoto 1988).

Tree paeonies, Mu dan pi, are also widely used in traditional Chinese medicine and Kanpo and are hardy, deciduous, ornamental shrubs. There are no European species although many varieties are cultivated in Europe. Botanical identification is complex because wild strains are variable in form, hybridize and interbreed with cultivated specimens (Page 2005). There are complexes (groups of very closely related species) such as *Paeonia spontanea* and *Paeonia delavayii*. The Feng Dan, Phoenix, group are the most widely grown for medicinal use. As these have been grown for centuries, these have been assigned the specific name of *ostii* but there is no definite finding of *Paeonia ostii* in the wild (McLewin & Chen 2006).

### Quality

Concentration of paeoniflorin is lower in boiled *Paeonia lactiflora*, Bai shao yao, Radix Paeonia alba (Cai et al 1994). According to Peng et al (2008) the term Radix Paeonia alba was not used to distinguish processed plant material until the 20th century whereas previous distinctions were based on the colour of either root or flower. The root is cultivated in different parts of China from Radix Paeonia rubra, Chi shao yao, and is sometimes treated with sulphur (Li et al 2009b).

## WHICH PAEONY?

Dioscorides (III 140) identified two forms of paeony used in medicine: the male, with leaves like those of walnut, the root the thickness of a finger, white and astringent to taste, and the female, with leaves split like those of Cretan Alexanders and a root with seven to eight tubers like acorns. These are good descriptions of *Paeonia mascula* and *Paeonia officinalis*, respectively. With the description of the pods on the top of the stems like almonds, containing red seeds like pomegranate and five or six black seeds tending to purple, we have a clear and unequivocal description of the medicinal plant. This description is also given by Ibn Sina.

THE WESTERN HERBAL TRADITION

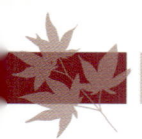

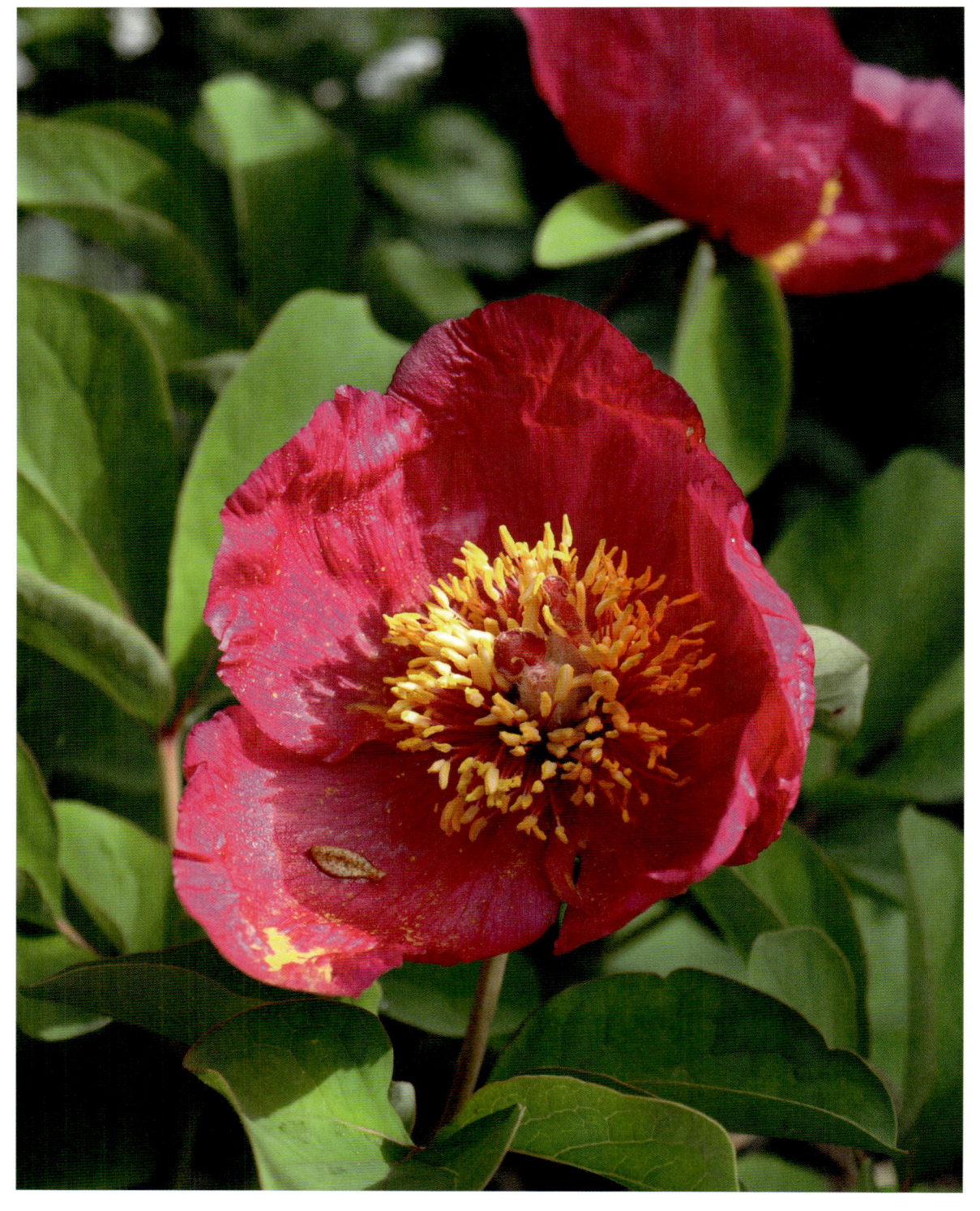

**Figure 23.1** *Paeonia mascula*, wild paeony (a garden in Yorkshire, May).

The Renaissance authors give similar descriptions and generally agree that the female paeony *Paeonia officinalis* is commonly grown but the male paeony is unusual. Turner records seeing the female paeony in England, Germany and Antwerp. Fuchs distinguishes the two types and states that they are mainly found in gardens but also occur in the wild in the mountains in France, Switzerland and from the Tyrol in northern Italy to northern Albania, which interestingly is the same as the distribution given by Halda (2004) for *Paeonia officinalis*. Mattioli confirms that it is usually the female paeony that is seen and that he had seen the male paeony only twice, one sent from Germany and one sent from the botanic garden at Pisa. Dodoens describes both paeonies as garden plants and his description is from observation as he likens the divided leaves of the female paeony to the leaves of angelica or lovage, and observes that the flowers of the female are a less intense red than those of the male paeony. He highlights the yellow threads or thrums (stamens), four great cods or husks which open when ripe, the red lining, polished black seeds and long, fragrant root.

According to Stern (1946), *Paeonia officinalis* and *Paeonia mascula* were the only species described until others were added by Charles de l'Ecluse. His descriptions of paeonies in *Rariorum Plantarum Historia*, published in 1601, include *Paeonia peregrina* and several more unnamed paeonies. His name was given to the white peony *Paeonia clusii* (Halda 2004), which was discovered by in Crete by Pierre Belon between 1546 and 1549. Stern gives a detailed account of the nomenclature of the paeony and explains that in 1753 Linnaeus considered the male and female paeony to be the same species. He named them *Paeonia officinalis* var. *feminea* and var. *mascula*. In 1768 Philip Miller described the male paeony as *Paeonia mascula* and this name has remained in use, and the female paeony retained the name *Paeonia officinalis*. There are three other subspecies, so the correct name is *Paeonia officinalis* subsp. *officinalis* but *Paeonia officinalis* will usually suffice (Burkhardt's Web Project 2006).

Gerard gives a similar description to Dodoens and describes the double red and pink varieties already being grown in London gardens. Parkinson gives accurate illustrations, and then discourses at length on how varied the progeny of seed from one plant can be as both single and double plants are produced. He also refers to the 'the doubtful female paeony', which has features of both *Paeonia mascula* and *Paeonia officinalis* and is probably a hybrid between the two. Parkinson comments on the attractive intermingling of the black seeds and 'crimson grains'. Culpeper gives a similar vivid description of the two species but is the only author to ascribe male and female properties to the respective plants. The authors make no distinction between the usage of the two types. In places, *Paeonia mascula* is preferred but Parkinson confirms the experience of Turner that it is mainly *Paeonia officinalis* that is cultivated and therefore is in common usage. Paeony fell out of use in Europe and there has been almost no analysis of the constituents of either *Paeonia mascula* or *Paeonia officinalis*.

## PAEONIA LACTIFLORA

The commercially available paeony in Britain is *Paeonia lactiflora*, Chi shao yao, Radix Paeonia rubra, a central herb in traditional Chinese medicine. It has been increasingly used by western herbalists in Britain in recent years. I began to use it in the 1990s partly as it was one of the herbs included in an eczema mixture that was investigated in children (Sheehan & Atherton 1992). In this context, the action 'to clear heat and cool blood' (Junying 1991) was particularly interesting as eczema, psoriasis and other hot skin conditions can be difficult to treat. I also use it for heat in, for example, hot flushes when the woman is a hot person. A further influence on usage in western herbal medicine is the recommendation by Trickey (1998) for use with liquorice *Glycyrrhiza glabra* in polycystic ovaries, endometriosis, failure of ovulation and menopausal symptoms. This can be associated with the action 'to remove stagnant blood' (Junying 1991) and paeony is therefore indicated for period pains, lack of periods, scant periods and polycystic ovary disease. It is not used in pregnancy or for period pains due to 'blood-cold'.

Like rose, paeony seems to be a herb which was widely used but then fell by the wayside. The sources on paeony build on the recommendations of Dioscorides and Galen but fade away in the 19th century. This must reflect diminished usage and indeed Cullen states that no writer or practitioner was found to testify to its virtues from their experience. Now that *Paeonia lactiflora* has entered into widespread usage, one can ask whether *Paeonia mascula* or *Paeonia officinalis* would be equally useful or even better as they could be sourced fresh. On the other hand, *Paeonia lactiflora* is obtainable from cultivation and has been the subject of a substantial body of research (Bone 1996).

## SEEDS, ROOTS AND FLOWERS

The decoction of root in wine is recommended by Dioscorides for 'belly aches', the jaundiced, kidney disease and 'those smarting in the bladder'. Astringency is referred to in the taste and Dioscorides states that boiled down in wine it stops diarrhoea, advice which is given by Galen too. The recommendation of an extract in wine is repeated by later authors. A compound medicine of 76 ingredients, including paeony, Potio sancti Pauli, is given in *The Trotula* for disease of the head and was used for 'epileptics, analeptics, cataleptics' with wine in which mixed paeony had been boiled (Green 2001). Pliny refers to use of paeony root as a food. He gives this after referring to a decoction in wine for the trachea and stomach, and with an astringent action on the bowels. Macer makes a similar suggestion of a mixture in honey water with powdered coriander for the stomach, spleen and kidney gravel. Macer and the Salernitan herbal suggest external use of the powder placed on the anus with a cloth for tenesmus caused by cold. Hildegard says that the crushed root in wine will chase away the tertian and quartan fevers, while the root in flour with lard or poppyseed oil as a porridge will act as a preventative.

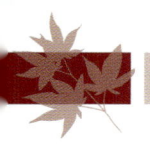

Dioscorides, Pliny and Ibn Sina make recommendations for use of the black seeds or the unfertilized red ovules in digestive and urinary problems, in menstrual problems and in nightmares. This is difficult to interpret as the yield of seeds would be small. In addition, there is no research on their constituents, and I have not felt comfortable about recommending the seed. It can be hard to decide whether later authors merely copied Dioscorides and Galen or had used these preparations. However, Culpeper states that powder of the black seeds could be purchased, and Miller lists the official preparations as syrup of flowers, Syrupus Paeoniae compositus, the simple water and the mixed water, and powders of both seed and root. The seeds were listed in a supplement to the German Pharmacopoeia in 1926 (Bisset & Wichtl 2001). Dioscorides and Ibn Sina recommend the seeds eaten to relieve gnawing in the stomach, and eaten or drunk to take away the beginnings of stones in the bladder in children (children can be subject to stones if dehydrated due to inadequate water supply). I have disregarded these indications as there are many common herbs that are more commonly used.

For paeony root and seed, Serapio gives the same qualities as Galen: that it is of subtle parts, a little astringent but with a sweetness that becomes sharp and biting on

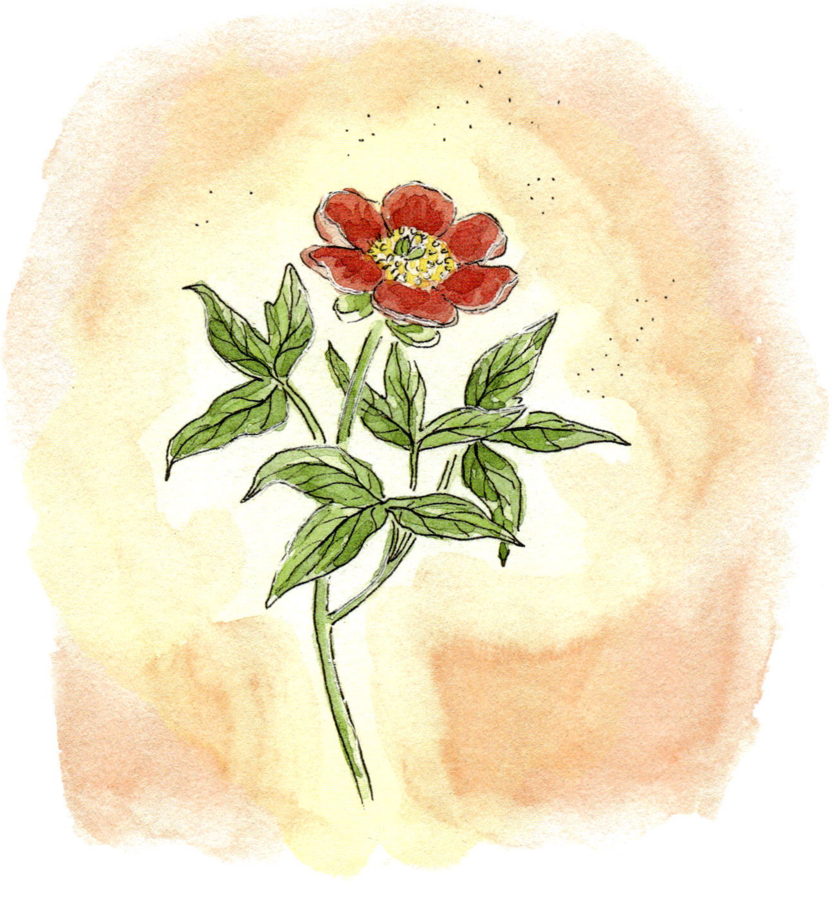

**Figure 23.2** *Paeonia* spp., wild paeony.

chewing. These same qualities are given by Fuchs and Parkinson, who both refer to Galen. Maybe using a different source, Serapio then describes paeony as slightly heating, strongly astringent and a herb which cleanses and strengthens. It is considered to treat the liver and kidneys because it is sharp and slightly bitter, and astringent so useful in fluxes. Ibn Sina describes the paeony as hot and dry, but not greatly, while the Salermitan herbal describes paeony as hot and dry in the second degree. Perhaps following Ibn Sina, paeony is described as dispersing and cleansing with the ability to dispel humours. Macer also describes it as hot and dry in the second degree and states that this derives from Hippocrates and Galen, but that others say the root is cold. The Salernitan herbal advises use of the decoction in wine when it is impossible to urinate, a use repeated by Fuchs.

Bauhin summarizes the texts of Dioscorides and Galen, and notes the action in clearing obstructions of the kidney and bladder. The indications given above may be the reasons underlying the long list of indications given by Commission E for paeony flower (Bisset & Wichtl 2001). Although it is included amongst unapproved herbs, it is listed for disease of the skin and mucous membranes, fissures, anal fissures associated with haemorrhoids, gout, arthritis, ailments of the respiratory tract, in combinations for nervous conditions, heart trouble and gastritis. The root is listed as antispasmodic but is used in combinations for arthritis, the gastrointestinal tract, the cardiovascular system, neurasthenia, neuralgia, migraine, allergy and in tonics. Bisset & Wichtl (2001) suggest that the flowers can be used to enhance the appearance of herbs teas but caution that they can only be stored for less than a year as they fade rapidly.

Other recent authors focus on the antispasmodic action. Cook refers to the 'showy paeonia of our gardens' whose root is mildly relaxing and antispasmodic. He advises an infusion of 1 oz in 1 pint of warm water taken freely in spasms and colics of children to remove flatus. He considers it too mild to fulfil its previous reputation for use in epilepsy and chorea. However, Wren gives it as tonic and antispasmodic and thus successfully employed in convulsive and spasmodic nervous affections such as chorea, epilepsy and spasms. Menzies-Trull gives the main action as antispasmodic but adds uses as a bitter and cholagogue with a blood thinning action. He gives the indications of menopause and fibroids. Chevallier discusses *Paeonia lactiflora* and focuses on the antispasmodic action and sedative action in whooping cough, nervous irritation and advises use as a suppository in intestinal and anal spasm.

Root and seeds are advised in excessive menstruation. Culpeper generally prefers the root. Dioscorides makes no distinction between the two types of paeony. He recommends the root for women 'not cleansed after childbirth'. He specifies a decoction of the amount of an almond to induce menstruation. This is repeated by Turner, who ascribes the same advice to Galen, adding that Galen recommended taking the root as a powder to bring on the menses. The version of Galen by Mattioli gives a preparation of the seed well crushed, sifted and sprinkled and the quantity of an almond in mead to provoke the menses. It is not clear whether the powdered seed is taken in mead or kept in mead and then taken when needed. This is analogous to use of *Paeonia lactiflora* and I would feel happier continuing with use of *Paeonia lactiflora* than seed. Dioscorides then advises up to 15 black seeds in hydromel or wine for suffocation of the womb and uterine pains. Pliny uses the phrase 'healing to the uterus'. Culpeper includes both root or powdered black seed for women not sufficiently cleansed after childbirth. In the Salernitan herbal the advice for use to cleanse the womb is as a fumigation. In this same text use in childbirth is more specific, suggesting 15 black seeds for 'deliverance of the bed of the child in her womb'. This must refer to deliverance of the afterbirth and could deserve further research to support this recommendation. Ibn Sina, however, who gives the dose as 600–900 mg, puts the indication differently as he suggests the seeds when menstruation does not return after childbirth.

## CONVULSIONS AND NIGHTMARES

Following its general 'cleansing' role and its specific use in menstruation, paeony has a more extraordinary application in the literature for nightmares and potential use in epilepsy. The name comes from a powerful god and suggests a deeper meaning to the herb. Paeon, an ancient god of healing, is famous for healing the wounds of the gods themselves when they foolishly become embroiled in the world of humans. When the gods took to the field in the Trojan war, he healed Ares, god of war, wounded fighting on the side of the Trojans. He gave Ares 'such sovereign medicines that as soon the pain was qualified … as fast as rennet curdles milk' and the sides of the wound were reunited (Nicoll 1956). Paeon used herbs to heal. In fact Macurdy (1912) argues that the word is associated with the Paioniae tribal group of northern Greece, who were designated herb-gatherers as they were from the north.

Both Dioscorides and Pliny refer to the familiar 15 black seeds. Dioscorides says simply for 'those who gasp from nightmares,' expressed by Turner as 'against the strangling of the nightmare'. Pliny, for the seeds taken in wine, has a more fanciful expression 'this plant also prevents the mocking delusions that the Fauns bring on us in our sleep'. The paeony growing on mountains, he says, was the first plant to be discovered by Paeon. Given the difficulty in interpreting the terms for diseases which were not described by our authors but have now fallen out of use, it is interesting that nightmares were considered to need description by a number of authors in this context. Dodoens describes the 'Night Mare' as, 'a disease wherein men seem to be oppressed in the night, as with some great burden and sometimes to be overcome with their enemies'. Parkinson reckons the powdered seed to be taken twice a day for nightmares, 'a suppressing both of voice and breath, and oppressing the body as it were, with some heavy burden, striving to be eased thereof, but seeming not to be able to call for help'. Fuchs refers to a high dose of 4 drachms (16 g) for 'the evil of the mind'. Dodoens adds a recommendation that it is 'good against melancholic dreams' and Parkinson, followed by Culpeper, advises paeony for melancholic people, who are more subject to nightmares than others, and for melancholic dreams. Ibn Sina gives the dose as 900 mg in honey water in this context. Gerard dwells at length on the question of one of the names given by Pliny, 'aglaophotis', which he says refers to the shiny seeds which make the plant visible at night so that it can be gathered then by shepherds. Apuleius also states that paeony is found mostly by shepherds in a far off place and the seeds are like a little lamp at night if the moon is bright. Pliny refers to collection at night lest the woodpecker of Mars attack the eye of the collector so as to protect the plant. The woodpecker was a bird of Roman augury so this may have had a more symbolic meaning. This tale is repeated from Pliny in the French version of Mattioli with the comment that the passage is invention and perhaps incorrectly transcribed. Gerard summarily dismisses the story as one of the fanciful tales of the ancients and assures us that paeony may be picked at any time of day or night. To conclude, root of paeony could be used for nightmares.

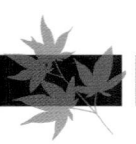

Quincy includes paeony with cardiacs and cephalics under nervous simples and considers it a good cephalic, while the flower is useful in all nervous distempers and convulsions in children. He acknowledges that the root has a broad action as an aperient and is therefore diuretic, detergent and alexipharmic and therefore included in the College Plague Water.

Paeony has a tradition for use in convulsions. Beginning with Galen, the external use of root and seeds is recommended in epilepsy. The term 'epilepsy' or the 'falling sickness' can be interpreted in various ways and maybe the term seizure is more useful. However, accounts were given of seizures which were recognized as separate from the convulsions associated with fever (Aronson 1999) and seizures were carefully described in ancient Mesopotamia (van de Goot & ten Berge 2001). Apuleius gives us the somewhat mysterious statement 'lie the lunatic down and place the herb on him, he will immediately get up healed'. Hildegard makes a similar claim. 'If the person goes out of his mind, as if he knows nothing and is lying deranged in ecstasy, dip the seed of the paeony in honey and put it on his tongue. The powers of the peony will ascend to the brain and stir it up, so that he will quickly return to his own mind and receive his understanding'. The Salernitan herbal quotes Galen as saying that it helps epilepsy if worn around the neck. Macer recommends the root in wine but agrees that the root hung about a person's neck 'will save him without doubt in 15 days'. Turner gives the original discussion by Galen of the use of root of paeony hung round the neck of children to prevent 'the falling-sickness'. Galen describes how a boy 'did not fall into the sickness' for 8 months until the paeony root fell off and he was ill again. Galen then carried out an experiment by removing the root. The boy was immediately ill again so Galen replaced it with a large piece of root, after which the boy had no more of the problem. Fuchs and Bauhin also give this account but it is Turner who goes on to say that he himself tried the experiment on two children, one in London and one at Syon House, the home of his patron Lord Somerset. Turner found it effective in children. Dodoens too refers to use of the root especially in children. Wood writes that 'several of my students have verified this usage with children, adults and even dogs'.

This example serves to highlight problems with translation and thus safe usage.

Other authors emphasize use of paeony root as a medicine. According to Turner, Galen ascribes the effectiveness of paeony to its drying power. Fuchs describes it as fiercely drying. Bauhin perceives the action of paeony as to disperse and consume the phlegm humour, which causes the collapse of the palate of the mouth. The idea has been cast aside that phlegm, the cold and moist humour, rises and accumulates in the brain, eventually disturbing the physiological balance and causing convulsions. Bauhin describes paeony as heating and drying and gives a dose of 2 drachms (8 g) in white wine for use in epilepsy. He further recommends the distilled water of the finely cut root taken in the morning before breaking fast. He points out the variable effectiveness of paeony because the disease may occur in different strengths and the herb will vary depending on where it was grown. Parkinson quotes Mattioli as wondering whether this is the same paeony as Galen used as it has not lived up to its powerful reputation. Parkinson, whose text is used by Culpeper, says he has not found it useful but has used it in older people with epilepsy. He gives a recipe, 'clean fresh male root, pound and infuse in Madeira or fortified wine for at least 24 hours, and take morning and night for a number of days before and after full moon'. He recommends taking paeony in a posset, a hot drink with milk and ale, with betony *Stachys officinalis*.

The recommendation of use hung about the neck reappears with Miller who gives the recommendation of root or seed used in this manner for convulsions during teething in infants. Quincy says the necklace is much esteemed by 'good women' for this purpose. Serapio explains this procedure works because, according to Abraham, the son of Solomon the Israelite, the fumigation cures epilepsy. In the version given by Mattioli, Galen argues that either 'certain parts flowing from the root and then attracted through inspiration, thus tend to the affected places, or the air from the root [is] changed and altered constantly'. We can agree with Galen, Serapio and Fuchs in looking for a rational explanation of this procedure. As Fuchs observes, the odour of fresh paeony root is characteristic and quite strong. However, unexplained diseases or events attract inexplicable remedies, in this case the use of paeony as an amulet (Domínguez-Rodríguez & González-Hernández 2007). Use of an amulet in seizures was advocated by John of Gaddesden in the 14th century when he said 'this species of devil is not cast out save by prayer and fasting. The patient should then write out this gospel and wear it about his neck and he will be cured' (Aronson 1999). The envious gaze or evil eye is invoked as the cause of inexplicable disease especially in young children (Lykiardopoulos 1981). This practice continues today with the current widespread usage of blue and white beads as amulets to protect from the evil eye in modern day Turkey. The shiny seeds of paeony might be threaded as a necklace but this cannot be advocated because the rational fear of infants eating seeds overrides any other considerations. Hippocrates would not have agreed with the use of amulets as he argued that that 'those using the divinity as a pretext and screen of their own inability to afford any assistance have given out that the disease is sacred' (Aronson 1999).

Control of seizures remains a challenge (Aylward 2008) and this is a condition where it would be valuable if herbal practitioners were able to work alongside medical practitioners as it may be that paeony could have an adjunctive role in epilepsy. It is noteworthy that paeony is used in traditional Chinese medicine in epilepsy alongside orthodox treatments but clinical trials were considered to be of poor methodology (Li et al 2009a). Investigating the safety profile of paeony, a study carried out in rats found that the absorption of phenytoin was slowed (Chen et al 2001). Whereas another study by the same team found no interaction between paeony and valproic acid in a crossover study on six volunteers (Chen et al 2000).

## RETURNING TO USAGE IN GYNAECOLOGICAL CONDITIONS

Chevallier discusses usage of *Paeonia lactiflora* in 'the four things soup', a women's tonic for cramps, pain and dizziness. A recent innovative study has looked at whether there is any pharmacological basis for the pairing of herbs in Chinese medicine (Yang et al 2009), which reminds us of the importance of considering the tradition from which *Paeonia lactiflora* arises. The use for women, which does have some parallels with the recommendations from the authors for use in menstrual problems, returns us to the main usage of paeony which is for gynaecological conditions: in endometriosis, polycystic ovaries, irregular periods and menopausal symptoms, particularly when the woman is hot and congested. Wood gives a thorough discussion of the herb and links the western concept of excess oestrogen with the eastern concept of excess heat. He specifically recommends paeony in acneiform sores on the chin, one of the symptoms of polycystic ovary syndrome that women find upsetting. I have used it in other skin conditions that are affected by the menstrual cycle such as herpes simplex. The further concept of stagnation seems particularly relevant in polycystic ovary disease and endometriosis.

A problem of the menopause can be anger, and I find paeony particularly useful for this. In a sense this might link back to the antispasmodic action of paeony and the use in nightmares. Rather than perceive menopausal symptoms as associated only with hormonal changes, they could be an expression of disruption within the body as a whole. It has been found that women often find the mood changes associated with the menopause more bothersome that the physical symptoms (Utian 2005). The anger or moodiness in the menopause can feel as if it is coming from deep inside, like the anger associated with premenstrual tension, and it is more useful to see it as disturbed energy rather than literally caused by hormonal changes. This leads to use of nervines, liver remedies, cooling remedies and paeony or *Astragalus membranaceus* for excess heat. I would agree with the assertion of Wood that it is useful in women in the menopause who are pink, warm and overweight. The link with liver stagnation is expressed by the way in changes in diet alone can result in substantial improvement in menopausal symptoms, while the idea of 'escaping yang' links with the way in which increased exercise, which keeps the blood moving, can lead to fewer hot flushes.

## RECOMMENDATIONS

- The recommendations are for use of *Paeonia lactiflora*, Chi shao yao, Radix Paeonia rubra.
- It is useful in menstrual problems particularly associated with inflammation, such as endometriosis, and with congested conditions, such as polycystic ovary syndrome.
- The cooling nature of paeony makes it particularly useful in eczema and psoriasis, and skin problems associated with the menstrual cycle such as herpes and acne.
- It is useful for menopausal symptoms and, given the discussion of nightmares, could be especially good for night sweats.

# THE WESTERN HERBAL TRADITION

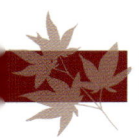

- It could have a role as an adjunct where epilepsy is proving difficult to control.
- There can be no recommendations whatsoever for use of seed without further research into their constituents.
- It would be useful to consider cultivation of *Paeonia officinalis*.

Dosage: Junying (1991) recommends 3–10 g as a daily dose.

## RECOMMENDATIONS ON SAFETY

- Do not use in pregnancy.

Authors since Dioscorides have recommended paeony for inducing periods and none of the species should be used in pregnancy although Trickey (1998) considers it safe in pregnancy.

## CONSTITUENTS

Reviews: *Paeonia lactiflora* (Bone 1996), *Paeonia lactiflora* (Tang & Eisenbrand 1992), *Paeonia lactiflora* and *Paeonia suffruticosa* (Williamson 2003).

### Volatile oils

*Paeonia mascula* subsp. *hellenica*, total 0.13%, *Paeonia clusii*, total 0.1%, *Paeonia parnassica*, total 0.14%: salicylaldehyde 74.6%, thymol, myrtanal. Paeonol in *Paeonia clusii* and *Paeonia parnassica* only (root, wild, Greece) (Papandreou et al 2002).

Paeonol is found in *Paeonia suffruticosa*. Most studies state that paeonol is not found in herbaceous species such as *Paeonia lactiflora* but it was found in *Paeonia veitchii* in one study (Lin et al 1996b).

### Monoterpene glycosides

*Paeonia lactiflora*, paeoniflorin 0.5–5.8%, albiflorin, benzoyl-paeoniflorin, oxypaeoniflorin and related compounds (Tang & Eisenbrand 1992).
*Paeonia lactiflora*, paeoniflorin 2.1% (Kamiya et al 1997), paeoniflorin 0.8% (Zhou et al 1998).
*Paeonia veitchii*, paeoniflorin 5.1%; *Paeonia lactiflora*, paeoniflorin 5.1–4.6% (12 samples extracted into water, Radix Paeonia rubra, commercial, Britain) (Cai al 1994).
*Paeonia veitchii*, paeoniflorin 1.26%, albiflorin, oxypaeoniflorin, benzoylalbiflorin (Lin et al 1996b).
In *Paeonia lactiflora*, paeoniflorin content was found to be highest in November (Yamamoto 1988) and concentration was higher in 1-year-old plants than in 3-year-old plants, and high in *Paeonia tenuifolia* (Tang & Eisenbrand 1992).

### Triterpenoids

*Paeonia lactiflora*, 0.025%, seven: oleanolic acid, hederagenin, betulinic acid (Kamiya et al 1997).

### Phenolic acids

*Paeonia veitchii*, benzoic acid 0.07%, gallic acid 0.06% (5 samples, commercial, Taiwan) (Lin et al 1996b).

### Gallotannins

Pentagalloylglupyranose 0–0.96% (Cai et al 1994).
*Paeonia suffruticosa*, paeonol 0.9–2.2%, gallic acid, paeoniflorin 0.3–1%, benzoylpaeoniflorin, oxypaeoniflorin (10 commercial samples) (He et al 2006).

## REFERENCES

Aronson SM 1999 He hath the falling sickness. Medicine and Health Rhode Island 82:151–152.

Aylward RL 2008 Epilepsy: a review of reports, guidelines, recommendations and models for the provision of care for patients with epilepsy. Clinical Medicine 8:433–438.

Bisset NG, Wichtl M (eds) 2001 Herbal drugs and phytopharmaceuticals, 2nd edn. Medpharm, Stuttgart.

Bone K 1996 Clinical applications of Ayurvedic and Chinese herbs. Phytotherapy Press, Warwick, Queensland.

Burkhardt's Web Project 2006 Paeonia – the peony database. Online. Available: http://www.paeon.de/name/kurz/wild.html.

Cai Y, Phillipson JD, Harper JI 1994 High performance liquid chromatographic and proton magnetic resonance spectroscopic methods for quality evaluation of *Paeonia* roots. Phytochemical Analysis 5:183–189.

Chen LC, Chou MH, Lin MF, et al 2000 Lack of pharmacokinetic interaction between valproic acid and a traditional Chinese medicine, *Paeoniae Radix*, in healthy volunteers. Journal of Clinical Pharmacy and Therapeutics 25:453–459.

Chen LC, Chou MH, Lin ME, et al 2001 Effects of *Paeoniae Radix*, a traditional Chinese medicine, on the pharmacokinetics of phenytoin. Journal of Clinical Pharmacy & Therapeutics 26:271–278.

Davis PH (ed.) 1965 Flora of Turkey, vol 1. Edinburgh University Press, Edinburgh.

Dharmananda S 2002 White peony, red peony, and moutan: three Chinese herbs derived from *Paeonia*. Online. Available: http://www.itmonline.org/arts/peony.htm. Accessed 20 July 2009.

Domínguez-Rodríguez MV, González-Hernández A 2007 Epilepsy in Thomas Phayer's The Boke of Chyldren (1546). Epilepsia 48:1664–1666.

Green MH (ed.) 2001 The Trotula. University of Pennsylvania Press, Philadelphia.

Halda JJ 2004 The genus *Paeonia*. Timber Press, Portland.

He Q, Ge ZW, Song Y, et al 2006 Quality evaluation of cortex Moutan by high performance liquid chromatography coupled with diode array detector and electrospray ionization tandem mass spectrometry. Chemical & Pharmaceutical Bulletin 54:1271–1275.

Junying G 1991 Medicinal herbs. New World Press, Beijing.

Kamiya K, Yoshioka K, Saiki Y 1997 Triterpenoids and flavonoids from *Paeonia lactiflora*. Phytochemistry 44:141–144.

Kuwacki T 1990 Chinese herbal therapy. Oriental Healing Arts Institute, Long Beach, CA

Li Q, Chen X, Zhou D 2009a Traditional Chinese medicine for epilepsy. Cochrane Database Systematic Review 8: CD006454.

Li SL, Song JZ, Choi FF, et al 2009b Chemical profiling of Radix Paeoniae evaluated by ultra-performance liquid chromatography/photo-diode-array/quadrupole time-of-flight mass spectrometry. Journal of Pharmaceutical Biomedical Analysis 49:253–266.

Lin W-C, Chunag W-C, Shue S-J 1996b HPLC separation of the major constituents in *Paeoniae Radix*. Journal of High Resolution Chromatography 19:530–533.

Lykiardopoulos A 1981 The evil eye: towards an exhaustive study. Folklore 92:221–230.

McLewin W, Chen D 2006 Peony rockii and Gansu Mudan. Cambridge Press, Wellesley, MA.

Macurdy GH 1912 The connection of Paean with Paeonia. The Classical Review 26:249–251.

Nicoll A (ed.) 1956 Chapman's Homer The Iliad. Princeton University Press, New Jersey.

Page M 2005 The gardener's Peony. Timber Press, Cambridge.

Papandreou V, Magiatis P, Chincu I, et al 2002 Volatiles with antimicrobial activity from the roots of Greek *Paeonia* taxa. Journal of Ethnopharmacology 81:101–104.

Peng HS, Wang DQ, Xu SJ 2008 The development and evolution of differentiation between Radix Paeoniae Rubra and Radix Paeoniae Alba. Zhonghua Yi Shi Za Zhi 38:133–136 (abstract).

Sheehan MP, Atherton DJ 1992 A controlled trial of traditional Chinese medicinal plants in widespread non-exudative atopic eczema. British Journal of Dermatology 126:179–184.

Stace C 1991 New flora of the British Isles. Cambridge University Press, Cambridge.

Stern FC 1946 A study of the genus Paeonia. Online. Available: http://www.paeon.de/h1/st/stern1.html.

Tang W, Eisenbrand G 1992 Chinese drugs of plant origin. Springer, Berlin.

Trickey R 1998 Women, hormones and the menstrual cycle. University of Queensland, St Leonards, New South Wales.

Van de Goot FRW, Ten Berge RL 2001 Historical perspective: a demon in the bathroom. Journal of Clinical Pathology 54:876.

Utian WH 2005 Psychosocial and socioeconomic burden of vasomotor symptoms in menopause: a comprehensive review. Health and Quality of Life Outcomes 3: 47 doi: 10.1186/1477-7525-3-47. Online. Available: http://www.hqlo.com/content/3/1/47.

Williamson E 2003 Potter's Herbal Cyclopaedia. CW Daniel, Saffron Walden.

Yamamoto H 1988 Paeonia spp: in vitro culture and the production of paeoniflorin. In: Bajaj YPS (ed.) 1988 Biotechnology in agriculture and forestry vol 4. Springer-Verlag, Berlin.

Yang WJ, Li DP, Li JK, et al 2009 Synergistic antioxidant activities of eight traditional Chinese herb pairs. Biological & Pharmaceutical Bulletin 32:1021–1026.

Zhou M, Cai H, Huang Z, et al 1998 HPLC method for the determination of paeoniflorin in *Paeonia Lactiflore* Pall. and its preparations. Biomedical Chromatography 12:43–44.

# CHAPTER 24
# *Potentilla erecta*, tormentil

## DESCRIPTION

**Family: Rosaceae**                                                                 **Part used: rhizome, root**

*Flora Europaea* gives 75 species in the genus (Tutin et al 1968) and Stace (1991) gives 17 species in Britain. *Potentilla* species are rather similar and distinguishing characteristics are emphasized by Gibbons and Brough (1995). The *Flora of Turkey* (Davis 1972) gives 53 *Potentilla* species, including *Potentilla erecta*, *Potentilla anglica* and *Potentilla reptans*.

*Potentilla erecta* (L.) Räuschel is a herbaceous perennial with a stout, hard rootstock. It is found throughout Europe on acid soils such as mountainous bog and moorland and upland meadows but also on dry sandy pinewoods and heathland. It is rare in the Mediterranean (Tutin et al 1968).

Procumbent and erect stems (10–25 cm) are non-rooting and the height is greater where the land is damp and not grazed by sheep. The alternate leaves are unstalked, toothed at the apex and hairy underneath. The leaves occur in groups of three with two stipules which resemble small leaflets so it appears to have five leaflets. The yellow flowers occur in summer in cymes and have four petals and many yellow stamens. There are four sepals and a four-sectioned epicalyx. All other *Potentilla* have five petals. The seed is an achene.

*Potentilla erecta* is used in botanical sources rather that the synonym *Potentilla tormentilla* Stokes. Stace (1991) distinguishes *Potentilla erecta* subsp. *erecta* from subspecies *strictissima*, which is taller with more dentate leaves, stem leaves which are serrate all round and larger flowers. As with other Rosaceae (see *Alchemilla vulgaris*), it can be apomictic so a population may be one clone. Hybrids occur: *Potentilla x suberecta* is a cross between *Potentilla erecta* and trailing tormentil *Potentilla anglica*, which has rooting stems. *Potentilla x mixta* is a cross between *Potentilla erecta* or *Potentilla anglica* and creeping cinquefoil *Potentilla reptans*, which has rooting, flowering stems (Stace 1991). Henriette's Herbal Homepage (2009) gives useful photographs of *Potentilla* species.

**Other species used**: Given the similarity between species it is probable that other species are collected, such as creeping cinquefoil *Potentilla reptans*, which is found throughout Europe (Tutin et al 1968). White cinquefoil *Potentilla alba*, which has white flowers, is used in a similar way (Oszmianski et al 2007). Silverweed *Potentilla anserina* is widely used in herbal medicines in Europe (Bisset & Wichtl 2001, Tomczyk & Latté 2009). It is a widespread perennial that spreads by stolons. The leaves are silver underneath and pinnate with 7 to 12 leaf pairs and the flowers are yellow with five petals.

## ASTRINGENCY IS THE THEME BUT WHICH *POTENTILLA*?

Tormentil is described by Weiss as the main vegetable astringent. Astringency in the widest sense must be the theme for this herb. Tannins have been identified as the astringent compounds in medicinal plants. They exert their effects through local action in the digestive tract in, for example, diarrhoea. The extent to which such large compounds are absorbed into the systemic circulation is a current topic of research but compounds which derive from tannins must be absorbed and be responsible for these actions (Rasmussen et al 2005). Tormentil can be of exceptional value as an astringent in heavy periods, and, although this action is not explained, it is one of those actions exerted by medicinal plants, of which perhaps the action of comfrey *Symphytum officinale* in bruising is the archetype, where once seen, always believed. 'Probatus est' as the old writers called it.

Dioscorides (IV 42) describes pentadactylon ('five fingers' in Greek) with five leaves on a petiole, saw edged all around, with a pale white flower, found growing in damp places and around water conduits. The *Potentilla* named pentadactylon by Dioscorides could be *Potentilla alba*, which has five white petals and five-fingered leaves that are only saw edged at the end. Beck gives *Potentilla reptans*, which is yellow like *Potentilla erecta*, for tormentil, which cannot be correct as Dioscorides describes a white flower. Dioscorides refers to a reddish root and, as red is the colour associated with tannins, this plant can be

THE WESTERN HERBAL TRADITION

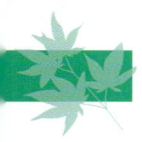

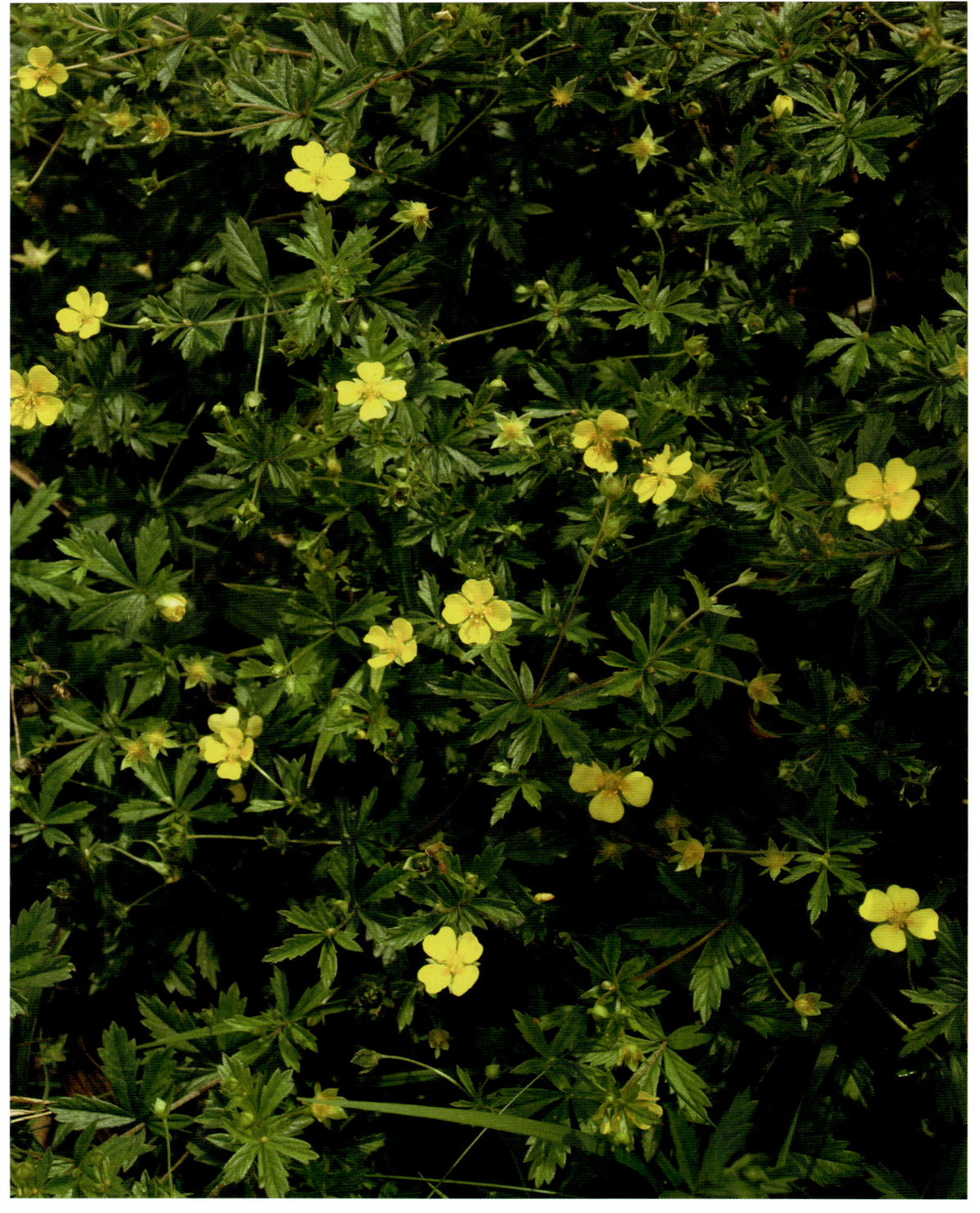

Figure 24.1 *Potentilla erecta*, tormentil (Wharfedale, Yorkshire, May).

identified as a *Potentilla* but is not tormentil. Fresh roots of tormentil are brown with a black surface but aqueous extracts and tinctures of *Potentilla* are a rich, deep red-brown. Dioscorides refers to uses in intermittent fevers and jaundice for the leaves; this usage is taken up by later authors mainly when discussing cinquefoil and must be associated with other *Potentilla* species.

Dioscorides says that pentadactylon is cut for religious ceremonies and purifications, which suggests a larger plant as he also refers to the sprays, which are a span long, like dry sticks and bear fruit. Pliny appears to be referring to the same herb when he describes cinquefoil with a red root which turns black on drying, 'commendable for the strawberries it bares' and used to bless a house against evil spirits. The possible identity is discussed at length by Parkinson, who reviews the names given for pentadactylon by the authors. As Turner argues, it must be a cinquefoil, also named quinquefolium, five-fingered grass or the five-fingered herb. Turner includes tormentil in his third volume, which covers herbs not found in Dioscorides. Galen refers to pentaphyllum, a five-leaved plant, cinquefoil, as very drying in the third degree with a minimum heat and little sharpness, so very useful. Dioscorides, Pliny, Galen and Theophrastus, according to Parkinson, all refer to a plant with a five-fingered leaf, which is therefore not tormentil but will be another *Potentilla* species, probably one of the cinquefoils.

Other *Potentilla* species are referred to by the Renaissance authors and it seems likely that various *Potentilla* species were used. Fuchs (1980) gives quinquefolium luteum maius which is five fingered and could be *Potentilla reptans* and quinquefolium luteum minor. Fuchs also gives argemone altera uel potentilla, which appears to be silverweed and states that it has the character of quinquefolium and therefore can be used when an astringent is required. Fuchs gives an illustration of 'heptaphyllum' that appears to be tormentil. Interestingly, Parkinson comments that tormentil is not found in Dioscorides yet has acquired the Greek name of heptaphyllum. Today, *Potentilla heptaphylla* is a mat-forming plant with tiny toothed leaves which is found in eastern Europe but not in Britain. Dodoens refers to tormentil as a plant with seven leaves on a stem, growing in dark and shadowy woods and green ways, which flowers all summer. He describes leaves with snipped, toothed edges and Dalechamps gives a very similar description. Parkinson discusses the plants suggested by other authors as being the pentaphyllum of Dioscorides and Theophrastus and disagrees with Tragus (Bock), who argues that tormentil must be equivalent as it is the 'best and most noble pentaphyllum', as he points out that the plant of Dioscorides had distinctive five-parted leaves and whitish flowers. Parkinson makes a long diversion into the question of leaves and argues that the leaves of *Potentilla* species are made up of leaflets as they wither and fall in one piece. As discussed below, Parkinson inherited the notes of de l'Obel and one wonders whether these are the words of de l'Obel, who studied leaves in depth having developed a classification system for plants based on leaf form (Pavord 2005).

Parkinson gives tormentil first but then states that the cinquefoils will do as well. He divides the cinquefoils into three categories: those with white flowers, those with yellow flowers which creep on the ground with a lax habit, and erect plants with yellow flowers. Parkinson recommends use of common cinquefoil, pentaphyllum vulgarissimum, which he describes as having yellow flowers, spreading by runners like strawberries, with toothed, five-fingered leaves, and blackish brown roots 'seldom as thick as the little finger' but spreading quickly by creeping along the ground. This could be *Potentilla reptans*. Parkinson states that Bauhin names it quinquefolium majus repens and Hill (1756) repeats the recommendation and lists this cinquefoil as Pentaphyllum vulgare stating that Gaspard Bauhin names it quinquefolium majus repens, and Jean Bauhin pentaphyllum vulgare repens. These names are confusing but are reproduced to show how much the Linnean binomial system was rooted in the labours of preceding authors (Louis 1980).

The conclusion thus far is that the authors refer to various *Potentilla* species and the roots are used interchangeably. Cultivation of these species would allow for more definitive recommendations. For this book we have selected herbs that are commonly used by herbalists, yet we have discovered enormous problems in both the identification of similar members of the same genus, and in the interpretation of recommendations where it is unclear which herb was originally used. One of the main aims of the Renaissance writers such as Turner, Fuchs, Dodoens, Mattioli and Parkinson was to determine the correct species. Yet as a profession we still have some way to go today in this matter because of the continuing wild collection of many medicinal plants (ISSC-MAP 2009). Parkinson expresses his frustration, while discussing hermodactylus (see below), at the 'shame of the physicians' who leave these matters to apothecaries and merchants. but should 'give orders that the unknown should be made more manifest'. Yet he feels that his admonitions will be pointless, 'but what do I in so saying run my Barke (ship) upon the Rockes and put her in danger of splitting'.

## USE IN 'ALL FLUXES'

It is the root of tormentil that is used, and we must start with recommendations for usage of root. Dioscorides advises a decoction of the root, reduced to one third, drunk for use in diarrhoea and dysentery and for suffering in the joints and hip ailments. He recommends the juice extracted when the root is soft for ills of the liver and lung and for deadly poisons. He gives a dose of 3 cyathoi (135 mL) for jaundice. Culpeper advises 4 fl oz of the juice for the same. However, use of the leaf is also recommended for jaundice. For example, Apuleius refers to the seven-leafed plant found in cultivated and sandy places and advises the herb for jaundiced people.

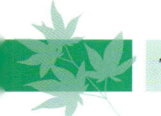

Fuchs, Turner, Dodoens and Parkinson suggest a mixture of powdered root, blended with egg white, and cooked in a terracotta pan, for biliousness or the desire to vomit. Dalechamps and Bauhin give a recipe: take powdered root and the same amount of oatmeal, with half as much egg white and nutmeg *Myristica fragrans*. Mix to make small cakes and cook 'in an iron spoon' (which could be adapted to a bun tin) to make small cakes. Take one daily, in the morning according to Parkinson, for fluxes, choleric humours, loss of appetite and vomiting, and what Culpeper describes as 'choleric belches and much vomitings with loathing in the stomach'. Dodoens suggests tormentil is 'good against the disease called choler or melancholy' and Dalechamps advises the decoction in an earthen vessel given to cholerics, who were considered to become peevish due to an overheated spleen.

The astringent qualities of tormentil lead to its use on 'all fluxes' of which the main one is diarrhoea, with or without blood in the stool. This cannot be separated from the recommendation for use in pestilence as infectious disease would have been a common source of uncontrollable diarrhoea. Turner advises a broth of the roots or stilled in a bain marie, for 'bloody flux' and pestilence. Culpeper gives recipes for distilling extracts from roots using a bain marie to avoid burning.

Dodoens states that tormentil opens and heals stoppings and hurts of the lungs and liver such as in jaundice.

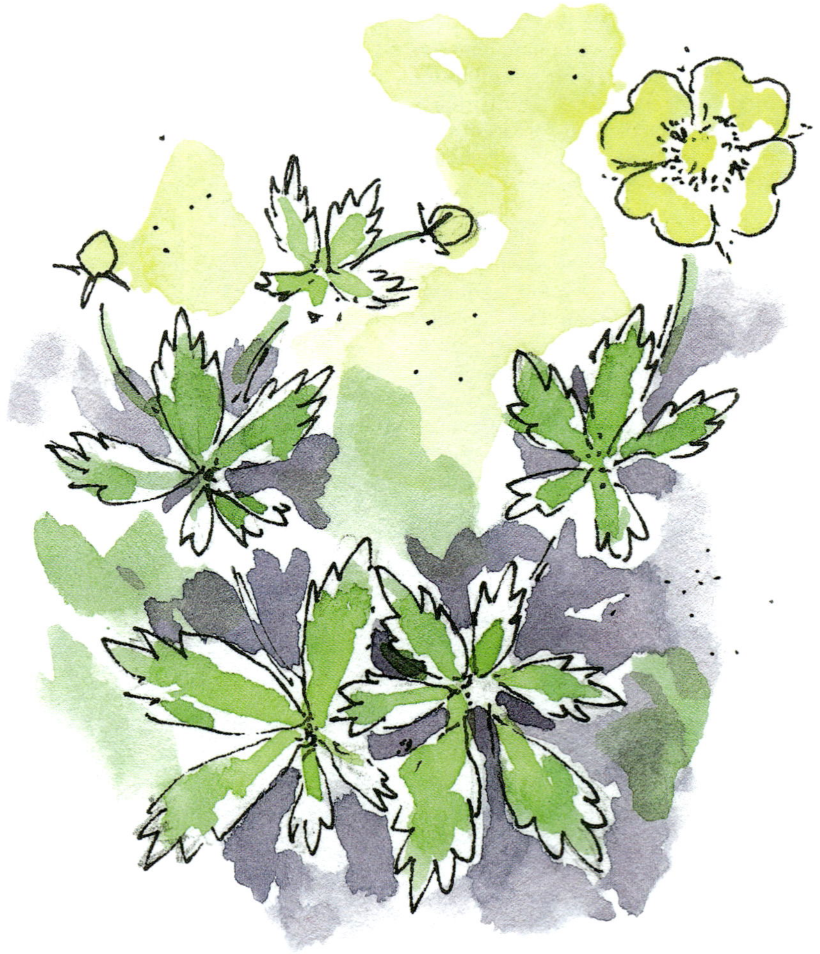

**Figure 24.2** *Potentilla erecta*, tormentil.

He recommends the dried root, powdered and drunk in wine when there is no fever and with water in which iron has been boiled, for bloody flux and all other fluxes. He suggests the leaf with the root, boiled in wine, or juice, or powdered root to provoke sweat and drive out venom from the heart in poison, plague and pestilence. The phrase 'provoke sweat and drive out venom from the heart' refers to alexipharmics.

## USE TO RESIST DISEASE

Pestilence refers to infectious disease, which may or may not be epidemic, of which the archetypal example is plague. The connection with the heart is that pestilence was considered to be carried by the air into the lungs where it would attack the heart and therefore corrupt the vital spirit. Ancient authors were aware of the infectious nature of disease (Nutton 1983), although not aware of the mechanism of infection. Later, Hildegard makes an explicit linkage between diarrhoea and food-borne infection. She describes the coldness of tormentil as effective against fevers that arise from noxious foods. She advises tormentil cooked in wine with a little honey added, strained, and drunk frequently at night on an empty stomach.

After the Black Death in the 1300s, it is hard to see that people cannot have been aware of the transmission of disease. According to Carmichael (1997) quarantine of ships where passengers were not allowed to disembark for a given period, began in 1377 in the Venetian port that is now Dubrovnik. Zuckerman (2004) gives an account of beliefs on contagion in the early 1700s when Richard Mead wrote a report for the British government on contagion and quarantine arrangements in response to the last outbreak of bubonic plague in Europe, in Marseille in 1720. Contagion was a problem for doctors, who retained some loyalty to the humoral system with its focus on the individual vulnerability of patients and places but this is probably over-represented in the texts which were written by educated people. Those with a less theoretical bent must have relied on observation and accepted that many diseases were contagious. However, it is impossible to cast one's mind back to the world views of the past and French (2003) gives a thought-provoking account of the changes in thought associated with the observation that syphilis was spread from person to person.

Dalechamps, perhaps citing Galen, notes that tormentil is without manifest heat and has the faculties of cinquefoil to resist poisons and suppress dysentery. Bauhin describes tormentil and cinquefoils stating that they expel poisons and plague by sweating by use of a warm decoction of a handful of leaves and roots, or 1 drachm (4 g) of powdered root. He also gives pastilles, powders, electuaries and drinks as useful in dysentery. Culpeper states that juice of the herb or root of tormentil resists all poison and venom of any creature, even pestilential fevers and the plague itself, and contagious disease such as the pox, measles and 'purples' by expelling the venom and infection from the heart by sweating. He also includes the distilled water of the herb and roots of tormentil in his list of antidotes.

The authors describe tormentil as dry in the third degree but opinions vary on its heat. Galen describes 'pentaphyllum' as without manifest heat. Parkinson gives it as cold in the second degree whereas Culpeper says it is hot in the first degree. This might be because of the discrepancies in the plant or part of the plant being discussed but use of aerial parts is definitely recommended in infection and fever. Use of the leaf is recommended by Dioscorides for intermittent fevers: the leaves of four sprays for quartan fevers, three sprays for tertian fevers and one spray for the quotidian. This is repeated by Culpeper in his entry for cinquefoil. He describes Dioscorides as 'full of whimsies' and says that a dose of 20 grains (1300 mg) of cinquefoil in white wine or white wine vinegar will cure agues of whatever type if given on three successive occasions. Culpeper describes cinquefoil as an especial herb in all inflammation or fever, 'whether infectious or pestilential'. Culpeper states that Andreas Vesalius (anatomist, 1512–1564) thought tormentil as good as lignum vitae *Guaiacum officinale* or china *Smilax* species in the 'French pox' (syphilis). This recommendation is also given by Grieve, who refers to tormentil as the English sarsaparilla.

Use in infection continues in the 18th century. Quincy states that tormentil is most noted for its binding qualities, yet is included amongst the alexipharmics particularly for 'malignant cases attended with any flux, either of the bowels or the womb'. Hill makes the same point, and suggests a larger dose of cinquefoil for intermittent fevers. Hill describes tormentil as cordial as well as astringent and that it 'operates by sweat' and so is useful in any fever associated with excessive diarrhoea Cullen (1772) considers tormentil as equivalent to cinquefoil in intermittent fevers used alongside *Gentiana lutea* and other bitters. Hill recommends it for loose bowels associated with measles and smallpox, and Cullen is more specific in that he uses astringents to promote suppuration and thus resolve disease.

## ASTRINGENCY IN MENORRHAGIA

Other usage of tormentil as a medicine is for the urinary tract, for heavy periods and for arthritic pain. Turner advises tormentil with juice of plantain for urinary incontinence both as a decoction and as an extract in vinegar 'held on the kidneys'. This usage is also given by Dalechamps, Gerard, Parkinson and Culpeper.

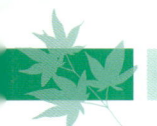

Tormentil is used today for heavy periods and it is interesting to trace this usage. Turner states that it stops women's flows if the woman sits in a broth up to the navel or the broken roots are laid on the belly with honey and spikenard. Parkinson recommends roots of either tormentil or cinquefoil for 'all fluxes in man or woman, whether the whites or the reds'. Parkinson states that many women use the distilled water of leaves and roots of tormentil 'as a secret, to help themselves and others, when they are troubled with an abundance of the whites or the reds, as they call them', both as a drink or injected with a syringe. This sentence is copied in some editions of Culpeper but not others. Bauhin also recommends the distilled water and juice for excessive menstruation.

Whilst herbal practitioners seek to prescribe for the individual, there can be situations where a prescription is effective for a particular symptom. Heavy periods are a debilitating problem and occur in the perimenopause as a result of anovulatory cycles (Apgar et al 2007). Orthodox treatment has limitations, while hysterectomy is now seen as a last resort (NICE 2007). The long-term prescription will address the constitution of the individual but it is useful to have a remedy to hand when the flow is unmanageable. I used a prescription successfully for perimenopausal heavy periods associated with uterine fibroids and have since used it again in other women. It is fluid extract of *Capsella bursa-pastoris* 30 mL and tinctures of *Potentilla erecta* 30 mL, *Achillea millefolium* 30 mL, *Aesculus hippocastanum* 10 mL, *Zingiber officinalis* 10 mL. The dose is 10 mL four times a day which is a large dose of alcohol so the patient must be warned of this. My extract is prepared from a strong decoction of tormentil which is allowed to cool and then ethanol and more water is added to achieve a 1:3 concentration before macerating the cold mixture in the normal manner. It is therefore stronger than some tinctures available from herbal suppliers.

Parkinson, followed by Culpeper, advises the powder or decoction as a drink or as a bath as an assured remedy against abortion in women if caused by the 'over flexibility or weakness of the inward retentive faculty'. I used tormentil thus in a woman of 40 with no children who had already had miscarriages but eventually gave birth to a health baby. She had bleeding at 10 weeks, at 12 weeks and again at 14 weeks and rested in bed when this occurred. A scan at 16 weeks showed a 6 cm fibroid. My concern was that she was struggling to support a healthy pregnancy and the prescription included a decoction of tormentil with lady's mantle *Alchemilla vulgaris* and tinctures of *Viburnum prunifolium* as an antispasmodic and *Alpinia galanga* as a circulatory stimulant.

## RHEUMATIC DISORDERS AND GOUT

Internal usage of root of tormentil for arthritic conditions goes back to Dioscorides, who advises a decoction of the root, reduced to one third, drunk for suffering in the joints and hip ailments. Beck usefully translates the Greek as 'hip disease' rather than draw inferences about the meaning of the words. This advice is repeated by Turner, Parkinson and Culpeper but yet it is not a common modern usage. Hip ailments is given by Turner as pain in the hucklebone called sciatica, under his entry for root of 'the herb five leaf'. Culpeper recommends the juice of the leaves and roots applied to sciatica, and states that it is effective against ruptures and bursting, bruises and falls both outward and inward. The entry in Culpeper is word for word from Parkinson, who refers to sciatica as hipgout. A recent review of five herbals found that the only Rosaceae recommended for rheumatic disorders were *Potentilla* species, given by Adam Lonitzer (Lonicerus) in 1557 and Jacob Theodor (Tabernaemontanus) in 1588 for pain. The corresponding modern terms given by the authors are 'polyarthritis' and 'gout of the feet' (Adams et al 2009).

The 1656 edition of Culpeper includes a tantalizing sentence that is not included in the modern edition. It is copied from Parkinson and reads, 'Lobel saith, that Rondelitus used it as Hermodactils for joint-aches'. Hermodactils or hermodactylus was an imported herb that, according to Parkinson, had not been identified but was most effective in purging phlegmatic, slimy and watery humours from the joints and therefore valuable in gout and other 'running joint aches'. Parkinson says some consider hermodactylus to be roots of '*Colchicum*, but they are dangerous if not deadly'. This designation seems unlikely to him partly because he says it was included in drinks with lignum vitae *Guaiacum officinale* and sarsaparilla *Smilax* species and also because he cites Mesue as stating that it was a finger-shaped root. Pereira (1853) had the opportunity to examine some material purchased as hermodactyl in India that he considered could be the underground parts of autumn crocus *Colchicum autumnale*, which is used in the treatment of gout. Pereira gives a quote from Paulus Aeginata, which may be referring to the use of *Colchicum*: 'some, in the paroxysms of all arthritic diseases, have recourse to purging with hermodactylus; but it is to be remarked that the hermodactylus is bad for the stomach, producing nausea and anorexia, and ought, therefore, to be used only in the case of those who are pressed by urgent business, for it removes rheumatism speedily, and after two days at most, so that they are enabled to resume their accustomed employment'. Another candidate is a Mediterranean member of the Iris family, *Hermodactylus tuberosus*, with a rootstock of 'finger-like tubers' (Grey-Wilson &

Mathew 1981). Whatever the identity of hermodactylus, the statement of Culpeper leads one to ask whether or not tormentil could be particularly useful in pain associated with arthritis.

Matthias de l'Obel (1538–1616) is influential in that he was a significant figure in the development of botany and transmission of knowledge (Louis 1980). He was born in Flanders but studied medicine in Montpellier. In the 16th century, the curriculum at the medical school in Montpelier was influenced by humanist ideas in that the study of original texts and of the living plants was encouraged (Reeds 1991). New Greek versions and translations direct from Greek into Latin were becoming available such as a Latin version of *De Simplicium Medicamentorum Facultatibus* by Galen, which was published in Paris in 1530 (Reeds 1976). Rondelitus is the latinized name of Guillaume Rondelet, who graduated in medicine at Montpellier in 1531 then returned as a lecturer. He was one of the pioneers of the use of Dioscorides and in 1545 he lectured on the books of Dioscorides. A translation into Latin from the Aldine Greek version published in 1499 had been published in Paris in 1516 by Jean Ruel (Reeds 1976). Rondelet pioneered field trips into the local countryside to address the thorny questions surrounding the sources of medicinal plants and the interpretation of the ancient authors. He travelled to Italy, where he saw the 'true Roman absynthium' in the ancient ruins and had contacts with Italian, Swiss and German scholars (Reeds 1991). Rondelet is important to this book as he taught two of our authors, Dalechamps and Jean Bauhin. He taught Charles de l'Ecluse, who translated the version of Dodoens which we have used from Flemish into French, and de l'Obel, to whom he left his papers at his death in 1566 (Arber 1986). De l'Obel was inspired to continue searching for wild plants throughout his life and, after graduating in 1565, he travelled in Europe with Pierre Pena. He came to Britain in 1569, returned to Antwerp until the early 1580s, then settled in London, where he died in 1616. His first book, *Stirpium Adversaria Nova*, was published in 1571 in London but an edited later version was published by Plantin in 1605 with the addition of *In G. Rondelletti Pharmaceuticum Officinam Animadversiones* (Lownes 1958). It could be that the comment that 'Lobel saith, that Rondelitus used it as Hermodactils for joint-aches' is taken from this book or from the papers of de l'Obel, which were edited by Parkinson. Some material from the papers was included in *Theatrum Botanicum*, published in 1640. Either way, the comparison with hermodactylus confirms the relative efficacy of tormentil. It also suggests that Rondelet used it in his own practice for joint pains and thus that the recommendation is not merely taken from Dioscorides. The point here is that when reading Culpeper we have a window into older usage as he copied Parkinson freely and Parkinson used many sources in the preparation of his material.

## EXTERNAL USE AS AN ASTRINGENT

Before moving to current practice, we can trace long usage of tormentil as an astringent in external remedies. Dioscorides advises the decoction of root, boiled down to one third, held in the mouth to relieve toothache, used as a rinse to control putrid humours in the mouth and as a gargle for hoarseness of the trachea. These are also given by Dodoens, who suggests the root and the leaf together. Dioscorides then gives a long list of indications and recommends a preparation of boiled root, ground up in vinegar to keep shingles in check, restrain herpes, disperse scrophulous swellings in glands, incurations, swellings, aneurysms, abscesses, erysipelas, fleshy excrescences in fingers, callous lumps and mange. Galen recommends pentaphyllum to dry wounds. Apuleius advises the juice of the herb bruised and mixed with egg yolk, rubbed on painful feet to take away the pain in 3 days. This usage also is given by Dalechamps and Bauhin, and reappears as a balm for the feet in Gloucestershire (Allen & Hatfield 2004). The Salernitan herbal refers to tormentil, which resembles cinquefoil, and recommends the juice of the root placed inside a fistula and the juice mixed with white wine applied for fleck in the eye. Turner finds it similar to bistort *Polygonum bistorta* and recommends it in running sores and the powder on a wound as a styptic and an extract in wine for 'green wounds without and within'. Green wounds may be taken to mean fresh wounds; this phrasing is similar to Culpeper's recommendation in ruptures within and without. Dodoens also advises leaves and root, decoction or juice, for wounds inwardly and outwardly. Dalechamps recommends juice of leaves to weeping fistulas, to the eyes to disperse blemishes and the herb and root chewed for putrescent ulcers. Bauhin advises tormentil for all wounds as a plaster or ointment or a wash decocted in water or wine for putrid wounds, hardnesses and swelling, especially around the ear. He then gives a preparation in vinegar for hip pain, haemorrhoids and scabies, a preparation with amber for defluxions (discharge) in the eyes and the fresh juice applied morning and evening for vertigo. Culpeper lists bruises, falls, ruptures, wounds, sores and ulcers of mouth and genitals, scabs, itches, scrophula and sciatica. Hill gives loose teeth, haemorrhages of nose and mouth, and falling of the uvula. Grieve proposes external use as a gargle for sore and ulcerated throat, in leucorrhoea, ulcers, long standing sores and the decoction, soaked in lint, regularly applied to remove warts. The modern authors also give a range of external usage. Wren describes tormentil as a tonic lotion in ulcers and old sores, and recommends the fluid extract as a styptic. The *National Botanic Pharmacopoeia* recommends a gargle for sore, relaxed ulcerated throat, to remove purulent mucus and as an injection for leucorrhoea (formerly referred to as the whites). The *British Herbal Pharmacopoeia* recommends use as a stypic and vulnerary, as a gargle for the mouth and mucous membranes of the throat and a lotion for haemorrhoids. Williamson advises usage in pressure sores and ulcers etc. Menzies-Trull recommends a poultice to ease pain and use in haemorrhoids with witch hazel *Hamamelis virginiana*. Chevalier advises use as a stypic and use in mouth ulcers and infected gums. Barker (2001) advises use of the powder as a stypic and up to 10 mL of tincture (1:5 45%) in sore throat, gingivitis and pyorrhoea, and use of a lotion in burns, warts and sunburn. Taken together, there is a substantial amount of external usage.

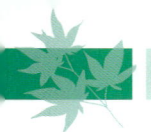

## 'THE MOST POWERFUL OF THE VEGETABLE ASTRINGENTS'

Returning to internal usage, the focus in later authors is clearly on astringency in diarrhoea. Cullen (1772) states that tormentil is the most powerful of the vegetable astringents. He argues that the qualities are not sufficiently extracted into water or alcohol and that it should be used as a material substance in the form of a powder. Hill recommends tormentil in bleeding piles but Cullen makes the point that haemorrhoids are often caused by 'costiveness' or constipation, and that this may be worsened by the use of astringent herbs. Coffin gives tormentil as a powerful astringent in diarrhoea, long-standing bowel complaints and the powder for external use to sprinkle on an old sore, or to stop bleeding.

Astringent herbs were important to the 19th century authors as they were used to cleanse the digestive tract of 'canker'. Robinson (1868) describes canker as 'a morbific state, tendency to disease in any locality, internal or external' which occurs in the throat, stomach or bowels and is caused by cold as 'when cold obtains power over the inward heat, the stomach and bowels become coated with canker'. Thomson emphasizes the cleansing of canker from the bowel walls by use of astringents and this formed the third stage, No. 3 of the Thomsonian course of treatment (Comfort 1859). The sequence in the course of treatment was to use lobelia *Lobelia inflata* as an emetic, followed by cayenne *Capsicum annuum* to heat and then astringents to heal the tissues. He writes that 'the canker is fixed on the inside and will ripen and come off in a short time, if the fever is kept up so as to overpower the cold' (Thomson 1832). Stevens (1847) lists Thomson's astringents then gives, as the eleventh astringent *Potentilla erecta*, and says that it was introduced to the list of tonic astringents and could be used equally as their substitute.

When discussing astringency Fox refers to canker as 'anything which corrupts, corrodes, destroys' and also recommends bayberry *Myrica cerifera* to 'detach morbid and vitiated matter'. Bayberry is the original herb given as No. 3 and it may be better than any substitute (Comfort 1859). It is certainly different in that it is a very peppery herb, which causes sneezing. Fox advises tormentil in all classes of bowel complaints, cholera, dysentery and diarrhoea associated with consumption. This last recommendation is also given by Robinson (1868), who ascribes the advice to Dr Graham. Fox calls tormentil 'the very best remedy for bloody flux'. He recommends half a cup every 30 minutes, as warm as convenient, of a tea made by pouring 1 pint of boiling water on 1 oz of herb. He notes that it often 'causes free perspiration'.

Robinson also recommends tormentil for all fluxes of blood at the dose of 1 drachm (3.5 mL) four times a day in an infusion of hops *Humulus lupulus*, which is also given by Grieve. He adds a recommendation from Dr George Fordyce for use in relaxed bowels, and recommends juice or decoction of herb and root to expel fever if the person is also laid to sweat. This appears to be the recommendation originally given by Culpeper. Robinson adds the recommendation of Dr Thornton for use in 'agues which had resisted the bark', leg ulcers turned away as incurable, scorbutic ulcers and long standing diarrhoea, and also recalls earlier authors in recommending it to open obstructions of the liver such as in jaundice.

Grieve rates tormentil highly as very astringent and gives a compound powder that is 'very reliable' in diarrhoea and other discharges. Infuse powders of tormentil, marshmallow root *Althaea officinalis* and galangal *Alpinia galanga* each at 1 oz with ginger *Zingiber officinale* 4 drachms (16 g) in 1 pint of water. Cool, strain and take 1–2 fluid drachms (3.5–7 mL) every 15 minutes and then reduce the dose to three times a day. The *National Botanic Pharmacopoeia* notes extensive use of the herb and root in diarrhoea and other abnormal discharges to nourish and support bowels and tone the uterus and whole uterine area.

## 20TH CENTURY USAGE IN DIARRHOEA

Of the modern authors, Weiss discusses the use of tormentil at length and recommends it highly. He gives a description which refers to *Potentilla erecta* and considers it the best astringent in chronic enterocolitis, summer diarrhoea, paratyphoid diarrhoea, acute and sub-acute enteritis and colitis although less useful in chronic cases of colitis. He recommends a good pinch of powder (500 mg) several times a day. Weiss also recommends one cup several times a day of a decoction prepared with 1–3 tablespoons of rhizome, steeped for 15 minutes in 500 mL water. He advises use with a carminative such as chamomile *Matricaria recutita*, lemon balm *Melissa officinalis* or peppermint *Mentha piperita*. Weiss considers the tincture less effective but gives a dose of 30–50 drops several times a day in peppermint tea. He gives a formula of tinctures of tormentil 30 mL, *Atropa belladonna* leaf 5 mL and carminative tincture 15 mL, 30 drops three times a day. The final dose of *Atropa belladonna* should be calculated before considering use of this formula. The *British Herbal Pharmacopoeia* gives the main actions as astringent and anti-haemorrhagic and recommends it for ulcerative colitis and diarrhoea, including acute diarrhoea and diarrhoea associated with anxiety. Barker (2001) suggests it in tormina and colic, and small doses in peptic ulcer. Wood describes another *Potentilla* as he refers to a plant which has deeply serrated leaves and pictures a *Potentilla* with five leaflets and five petals. He finds the plant very similar in action to agrimony *Agrimonia eupatoria*, which one recalls is another Rosaceae used in problems of the digestive tract.

Chevalier recommends tormentil in irritable bowel syndrome, colitis, ulcerative colitis, dysentery and rectal bleeding. Low grade mucosal inflammation has been identified as a factor in the pathogenesis of irritable bowel syndrome (Hammerle & Surawicz 2008) and the indication given by all the authors for use in diarrhoea and blood in the motions suggests usage in inflammatory bowel disease such as ulcerative colitis and Crohn's disease where orthodox treatment remains of limited effectiveness (McFarland 2008). The use of tormentil in inflammatory bowel disease and in irritable bowel syndrome where diarrhoea is the predominant symptom has been linked to the antioxidant activity of polyphenols. Tormentil and other astringent herbs have been investigated as researchers have asked whether astringency depends on the overall concentration of polyphenols or on the concentration of particular polyphenols. For example, root of *Potentilla alba* was shown to have a high level of condensed tannins and a high antioxidant activity in vitro (Oszmianski et al 2007). Bos et al (1996) investigated tormentil and found that the dimers and trimers inhibited lipid peroxidation and pentamers and hexamers inhibited the enzyme elastase. A study of antioxidant activity (superoxide formation) using the same extract found that the larger procyanidin pentamers and hexamers were the most active (Vennat et al 1994). Condensed tannins are common in foods (Hammerstone et al 2000) and there is a high procyanidin concentration in foods from the Rosaceae family, such as apples and medicinal herbs such as hawthorn *Crataegus monogyna*. One could therefore conclude that particular compounds are responsible for the effectiveness of tormentil as an astringent rather than the overall content of procyanidins.

An in vitro study of herbs used in inflammatory bowel disease investigated their antioxidant activity as reactive oxygen metabolites are found in excess in colonic mucosa. Tormentil extract was found to inhibit superoxide and peroxyl formation and it was further found that incubation of inflamed tissue from human colorectal mucosal biopsies in a 1:1000 dilution of tormentil resulted in decreased formation of reactive oxygen metabolites (Langmead et al 2002). There is some evidence in clinical usage from a pilot study in 16 patients. The participants had active ulcerative colitis, mainly left-sided, and continued with orthodox treatment alongside three doses of tormentil extract each for 3 weeks with washout periods of 4 weeks. Scores on the Rachmilewitz colitis activity index decreased during each treatment phase and a dose of 2400 mg was found to be most effective. Stool frequency and blood in the stool decreased (Moss & Chefetz 2007). Tests showed that the tannins were not systemically absorbed.

An unusual clinical trial was undertaken in Russia where children are routinely admitted to hospital with diarrhoea to avoid further spread in the community so a clinical priority is to stop the intensity of the diarrhoea. Forty children were included who were admitted with diarrhoea and whose stool samples were positive for rotavirus antigen. The children were given 3 drops of tincture per year of age three times a day of either tormentil or a placebo. The 1:10 tincture was made from dried root using 40% ethanol. The treatment group was aged 4–79 months (median 23.5) and the control group 3–60 months (median 24.5). Both groups were also given oral rehydration therapy. The outcome for the treatment group was significantly better as regards volume of parenteral rehydration required, duration of abnormal stool consistency and duration of hospitalization. For example, after 48 hours diarrhoea had ceased in 8 of 20 in the treatment group but in only 1 of 20 in the control group. Tormentil did not reduce the rate of vomiting (Subbotina et al 2003). This study is useful as it is a study whose results can be applied in normal herbal practice as the dose and the preparation is clearly stated. The results are all the more interesting as the placebo was a tincture of Indian tea. Indian black tea has been shown to inhibit bovine rotavirus in vitro and is used to treat diarrhoea (Palombo 2006).

## RECOMMENDATIONS

- Tormentil has been consistently advised for use in diarrhoea, blood in the stools and 'all fluxes' and could be particularly useful in ulcerative colitis. There is a consistent tradition of use in dysentery and infectious disease.
- Aerial parts of other *Potentilla* species, including cinquefoil and silverweed, were used and continue to be used in Europe and could be integrated into herbal practice.
- Use of the powder is recommended. Then large doses could be given in, for example, ulcerative colitis without giving a large amount of alcohol. Equally, the randomized controlled trial described above found that quite small doses of tincture were

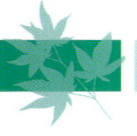

effective in diarrhoea associated with rotavirus infection in children.
- Tormentil has a more recent use in heavy periods. It has been recommended both for excess bleeding and leucorrhoea and in urinary incontinence.
- Usage internally for arthritic pain, and possibly for gout, and external usage for a wide range of indications is strong throughout the tradition. These usages are now less common but could be reintroduced into current practice.

Dosage: The *British Herbal Pharmacopoeia* recommends 2–4 g three times a day of dried rhizome.

## RECOMMENDATIONS ON SAFETY

- Use caution in dosage in long-term use, particularly of a decoction or powder.

Other herbs such as agrimony and raspberry leaf could be more suitable for long-term use both because they are a more pleasant tea and because they are less astringent. Tannins have been shown to complex with proteins and minerals (Haslam 1996) and absorption of non-haem iron has been found to be significantly reduced by concurrent consumption of tea (Thankachan et al 2008). There is concern about the long-term use of tannins, especially where total intake of proteins and iron may be low, such as in vegans. A recent review found that many factors are relevant in iron status but recommended that where iron status may be low, tea should not be consumed with meals and at least an hour should elapse after eating (Nelson & Poulter 2004). The advice would the same for tannin-containing herbs, as herbal teas have also been shown to reduce non-haem iron absorption (Hurrell et al 1999).

## CONSTITUENTS

Reviews: Bisset & Wichtl (2001), Mills & Bone (2005), Tomczyk & Latté (2009), Williamson (2003), WHO (2002).

### Triterpenoid saponins

Total 1.7%, euscaphic acid glycoside, tormentic acid glycosides: tormentoside (isomer of rosamultin) and isomers: kaji-ichigoside F1 & arjunetin (cultivated, Poland) (Stachurski et al 1995).
*Potentilla tormentilla*, euscaphic acid, tormentic acid (commercial) (Kite et al 2007).
*Potentilla tormentilla*, nine glycosides: euscaphic acid, tormentic acid, ursolic acid, kaji-ichigoside F1, arjunetin, rosamultin and newly isolated glycosides (commercial) (Bilia et al 1994); pomolic acid glycoside (commercial) (Bilia et al 1992).

### Tannins

Mainly condensed tannins which are proanthocyanidin polymers, also hydrolysable tannins (Bruneton 1999).

### Condensed tannins

Mainly procyanidins: dimers, trimers, tetramers, pentamers, hexamers (Vennat et al 1994).
Total 15–20% type B proanthocyanidins: mainly dimers and trimers (Tomczyk & Latté 2009).
*Potentilla alba* Total 8% proanthocyanidins mainly polymers of (−) epicatechin (cultivated, Poland) (Oszmianski et al 2007). (+)-catechin gallate and B3 dimer (wild, Russia) (Omurkamzinova & Erzhanova 1986).

### Hydrolysable tannins

Ellagitannins: pedunculagin 1%, agrimoniin 3.5%, laevigatin B, laevigatin F (commercial, Germany) (Geiger et al 1994).
*Potentilla alba*, ellagic acid, *p*-coumaric acid (cultivated, Poland) (Oszmianski et al 2007).

## REFERENCES

Adams M, Berset C, Kessler M, et al 2009 Medicinal herbs for the treatment of rheumatic disorders – survey of European herbals from the 16th and 17th century. Journal of Ethnopharmacology 121:343–359.

Allen DE, Hatfield G 2004 Medicinal plants in folk tradition. Timber Press, Portland.

Apgar BS, Kaufman AH, George-Nwogu U, et al 2007 Treatment of menorrhagia. American Family Physician 75:1813–1819.

Arber AR 1986 Herbals, their origin and evolution, 3rd edn. Cambridge University Press, Cambridge.

Barker J 2001 The medicinal flora of Britain and Northwestern Europe. Winter Press, West Wickham, Kent.

Bilia A R, Catalano S, Fontana C, et al 1992 A new saponin from *Potentilla tormentilla*. Planta Medica 58:A723.

Bilia AR, Palme E, Catalano S, et al 1994 New triterpenoid saponins from the roots of *Potentilla tormentilla*. Journal of Natural Products 57:333–338.

Bisset NG, Wichtl M (eds) 2001 Herbal drugs and phytopharmaceuticals, 2nd edn. Medpharm, Stuttgart.

Bos MA, Vennat B, Meunie M, et al 1996 Procyanidins from tormentil: Antioxidant properties towards lipoperoxidation and anti-elastase activity. Biological and Pharmaceutical Bulletin 19:146–148.

Bruneton J 1999 Pharmacognosy, phytochemistry, medicinal plants, 2nd edn. Intercept, London.

Carmichael AG 1997 Bubonic plague: the black death. In: Kiple KF (ed.) Plague, pox & pestilence. Weidenfeld & Nicholson, London.

Comfort JW 1859 The practice of medicine on Thomsonian principles. Lindsay & Blakiston, Philadelphia. Online. Available: http://books.google.com.

Cullen W 1772 Lectures on the materia medica, as delivered by William Cullen. Lowndes, London. Eighteenth Century Collections Online. Available: http://library.wellcome.ac.uk/eresources.

Davis PH (ed.) 1972 Flora of Turkey, vol 4. Edinburgh University Press, Edinburgh.

French RK 2003 Medicine before science. Cambridge University Press, Cambridge.

Fuchs L 1980 Holzschnitte, die historischen Taschenbücher. Konrad Kölbl, Grünwald bei München.

Geiger C, Scholz E, Rimpler H 1994 Ellagitannins from *Alchemilla xanthochlora* and *Potentilla erecta*. Planta Medica 60:384–385.

Gibbons B, Brough P 1996 Wild flowers of Britain & Northern Europe. Chancellor Press, London.

Grey-Wilson C, Mathew B 1981 Bulbs. Collins, London.

Hammerle CW, Surawicz CM 2008 Updates on treatment of irritable bowel syndrome. World Journal of Gastroenterology 14:2639–2649.

Hammerstone JF, Lazarus SA, Schmitz HH 2000 Procyanidin content and variation in some commonly consumed foods. Journal of Nutrition 130:2086S–2092S.

Haslam E 1996 Natural polyphenols (vegetable tannins) as drugs: possible modes of action. Journal of Natural Products 59:205–215.

Henriette's Herbal Homepage (2009) Image Galleries. Online. Available: http://www.henriettesherbal.com.

Hill J 1756 The British herbal. London, printed for T. Osborne and six others Eighteenth Century Collections Online. Available: http://library.wellcome.ac.uk/eresources.

Hurrell RF, Reddy M, Cook JD 1999 Inhibition of non-haem iron absorption in man by polyphenolic-containing beverages. British Journal of Nutrition 81:289–295.

ISSC-MAP 2009 International standards for sustainable wild collection of medicinal and aromatic plants. Online. Available: http://www.floraweb.de/map-pro.

Kite GC, Porter EA, Simmonds MS 2007 Chromatographic behaviour of steroidal saponins studied by high-performance liquid chromatography-mass spectrometry. Journal of Chromatography A 1148:177–183.

Langmead L, Dawson C, Hawkins C, et al 2002 Antioxidant effects of herbal therapies used by patients with inflammatory bowel disease: an in vitro study. Alimentary Pharmacology & Therapeutics 16:197–205.

Louis A 1980 Mathieu de l'Obel. Editions Story-Scientia, Ghent-Louvain.

Lownes AE 1958 Persistent remaindering (Pena and de l'Obel's adversaria, 1570–1618). The Papers of the Bibliographical Society of America 52:295–299.

McFarland LV 2008 State-of-the-art of irritable bowel syndrome and inflammatory bowel disease research in 2008. World Journal of Gastroenterology 14:2625–2629.

Mills S, Bone K 2005 The essential guide to herbal safety. Churchill Livingstone, St Louis.

Moss AD, Chefetz AD 2007 Tormentil for active ulcerative colitis. Journal of Clinical Gastroenterology 41:797–798.

Nelson M, Poulter J 2004 Impact of tea drinking on iron status in the UK: a review. Journal of Human Nutrition and Dietetics 17:43–54.

NICE 2007 Heavy menstrual bleeding. National Institute for Health and Clinical Excellence. Online. Available: http://guidance.nice.org.uk/CG44.

Nutton V 1983 The seeds of disease: an explanation of contagion and infection from the Greeks to the Renaissance. Medical History 27:1–34.

Oszmianski J, Wojdylo A, Lamer-Zarawska E, et al 2007 Antioxidant tannins from Rosaceae plant roots. Food Chemistry 100:579–583.

Omurkamzinova VB, Erzhanova MS 1986 Flavans of the rhizomes of *Potentilla erecta*. Chemistry of Natural Compounds 22:350.

Palombo EA 2006 Phytochemicals from traditional medicinal plants used in the treatment of diarrhoea: modes of action and effects on intestinal function. Phytotherapy Research 20:717–724.

Pavord A 2005 The naming of names: the search for order in the world of plants. Bloomsbury, London.

Pereira J 1853 The elements of materia medica and therapeutics, 3rd edn, vol 2. Online. Available: http://www.henriettesherbal.com.

Rasmussen SE, Frederiksen H, Strunze Krogholm K, et al 2005 Dietary proanthocyanidins: occurrence, dietary intake, bioavailability, and protection against cardiovascular disease. Molecular Nutrition and Food Research 49:159–174.

Reeds KM 1976 Renaissance humanism and botany. Annals of Science 33:519–542.

Reeds KM 1991 Botany in medieval and Renaissance universities. Garland, New York.

Robinson M 1868 The new family herbal and botanic physician. William Nicholson, London.

Stace C 1991 New flora of the British Isles. Cambridge University Press, Cambridge.

Stachurski L, Bednarek E, Dobrowolski JC, et al 1995 Tormentoside and two of its isomers obtained from the rhizomes of *Potentilla erecta*. Planta Medica 61:94–95.

Stevens J 1847 Medical reform, or physiology and botanic practice, for the people. John Turner, Birmingham & Whittaker, London.

Subbotina MD, Timchenko VN, Vorobyov MM, et al 2003 Effect of oral administration of tormentil root extract (*Potentilla tormentilla*) on rotavirus diarrhea in children: A randomized, double-blind, controlled trial. Pediatric Infectious Disease Journal 22:706–710.

Thankachan P, Walczyk T, Muthayya S, et al 2008 Iron absorption in young Indian women: the interaction of iron status with the influence of tea and ascorbic acid. American Journal of Clinical Nutrition 87:881–886.

Thomson S 1832 New guide to health; or, botanic family physician, 8th edn. Pike, Platt, Columbus. Online. Available: http://books.google.co.uk.

Tomczyk M, Latté KP 2009 *Potentilla* – a review of its phytochemical and pharmacological profile. Journal of Ethnopharmacology 122:184–204.

Tutin TG, Heywood VH, Burges NA, et al 1968 Flora Europaea, vol 2. Cambridge University Press, Cambridge.

Vennat B, Bos MA, Pourrat A, et al 1994 Procyanidins from tormentil: fractionation and study of the anti-radical activity towards superoxide anion. Biological and Pharmaceutical Bulletin 17:1613–1615.

WHO 2002 WHO monographs on selected medicinal plants, vol 2. World Health Organization, Geneva.

Williamson E 2003 Potter's herbal cyclopaedia. CW Daniel, Saffron Walden.

Zuckerman A 2004 Plague and contagionism in eighteenth-century England: the role of Richard Mead. Bulletin of the History of Medicine 78:273–308.

# CHAPTER 25
# *Rosa damascena*, damask rose

## DESCRIPTION

**Family: Rosaceae**      **Part used: flower petals, hips**

Forty-seven species within the *Rosa* genus are found wild in Europe, including *Rosa gallica* L., with *Rosa sempervirens* L. in more southern areas and the *Rosa canina* L. group in more northerly areas (Tutin et al 1968). The species have some common characteristics: firm stems, which are usually prickly, and bear pinnate leaves with stipules, which are usually deciduous. Terminal flowers are often white or pink and single or borne in corymbs. The roots are stout and roses are generally very hardy. Innumerable hybrids are cultivated in gardens and their ancestry can be complex mixtures of European and east Asian species (Tutin et al 1968). The complex history of the cultivation of roses is discussed by Shepherd (1954, 1978). 'Old roses' is the term used for the groups of roses which existed before 1867 when the first hybrid tea rose cv. La France appeared (Joyaux 2005). The following four groups are significant and examples are given of varieties.

*Rosa* × *damascena* Mill. is a pink rose that is a cultivated hybrid and is therefore correctly written as *Rosa* × *damascena*. It is argued that it developed in Iran as a cross between *Rosa moschata* Benth., *Rosa gallica* L. and *Rosa feldschenkoana* Regel (Iwata et al 2000). *Rosa moschata* is thought to have originated in India or southern China, *Rosa gallica* is found in Europe and western Asia, and *Rosa feldschenkoana* is from central Asia (Shepherd 1954, 1978). The development of this rose is discussed below.

*Rosa gallica* var. *officinalis*, the Red Rose of Lancaster, spreads vegetatively and by seed. The early breeding of roses was by seed and thus determining the parentage of varieties of old roses from before the 19th century is often impossible. Examples are cv. Tuscany, which is known to be an old variety, cv. Sissinghurst Castle, which is thought to be a very old selection, and cv. Charles de Mills. The earliest striped rose cv. Rosa mundi was described by de l'Obel in 1581 but may be older (Joyaux 2005).

*Rosa* × *centifolia* L. is thought be a very old hybrid possibly including *Rosa gallica*, *Rosa phoenicia*, *Rosa moschata* and *Rosa canina*. It was described by de l'Obel in 1597. Flowers are usually pink although sometimes white. An example is cv. Fantin-Latour (Joyaux 2005).

*Rosa* × *alba* is thought to be a natural hybrid, probably cultivated in Roman times. Examples include cv. Cuisse de Nymph, cv. Céleste and cv. Felicité Parmentier (Joyaux 2005).

Rosehips: The red fruit is a pseudocarp that encloses numerous achenes. Rosehips are collected from wild rose species such as the dog rose *Rosa canina*.

## Quality

Usage of cultivated roses in Britain for the preparation of medicines should be restricted to certain old rose cultivars as they have equivalent volatile oils to *Rosa damascena* but other rose cultivars may have none of the typical constituents (Brunke et al 1992) so should not be used to make preparations. Hybrid tea roses should not be used as they were not bred until the 19th century and have a different parentage.

It is thought that cultivation of *Rosa damascena* originally developed in the Lyzangan Valley near Fars in Iran (Kiani et al 2008). A study of 40 accessions, both cultivated and wild, from 28 provinces of Iran, identified nine genotypes and the authors argue that this shows Iran to be the centre of diversity for the damask rose (Babaei et al 2007). A study of 40 accessions from five rose-growing areas in Iran also found genetic diversity and six of these had a separate genetic background (Kiani et al 2008).

Cultivars were taken from Iran to Bulgaria in the 17th century and the genotype in Isfahan, the main production area of Iran, was found to be identical to the Bulgarian genotype (Babaei et al 2007). A study of 24 *Rosa damascena* plants cultivated in Kazanluk, Bulgaria found that the plants had a very narrow gene pool (Rusanov et al 2005). Cultivation was also developed in Turkey from the 1880s. The largest producers of rose oil today are Bulgaria and Turkey (Bayrak & Akgül 1994). A study of cultivated material from 15 sites in Isparta, the main area of rose-growing in Turkey, showed that all *Rosa damascena* samples were genetically identical (Baydar et al 2004).

THE WESTERN HERBAL TRADITION

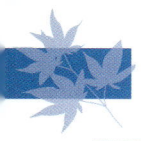

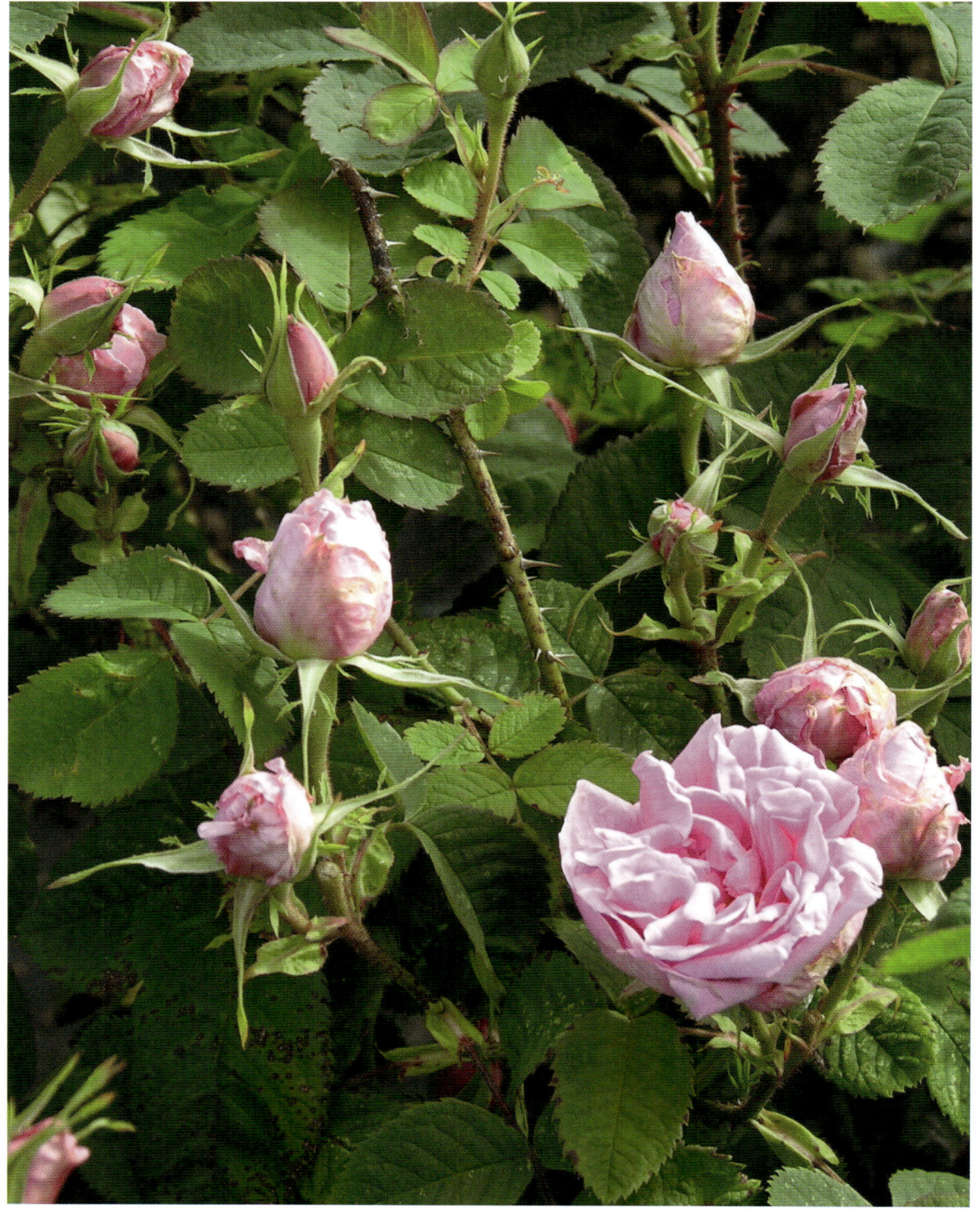

Figure 25.1 *Rosa damascena*, damask rose (Ceredigion, Wales, June).

*Rosa damascena*, damask rose | Chapter | 25

> The study above on Bulgarian roses also studied 13 garden damask roses and found that the old roses Kazanlik, Quatre Saisons and York & Lancaster are identical with the Bulgarian roses (Rusanov et al 2005). A genetic study of the four oldest damask roses in Europe (cv. Kazanlik, cv. Quatre Saisons, cv. Quatre Saisons Blanc Mousseux and cv. York & Lancaster) found that their common ancestors were *Rosa moschata* and *Rosa gallica*, which probably formed a natural hybrid that was then crossed with *Rosa feldschenkoana*. The authors suggest that *Rosa feldschenkoana* could have contributed the glaucous leaf colour and shape of the hips to these roses (Iwata et al 2000). These four roses can therefore be used for medicine. Other damask roses that are likely to be suitable are cv. Ispahan, cv. Omar Khayam and cv. La Ville de Bruxelles. In addition, *Rosa × alba* cv. Felicité Parmentier, *Rosa × gallica* cv. Charles de Mils and hybrid perpetual cv. Ferdinand Pichard were shown to have similar components to *Rosa × damasacena* (Antonelli et al 1997) as was the Austin rose cv. Othello (Brunke et al 1992).
>
> Damask rose varieties are discussed by Katzer (2003). Useful books on the cultivation of roses are Thomas (2004) and Joyaux (2005). The national rose collection is held at Peter Beales Rose Gardens (2009) and the Royal National Rose Society (2009) has a substantial collection.
>
> Other species cultivated for rose oil in France and north Africa are *Rosa centifolia*, *Rosa gallica*, and, in China, *Rosa rugosa* (Baydar et al 2004) but, as the above cultivars are widely available, then they are recommended for cultivation.

## HERITAGE AND IDENTITY

The rose has an ancient heritage. Fossils have been found across the northern continents of Europe, America and Asia dating back to the Miocene period, 7–26 million years ago. From an easy tendency to hybridization, chance mutation and human inclination to encourage these processes dating back to the earliest civilizations, we have the joyous variety of current blooms. The breeding of roses appears to have originated in three main areas – Iran, Iraq and China. Clements et al (1979) write of rose gardens in China possibly as far back as 2700BC, and certainly in imperial Peking in the 4th and 5th centuries BC. In Persia early references are found, one of the earliest to 2200 BC in Sumeria, and as official symbol of King Kyros II in the 6th century BC. Medicinal rose plants can be found among the predecessors of our cultivated old garden roses, from early western hybrids, developed through a long history of successive civilizations from mainly Persian descent, and carried to the West. The development of our modern tea roses owes its heritage to aspects of Chinese antecedents and these were developed in Europe relatively recently in the 19th century. There is evidence of roses in Egypt and mention in Homer, Herodotus and Pindar among early authors. The Romans appear to have taken rose use to extremes with stories of revellers suffocating in rose petals at banquets, culminating in Nero spending a fortune covering a beach with rose petals for one of his celebrations. Clements et al (1979) report the Roman poet Horace complaining that instead of the necessary food crops, the grain fields and orchards were planted with roses because the rose culture was so lucrative.

*Rosa gallica* is described as the 'European prototype'. By the 17th century, Clements et al (1979) assert, Europe had developed varieties of roses descending largely from this rose. Varieties were also based on the three hybrids: *damascena*, *alba* and later *centifolia*. Grieve says the Ancients were familiar with at least the *Rosa gallica*, that is the red Provins rose or apothecaries rose, mistakenly called the Provence rose, although the varieties were limited. Provins is the town southeast of Paris where roses were cultivated. Dioscorides specifies no type, nor even colour, nor offers description nor comment of any kind in this direction, Galen neither. Pliny, on the other hand, gives us 11 names and appends at least some description to each, but not enough detail to allow any definitive, or necessarily useful, comparison with later blooms, although of course a number of authors have made more or less informed guesses as to their identity. Parkinson and Mattioli cite Pliny that the Romans esteemed greatest the praestinian, campanan and milesian, this latter held to be the best red rose and of the brightest colour. The tracynian, less red, and the alabandican, the least one, with white petals, follow. Most useful of all, but the smallest, is spineola. There is a centifolia and a variety of moscheuton, of which Pliny's coroneola is generally agreed, says Parkinson, to be the double musk rose. The Renaissance authors, not unexpectedly of course, have a field day enumerating the varieties familiar to their own experience and comparing these to Pliny and to each others' views on this matter with commendable fastidiousness. Gerard discusses six garden roses, eight musks and four wild types. Dodoens offers 10, including musk and wild, Bauhin covers 12 and is particularly detailed on discussion of who says which rose is which, while Parkinson excels with 24. Their opinions and descriptions do not always coincide, particularly on which might correspond to Pliny.

Dodoens' 10 roses, as example, cover, briefly, (1) rosa alba, the white rose, called (confusingly) in Italy the damask rose, possibly the campana of Pliny; (2) rosa rubra, the red rose, Pliny's trachinias, amongst which rosae milesiae are the deepest red; (3) rose de Provinces, called in English also damask rose, perhaps Pliny's alabandicas; (4) rose de Provins, perhaps the rosae milesiae of Pliny;

255

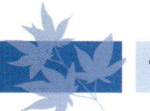

(5) the civet rose or bastard muske rose, possibly the rosa praenestina of Pliny; (6) rosa coroneola of Pliny, the muske rose; (7) rosa canina, the brier bush or hep tree; (8) the kunosbatos of the Greeks, Pliny's rosa spinosa; (9) the yellow rose; (10) eglantine, rosa Graeca in Latin. Of garden roses Gerard details the white rose, the red rose, the common damaske rose, the lesser Province rose, the rose without prickles, and the Holland or Province rose.

There are nevertheless many points of similarity through the Renaissance authors, particularly concerning the main varieties used in medicine. All of their texts seem to have some version of the later recognized varieties: *Rosa gallica* also known as Provins or Apothecaries rose, of a deep crimson colour; the white rose; the damask rose, which is pink to light red, and *Rosa centifolia* or Provence rose, which is also pink. It is doubtful whether they had the

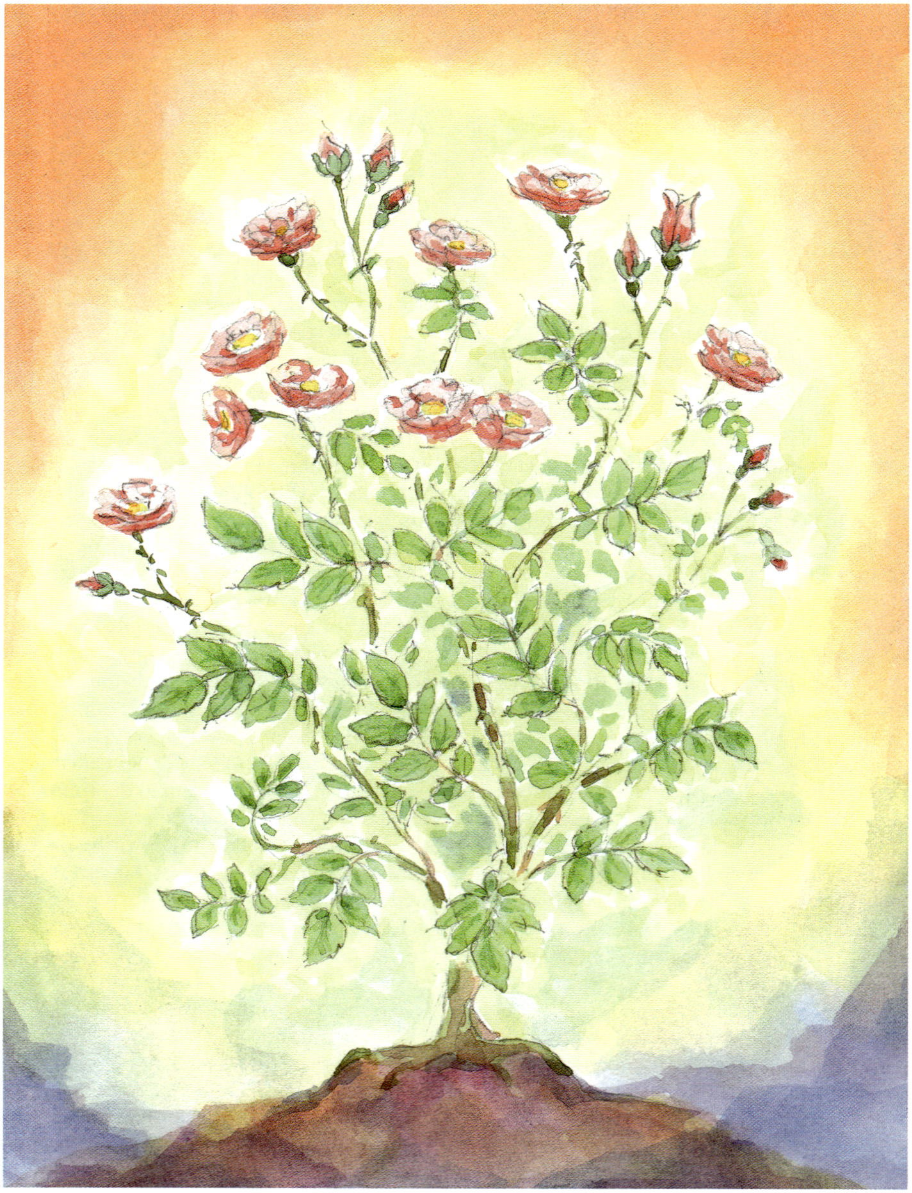

**Figure 25.2** *Rosa damascena*, damask rose.

damask rose in the Roman era, since it may not have reached the West by then. Mattioli includes a suggestion that Mesue might not have been familiar with the damask, since it had only recently been introduced into Italy in Mattioli's time, but Mesue, I would have thought, being Persian, is possibly rather more likely to have been acquainted with it than not.

As a flower of perfection, the symbol of love, famed in many mythologies, highly prized by poets and holding a central position through many traditions and ages, the rose as a medicinal plant has a less uniformly sustained history. It begins its journey in our sources with appreciable use in Dioscorides and Pliny. It then seems to parallel the relative constraint to local resource of all cultural activity in Europe, following the fall of the Roman empire, with many records limited to wild rose use. By the 12th century however, we find Hildegard extolling its use as addition to any medicine 'Rose is also good to add to unguents and all medications. If even a little rose is added, they are so much better, because of the good virtues of the rose'. In the meantime, again pacing cultural development, the rose takes a significant leap forward in Arabic hands, both horticultural and medical, and in recorded form. This serves then the crescendo to the Renaissance with its explicit recognition as one of the most useful herbs and its detailed recorded use, where its medical applications were arrayed in a fine appreciation of the niceties of internal and external treatment through many different preparation choices. Parkinson says 'The rose is of exceeding great use with us'. Mattioli says 'clearly roses are to be esteemed highly…not only because they are an embellishment to pleasure gardens…but because they are useful as the most outstanding medicines by which human life is aided'. It then sinks gradually into relative obscurity with the perfunctory 'almost entirely overlooked as a medicinal plant' of the *National Botanic Pharmacopoeia* of 1921 and an unprepossessing role as adjunct to make other medicines taste better. It appears only as rosehip in the 1983 *British Herbal Pharmacopoeia*, and is missing entirely from many later herbals. There are encouraging signs of its rehabilitation among current authors and herbalists, but it merits a more serious reappraisal of its virtues.

## PARTS OF THE ROSE

It might be illuminating to follow the example of some of the Renaissance authors and precede any discussion of the virtues of rose with a brief enumeration of the various sections of the plant noted by the Ancients, and later writers, and considered to have different properties, 'worthy to know and useful in medicine' says Mattioli, although he complains 'though there are few apothecaries who place them separately'. There are six parts according to Mattioli, eight for Bauhin, since he includes the hips in his counting. Dodoens lists six, including the hips, and Parkinson five, but these latter are just not so detailed. There are two parts to the petals – confusingly written 'folia' in Latin which also translates as 'leaf' – the nails or 'ungues', the white inner parts to the petal where it joins the stem, and the rest of the petal. The 'yellow haire' in the centre, Dodoens explains, is called 'anthos' (plural anthera) in Greek, and 'flos' in Latin, and these terms give rise to even more confusion. 'Flos' usually translates as 'flower', while 'anthera' is sometimes applied to the yellow centre, but more often referred to a certain composite medicine, according to Celsus, Galen and Paulus, Mattioli tells us, of frequent use among the Ancients for ulcers of the mouth, cracks of the feet and pterygia, a growth of flesh over the nails of the hand. These yellow centres were called the 'blowing of the rose' by the Arabic writers. Mattioli distinguishes two parts to these centres, the thin hairs and the parts like minute seeds on top of them. The next two parts Bauhin is clearest about. The calyx, by which name, he says, some call the ball with all the petals before it opens (and this is Dodoens version), but by Bauhin's fuller account it is the pedicle which holds the flower and ends in the solid head, covered in a kind of down, laying under the petals and flowers as the base sustaining the whole rose. This is followed by the cortex or cortices rosarum, 'the five little leaves that stand around the bud'; that is to say the 'shels or pils of roses', Dodoens explains, also called the five brothers (see below for Albertus Magnus' poem on this point). Finally, come the hips of which Mattioli lists three parts – the flesh, the down and the seeds. The latter two are Bauhin's final two categories. Some authors, including Dodoens, go further and extend the coverage to the rose gall of wild roses, 'the rough spongious bawle or excrescence that growth in the wilde rose bush' as good against stone and strangury, they say. Again there is some controversy since some authors refer to this as the bedeguar, and Parkinson at least insists the bedeguar is a thistle. And still further, Culpeper refers to the worms in the gall, which 'dried, powdered and drunk' are good against worms of the belly 'found by long experience of many'.

## ANCIENT USE

Dioscorides (I 99) records modest use. He tells us that roses (rodon, plural roda in Greek) cool and contract, but dried roses contract more strongly. He is precise about the preparations and the parts used. In preparing the juice, the 'nails' of the roses are first removed. The remainder of the petals, and they should be from young roses, are then squeezed and pounded in a mortar, compressed into a ball and stored to make ointment for eyes. Roses have to be dried carefully in the shade and turned frequently to avoid mould. The expressed juice of dried roses boiled in wine is good for headaches, ear aches, sore eyes, painful gums, and for anal and uterine pain – for the latter when 'applied with a feather brush' and 'used as a wash' (Beck), thus presumably massaged onto the abdomen or used as a douche or pessary. Osbaldeston's version records perineum, intestine, rectum and vulva, here. For inflammations of the hypochondrium (Parkinson has 'region of the heart'), for excess fluids in the stomach and for erysipelas roses should be used as a plaster. The preparation here is ambiguous. Beck reads 'The roses themselves, chopped up without being squeezed …' which could refer either to the previous preparation of dried roses boiled in wine, or simply to fresh roses. Parkinson's interpretation is for the former, since he translates 'the same decoction, with roses remaining in them…' Dioscorides continues that dried roses, ground up finely to powder are used on the inside of the thighs. Beck suggests here an interpretation of antiperspirant and deodorant, since roses contract the pores. Turner's wording is very resonant 'when as they are dried and broken they are sprenched amongst the thighs or shares'. The same preparation can be mixed with lip salves, wound medications and antidotes. Dried roses, burnt, make a paint for eyelids and eyelashes. The yellow centre, the 'flower', has its own specific use, dried and applied for discharges of the gums. Rose hips (although an argument could be made that this is the unripe head of the rose) control diarrhoea and the spitting of blood. These need to be drunk, Dioscorides says, but he gives no specific preparation. He finally gives a recipe for making 'rhodides', disks or beads which women hang round their necks to counter perspiration or they are made into powders for use after baths or in ointments. The recipe runs: 40 drachms (160 g) of fresh dried roses, 5 drachms (20 g) of Indian spikenard *Nardostachys jatamansi*, 6 drachms (24 g) myrrh *Commiphora molmol*, ground together and mould into small disks, dry and store in a sealed jar. Some add, he says, 2 drachms (8 g) of costus root, 2 drachms (8 g) of Illyrian iris, mixed with honey and Chian wine.

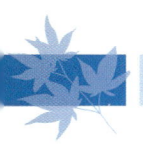

Beck includes an earlier entry, (I 94) as kynosbatos, *Rosa sempervirens* L. the white rose, which, Dioscorides says, 'some call oxyacantha'. He describes it as 'a tree-like shrub, much bigger than a bramble. It bears leaves broader than the myrtle's, strong thorns around its twigs, a white flower, and fruit that is oblong, resembling an olive pit, growing red as it ripens and having its insides woolly'. The dried fruit, with woolly interior removed (as it is bad for the trachea), boiled in wine and taken internally will stop diarrhoea. There is more controversy over this plant. Mattioli, for example, treats it only as oxyacantha with no mention of kynosbatos, although with further actions and a long discussion of what it might be. Parkinson argues it is more likely hawthorn saying: 'Tragus and Dodonaus because they would not confound Cynosbatos with Cynorrhodon, the descriptions being so different both in Dioscorides and Theophrastus, referred the Cynosbatos… to the white thorne or Hawthorne and the Cynorrhodon to the wilde Rose… and yet many even to this day doe referre the Cynosbatos to the wilde Rose'.

Pliny on rose reads much like Dioscorides, although with additions. Fuchs and Dalechamps, citing Pliny, include the use of rose in fever by itself or with vinegar, and for sleep and sickness. Roses have the capacity to penetrate deeply. They inhibit fluxions of women, especially 'the whites', i.e. leucorrhoea, and menorrhagia, with vinegar and water. The flowers (yellow centres?) help sleep. The saffron-coloured seed is best dried in shade and no older than a year. It heals toothaches and excites urine. It purges the head if put under the nostrils, presumably thus as snuff. The nails are good for ulcers of the eyes applied with bread. The petals are good for weakness of the stomach, corrosions and weak bowels and intestines, and very healing for the praecordia. This word 'praecordia' perhaps deserves a comment. Is Pliny suggesting here this is a topical remedy for the heart? Roses are used as seasonings in food. Wild rose with bear's fat 'heals alopecia wonderfully'. Finally Parkinson relates Pliny's commendation of the root of wild rose for the bite of a mad dog which was discovered 'by a miracle [other sources say an 'oracle']…but how wee may beleeve him I know not'.

Galen is succinct; the rose possesses heat in a watery substance, mixed with two other qualities, astringency and bitterness. The flowers are more astringent. Parkinson's rendition suggests this reference to 'flowers' is to the yellow centres.

## MEDIEVAL CONTRACTION

The *Old English Herbarium* includes only the sweet briar or eglantine *Rosa canina* or *Rosa rubiginosa*, the 'plant called cynosbatus'. It is 'harsh on the throat and disagreeable before meals, but nevertheless, it will purge the chest, and anything sour or bitter; although it harms the stomach, it benefits the spleen greatly. If the flowers of this plant are drunk, they affect a person in a way so that the intestines and urine will take out disease. It also purifies bleeding.' The bark can be used as external application for the spleen. Without the richness of cultivated roses, the uses here appear rather restricted and do not attain the breadth of Arabic or Renaissance sophistication, although application to the chest is notable, reflecting somewhat Dioscorides' spitting of blood and reappearing in Culpeper's later use for TB.

Hildegard may have had access to better stock or wider sources, but her applications are still not wide and there is no specific reference to internal use, or wider external use. Rose is cold, she says, and this coldness contains moderation which is useful. Rose petals placed on the eyes in the morning will draw out the humour and clear them. The mucus of small ulcers on the skin can be drawn by rose petals. A person who is 'inclined to wrath' should make a powder of rose and sage, less sage than rose, and take as snuff, 'hold this powder to his nostrils', for the sage eases the wrath and the rose cheers. An ointment can be made from the same two plants cooked in lard for rubbing on cramps and paralysis.

*The Trotula* (Green 2001) has a few uses for rose, variety unspecified, and they are all cooling remedies. A very practical one is for pain of the womb coming from heat, for instance made hot from the 'use of Venus' when marshmallow, herb of violets, roses and root of rush should be cooked in water, fomented and applied. If the feet swell in pregnancy, rub with rose oil and vinegar. A plaster which mitigates pain and restores strength for a lesion of the womb from a hot cause might include juice of purslane, houseleek, fleawort, great plantain, prickly lettuce and rose oil.

A most interesting entry in a later section of *The Trotula* is the recipe for oleum rosaceum or oleum rosatum, since it shows clear influence, albeit limited, from earlier, presumably Arabic, texts. 'The oleum has a cold and styptic power', the recipe says, 'and this is the best thing for head pains from fever or heat of the sun'. It will remove burning and heat from a bilious stomach and when its windiness [of the stomach] fills the head. Pain in the head or part of the head is eased if anointed with this oil. For pains in the stomach or intestines from 'sharpness of the humors' it should be applied mixed with mastic and wax. It is good for erysipelas that does not appear on the surface of the skin and other similar conditions. This oleum rosaceum, typically for this time an infused oil, not a distilled one, is made thus; 1½ lb slightly crushed fresh roses are placed in 2 lb of common '(and in our opinion cleaned)' oil; these are put in a pot in a bain marie and boiled until reduced to one third of the quantity, pressed and the liquid saved. There is a further recipe for rosata novella which rids vomiting and upset stomach, counters weakness and thirst and eases a long sickness: Take 1 oz, 1 drachm (4 g) and 2½ scruples (38 g) each of rose, sugar and liquorice; 2 drachms, 2 scruples and 2 grains (10.5 g) cinnamon; 1 scruple and 8 grains (1.8 g) each of clove, spikenard, ginger, galangal, nutmeg, zedoary, storax, watercress and wild celery and honey as needed. Take morning, noon and night in cold water.

## SOME EXPANSION

The Salernitan herbal, as might be expected, echoes earlier texts a little more fully and introduces the less material effects too. The rose is hot in the first degree and dry in the second. The water binds and fortifies. A recommendation of breathing the scent of dried roses to fortify the brain and heart and restore the spirits appears to be translated into more material benefit as those with a weak heart and tendency to faint should take rose water or decoction of the powder and egg white. Use for the stomach and intestines is repeated and further suggestions follow: rose honey with senna and salt for cold humours in the stomach; for diarrhoea and vomiting rose water cooked with mastic and one clove; for diarrhoea when the intestines are scratched (is this Pliny's 'corrosions'?) and vomiting hot humours and strange liquids: rose oil, put on the forehead and temples, heals the liver and headache from heat; rose juice cooked in water is applied for redness and burns; and washing the face in rose water firms, freshens and gives a good colour.

The Arabic writers appear to take up the Ancients' recommendations readily and add experience of their own, being clearly familiar with cultivated roses. Ibn Sina says it is often used. Serapio mainly repeats Galen, Dioscorides and Pliny. He adds rose flowers shaken with vinegar and applied to the head will ease pains due to heat of the sun; they can be used to treat bloody abscesses and dried roses can be included in many medicinal powders for curing ulcers. Ibn Sina too echoes the Ancients. Galen's qualities are explored: its strength is composed of a water and earthy substance, but it has a causticity and ability to bind, also a bitterness and astringent quality together with a little sweetness. Ibn Sina appears to account for Pliny's penetrating qualities: its wateriness, he says weakens its warmth by reason of that principle which makes it sweet and bitter. In it is a rarefaction, facilitating a penetration of its binding qualities. He notes, however, a consequence of this, for it often brings on a cold in the head. Roses are cold in the first degree and dry in the second. He repeats the difference between fresh and dried roses, how they open and cleanse, the seeds and bits of fluff within binding more strongly. How all parts strengthen internal organs but bind no further than to prevent dissolution. He cites uses through the body and for various purposes: as cosmetic he repeats Dioscorides' recipe for a necklace with nard and myrrh against the smell of sweat. For the skin, the boiled petals will resolve hot swellings and erysipelas, restore flesh in old ulcers and draw out arrow tips and thorns. Ibn Sina's interpretation of Dioscorides' application on the thighs and in the groin is to prevent abrasions there. For the head, fresh and distilled roses ease pain; roses cause sneezing in those whose brain is hot. Uses for the eyes, gums and ears are rehearsed. Fainting, spitting of blood, digestive and uterine applications all appear here too. He includes a recommendation for pains of the colon and the decoction as enema for ulcers of the intestines. To sleep on a bedding of roses, he says, pacifies lust, although Nero perhaps would not agree. The wild rose Ibn Sina treats separately. Hot and dry in the second degree, it is good for cold in the nerves, kills worms in the ears, helps ringing in the ears and is useful for tooth pain. It is used for swellings in the throat and tonsils, to open obstructions in the nostrils and to calm head pain.

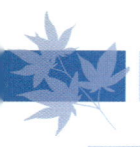

## ABUNDANCE

Mesue has much to say and it appears to be mainly his text, rather than that of Ibn Sina, plus those of the Ancients, presumably also stimulated by a flourishing of professional interest in roses consequent on the developing of different varieties, that produce the acme of expertise in all things medicinally rose achieved among the Renaissance authors. Turner, Mattioli, Gerard, Parkinson, Dodoens, Culpeper and Bauhin, for example, all devote many pages to the rose, Bauhin in the greatest detail with contrasting opinions carefully summarized and weighed. They address the topics in more or less similar vein. Within this rich Renaissance context I first look at the nature of the rose and its qualities, then put a toe into the water of whether red or white, dried or fresh, bud or open are better. Then having established beyond doubt the gentle nature of the rose, I plunge into the deeper water of general applications, the specific use of the separate parts, the vast array of preparations and one or two recipes from the time.

Turner and Mattioli consider Mesue's expansion of Galen's qualities into his thoughts on the nature of roses. The rose is cold in the first degree and dry in the second, says Mesue, compounded of various parts of different natures. The first is a material and binding, substantial faculty from the watery and earthy; then there is the airy, which is sweet and fragrant, along with the fiery from which comes the bitterness, the redness and, says Turner, the perfection and the form or beauty. There is more heat in the red than in those which are only reddish, says Mattioli; but then Bauhin cites Galen that you cannot tell the temperature of a plant by its colour. But the bitterness, continues Mesue, among these fiery qualities, is the weakest faculty, since it is easily lost, disappearing even with simple drying of the flower. Since it is the bitterness which purges, then fresh roses are more bitter, and hence laxative, while the dried are more astringent, binding and drawing together. Mattioli says on this point 'from this it is learned that the laxative faculty…comes as much from their bitterness (which faculty the Greeks had not noticed) since the fresh draw down the belly but the dried not at all'. Turner puts it only slightly differently 'Yet green roses are more bitter than binding, and by reason of this bitterness green or moist roses purge and that chiefly with their juice, but when they are dried, the heat being resolved which maketh the bitterness, they show a substance binding or drawing together'.

Turner continues with Mesue's estimation of the juice of roses as hot almost in the first degree, which other authors, even those citing Mesue, choose to ignore, except for Bauhin, who occupies a whole column of text taking Mesue to task for his error that anything about the rose can be heating. Dalechamps gets involved to some extent saying 'my manuscript codex says: it heats if applied to the body'. He records it is held that the oil is cold in the first degree but the juice is more temperate than this. His own opinion suggests that it is balanced between heat and cold.

## RESOLUTION?

Culpeper follows Parkinson throughout, almost word for word, but his introduction, and he was obviously in jocular temper when he wrote it, is to the point: 'What a pother have authors made with roses! What a racket they have kept! I shall add red roses are under Jupiter, Damask under Venus, white under the Moon, and Provence under the King of France. The white and red roses are cooling and drying and yet the white is taken to exceed the red in both the properties, but is seldom used inwardly in any medicine. The bitterness in the roses when they are fresh, especially the juice, purges choler and watery humours; but being dried…they have then a binding and astringent quality. Those also that are not full blown do both cool and bind more than those that are full blown and the white rose more than the red'. Turner cites Mesue with different emphasis 'The white roses purge nothing at all or else very little, but they bind and strengthen more than the red do. The juice of them that are fully ripe is better, and so is the water wherein the ripe roses are steeped'.

The juice of the best quality is made from red roses, says Mattioli, then the pink, but it is of much weaker quality. Rhodopharmacum, a harmless laxative, is made from the leaves (petals) of pink roses, but damask are far better. But Mattioli says damask roses are white. It raises the question then whether his reference is to white damask roses or simply the white roses which Dodoens tells us the Italians call damask. Twenty such leaves, Mattioli says, eaten, draw the bowels quickly and harmlessly. These 20 petals appear again in Parkinson but not ascribed to Mattioli. Parkinson is considering whether the simple or double roses are better and it is to Camerarius he refers the recommendation 'The Muske Roses both single and double doe purge more forceable then the Damaske, and the single is he'd to be stronger than the double, for although none of the Greek writers have made any mention thereof, yet Mesues especially of the Arabians doth set it down: twenty of the leaves of the single rose must be taken saith Camerarius but more of the double kinde to open the belly and purge the body'. But although they purge, Culpeper reassures us, roses leave a binding property. Is this perhaps another example of balance?

## GENTLENESS AND BREADTH OF USE

All Renaissance authorities seem to agree on the gentleness of rose. For example, Dodoens says 'the juyce of roses, especially of them that are reddest, or the infusion or the decoction of them is of the kind of soft and gentle medicines which loose and open the belly, and may be taken without danger. Gerard similarly writes 'The juice, infusion or decoction of roses are to be reckoned among those medicines which are soft, gentle, loosing, opening and purging gently the belly, which may be taken at all times and in all places, of every kinde or sex of people both old and young, without danger or perill'. Mattioli notes how 'modern doctors' credit a rose syrup preparation for loosening the bowels among the medicines termed 'Benedicta'.

Most authors give a summary, and they mainly coincide, of the main uses of rose, familiar from Dioscorides, Pliny and Mesue. Gerard's list is typical: (1) they strengthen the heart and help its trembling and beating. Dodoens explains on this point 'for it dryveth forth, and dispatcheth all corrupt and evill humors, in and about the veynes of the heart'. (2) They strengthen the liver, kidneys and other weak 'intrails'; they dry and comfort a weak and moist stomach; stop leucorrhoea and excessive menstrual flow; staunch all bleedings in the body, stop sweating, bind, loosen and moisten the body. Dodoens adds of the juice that 'it purges downwards choleric humours and opens stoppings of the liver, strengthening and cleansing it. It is also good against hot fevers and the jaunders'. (3) Roses can be added to antidotes and similar, internally or externally to which they will add a strengthening and binding quality. (4) Honey of roses, mel rosarum, is very good for cleansing and drying wounds, ulcers, 'issues' and other similar lesions. (5) The oil reduces all heat and will help and ease inflammations and hot swellings.

Dodoens adds to Dioscorides' reference to heat of stomach, St Anthony's fire and erysipelas an application of roses 'pound and beaten small' for inflammation or swelling of the breasts or paps and serpigo. Turner alone cites Mesue that they 'make a man sleep but they provoke a man to nese [sneeze] and steer a man to the pose and are evil for rheumatic persons'. However, they fasten the uvula and 'thropple or throat' and they take drunkenness away.

Culpeper in the *Pharmacopoeia Londinensis*, writing of sugar of roses, summarizes its actions 'it strengtheneth the heart, the stomach, the liver and the retentive faculty; is good against all kinds of fluxes, prevents vomitings, stops tickling coughs and is of service in consumption'. This is one of the few references in our texts to coughs, perhaps an expansion of Dioscorides' spitting of blood.

## USE OF PARTS

In a number of authors, there is a further consideration of the virtues of the separate parts. For example, Gerard begins with 'yellow haires and tips' which bind and dry;

then he mentions, almost in parenthesis, 'fluxes at sea', which may refer to Pliny's 'nausea(s)' which can mean both sickness and sea-sickness: 'the cups and beards are of the same temperature, but since none of them has a sweet smell they are not so useful, except in fluxes at sea for which they are more useful than on land'. The anthera, dried and beaten to a powder, stay fluxes on land as well as at sea, he says, and also both white and red flux in women, 2 scruples (2.6 g) in red wine with some powdered ginger. Mattioli adds Dioscorides' defluxions of the gums here. For Culpeper, the stamens, powdered, should be drunk in distilled water of quince for overflowing of women's courses and defluxions of rheums on gums and teeth. The nails, says Gerard, are good for watering eyes. Mattioli says they are useful incorporated into lotions and clysters for stopping fluxes. The heads or buttons staunch bleeding and stop the laske (diarrhoea), continues Gerard while Mattioli talks of the calyx with the remaining part of the base, stopping flux of the bowels and coughing of blood. The hips astringe, he says, and are a remedy against diarrhoea, abundance of flow in women of whatever kind and are particularly powerful against gonorrhoea/urethral flux. Culpeper adds more on rosehips 'hips are grateful to the taste and a considerable restorative, fitly given to consumptive persons, the conserve being proper in all distempers of the breast and in coughs and tickling rheums. The pulp, powdered, breaks the stone and helps colic'.

## PREPARATIONS AND THEIR APPLICATION

Parkinson, copied by Culpeper, then details the various preparations and their uses, and this list is very impressive. He begins with red roses which, as we now know, 'strengthen the heart, stomach, liver and retentive faculty', so they 'mitigate pains from heat, assuage inflammations, procure rest and sleep, stay whites and reds, gonorrhoea, running of the reins (incontinence or frequency?) and flux of the belly'.

The electuary: purges choler, is good in hot fevers and pains in the head and joint ache from hot choleric humours, and for heat in the eyes and jaundice. It is a 'competent' purger for weak constitutions. Up to 6 drachms (24 g) can be taken according to the quality and strength of the patient.

The moist conserve is very useful for both binding and as cordial; when it is young it is more binding, when over 2 years old it is more cordial. So the young conserve, with Mithridatum, is good for distillations of rheum from the brain to the nose and defluxions of rheum into the eyes, fluxes and lasks of the belly. It can be taken with mastich for gonorrhoea (this is Culpeper's word, Parkinson has 'running of the reins') and looseness of humours. The old conserve is taken with Diarrhodon Abbatis or Aromaticum Rosarum (see *Pharmacopoeia Londinensis* for recipes) as a cordial for faintings, swoonings, weakness and tremblings of the heart. It strengthens the heart and a weak stomach, helps digestion, stays castings (vomiting) and is a good preservative in time of infection.

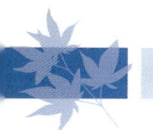

The dry conserve or Sugar of Roses is very good as a cordial to strengthen the heart and spirits and stay defluxions.

The syrup of dried red roses strengthens a stomach given to casting, cools an overheated liver and the blood in agues, comforts the heart, resists putrefaction and helps stay lasks and fluxes.

Honey of roses is much used in gargles and lotions to wash sores of the mouth, throat and other parts, to cleanse and heal, and to stay fluxes of humours in these parts. It is used in clysters (enemas) to cool and cleanse.

The cordial powders Diarrhodon Abbatis and Aromaticum Rosarum comfort and strengthen the heart and stomach, prepare appetite, help digestion, stay vomiting, are very good to strengthen and dry up slippery bowels.

Red rose water, well known and of familiar use, is better than Damask rose water. It is cooling, cordial, refreshing, quickening weak and faint spirits, used in meat and broths, to wash the temples and to smell at the nose from perfuming or a hot fire shovel. Also for red and inflamed eyes and pain in the temples.

Vinegar of roses is used as rose water for pain and ache in the head, and to procure rest and sleep, often applied overnight with rose cake, heated in a cloth together with nutmeg and poppy seed.

Ointment of roses counters heat and inflammation in the head and is applied to the forehead and temples and for rest. Mixed with some populeon it is also used for heat of the liver, back and reins, to cool and heal pushes, wheals and pimples.

Oil of roses is used by itself to cool hot swellings and inflammations and to dry sores, and is added to other ointments and plasters to cool, bind and restrain flux.

Rose leaves (petals?) and mints are heated and applied externally to help a weak stomach, cool the liver and heart and, applied to the head, ease overhot spirits which allow no rest.

And this is just the red rose!

Not so many preparations, however, are made of the damask rose, says Parkinson, but more are used than the red roses 'so much hath pleasure outstripped necessary use'. He lists the preparations, usually termed 'solutive', of damask rose and their uses. The simple solutive syrup is a safe, gentle and easy medicine which purges choler. He remarks how strange it is then that the distilled water of this syrup rather binds the belly. The syrup is stronger if used with 'Agoricke' and works as much on phlegm as on choler. The compound syrup is stronger for melancholy humours and can be used against leprosy (the word lepra means a scaly condition of the skin in Greek), itch, tetters (any number of skin conditions characterized by eruptions and itching) and the French disease (venereal disease).

Honey of roses solutive works as the sugar syrup in purging, but is given more often to phlegmatics than cholerics, and more often used as enemas than potions.

The simple water is used rather in cooking and perfuming and little used in physic but has some purging quality.

## RECIPES

To complete the instruction for the reader some authors offer recipes.

Gerard's syrup of the infusion of roses says: 'Take two pounds of roses, the white ends cut away, put them to steepe or infuse in six pintes of warm water in an open vessel for the space of twelve hours: then straine them out, and put thereto the like quantitie of roses, and warm the water again, so let it stand the like time: do thus foure or five times; in the end adde unto that liquor or infusion, foure pound of fine sugar in powder; then boyle it unto the forme of a syrup, upon a gentle fire, continually stirring it until it be cold; then straine it, and keepe it for your use, whereof may be taken in white wine, or other liquor, from one ounce unto two'.

Gerard's syrup of the juice is made thus: 'Take roses, the white nails cut away, what quantitie you please, stampe them, and straine out the juice, the which you shall put to the fire, adding thereto sugar, according to the quantity of the juice: boiling them on a gentle fire unto a good consistence'.

Three recipes from Culpeper follow:

Sugar of roses: 'Take of red rose leaves (petals), the whites being cut off, and speedily dried in the sun an ounce, white sugar a pound, melt the sugar in rose water and juice of roses of each two ounces which being consumed by degrees, put in the rose leaves in powder, mix them, put it upon a marble, and make into lozenges according to art'.

Rose vinegar: 'Take of red rose buds, gathered in a dry time, the whites cut off, dried in the shade three or four days, one pound, vinegar eight sextaries, set them in the sun forty days, then strain out the roses, and repeat the infusion with fresh ones'. Taking a sextary as equivalent to a sextarius, eight sextaries would be 4320 mL. Estimates of a sextary vary from just under a pint to a pint (568 mL) to a pint and a half.

Honey of roses solutive: 'Take of the often infusion of damask roses five pounds, honey rightly clarified four pounds, boil it to the thickness of honey…after the same manner is prepared the honey of the infusion of red roses'.

## 18TH CENTURY AND LATER

In the 18th century Miller and Quincy present quite a contrasting picture to each other. Quincy classes the rose under Cardiacs and Cephalics, class one of Nervous Simples. Within his very detailed account of how such medicines achieve their effects, he suggests that 'whatever is cordial must be cephalic as the head hath a principle share in agreeable sensations', while cathartics and other evacuants will depress the spirits. Whatever 'raises the spirits and gives sudden strength and cheerfulness' is accounted cardiac or cordial, comforting the heart. The more spirituous anything is which enters into the stomach, the sooner a person feels its cordial effects. Common foods take a long time to achieve a sufficient fineness to reach the nerves, but a 'spirituous substance' is more readily available since 'it is so fine and subtle in all its parts before it is taken, that it seems to enter or soak into the nerves as soon as it touches them; whereupon their vibrations are 'invigorated' and all sense of faintness is removed'. Rose, however, having been introduced as belonging to this category, is summarily dismissed among Quincy's materia medica, its entry containing only a reference to orange and jessamy (jasmine) as being of greater efficacy. It is worth considering whether Quincy is influenced by Ibn Sina here, who says in reference to wild rose that in its essence it is similar to jasmine but weaker (and similar to narcissus); that by its strength the oil of this rose is close to jasmine oil but weaker.

Miller, on the other hand, shows us that rose still constituted a valued medicine at that time, albeit apparently not on the same scale as in the Renaissance. Miller writes of white, damask, red and canina roses. The only preparation from white rose flowers, being drying, binding and cooling, is the white rose water, used in collyriums for sore and inflamed eyes, but he designates this preparation 'much used'. The damask, as gentle, and purging choleric and serous humours, is given to children and weakly persons and mixed frequently with stronger cathartics. He notes a few preparations: syrupus and succo rosarum (syrup and juice of roses); syrupus infusionis rosarum (infused syrup of roses); aqua rosarum Damascenarum (damask rose water); and the electuarium and succo rosarum (electuary (a thick syrup) and juice of roses). The red rose is still distinguished as more binding and astringent than any other species. The applications echo Culpeper/Parkinson, as good against fluxes of all kinds, they strengthen the stomach, prevent vomiting and stop tickling coughs by preventing defluxion of rheum, and are of good service in consumptions. Miller notes the potential of 'antherae or apies' as cordial, 'though they are but seldom used'. The preparations of red roses are: simple water; conserva rosarum (conserve of roses); sacharum rosarum (sugar of roses); syrupus de rosis siccis (syrup of dried roses); mel rosarum (honey of roses); ol rosarum (oil of roses); unguentum rosarum (ointment of roses); tinctura rosarum (tincture of roses) and aromaticum rosarum (a cordial powder). The wild rose flowers, Miller says, are more restringent than garden ones and are reckoned by some a specific for the catamenia (menses). The pulp of the hips is tasty, strengthens the stomach, cools fevers, is pectoral, good for coughs, spitting of blood and the scurvy – again very like Culpeper. The only preparation is conserva cynosbati (conserve of rosehips). Miller carries the familiar addendum that the seed is 'accounted extraordinary good' for stone and gravel, as is the bedeguar.

Hill, like Miller, is clearly a fan of rose and writes enthusiastically about the dog rose, damask, white and red. He defends the dog rose with vigour 'The fruit is the only part used…this is a pleasant medicine and is of some efficacy against coughs. Though this is the only part that is used, it is not the only that deserves to be; the flowers gathered in the bud, and dried, are an excellent astringent, made more powerful than the red roses that are commonly dried for this purpose. A tea, made strong of these dried buds, and some of them given with it twice a day in powder, is an excellent medicine for overflowings of the menses, it seldom fails to effect a cure. The seeds separated from the fruit dried and powdered, work by urine and are good against the gravel, but they do not work very powerfully'. He continues with the bedeguar as astringent used against fluxes, but with reservations; 'they re said to work by urine, but experience does not warrant this'. The damask he records as being best used as a syrup, as an excellent purge for children, and adults too 'there is not a better medicine for grown people who are subject to be costive. A little of it taken every night will keep the body open continually'. He adds though the later binding action as noted in Culpeper. The white roses are used as fresh or dried buds in strong infusion for overflowings of menses and bleeding of piles. The red roses are used as buds, and with the white bottoms removed. The dried have more virtue, he says. They are given as infusion and sometimes in powder against profuse menses and all other bleedings. The central ground seems covered here but there is no reference to its earlier cordial effects nor more material actions on the heart. The antiinflammatory and febrifuge properties are also notably lacking, as is external use.

Cullen was not so impressed. He seems to have only one sentence on the rose, and this with violet too; 'of violets and pale roses the purgative value is little to be depended upon'.

Cook, in the USA, indicates little medicinal use for rose. He says they are 'occasionally used in medicine, though more as a grateful flavour than as a remedy'. He nevertheless deems it worthy of a recipe or two. He begins with rosa centifolia, 'the most fragrant' and its use for rose water, as 'addendum to mild syrups and some external washes designed for diseases of the scalp or irritable diseases of the skin'. It is made by distilling two gallons of water from 8 lb fresh, 10 lb dried petals, the petals normally having been preserved with one third their weight of common salt. The syrup of roses is a very gentle laxative, Cook says, sometimes used for children, but mainly used for confection of senna and scammony. Scammony *Convolvulus scammonia* is no longer used as it is a fierce cathartic. This 'syrup is made by maceration of 7 oz petals in 3 pints water for 12 hours, it is then gently heated and strained, evaporated to 2 pints and 3 lb white sugar and 5 oz diluted alcohol added. *Rosa gallica* is only used as syrup or confection to make palatable more unpleasant, powerful, powdered astringents. Hips of *Rosa canina* he refers only to European use as confection. Ellingwood has no entry under rose.

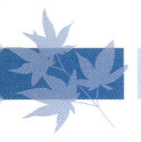

## MORE MODERN THOUGHTS – DECLINE AND RESURRECTION

Grieve gives a fine account of the development of rose oil production. How Avicenna first produced rose water in the 10th century, yet the distilled oil did not appear until the late 1500s or early 1600s. She tells the story of the wedding feast of Akbar's son, when a canal was dug circling the wedding garden and filled with rose water. How then in the hot sun the oil separated from the water and its exquisite perfume was realized, captured and shortly afterwards manufactured. Medicinal use in Grieve's time seems to have come more or less to a stop, or at least has dwindled into relative obscurity. She records rose petals as official in nearly all pharmacopoeias but in very limited use 'though formerly employed for their mild astringency and tonic value, they are today used almost solely to impart their pleasant odour to pharmaceutical preparations'. She mentions the confection of 1 lb fresh red rose petals beaten in a stone mortar with 3 lb sugar, used for pill making, though formerly prescribed, she says for haemorrhage of the lungs and for coughs and the acid infusion employed for treatment of stomatitis and pharyngitis is no highly rated preparation owing its action more to its sulphuric acid content. A simple infusion is used for ophthalmia. She mentions syrup of red rose and honey of roses and their use in the past. Rose vinegar is specific on the Continent, she says, for headache caused by a hot sun, when cloths, soaked in the vinegar in which the rose petals have been steeped, but not boiled, are put on the head. *Rosa centifolia* is also not official in British pharmacopoeias at that time, used again only as a vehicle for other medicines, an eye lotion and in cold cream. Grieve gives a recipe for the latter: 3 oz of waxes melted with 9 oz almond oil, mixed with 7 fl oz rose water and 8 minims (0.5 mL) oil of roses added. The only use in 'modern herbal medicine' noted by Grieve is that of dried red rose flowers in infusions, or sometimes as powder, for haemorrhage, or the tincture for strengthening the stomach and a pleasant remedy for haemorrhage. Rose hips, while long official in the *British Pharmacopoeia*, Grieve continues, as refrigerant and astringent, had by then been omitted and only used for confection with other drugs.

The *British Herbal Pharmacopoeia* of 1983 has no entry for rose itself, only for rose hips for gastritis, polydipsia and avitaminosis C. In a number of modern texts it does not appear at all. Such a journey from its Renaissance heyday! Weiss writes on rose briefly; the use of the seeds as a 'family tea' being mildly diuretic, and the hips for colds and flu and in larger amounts as diuretic when necessary. He mentions rose honey from the petals for coughs and its strengthening effect, and the pureed pulp of the hips as use for food. Rose was not covered in the curriculum when I trained as a herbalist at the School of Herbal Medicine in the 1980s. Its coverage by some modern authors demonstrates encouraging sign of some recovery since then. Menzies Trull records two preparations, tincture of flowers and rose water, along with the broad historical uses.

Barker (2001) covers apothecaries rose for diarrhoea, especially in children and for afflictions of the mouth and throat, with infusion or syrup as preparations, and the hips of the dog rose for diarrhoea, vitamin deficiency, convalescence, lassitude and debility, and those prone to infection, again through infusion and syrup. Wood in the USA records traditional use, particularly for consumption, and notes indication of the petals and hips, although not as separate preparations, for acute inflammatory conditions of the respiratory tract, chronic inflammation and use in convalescence, old age and for delicate children, also its use in digestive tract, menstrual problems and yeast infection. He cites Messegue's recommendation against the ill effects of antibiotics on intestinal flora. He notes, however, that most frequent use today is made of the hips.

Chevallier goes as far as to suggest that though there is little current use of rose, 'it is probably time for a re-evaluation of its medicinal benefits'. He records the mild sedative, antidepressant and antiinflammatory properties of rose petals and use of rose water for inflamed eyes, and the use of hips of dog rose for their vitamin content, as a diarrhoea remedy and capacity to reduce thirst and ease gastric inflammation. This is at least a beginning.

As noted, the recording of modern uses in these herbals indicates some, and in my view most merited, return to grace of the rose. I am encouraged by a very recent conversation with a reputable and busy current herbal supplier that he sells more tincture of fresh damask rose than any other plant. Perhaps the herbals are already out of date and rose needs a fuller coverage to reflect modern need.

In contrast to the European decline, rose remains important in the Middle Eastern tradition, supported by encouraging scientific research, revealing very modern applications. For example a study of six samples of

'Zahraa', a Unani herbal tea widely consumed in Syria, identified 6–12 ingredients, but all included flowers of *Rosa damascena* 11–50%, lemon verbena *Aloysia triphylla* 4–9% and a hollyhock *Alcea damascena* 15–29% (Carmona et al 2005). The samples were purchased in the central market in Damascus. A study on hot water infusions found that the antioxidant activity in vitro was higher for *Rosa damascena* than for green tea. The authors review other studies on the antioxidant activity of *Rosa* cultivars. They correlate this with the concentration of phenolic compounds and suggest that roses would be a valuable addition to herbal tea mixes (Vinokur et al 2006).

## MYTHOLOGY, SYMBOLISM AND DEEPER APPRECIATION

The rose has a rich history in its more esoteric relationship with humans, holding a central place in the mythology of many traditions and celebrated throughout as a symbol of love in its many forms, and of beauty and perfection. Many sources (Dodoens, De Cleene & Lejeune (2003), Clements et al (1979)) record these stories. The rose was dedicated to the goddess Ishtar in Babylonia, for the ancient Egyptians it belonged to Isis, for the Greeks, Aphrodite, and the Romans, Venus. In Islam the rose is said to come from the sweat and tears of the prophet Mohammed and obtained its red colour from his blood. The Greek myths hold many versions of the rose's story, among them that as Aphrodite, the goddess of love, emerged from the sea, roses grew from the foam. A yet more romantic story tells how Aphrodite ran, in vain, to save her lover, Adonis, from a wild boar sent by jealous Ares to kill him. She became entangled in thorn bushes in her haste and roses grew from her spilt blood. In a Christian context roses are strongly associated with the Virgin Mary, the Mystic Rose, depicted in many paintings, particularly by artists in the Middle Ages, for example Schongauer's Madonna in the rose bower, held in a Colmar church. She is drawn among roses after the birth of Christ as a symbol of perfected love. The rose is associated with Christ too, representing attainment of perfect love through suffering. The Rosicrucians have as their emblem red roses on a black cross in recognition of this. Prayer beads are called rosaries. Dante gave paradise the shape of a rose, but it is intriguing why one plant should inspire such consistent imaginative interpretation as an almost universal response, and whether there is a link with rose's reputation as a gentle balanced medicine, used specifically as a cordial.

Pelikan and Grohman (1989) take their studies of the rose into some appreciation of this response. The two authors witness the remarkable nature of the Rosaceae as a family and the rose as central ornament within it. They speak of the beauty and perfection of the rose, and of the Rosaceae family as a whole having an innate balance and clarity of form. The Rosaceae appeal to our sense of beauty, says Pelikan. He speaks of the balance between form and substance, whether in a tormentil, silverweed, dog rose, mountain ash, cherry or apple tree. 'In every case, the impression is one of brimming fullness, copious riches without ever going beyond the bounds of form and measure, and it is this which gives the impression of utter wholesomeness'. Their essential nature, he says, is 'bounteous grace'. Grohman (1989) illustrates this harmony and bounty and finds it in every aspect of the plant. He speaks of the Rosaceae as holding a central position among the dicotyledons, as the lilies do among the monocotyledons. In Kranich's (1976) spectrum of dicotyledons (see introduction), he begins with waterlilies and develops his study through the bindweed, cabbage and buttercup families to the Rosaceae. Following these are the carrot, pea, deadnettle and daisy families. Considering the properties of the families the Rosaceae have neither the 'undefined and changeable nature' of the 'watery' ranunculaceae with their endless capacity to metamorphose, nor the airy nature of the umbellifers, nor the fire of the labiates described in Pelikan. The Rosaceae hold the centre, the balance within the spectrum. Grohman (1989) explains, 'In the Rosaceae the calyx is always a real calyx, the corolla a real corolla, etc.'. The Rosaceae have stability, firmness and clarity of form, he says. There are no irregular or bilaterally symmetrical flowers in the family, they are always sun-like. They have a strong root principle, which allows them to take hold of the earth and make woody plants and trees. There are hardly any annuals. They have a close connection with the 'mineralising, hardening forces of the earth', that gives them 'an enduring quality', he says. Grohman (1989) and Pelikan comment on the rose family's capacity for great variety, Grohman in the form of its fruits, since cherry, plum, strawberry, raspberry, sloe, almond, apricot, peach, apple, pear, medlar, quince, damson, hawthorn, mountain ash all belong to this family; Pelikan in its 2000 and more species and its 'sheer limitless number of variants' in species like bramble, rose and apple. Moreover the rich flowering process, says Pelikan, links the Rosaceae to the sphere above the plant and balances the strong root process linking to the earth. He says 'a mighty astral sphere desires to combine in the flowering process with the etheric principles of vegetative plant nature. However, moderation is once again masterly; the etheric is not overpowered by the astral for that would lead to the development of poisons, especially alkaloids. The etheric element is always strong enough to withstand the onslaught of the astral'.

Then Grohman (1989) considers the nature of the rose itself, whose value lies in its beauty, how it stands right at the centre of the Rosaceae, betraying perfection and balance in all its parts. 'Wherever we look at it, we meet with harmony', he says, 'form and substance in equilibrium'. The scent is noble and well balanced, containing strength and gentleness, 'nothing of a desire nature…nothing sickly or repulsive…a flowery fragrance… with a satisfying heavier perfume'. The dog rose, in its shape, might stand centrally within the rosaceae, holding a position between shrub and tree with its graceful, arching stems, putting the rose right at the centre, the heart, of the flower world. Grohman (1989) discusses too the principle of the pentagram within the rose. Although this principle pervades the dicotyledons as a whole (compare the six-fold monocolyledons) it sits more strongly in the rose than in other flowers. The arrangement of the leaves as they spiral up the stem begins the theme. 'They exactly correspond', he says, 'to the five angles of a regular pentagram', and 'the angle between successive leaves equals two fifths of the circumference of the stem'. The flower has the same five-fold nature. And the consistency shown in the rose in both leaf and flower following the same numerical principle is noteworthy, Grohman points out, since most plants do not. The calyx in the rose is remarkable too and also carries the pentagram principle in the unfolding two-fifths sequence of the metamorphosis of the sepals, of which some are bearded and some not. The unusual nature of such a metamorphosis was even deemed by Albertus Magnus to merit a verse:

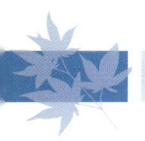

> *Quinque sunt fratres*
> *Duo sunt barbati*
> *Duo sine barba nati*
> *Unus e quinque*
> *Non habet barbam utrimque*

Grohman translates:

> *Five are brothers*
> *Two are bearded*
> *Two are born without beards*
> *One of the five*
> *Is not bearded on both sides*

Finally Grohman (1989) considers how the rosehip falls centrally in form between the cherry and the apple, and is the direct opposite of the strawberry. (It is a wonderful Goethean exercise to metamorphose the fruits of the rose family from cherry to apple in imagination). In the cherry the ovary itself becomes the fruit and rests on the receptacle, which plays no part in the fruit formation; the apple, at the other end of the scale, is formed from the receptacle swelling round the five-fold ovary embedded within it and growing together with it. In the rose hip, the jug-shaped receptacle swells to form the flesh of the hip but does not fuse with the contained stony pips, each of which corresponds to a whole cherry, so the rosehip is a fruit within a fruit and again maintains a middle position between two poles. The strawberry is the opposite of the rosehip in that it is the cushion of the receptacle that swells, pushing the ovaries to the outside surface.

There is a further link between the pentagram and the rose with the planet Venus, perhaps fanciful to some, but interesting nevertheless. Kranich (1976) records how the relationship of the planet Venus to the earth in space is based on Venus' synodic cycle of 584 days, $1^3/_5$ years, which results in five upper and five lower conjunctions with the sun in 8 years from an earth perspective, forming a 'Venus pentagram'. Murrell (2007), having mapped this pattern out through the alternating appearance of Venus as morning and evening star, says 'The relationship in space of Venus to the earth can be drawn by rotating an octogram around a pentagram. By joining the points made by this double rotation we find a graceful curving of the planet towards and away from the earth. The path is recognisably heart shaped – it is a mathematical curve called a cardioid'. See figure 25.3.

Kranich (1976) writes of the facility of seeing plants as the interpretation of inner soul qualities in outer pictorial form, and it is perhaps possible to see the gesture of the rose as expression of the deepest soul quality. One might also contemplate the alchemists moving from the hexagon of wisdom to the pentagon of love, but this is well beyond the bounds of this text.

Pelikan discusses the pharmacological activity of the Rosaceae having sugar, tannic and cyanide processes, and links the actions of the dog rose to these. He includes rose petals for checking diarrhoea and internal haemorrhage through the tannins, the fruit acids for stimulation of sluggish metabolism and tea from the seeds for diuresis counteracting stone formation due to their silica content. It is interesting to contemplate, in the light of Grohman's (1989) observations on the hip and the strawberry, Pelikan's noting of the opposite directions of the silica process in the strawberry which will send the blood process outwards from within, while the rosehip eliminates through the kidney, reversing the direction.

So the question remains that if appreciation of the rose mirrored cultural shifts in history, does its gradually fading fortune from the glory of the Renaissance to the languor of the relatively recent past match a gradual loss of balance and a lack of heart, or soul or centre, in our modern approach to healing? Perhaps the rose, while at ease with humoral and 'felt' approaches to treatment, and those with at least some spiritual or soul dimension, was too 'effeminate' and hardly robust enough to hold a place in a purely materialist and ontological approach to disease, and was relegated to a role either of sweetener, or only worthy of use in cosmetics. Is it too fanciful now to read the spontaneous rally reflected in renewed enthusiasm for the rose as a medicine as a clear soul response and a heart of sorts returning to herbal treatment in these troubled times when a viable marriage of the rational and the spirit is very much needed.

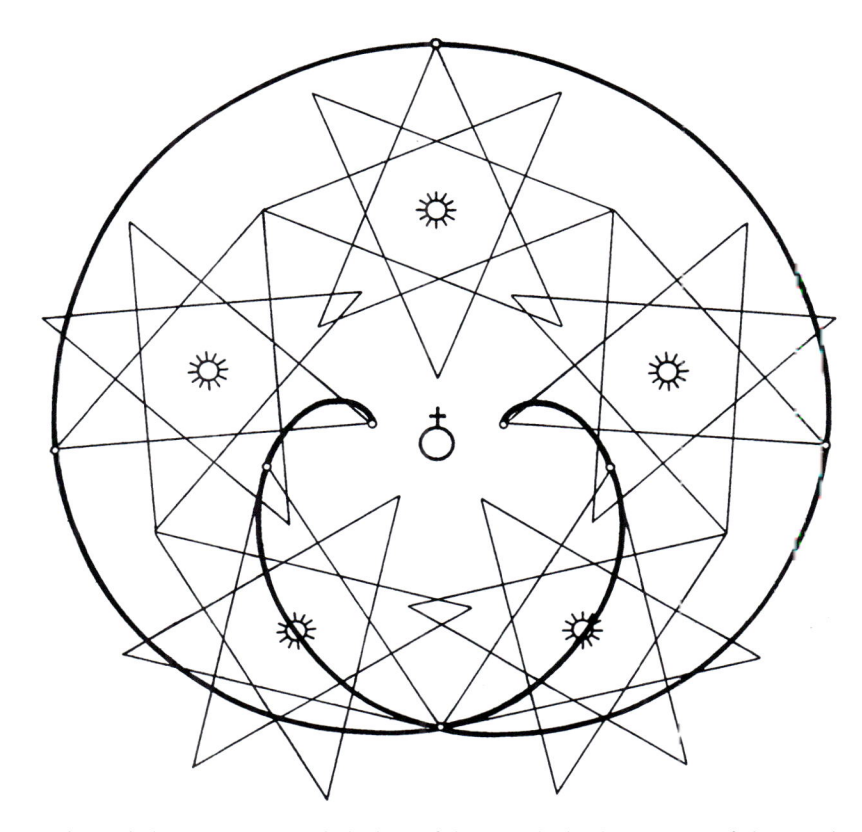

**Figure 25.3** From Joachim Schultz, *Movement and Rhythms of the Stars*, by kind permission of Floris Books.

## RECOMMENDATIONS

Renewed exploration of the virtues of the rose and their various preparations are to be encouraged. It would be interesting to discover the nature of *Rosa gallica* again and compare it with the damask. To what extent is a preparation from dried red roses more binding than one of damask? Are the damask preparations more amphoteric in their effects? Would sugary concoctions be acceptable in these days of obesity awareness? There are many explorations to be made if we wish to approach Renaissance expertise in these matters. Nevertheless, from the literature general recommendations can be made:
- To strengthen the heart, in palpitations, fainting.
- To lift the spirits in melancholy (internal and external preparations).
- To strengthen a 'weak' stomach, liver and bowels.
- For vomiting and diarrhoea.
- For constipation in children and adults.
- For cooling hot fevers, hot headache and joint ache (internal and external preparations).
- For menorrhagia and leucorrhoea, and for use in menopause.
- For sore mouth and throat, and for coughs, especially as honey of roses.
- Hips for diarrhoea, menorrhagia and as source of vitamin C.
- Seeds as diuretic and for stones.

As external use:
- Rosewater as eye wash for sore eyes.
- Honey of roses for wounds, ulcers, sores, inflammations and swellings.
- Rose vinegar for headache from sunburn.
- Rose vinegar or ointment for insomnia.

Dosage: We are currently using an excellent 1:1 specific tincture of *Rosa damascena*, distilled and macerated, as a cordial and calming digestive astringent in doses of 5–10 mL per week. Culpeper recommends 1–4 oz of the syrup of roses solutive as a single dose. Honey of roses, he says, is made of the same infusion and works the same effect but it is more commonly given to phlegmatic subjects than to choleric.

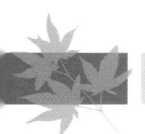

Regarding the prescribing of these preparations today, the dosage for honeys, syrups and electuaries is likely to be limited as much by concerns for the quantity of sugar used as by the amount of fresh rose petals required.

## RECOMMENDATIONS ON SAFETY

No safety concerns are documented.

## CONSTITUENTS

Reviews: none.

### Volatile oil

Total 0.017–0.035% (means at 13 sites, 40 samples, Iran) (Tabaei-Aghdaei et al 2007).
Rose oils are complex and 95 compounds were identified (94.75% of the oil), monoterpene alcohols: beta-citronellol 26%; oxides; ethers; aldehydes: geranial; hydrocarbons: eicosane 30%, docosane 14%, 1-nonadecene 7% (cultivated, Iran) (Jalali-Heravi et al 2008).
Monoterpene 'rose' alcohols: 18 alcohols, citronellol 24–43%, geraniol 2–18% and its cis-isomer nerol 0.7–18% (15 rose oils, Turkey) (Bayrak & Akgűl 1994).
Rose alcohols 96%: citronellol and nerol 24%, geraniol 21%, linalool 23% (oil redistilled from rose water, cultivated, India) (Babu et al 2002).
Monoterpene alcohols: geraniol 0.1–30.6%, nerol 0.01–18.6%, very low citronellol; hydrocarbons 7–28% (24 old roses, Italy) (Antonelli et al 1997).
Other alcohols: 2-phenylethanol 12–90% (over 50% in 19/24 samples), benzyl alcohol 0.3–34.2%, (24 old roses, Italy) (Antonelli et al 1997).
Relative yield of oil depends on the extraction conditions. Babu et al (2002) argue that extraction at atmospheric pressure produces a better oil and their study of field distillation in India found that the rose alcohol content was higher in rose water than oil. Water-soluble constituents such as 2-phenylethanol are partially extracted during distillation but are significant components in rose water (Eikani et al 2005). Ethanolic tinctures would also contain more alkanes than rose oil. This is suggested by a study of rose concrete, a quasi-solid extract, treated with ethanol as solvent, which found citronellol 4.7%; 2-phenylethanol 25%; alkanes: n-nonadecane 13%, heneicosane 12%, n-trixcosane 7% (Reverchon et al 1997). A detailed review of rose oils, rose waters and rose concrete found substantial complexity in the constituents, and variation between samples. It also reviewed studies on rose oils cultivated in India and a new cultivar Ranisahiba developed in India (Lawrence 2005).
Fragrance is associated with characteristic components of the volatile oil such as *cis* and *trans* rose oxides (Bayrak & Akgűl 1994) or damascenone (Demole et al 1970). A study of the changes in fragrance of rose oil over 5 hours on the skin of volunteers suggests that whilst the rose oxides and damascenone are very important, the compounds which are characteristic of rose oil, namely citronellol, geraniol, nerol, geranial, 2-phenylethanol contribute significantly to the fragrance, and the hydrocarbons have a fixative effect which results in a longer-lasting fragrance when applied to the skin (Jirovetz et al 2005). A study showed that volatile oil content and aroma was highest just as the petals open, which confirms the practical experience of growers (Oka et al 1999).

### Phenolic acids

Total 8% measured as gallic acid equivalents (total 6% in green tea). The rose teas were rich in free gallic acid. (Vinokur et al 2006).
Gallic acid (cultivated, northern India) (Kumar et al 2008).
Glycoside of 2-phenylethanol (see other alcohols above), ester of glycoside of 2-phenylethanol with gallic acid (Pakistan) (Mahmood et al 1996).

### Flavonoids

#### Flavonol glycosides

Quercetin glycosides: rutin, quercitrin; myricetin; kaempferol (Kumar et al 2008).
Quercetin glycosides; kaempferol glycosides (Mahmood et al 1996).
Quercetin glycosides; kaempferol glycosides (cultivated, Turkey) (Velioglu & Mazza 1991).

#### Anthocyanins

Total 2.85%: cyanidin 3,5-diglucoside 95% (fresh flowers, cultivated, Turkey) (Velioglu & Mazza 1991).

# REFERENCES

Antonelli A, Fabbri C, Giorgioni ME, et al 1997 Characterization of 24 old garden roses from their volatile compositions. Journal of Agricultural and Food Chemistry 45:4435–4439.

Babaei A, Tabaei-Aghdaei SR, Khosh-Khui M, et al 2007 Microsatellite analysis of Damask rose (*Rosa damascena* Mill.) accessions from various regions in Iran reveals multiple genotypes. BMC Plant Biology 7:12 Online. Available: http://www.biomedcentral.com/1471-2229/7/12 30 Mar 2009.

Babu KGD, Singh B, Joshi VP, et al 2002 Essential oil composition of Damask rose (*Rosa damascena* Mill.) distilled under different pressures and temperatures. Flavour and Fragrance Journal 17:136–140.

Barker J 2001 The medicinal flora of Britain and Northern Europe. Winter Press, West Wickham.

Baydar NG, Baydar H, Debener T 2004 Analysis of genetic relationships among *Rosa damascena* plants grown in Turkey by using AFLP and microsatellite markers. Journal of Biotechnology 111:263–267.

Bayrak A, Akgül A 1994 Volatile oil composition of Turkish rose (*Rosa damascena*). Journal of the Science of Food and Agriculture 64:441–448.

Brunke E-J, Hammerschmidt F-J, Schmaus G 1992 Scent of roses – recent results. Flavour and Fragrance 7:195–198.

Carmona MD, Llorach R, Obon C, et al 2005 Zahraa, a Unani multicomponent herbal tea widely consumed in Syria: components of drug mixtures and alleged medicinal properties. Journal of Ethnopharmacology 102:344–350.

Clements J, Gregory T, Gregory D, et al 1979 The rose. Mayflower Books, New York.

De Cleene M, Lejeune M C 2003 Compendium of symbolic and ritual plants in Europe. Man and Culture Publishers, Ghent.

Demole E, Enggist P, Säuberli U, et al 1970 Structure et synthèse de la damascénone (triméthyl-2,6,6-trans-crotonoyl-1-cyclohexadiène-1,3), constituant odorant de l'essence de rose bulgare (*Rosa damascena* Mill.) Helvetica Chimica Acta 53:541–551.

Eikani MH, Golmohammad F, Rowshanzamir S, et al 2005 Recovery of water-soluble constituents of rose oil using simultaneous distillation-extraction. Flavour and Fragrance Journal 20:555–558.

Green M H (ed.) 2001 The Trotula. University of Pennsylvania Press, Philadelphia.

Grohman G 1989 The plant vols 1 and 2. Bio-dynamic Farming and Gardening Association, Kimberton.

Iwata H, Kato T, Ohno S 2000 Triparental origin of Damask roses. Gene 259:53–59.

Jalali-Heravi M, Parastar H, Sereshti H 2008 Development of a method for analysis of Iranian damask rose oil: Combination of gas chromatography–mass spectrometry with chemometric techniques. Analytica Chimica Acta 623:11–21.

Jirovetz L, Buchbauer G, Stoyanova A 2005 Solid phase microextraction/gas chromatographic and olfactory analysis of the scent and fixative properties of the essential oil of *Rosa damascena* L. from China. Flavour and Fragrance Journal 20:7–12.

Joyaux F 2005 Nouvelle encyclopédie des roses anciennes. Ulmer, Paris.

Katzer G 2003 *Rosa damascena* Miller. Online. Available: http://www.uni-graz.at/~katzer/engl/Rosa_dam.html#part 15 June 2009.

Kiani M, Zamani Z, Khalighi A, et al 2008 Wide genetic diversity of *Rosa damascena* Mill. germplasm in Iran as revealed by RAPD analysis. Scientia Horticulturae 115:386–392.

Kranich E 1976 Pflanze und Kosmos. Verlag Freies Geistesleben, Stuttgart. Also available in English as Kranich E 1986 Planetary influences upon plants: cosmological botany Chelsea Green, White River Junction.

Kumar N, Bhandari P, Singh B, et al 2008 Reversed phase-HPLC for rapid determination of polyphenols in flowers of rose species. Journal of Separation Science 31:262–267.

Lawrence BM 2005 Progress in essential oils. Recent research on the composition of the essential oils of *Rosa damascena*, grown commercially in Bulgaria, Turkey, India and Morocco, is reviewed. Perfumer & Flavorist 30:60–74.

Mahmood N, Piacente S, Pizza C, et al 1996 The anti-HIV activity and mechanisms of action of pure compounds isolated from *Rosa damascena*. Biochemical and Biophysical Research Communications 229:73–79.

Murrell A 2007 Venus: Evening star – morning star – sun. New View 45:36–42.

Oka N, Ohishi H, Hatano T, et al 1999 Aroma evolution during flower opening in *Rosa damascena* Mill. Zeitschrift für Naturforschung 54c, 889–895.

Peter Beales Rose Gardens 2009 National collection of Rosa species. Online. Available: http://www.classicroses.co.uk 4 April 2009.

Reverchon E, Della Porta G, Gorgoglione D 1997 Supercritical $CO_2$ extraction of volatile oil from rose concrete. Flavour and Fragrance Journal 12:37–41.

Royal National Rose Society 2009 Garden of the rose. Online. Available: http://www.rnrs.org/about_the_garden 4 April 2009

Rusanov K, Kovacheva N, Vosman B, et al 2005 Microsatellite analysis of *Rosa damascena* Mill. accessions reveals genetic similarity between genotypes used for rose oil production and old Damask rose varieties. Theoretical and Applied Genetics 111:804–809.

Shepherd RE 1978 History of the rose (facsimile reprint of 1954 edition) Heyden, London.

Tabaei-Aghdaei SR, Babaei A, Khosh-Khui M, et al 2007 Morphological and oil content variations amongst Damask rose (*Rosa damascena* Mill.) landraces from different regions of Iran. Scientia Horticulturae 113:44–48.

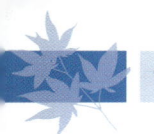

Thomas GS 2004 The Graham Stuart Thomas rose book. Frances Lincoln, London.

Tutin TG, Heywood VH, Burges NA, et al 1968 Flora Europaea, vol 2. Cambridge University Press, Cambridge.

Velioglu YS, Mazza G 1991 Characterization of flavonoids in petals of *Rosa damascena* by HPLC and spectral analysis. Journal of Agricultural and Food Chemistry 39:463–467.

Vinokur Y, Rodov V, Reznick N, et al 2006 Rose petal tea as an antioxidant-rich beverage: cultivar effects. Journal of Food Science 71:S42–S47.

# CHAPTER 26
# *Rubus idaeus*, raspberry

## DESCRIPTION

**Family: Rosaceae**  **Part used: leaves, fruits**

The *Rubus* genus is large and diverse and *Flora Europaea* lists 75 species (Tutin et al 1968). It includes deciduous or semi-evergreen perennial herbs or shrubs, which are often spiny (Stace 1991) with a characteristic fruit formed of a head of one-seeded drupelets. The genus is divided into subgenera of which the largest, *Rubus*, contains the brambles and blackberries (Alice & Campbell 1999).

*Rubus idaeus* L. is in the *Idaeobatus* subgenus, which has biennial stems and a fruit that separates from the convex receptacle when ripe. It is a very hardy perennial found throughout temperate Eurasia and North America but only found on mountains in southern Europe (Tutin et al 1968).

Large stands (to 10 m$^2$) of erect stems, which are rough or smooth with weak prickles bear ovate, pinnate leaves with three to seven leaflets, which are white and tomentose on the underside. The perennial rootstock sends out biennial stems, which produce leaves in the first year and flowering side shoots in the second year. Racemes of five-petalled white flowers (4–7 mm) occur in summer. The fruit is usually red but rarely yellow and separates from the receptacle at maturity. The fruit is an aggregate of drupelets each containing a small seed. Raspberry is propagated vegetatively or by seed.

**Other species used:** Bramble *Rubus fruticosa* is a largely apomictic species with over 400 microspecies (Stace 1991). Hybrids occur with *Rubus idaeus* and dewberry *Rubus caesius*, of which some have developed into new species (Alice et al 2001). The American red raspberry occurs throughout North America and is considered either as a separate species, *Rubus strigosa* Michx. or as a subspecies, *Rubus idaeus* L. subsp. *strigosa* (Michx.) Focke (USDA 2009).

### Quality

Raspberry leaves can be collected from wild stands or cultivars. In a study of 13 cultivars, the concentration of tannins and ellagic acid in the leaves was found to be highest in the cultivar Tulameen (Gudej & Tomczyk 2004), which is also a good cropper over a long season. A study of samples from 78 sites in Scotland found that plants from higher altitudes in the glens tended to be shorter and to flower later, but there was substantial variation in characteristics between all the populations (Jennings 1964). The raspberry has been domesticated for fruit production and there are many cultivars. Stands in the wild may be escapes from cultivation but a study of 103 samples from seven sites in Tayside, Scotland, which is a centre of raspberry cultivation, suggested that interbreeding between wild and cultivated plants is limited (Marshall et al 2001).

The epicuticular leaf waxes vary and their composition may be associated with resistance to the large raspberry aphid *Amphorophora idaei*, which is the main vector for viruses that infect raspberry leaves (Shepherd et al 1999). Aphid-resistant cultivars should be chosen for cultivation of leaves.

## RASPBERRY AND BRAMBLE

Raspberry is mainly used as an astringent, both internally and externally, and is often used alongside other astringent plants. Raspberry leaf is commonly used by herbalists today but bramble *Rubus fruticosus* is more commonly discussed by the authors. Sometimes the recommendations for each plant cannot be separated, especially as the part used may be leaf, aerial parts, including stems, flower, unripe fruit and ripe fruit, or root. Raspberry is notable in that it is widely self-prescribed in preparation for childbirth. This usage is first given by Thomson and this tradition will be discussed as well as more recent research into the use of raspberry for this purpose. Raspberry vinegar is a traditional remedy which uses the fruits and usage of the fruit will be included.

That the genus includes many similar species was recognized by Theophrastus. Mattioli cites Theophrastus as stating that some grow in the woods and others on the mountains and some grow like trees, some grow to a height, others are entwined in hedges, fences and bushes, and some creep on the ground and strike roots like grass.

THE WESTERN HERBAL TRADITION

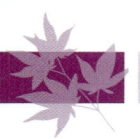

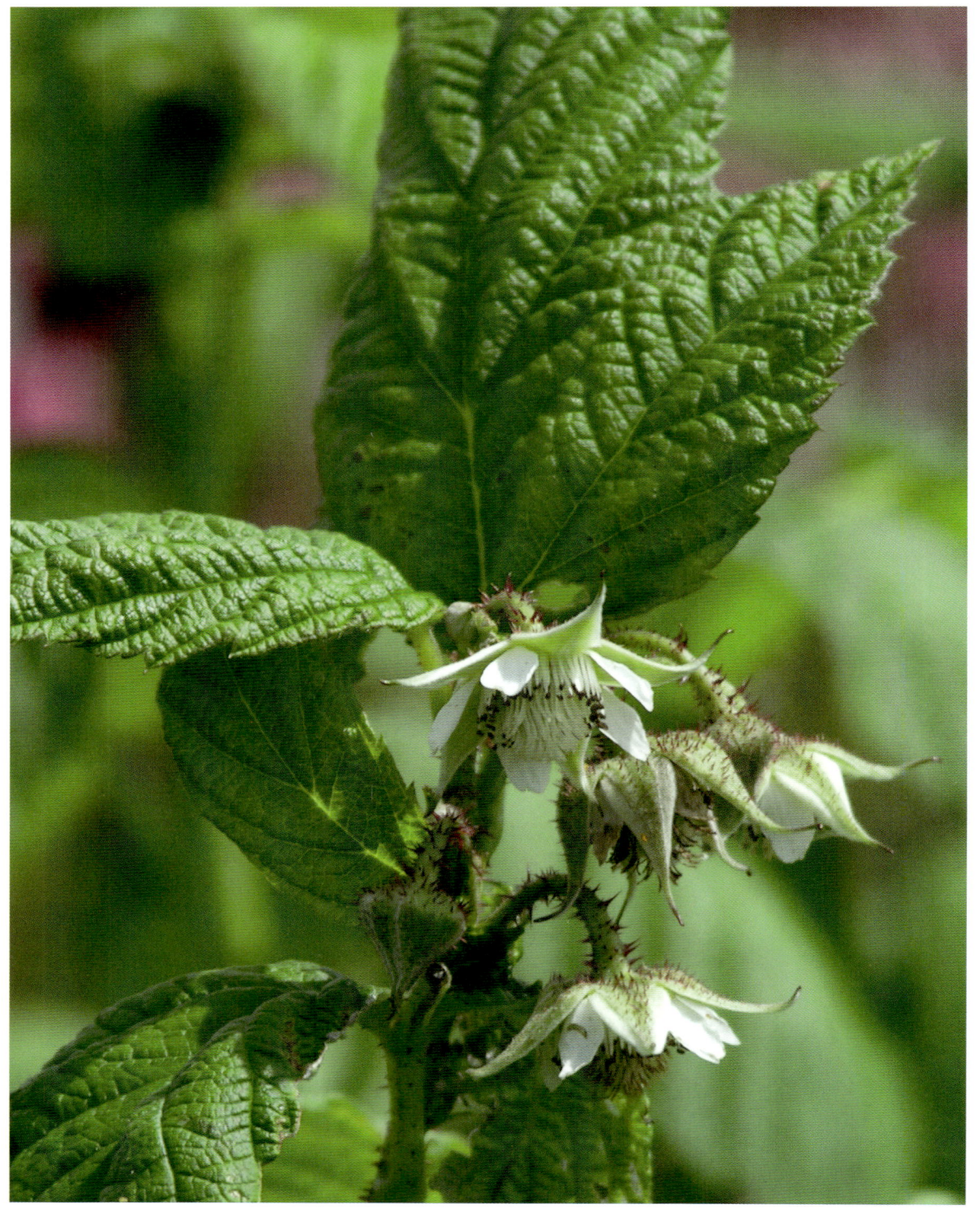

**Figure 26.1** *Rubus idaeus*, raspberry (an allotment in Horsforth, Yorkshire, July).

These features are similar to those given in a modern review (Alice & Campbell 1999). Dioscorides (IV 38) refers to the Idaian bramble, raspberry, as used for similar indications as bramble (IV 37) and describes it as softer and with or without prickles. Theophrastus makes 22 references to Mount Ida in northwestern Turkey and to information given him by local people. He spent 3 years (347–344 BC) with Aristotle in the coastal city of Assos, which is very close to the mountain. According to Thanos (2001) he refers mainly to trees but unfortunately not to *Rubus idaeus*.

The descriptions of Dioscorides show that he was referring to two species of *Rubus*. Dioscorides states that the Idaian bramble can treat the same conditions as bramble, including use of the flower in wine for diarrhoea, but that the flowers are far more useful than those of bramble for eye inflammation when macerated with oil and smeared on the eye. This poses the question of whether Dioscorides was referring to *Rubus idaeus*, which has small white flowers, or a bramble or raspberry with larger flowers. Pliny states that the Idaian bramble was so-called because no other grows on Mount Ida. He describes it as more delicate than other brambles, smaller, with canes further apart and less prickly, and growing under the shade of trees. His list of indications, which includes the flower with honey for discharges from fluxes of the eye and erysipelas and as a drink in water for a disordered stomach, reads similarly to that of Dioscorides. They appear to have used the same source, so we have no evidence that either of them visited Mount Ida and saw the bramble. Historians continue to rely on the work of Wellmann (1889), who argued that Dioscorides and Pliny had used a common source, probably Sextius Niger, who was a Roman writing in Greek in the 1st century AD (Scarborough & Nutton 1982). Stannard (1965) supports this by showing, as we have found, that their accounts, while similar, are not identical, which suggests that each author chose different points from the same text.

Later authors debated the identity of the Idaian bramble. Turner dwells at length on the statement of Dioscorides that raspberry grows abundantly on Mount Ida. He discusses Mattioli's commentary on Dioscorides and Mattioli's comments on other authors. The point at issue is whether raspberry grows only on Mount Ida or plentifully on Mount Ida but also in other places. Turner describes raspberry growing in many gardens in England, in the wild in the high hills above Bonn in Germany and in East Friesland, Holland. Turner and Mattioli both discuss the meaning of the Latin text and Turner suggests that Mattioli wrongly argues that the correct species grows only on Mount Ida. However, the edition of Mattioli which we have used only records the opinion of Dioscorides and Pliny that it grows plentifully on Mount Ida.

In the same section, Mattioli comments on another plant as he discusses a type of *Rubus* called 'ampomele', which has red berries not unlike strawberries and is found in the mountains and eaten by bears. It has 'no small bones inside', which can be read as no seeds inside. He states that there are recent authors who think this species is for certain the Idaian bramble but there is no firm evidence to confirm or disprove the claim. One wonders whether this could be an alpine strawberry *Fragaria vesca* and have been chosen because botanists were searching for a plant associated with mountains. In fact, Mattioli wonders whether the word 'idaean' is used by Dioscorides to refer to mountains rather than just Mount Ida. It could be that this is solved by a note in Tutin et al (1968), which states that in southern Europe *Rubus idaeus* grows only on mountains. So, Dioscorides and Pliny take care to associate raspberry with mountains, whereas the Renaissance authors question this as they observe that raspberry grows more widely. For example, Gerard describes it as growing in gardens and has seen it growing wild near Harwood in Lancashire. To conclude, there appears to be no evidence of use of *Rubus idaeus* before the Renaissance whereas there is evidence for the use of bramble *Rubus fruticosus*. One of the most delightful illustrations in the *Juliana Anicia Codex* is of a robust and very prickly bramble. This version of Dioscorides is now kept in Vienna but was copied and given to the imperial princess Juliana Anicia in gratitude for the building of a church in Constantinople in about 512 AD (Collins 2000).

The debate illustrates the struggles for the early botanists who had limited means of transport, poor maps and few reference books. Pavord (2005) gives a vivid account of the adventures of Thomas Johnson in 1629 as his group was caught in a storm on a boat trip from London into Kent to identify the wild flora. This trip occurred almost 2000 years after Theophrastus made his trips up Mount Ida. Yet it is hard for the reader today to imagine trips made without the aid of trains, cars and maps. Botanical identification of wild plants remains a challenge today even when coloured drawings, photographs, herbarium samples and reference books have been consulted. *Rubus* remains a problematic genus and botanists still do not agree on classification in this genus as phylogenetic studies of *Rubus* have led to different approaches to the subdivisions and number of species of bramble (Alice & Campbell 1999).

A further complication arises in that there are two mountains called Mount Ida, the name denoting a densely wooded mountain (Thanos 2001). One is in Crete and one is south of Troy, in northwest Turkey. Mount Ida in northwest Turkey has mythological associations. It was the place where Paris, son of King Priam of Troy, had to make his famous judgement and choose between the beauty of three goddesses: Athena, Aphrodite and Hera, the wife of Zeus. Paris chose Aphrodite, who promised him Helen the wife of Menelaus, King of Sparta. The ensuing abduction of Helen led to the Trojan war. Zeus is said to have watched the siege of Troy from the mountain top, while the slopes provided the wood for the Trojan horse and for the ships in which Aeneas and his followers escaped. This story from

# THE WESTERN HERBAL TRADITION

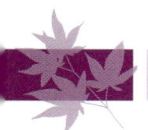

far distant times weaves between gods and mortals, but it reminds us how some of the Latin words which we use to describe plants give a window into history.

## STARTING WITH BRAMBLE

Dioscorides (IV 38) sets the scene for all later authors and compares raspberry to the preceding entry for bramble or blackberry. He states that bramble (IV 37) contracts and dries, and recommends a decoction of the branches of bramble for diarrhoea and leucorrhoea, but argues that the juice of the leaves and stems, dried in the sum is stronger. Pliny, Turner, Mattioli, Dodoens, Bauhin, Gerard and Parkinson refer to this preparation. Dioscorides recommends the leaves of bramble chewed to strengthen the gums and heal the thrush, and external use of the leaves as a plaster for shingles, head scurf, 'prolapses of the eye', callous lumps, haemorrhoids and ground up externally for those with stomach and heart ailments. For bramble, the authors give prominence to the recommendations of Pliny, which are similar to those of Dioscorides but more detailed, and of Galen, who reads like a summary of Pliny with some added material on the temperament of bramble.

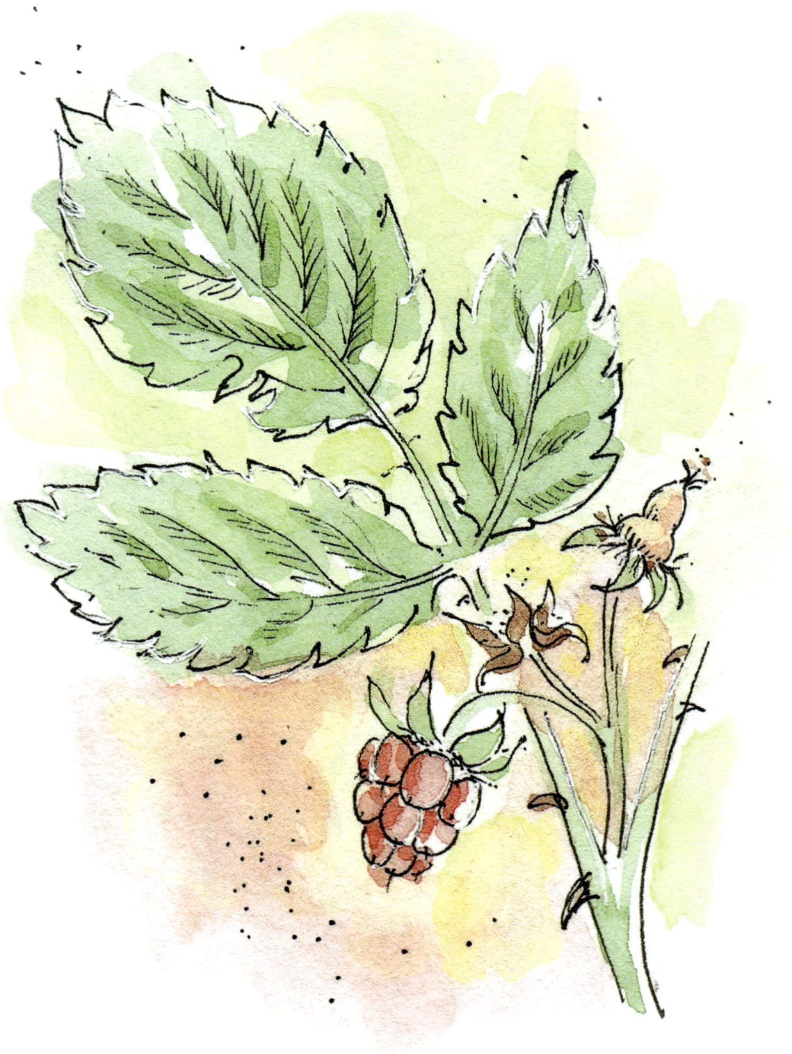

**Figure 26.2** *Rubus idaeus*, raspberry.

The following section is a summary of the recommendations for bramble, as raspberry is considered appropriate for the same uses. For example, Fuchs refers only to bramble and Dodoens gives a full description of brambles. Dodoens identifies the raspberry as growing widely and useful for the same uses as bramble but his recommendations for raspberry do not add to those of Dioscorides.

The authors differ in their emphasis on the parts of brambles: leaves, seeds, flowers, fruit and root, but it is the text of Pliny which appears to be the source of much of the information. Some sections of his text identify the part used and some do not. Galen states that brambles have an astringent quality 'and these not obscurely'. He observes that the new leaves are more watery and so less astringent whereas Dodoens considers them more astringent, cold and dry almost in the third degree. Galen can be read as stating that the new leaves are useful to chew to heal ulcers of the mouth and 'have the strength to glue together other wounds' for their 'temperature is of an essence both earthy and cold, and watery and warm'. Pliny states simply that 'they close wounds without any gatherings'. Mattioli, Bauhin and then Parkinson all give the text of Galen.

Pliny gives a usage of bramble for the digestive tract: applied externally near the left breast for heartburn or to the stomach for stomach ache. He then advises the tender shoots for looseness of the bowels, dysentery and discharges of blood, and the berries for heartburn. This is very similar to the text of Mattioli, citing Galen, who advises the flower as similar to the immature fruit, and suitable for dysenteries, flux of the belly, lost strength and spittings of blood. Serapio recommends external use of the powdered herb for a weak stomach 'full of humours' but also mature fruits to astringe the stomach or the flower drunk in wine. Similar advice for use in 'queasy stomachs' is given by Turner and, in varying terminology, Dodoens, Mattioli, Parkinson, Culpeper and Bauhin. Gerard describes raspberries as similar but less drying and the fruit particularly useful for weak stomachs.

Dioscorides advises the ripe fruit of raspberry for mouth ailments. Pliny recommends the chewed leaves of bramble for affections of the mouth but then states that the blackberries are a better 'mouth-medicine' than even the cultivated mulberry. Serapio refers to use of the chewed leaf of bramble in mouth ulcers, which is also given by Gerard and Parkinson. Pliny then recommends the tender shoots of bramble, eaten as a vegetable, or as a decoction in white wine, to strengthen loose teeth. Pliny gives the same preparation as a quick remedy for 'affections of the uvula' and this is repeated by the Salernitan herbal, and by Dodoens, Gerard, Parkinson and Culpeper.

Looking at external uses, Pliny states that nothing is more effective as a styptic than the root 'of a blackberry bearing blackberries' decocted in wine and reduced to a third, especially for sores in the mouth and the anus and it is 'so powerful that the very sponges used become hard as stone'. Hildegard recommends the powdered stems of the bramble for external treatment of flesh, where worms are eating, to kill the worms. Turner refers to use of bramble for itching of the head and running sores in the head. This is given by Dodoens, Parkinson and Culpeper. Turner and Dodoens recommend powdered leaf of bramble for cancerous and spreading sores. The Salernitan herbal gives a recipe from Constantine for the young shoots with egg white to be used for hot abscesses, and with rose water for burns.

Pliny offers a recipe for a preparation made from the young stalks, pounded and the juice extracted, dried in the sun until the thickness of honey and taken by mouth or applied as an ointment. He describes this as a specific for affections of the mouth or ears, spitting of blood, quinsy, troubles of the uterus or anus, and for intestinal afflictions. Parkinson quotes Pliny on the value of the juice, describing troubles of the anus as 'sores of fundament and piles'. Bauhin says that Erasistratus, a Greek and putative founder of the first medical school in Alexandria in the 2nd century BC (Fraser 1972), healed his own mouth ulcer with the thickened juice. Whether juice was always prepared from stems is impossible to know. Serapio recommends juice from the leaves and tops for the same indications. He is also one of the few authors to make further mention of the womb, recommending this plant to 'remove chronic humours of the womb'.

Gerard quotes Galen as stating that root is binding and contains a thin substance 'that wasteth away kidney stones'. Turner, Dodoens, Mattioli and Bauhin agree. Gerard suggests that the berries and flowers are diuretic and a decoction is useful against kidney stones. He ascribes this advice to Pliny although we did not find this reference. Given that both brambles and raspberry are discussed by the authors and that so many plant parts are recommended, this has been a most difficult herb to describe. The reading may still be open to interpretation but it is interesting that Pliny appears to be the main source for all the authors. The entry for blackberry in an ethnographic survey of usage in Britain and Ireland (Allen & Hatfield 2004) shows how the usage given by the ancients has been transmitted to the 20th century. Alongside the usage for diarrhoea is chewing the tip of a shoot for heartburn and external application for sore eyes, shingles, sores and tumours. One has to conclude that, although brambles are not generally used today, they may deserve a renaissance, especially as they are such a prolific and vigorous native plant.

## FRUITS AND CORDIALS

The fruit has been mentioned and the next section looks at usage of fruits. The Salernitan herbal describes the unripe blackberries as sour, firm, cold and dry, and thus strengthening to the stomach and intestine, 'binding the belly' and for dysentery, especially due to bilious humour.

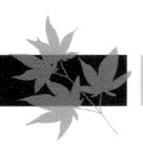

The Salernitan herbal discusses mulberries at more length but refers back to Galen as describing blackberries as restraining, dispersing and separating humours by their sharpness and acidity. Hildegard describes the fruit of blackberry as easily digested but not a medicine. Parkinson quotes Galen on the value of the unripe fruits as an astringent to the digestive tract. Bauhin gives a thorough overview of previous authors and recommends raspberry wine for all uses, especially the stomach and the mouth. He notes that the ancient authors were not referring to raspberries but that raspberries grow everywhere in Germany. He says that Galen found that overeating blackberries causes headaches but that he himself has often eaten many raspberries without harm, despite having a cold, damp and phlegmy stomach.

By the 18th century there is more direct reference to raspberry. Cullen, possibly because he was writing in Edinburgh, describes raspberries as tender, sweet and innocent. Miller describes the fruit as pleasant with a grateful smell and taste, and refers to the cordial as somewhat astringent, strengthening to the stomach and resisting vomiting. Quincy includes the raspberry fruit in Class 2 of the strengtheners, the astringents, and compares them to mulberries but finds them more fragrant, pleasant and cooling as a syrup in vomiting and loose bowels or as a gargle. Hill advises the juice of the ripe fruit, boiled with sugar for a syrup, which is agreeable to the stomach and good for sickness and retching.

Raspberry vinegar and raspberry cordial continue to be used as home remedies for digestive upsets and sore throats. Grieve advises the vinegar added to water as an excellent cooling drink in summer that is also suitable in fever and as a gargle for a relaxed, sore throat. The recipe given is for 2 lb of raspberries in 1 pint of white wine vinegar. Grieve also quotes a recipe from a cookery book where similar proportions are used but first 1 lb is added to the vinegar and then another 1 lb after 24 hours' maceration. The vinegar is then made into a syrup at the usual proportion of 1 lb sugar to 1 pint of liquid. The dosage given is a large spoonful or two in a tumbler of water, which makes a 'refreshing beverage of singular efficacy in complaints of the chest'. Fox gives a recipe for raspberry syrup that is 'particularly good' for asthma, croup, whooping cough and dry coughs. Boil 8 oz of honey with a cup of water, remove the scum and pour boiling hot onto $\frac{1}{2}$ oz lobelia *Lobelia inflata* herb and $\frac{1}{2}$ oz cloves *Syzygium aromaticum*. Mix, strain and add half a pint of raspberry vinegar. The dose is given as 1 teaspoonful or dessertspoonful, four times a day. This is an example of a traditional recipe where close attention to yield and thus dosage is required as it includes *Lobelia inflata*.

According to Ryan et al (2001), raspberries remain in usage in Australia. They investigated raspberry juice prepared from frozen raspberries and raspberry juice cordial as they are widely used to prevent gastroenteritis in humans, farm animals and caged birds. The in vitro study found that the 1:5 dilution juice and the cordial inhibited 11 bacteria, including *Salmonella enteritidis*, a common cause of diarrhoeal infections (Ryan et al 2001). The study found that raspberry leaf was inactive and it could be that this antibacterial activity is associated with the volatile components of the fruits (Robertson et al 1995). A study in Finland on eight berries found that raspberry and cloudberry were the best inhibitors of bacteria, and the ellagitannins inhibited *Staphylococcus*, whereas organic acids inhibited *Salmonella enterica* (Puupponen-Pimiä et al 2005). Another in vitro study of the fruit found poor antibacterial activity but this did not include *Salmonella* (Rauha et al 2000).

There has been substantial research into the health benefits of berry fruits and this is considered to be associated with the concentration of phenolic compounds and thus antioxidant activity (Scalbert et al 2005). Components in raspberry fruits are reviewed by Anttonen & Karjalainen (2005), who discuss the variation between cultivars and the effects of environment, storage and processing. Quercetin content ranged from 0.32 to 1.55 mg/100 g fresh weight, ellagic acid content was 38–118 mg/100 g and anthocyanin concentration was 0–51 mg/100 g. The highest total phenolic concentration was in the cultivar Gatineau and the lowest was in yellow fruits.

Beekwilder et al (2005b) compare different methods of analysis of antioxidants and argue that raspberry fruits are a rich dietary source of ellagitannins and thus antioxidants. In an earlier study, they found that ellagitannins, mainly sanguiin H6 and lambertianin C, were the dominant antioxidants in ripe fruits of 14 cultivars and contributed over 50% of total antioxidant activity (Beekwilder et al 2005a). The degree of absorption and thus activity of ellagitannins is unclear, whereas the anthocyanins have been shown to be absorbed. The anthocyanins are mainly cyanidin glycosides and contribute about 25% of the oxidant activity (Beekwilder et al 2005b). The other main antioxidants were vitamin C which contributed 20% of total capacity, and some minor proanthocyanidins. In another study, on cultivar Glen Ample, the authors note the contribution to the antioxidant activity of the full range of ellagitannins (Mullen et al 2003). Compounds isolated were high concentrations of ellagitannins, mainly sanguiin H-6 and lambertianin C, traces of ellagic acid and its sugar conjugates, 11 anthocyanins, including cyanidin and pelargonidin glycosides, and quercetin and kaempferol glycosides. As Russell et al (2009) argue, it is easy to ignore the relative health benefits of fresh local Scottish produce over than imported fruits.

## THE ASTRINGENT LEAF

From the 19th century, the authors recommend use of raspberry leaf and for this we need to discuss the concept of astringency. Samuel Thomson (1832) recounts how he was in Eastport, Maine looking for an astringent herb and discovered raspberry by taste. He describes suitable astringents if chewed as leaving the mouth feeling clean, but not rough and dry. Raspberry is native throughout North America and Thomson later made it his main astringent. Astringents were the basis of No. 3, the third stage in a Thomsonian course of treatment. The sequence in the course of treatment was to use lobelia *Lobelia inflata* as an emetic, followed by cayenne *Capsicum annuum* to heat and then astringents to heal the tissues. The third stage was designed to cleanse the stomach and bowels of 'canker', thus fully resolving the disease process. The aim was to 'scour the stomach, promote perspiration, repel the cold' (Haller 2000). Thomson defined canker as 'the coating which prevents the resolution of disease as it prevents the little vessels working' which is caused by cold overcoming the natural heat of the body. Haller (2000) describes canker as 'the term both regulars and sectarians used to refer to the hard, greyish substance that lined the stomach and intestines in the state of disease'. This was ascribed to cold, which leads to a vitiated state of the secretions which become thicker and harder and so prevent the proper absorption of food.

Thomson claims that raspberry '…answered every purpose wished. I gathered a large quantity of the leaves, and dried them, and have been in constant use of it as a medicine ever since, and have found it an excellent article, both for canker and many other complaints'. He found it the best remedy he had used for loose bowels in children as a tea and as an enema. Cook makes the point that as it is soothing to the stomach, it is useful in nausea and vomiting but also has a mild action which lessens diarrhoea and subacute dysentery without being too abrupt. This is similar to the earlier recommendation in 'queasy stomachs', a term which remains in common parlance but not in medical terminology. Coffin recommends raspberry for dysentery and instead of ordinary tea or coffee for chronic diarrhoea and claims that 'the patient need never be afraid of taking too much'. Fox recommends a strong infusion for looseness of bowels and summer complaints of children. Hool takes up the connection of diarrhoea with infection and claims that it is 'invaluable for removing canker, from the mucous surfaces of the body, cleansing the system of all filthy material, gives nature the opportunity to bring about complete restoration of health.' He uses it for diarrhoea in children, fevers, measles, smallpox, chickenpox and dysentery but also in children to temper a more laxative medicine. Grieve claims that it 'never fails to give immediate relief' in cold and extreme laxity of bowels. A review of the use of raspberry by 16 Members of the National Association of Medical Herbalists (Fletcher-Hyde 1942) notes its tonic and mild astringent action in gastric atony, white furred tongue, summer diarrhoea and atonic bowel in children. The *British Herbal Pharmacopoeia* gives the main action of raspberry as astringent indicated for diarrhoea, with agrimony *Agrimonia eupatoria* and wood avens *Geum urbanum*. Priest & Priest describe it as a mild soothing astringent tonic which allays nausea, sustains the nerves and tones mucous membranes. Wren refers to the summer complaints of children. Menzies-Trull advises larger doses where an antidiarrhoeal action is sought. He advises it in relaxed intestine with diarrhoea, dysentery, gastrointestinal haemorrhage and for diverticular disease with agrimony *Agrimonia eupatoria* and marshmallow *Althaea officinalis*. Hoffmann gives the above indications and includes too the bark of bramble root for diarrhoea in adults and children and as an external remedy.

External usage continues to be recommended highly by later authors. Thomson recommends a tea of raspberry for sore nipples, with the addition of slippery elm *Ulmus rubra* if very sore. Coffin states that it is unequalled for removing scurf or canker from tongue. Skelton (1853) advises washing the mouth with a tea three to four times a day for oral thrush in infants. Wren advises an infusion of leaves or fruits as a gargle for sore mouth and 'canker of the throat'. Preparations recommended by herbalists include a gargle for stomatitis, laryngitis and a wash for tonsillitis (Fletcher-Hyde 1942). Priest & Priest suggest a gargle with dilute vinegar in sore throat and hoarseness. The *British Herbal Pharmacopoeia* advises a mouthwash for tonsillitis with sage *Salvia officinalis* and a lotion for conjunctivitis with eyebright, *Euphrasia* species.

## IN PREPARATION FOR BIRTH

Raspberry may not now be amongst the herbs most commonly used as an astringent, but it is very widely used as a 'partus praeparator', to prepare for birth. Although it is considered to have been used 'since ancient times' (Braun & Cohen 2005), references to use by women are few in the older authors. The *Old English Herbarium* gives ripe blackberries for 'a woman's menstrual flow,' 'three times seven', simmered down in water by two thirds, made daily and taken on an empty stomach for 3 days. Dodoens recommends the juice of brambles for heavy menstrual flow. Gerard refers to the use of the decoction in all bleeding, and Parkinson, followed by Culpeper, recommends the decoction of the leaves and dried blackberry stems for heavy menstrual flow. Miller says it is considered good in miscarriage. However, there is an association between astringency and strengthening of the tissues and this provides a linkage to the recommendation of raspberry as a 'partus praeparator'. Quincy includes astringents under strengtheners; substances which maintain the solids in a condition ready to exert themselves into action when needed. Strengtheners include substances which crisp and corrugate the fibres into a more compacted tone' and substances which absorb and dry up superfluous humidity, which are the astringents, but they strengthen too as too much moisture may contribute to relaxation. Hoffmann describes raspberry as strengthening and toning the tissue of the uterus and suggests an infusion of 1 cup of boiling water poured over 2 teaspoons of dried herb and infused for 10–15 minutes. Trickey describes raspberry as improving uterine muscle tone and makes the practical point that raspberry is light and fluffy when dried, so may need a larger volume than other dried herbs. Coffin gives an account of the treatment of two women, aged 20, in Troy, Ohio. One had not had a period for 7 months and one suffered from flooding. He gave each woman the same treatment: composition powder in a strong raspberry leaf tea for 2 days, then a vapour bath and lobelia *Lobelia inflata* emetic every other day for 3 weeks, stomach bitters in raspberry leaf tea daily, and an injection of oak bark *Quercus robur*, valerian *Valeriana officinalis* and cayenne *Capsicum annuum*. Treatment was successful, in both cases and he uses this example to support the principle of heating and equalizing the circulation (Coffin 1866). While this robust course of treatment would be considered too intense today, it serves to illustrate the point that herbs cannot be categorized merely by indication.

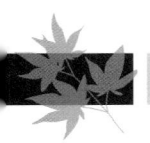

Thomson (1832) is our first advocate of the use of raspberry in pregnancy or labour. He states that a tea made of the leaves, with milk and sweetened, is very pleasant and may be used freely. 'It is the best thing for women in travail of any article I know of. Give a strong tea of it, with a little of No. 2 capsicum, sweetened, and it will regulate everything as Nature requires. If the pains are untimely, it will make all quiet; if timely and lingering, give more No. 2.'

Raspberry is further endorsed by Coffin, who recommends it in 'obstruction of menses', premature labour pains and to promote progress of labour. He includes raspberry in a tea for sickness in early pregnancy but does not appear to advocate its use in preparation for birth. Coffin is at pains to emphasize that childbirth is a natural process and gives an account of the anatomy and physiology of the process. The first edition was written in 1849 and this account reflects his desire to promote knowledge. He advocates temperance, regular meals, loose clothing and no tight corsets, free pure air and 'everything needed to keep the mind composed and happy'. In the management of labour, he was speaking from experience as he describes difficult births at which he was in attendance. In normal births, Coffin recommends an enema to ensure that the bowels are active, and to have a very strong decoction of raspberry leaves ready. At the onset of pains, the woman should take a wineglassful (60 mL) sweetened, as hot as can be borne, at intervals, occasionally adding as much cayenne *Capsicum annuum* as will lie on the end of a common teaspoon (Coffin 1866). Both Thomson and Coffin discuss the use of raspberry during labour rather than in preparation for labour.

Cook quotes Thomson and states that raspberry has a fine influence on the uterus, when flagging in labour, anticipates flooding and relieves after-pains. Fox suggests it is an excellent remedy in profuse and painful menstruation and to regulate labour pains in childbirth. Fox advises a teacupful of strong tea, in which the juice of an orange has been pressed, three times a day in the last month of pregnancy to prevent pain and render labour easy when the hour of parturition has arrived. This is repeated in Wren as 'rendering parturition speedy and easy, take freely before and during confinement, with composition essence, always take warm'. Trickey (1998) gives the same recommendation as Fox 'in the last months of pregnancy'. Grieve states that it is 'unequalled as a warm infusion drunk before and during childbirth' and recommends it for menorrhagia, flooding and miscarriage. Hool recommends use of a warm infusion with a pinch of composition essence as valuable for women in labour, for quieting untimely pains and rendering them more efficient if labour has commenced. He advises 1 teacupful of infusion every hour until labour is completed but also that 'it may be taken, with grateful results, for several months before the expected event. If this herb were generally used instead of ordinary tea, haemorrhage would rarely occur after confinement and instruments would rarely be required'. Priest & Priest also note its use in heavy periods and to prepare for childbirth. All 16 collaborators in a review of the use of raspberry mention its role in preparation for childbirth. The dosage given is 3–4 pints per week in the last 3 months and a full pint of hot tea with 2 teaspoons of composition essence when labour begins (Fletcher-Hyde 1942).

Raspberry leaf is one of the few herbs which continue to be self-prescribed and surveys have found that self-prescribing is common in pregnancy (Ernst 2002, Forster et al 2006). A survey of all women who visited an antenatal clinic at around 37 weeks in Melbourne, Australia found that 36% of the 588 women were taking a herbal supplement and 14% of the 588 were taking raspberry leaf (Forster et al 2006). In interviews with 201 women in Adelaide, Australia, 9% took raspberry leaf in the last trimester in preparation for labour, usually on the recommendation of friends or relatives (Maats & Crowther 2002). A survey of 500 nurse-midwives in the USA found that, of the 90 who replied, 63% used red raspberry leaf to 'stimulate labour' in particular in home births or birth centres. 69% of the midwives had learned about the use of raspberry from colleagues and only 22% included use of herbs in their written protocols (McFarlin et al 1999). In an observational study of 55 women in Australia, 32 drank the tea with 75% taking up to 3 cups a day, and 23 took tablets at a dose of 1–8 tablets of which 43% took 6 tablets a day (Parsons et al 1999).

It would be useful to have more guidance on dosage, effectiveness and safety but this raises some of the problems in investigating herbal medicines. 'Preparation for labour' is not a disease entity and planning the methodology and gaining ethical approval for a clinical trial would raise complex issues. For an estimate of the safety of any herb or drug, very large surveys are required to make statistical inferences and this would be difficult to organize. Equally, it is not possible to merely assume that raspberry leaf is safe because it is widely used as surveys show that there is low reporting of use of herbs to healthcare professionals (Conover 2003). Adverse events in pregnancy and labour are unpredictable and multifactorial, and a history of use of herbal medicines may not be investigated. There is little evidence on the effectiveness or safety of raspberry and so Ernst (2002) and Barnes (2003) advise that it should not be taken during pregnancy. However, this recommendation could not be enforced, even if one supported it, and it is useful to review the evidence such as it is. Women are mainly taking raspberry on personal recommendation in an 'underground' way (Holst et al 2009) and would like more guidance from healthcare professionals. Lowdog (2005) reviews the evidence and suggests that raspberry is safe but takes a similar view to Coffin that the preparation of the psyche is most important.

What evidence is there for efficacy, effectiveness and safety? Regarding efficacy or mechanism of action, there have been in vitro studies on rat and human uterine tissues. Studies on animals or animal tissues are widely used to support the traditional usage of herbal medicines with the implicit assumption that that the action will be found in human studies. For example, Trickey (1998) uses the statements made by Bamford et al (1970), who propose that raspberry leaf would prevent or reduce the risk of incoordinate uterine action by regulating the action of uterine muscle. This publication was a poster only (Bamford et al 1970). Contractions in strips of uterine tissue from pregnant rats were inhibited, and contractions were stimulated in strips of human uterine tissue (1–16 weeks of pregnancy). In both tissues, normal contractions were resumed and became less frequent but more regular over 20 minutes. Criticisms of this study are the sparse experimental detail given and that contractions during labour are influenced by oxytocin release and thus this study may have no relevance to labour. There have been other in-vitro studies but the results are inconclusive and are discussed in detail by Bradley (2006), Mills & Bone (2005), Braun & Cohen (2005) and Williamson (2003).

There has been one study of the safety of raspberry leaf. A study on 40 Wistar rats who were given an oral dose of raspberry leaf (10 mg/kg per day), quercetin, kaempferol or control, found no differences in the birthweight or survival of the offspring but found a significant lengthening in gestation and a reduction in the number of live births in the raspberry group. It also found that the females in the next generation of offspring had a significantly earlier puberty (Johnson et al 2009). The relevance of these findings is limited as there were only 10 rats in each group and because normal practice is to take raspberry only in the last weeks of pregnancy rather than from conception.

There have been two studies of the effectiveness of raspberry leaf. An observational study in Australia compared 57 women who had consumed raspberry leaf products with 51 women from the same hospital who had not, and found no significant differences in outcome for the baby and a possible association between raspberry leaf consumption and normal delivery without interventions (Parsons et al 1999). On the basis of this study, a double-blind, randomized, placebo-controlled trial was carried out in a hospital in Sydney, Australia. Two hundred and forty low-risk women who were expecting their first baby were entered into the trial. There were 48 withdrawals for medical and non-medical reasons which are not given in complete detail. The results were analysed for the 192 women who continued with the trial until labour. They took raspberry leaf tablets (1.2 g per day) or placebo from 32 weeks until birth. The women were carefully monitored. An important finding is that there were no major differences in outcome between the two groups. There was no shortening of the first stage but there was a shortened second stage of labour (mean difference 9.6 minutes) and a lower rate of forceps deliveries in the treatment group (19% treatment/30% placebo). There was no difference in mean length of gestation or in the rate of spontaneous labour (48% treatment/51% placebo), medical augmentation of labour (31% treatment/28% placebo), induction (20% treatment/21% placebo) or emergency caesareans (18% treatment/19% placebo) (Simpson et al 2001). The study did not show a significant benefit of raspberry and the authors discuss whether they were too cautious with the dosage. A weakness of the study is that the results are not presented as an intention-to-treat analysis, which tends to make the treatment seem comparatively more effective than it was. A second weakness of the study is that the reasons for withdrawal are not given in complete detail (Barnes 2003). Finally, of the 240 women initially recruited, 4% from the raspberry group and 2% from the placebo group developed pregnancy-induced hypertension and pre-eclampsia. Six of these 15 women remained in the study. This has raised concerns (Bayles 2007) about a possible association with hypertension but others have not taken this view (Mills & Bone 2005, Braun & Cohen 2005). The trial shows that, apart from this possibility, taking raspberry was not associated with any increase of adverse events in labour in this group of 192 women. Randomized controlled trials can flag up concerns but the numbers are too small to draw firm inferences on questions of safety.

Thomson did not admit that his practice was influenced by Native American usage, but Coffin (1866) claims that Native American women gave birth with ease. De Bairacli-Levi (1966) claims that raspberry is useful as a tonic throughout pregnancy and in labour, and advises 2 teaspoonfuls of leaves as a tea every 2–3 hours in labour. She states that 'it would be rare for a gypsy woman to go through pregnancy without having taken raspberry leaf teas from the first weeks of knowledge of conception. And the true nomad gypsy gives birth to her children with the ease of a wild vixen'. This potent image is attractive but deeply flawed as it arises from the myth of the 'noble savage' (Jasen 1997) but yet, excessively cautious safety concerns are disempowering to women. We may conclude that in contrast to some other herbs recommended for use in pregnancy (McFarlin et al 1999), raspberry has been shown to be safe (Mills & Bone 2005). Menzies-Trull adds a caution that it should not be used in 'athletic typology pregnancies,' or where there is a history of precipitate labour and should be discontinued if there are early labour pains.

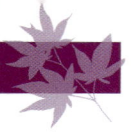

## RECOMMENDATIONS

- Brambles have a substantial traditional usage as an astringent for digestive tract problems and externally for healing inflammation and wounds. Although the authors find the herbs similar, it may be that bramble is more astringent and styptic. The external usage of powdered bramble leaf for spreading, cancerous sores deserves further investigation.
- Raspberry leaves are considered mild and useful for diarrhoea, especially in children.
- Leaves of both are recommended for oral thrush, mouth ulcers and gum infections. This recommendation dates back to Pliny and raspberry could be used more in these indications.
- Raspberry fruit cordials and vinegar remain in popular usage and are examples of the close association between use of plants as foods and as medicinal herbs. Raspberry syrups provide a useful vehicle for remedies for the respiratory and upper respiratory tract as in the example given by Fox.
- Raspberry is widely used to prepare for birth, and could be used more under the supervision of midwives in the management of normal pregnancy as proposed by Thomson and Coffin.

Dosage: the British Herbal Pharmacopoeia recommends 4–8 g three times a day. Braun & Cohen (2005) recommend use in the last 6–8 weeks of pregnancy and this appears a sensible compromise.

## RECOMMENDATIONS ON SAFETY

- Monitor use in pregnancy.
  No safety concerns are documented for raspberry, but the evidence on usage and dosage in preparation for birth is discussed above. Use of raspberry in pregnancy appears to be safe as it is used by large numbers of women, and it is compatible with breastfeeding (Mills & Bone 2005).

### CONSTITUENTS (RASPBERRY LEAVES)

Reviews: Barnes et al (2007), Bradley (2006), Braun & Cohen (2005), Patel et al (2004), Williamson (2003).

#### Flavonoids

#### Flavonol glycosides

Total 0.44% (mean), maximum 0.57% in cv. Malling Promise: quercetin glycosides mainly hyperoside, kaempferol glycosides (1 wild, 12 cultivars, Poland) (Gudej & Tomczyk 2004).

#### Tannins

Total 4.6% (mean), maximum 6.9% in cv. Tulameen (1 wild, 12 cultivars, Poland) (Gudej & Tomczyk 2004). 0.5–1.2% phenolic compounds (41 samples, wild, Lithuania) (Venskutonis et al 2007). Samples were taken from April to November but concentration did not correlate with season.

#### Hydrolyzable tannins

Ellagic acid 3.18% (mean), maximum 4.2% in cv. Tulameen (1 wild, 12 cultivars, Poland) (Gudej & Tomczyk 2004). Ellagitannins: sanguiin H6, lambertianin C, lambertianin D (Patel et al 2004).

## REFERENCES

Alice LA, Campbell CS 1999 Phylogeny of *Rubus* (Rosaceae) based on nuclear ribosomal DNA internal transcribed spacer region sequences. American Journal of Botany 86:81–97.

Alice LA, Torsten E, Bente E, et al 2001 Hybridization and gene flow between distantly related species of *Rubus* (Rosaceae): evidence from nuclear ribosomal DNA internal transcribed spacer region sequences. Systematic Botany 26:769–778.

Allen DE, Hatfield G 2004 Medicinal plants in folk tradition. Timber Press, Portland, Oregon.

Anttonen MJ, Karjalainen RO 2005 Environmental and genetic variation of phenolic compounds in red raspberry. Journal of Food Composition and Analysis 18:759–769.

Bamford DS, Percival RC, Tothill AU 1970 Raspberry leaf tea: a new aspect to an old problem. British Journal of Pharmacology 40:205–216.

Barnes J 2003 Complementary therapies in pregnancy. The Pharmaceutical Journal 270:402–404.

Barnes J, Anderson LA, Phillipson JD 2007 Herbal medicines, 3rd edn. Pharmaceutical Press, London.

Bayles BP 2007 Herbal and other complementary medicine use by Texas midwives. Journal of Midwifery & Women's Health 52:473–478.

Beekwilder J, Jonker H, Meesters P, et al 2005a Antioxidants in raspberry: on-line analysis links antioxidant activity to a diversity of individual metabolites. Journal of Agriculture and Food Chemistry 53:3313–3320.

Beekwilder J, Hall RD, De Vos CHR 2005b Identification and dietary relevance of antioxidants from raspberry. Biofactors 23:197–205.

Bradley PR 2006 British herbal compendium, vol 2. British Herbal Medicine Association, Bournemouth.

Braun L, Cohen M 2005 Herbs and natural supplements. Churchill Livingstone, London.

Coffin A I 1866 (1995 reprint) Treatise on midwifery and the diseases of women and children, 13th edn. Yesterday's Books, Windsor.

Collins M 2000 Medieval herbals. The British Library, London and University of Toronto Press.

Conover EA 2003 Herbal agents and over-the-counter medications in pregnancy. Best practice and research. Clinical Endocrinology and Metabolism 17:237–251.

De Bairacli-Levi J 1966 A herbal handbook for everyone. Faber & Faber, London.

Ernst E 2002 Herbal medicinal products during pregnancy: are they safe? British Journal of Obstetrics and Gynaecology 109:227–235.

Fletcher-Hyde F 1942 Rubus idaeus. The Herbal Practitioner 3:4–5.

Forster DA, Denning A, Wills G, et al 2006 Herbal medicine use during pregnancy in a group of Australian women. BMC Pregnancy and Childbirth 6:21. Online. Available: http://www.biomedcentral.com/bmcpregnancychildbirth/.

Fraser PM 1972 Ptolemaic Alexandria. Oxford University Press.

Gudej J, Tomczyk M 2004 Determination of flavonoids, tannins and ellagic acid in leaves from *Rubus* L. species. Archives of Pharmacal Research 27:1114–1119.

Haller JS 2000 The people's doctors: Samuel Thomson and the American botanical movement, 1790–1869. Southern Illinois University Press.

Holst L, Wright D, Nordeng H, et al 2009 Use of herbal preparations during pregnancy: focus group discussion among expectant mothers attending a hospital antenatal clinic in Norwich, UK. Complementary therapies in clinical practice, In Press, Corrected Proof, Available online 22 May 2009 doi: 10.1016/j.ctcp.2009.04.001

Jasen P 1997 Race, culture, and the colonization of childbirth in Northern Canada. Social History of Medicine 10:383–400.

Jennings DL 1964 Some evidence of population differentiation in *Rubus idaeus* L. New Phytologist 63:153–157.

Johnson J, Makaji E, Ho S, et al 2009 Effect of maternal raspberry leaf consumption in rats on pregnancy outcome and the fertility of the female offspring. Reproductive Sciences 16:605–609.

Lowdog T 2005 Women's health in complementary and integrative medicine. Elsevier, Philadelphia.

Maats FH, Crowther CA 2002 Patterns of vitamin, mineral and herbal supplement use prior to and during pregnancy. Australian and New Zealand Journal of Obstetrics and Gynaecology 42:494–495.

McFarlin BL, Gibson MH, O'Rear J, et al 1999 A national survey of herbal preparation use by nurse-midwives for labor stimulation. Review of the literature and recommendations for practice. Journal of Nurse-Midwifery 44:205–216.

Marshall B, Harrison RE, Graham J, et al 2001 Spatial trends of phenotypic diversity between colonies of wild raspberry *Rubus idaeus*. New Phytologist 151:671–682.

Mills S, Bone K 2005 The essential guide to herbal safety. Churchill Livingstone, St Louis.

Mullen W, Yokota T, Lean ME, et al 2003 Analysis of ellagitannins and conjugates of ellagic acid and quercetin in raspberry fruits by LC-MS. Phytochemistry 64:617–624.

Parsons M, Simpson M, Ponton T 1999 Raspberry leaf and its effect on labour: safety and efficacy. Australian College of Midwives Incorporated Journal 12:20–25.

Patel AV, Rojas-Vera J, Dacke CG 2004 Therapeutic constituents and actions of Rubus species. Current Medicinal Chemistry 11:1501–1512.

Pavord A 2005 The naming of names: the search for order in the world of plants. Bloomsbury, London.

Puupponen-Pimiä R, Nohynek L, Hartmann-Schmidlin S, et al 2005 Berry phenolics selectively inhibit the growth of intestinal pathogens. Journal of Applied Microbiology 98:991–1000.

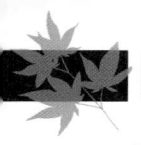

Rauha JP, Remes S, Heinonen M 2000 Antimicrobial effects of Finnish plant extracts containing flavonoids and other phenolic compounds. International Journal of Food Microbiology 56:3–12.

Robertson GW, Griffiths DW, Woodford JAT 1995 Changes in the chemical composition of volatiles released by the flowers and fruits of the red raspberry (*Rubus idaeus*) cultivar Glen Prosen. Phytochemistry 38:1175–1179.

Russell WR, Labat A, Scobbie L, et al 2009 Phenolic acid content of fruits commonly consumed and locally produced in Scotland. Food Chemistry 115: 100–104.

Ryan T, Wilkinson JM, Cavanagh HMA 2001 Antibacterial activity of raspberry cordial in vitro. Research in Veterinary Science 71:155–159.

Scalbert A, Manach C, Morand C 2005 Dietary polyphenols and the prevention of disease. Critical Reviews in Food Science and Nutrition 45:287–306.

Scarborough J, Nutton V 1982 The preface of Dioscorides' materia medica: introduction, translation, and commentary. Transactions and Studies of the College of Physicians of Philadelphia 4:187–227.

Shepherd T, Robertson GW, Griffiths DW, et al 1999 Epicuticular wax composition in relation to aphid infestation and resistance in red raspberry (*Rubus idaeus* L.). Phytochemistry 5:1239–1254.

Simpson M, Parsons M, Greenwood J. et al 2001 Raspberry leaf in pregnancy: its safety and efficacy in labor. Journal of Midwifery and Women's Health 46:51–59.

Skelton J 1853 A plea for the botanic practice of medicine. J Watson, London.

Stace C 1991 New flora of the British Isles. Cambridge University Press, Cambridge.

Stannard J 1965 Pliny and Roman botany. Isis 56:420–425.

Thanos CA 2001 Mt Ida in mythology and classical antiquity – a plant scientist's approach. Online. Available: http://www.biology.uoa.gr/~cthanos/Papers/MtIda.pdf 24 May 09.

Thomson S 1832 New guide to health, or, botanic family physician, 8th edn. Pike, Platt, Columbus.

Trickey R 1998 Women, hormones and the menstrual cycle. Allen & Unwin, St Leonards, New South Wales.

Tutin TG, Heywood VH, Burges NA, et al 1968 Flora Europaea, vol 2. Cambridge University Press, Cambridge.

USDA 2009 Plants database. Online. Available: http://plants.usda.gov/java/profile?symbol=ruids2)USDA 25 May 09.

Venskutonis PR, Dvaranauskaite A, Labokas J 2007 Radical scavenging activity and composition of raspberry (Rubus idaeus) leaves from different locations in Lithuania. Fitoterapia 78:162–165.

Wellmann M 1889 Sextius Niger. Hermes 24:530–569.

Williamson E 2003 Potter's herbal cyclopaedia. CW Daniel, Saffron Walden.

# CHAPTER 27
# *Ruta graveolens*, rue

## DESCRIPTION

### Family: Rutaceae
### Part used: aerial parts

The genus includes six species found in Europe (Tutin et al 1968). The *Flora of Turkey* (Davis 1967) gives two *Ruta* species, not including *Ruta graveolens*.

*Ruta graveolens* L. is a native of southeastern Europe but is widely naturalized in southern Europe and cultivated worldwide. It is a shrubby perennial with a distinctive smell. Smooth erect stems (14–45 cm) bear alternate, stalked bluish-grey-green pinnate leaves with deeply lobed obovate leaflets. Shiny yellow flowers with four spoon-shaped petals occur in terminal umbel-like groups in June–August. A smooth green capsule containing many seeds develops in each flower while other flowers around are still coming into flower.

**Other species used:** *Ruta angustifolia* Pers. and *Ruta chalepensis* L. are found in southern Europe and are similar but with fringed cilia on the petal edge (Tutin et al 1968).

### Quality

All *Ruta* species are associated with phytophotodermatitis (see below) and plants should not be touched with bare hands, especially on sunny days.

Rue is included among the plants discussed in this book not because we ourselves use it, but because of its reputation as a great healing medicine in the Western herbal tradition and the suspicion that it is a neglected remedy. Its application extends even to culinary purposes – rue belongs to the citrus family – but it is said no longer to suit the modern palate. From this it may be thought that rue is a relatively innocuous herb, but current concerns about the risks involved in its administration coupled with a lack of a modern evidence base for its therapeutic benefits has led to calls for rue to be withdrawn from over-the-counter sale for safety reasons. If it is to remain in the repertoire of registered herbal practitioners, then they require a better understanding of its recorded actions and uses in order to weigh this against potential toxicity and safety concerns so that a judicious decision on the reasons for employment and method of administration may be properly reached.

In a section headed 'Causes of contention' and subtitled 'False alarms?', Mills & Bone (2000) record rue appearing on a list of herbs circulated in 1992 by the European Commission Committee for Proprietary Medicinal Products which, in the committee's opinion, should be withdrawn from sale. It is, say Mills & Bone, one of a number of herbs on the list that are widely used and popular among practitioners. They bemoan the fact that there is too little representation of herbal expertise on such controlling bodies, making the herbal profession vulnerable to legislative decisions restricting the availability of medicinal herbs. This can happen because 'it may be easier to publish reports in medical journals on the risks of herbal remedies than it is to prepare a publishable account of their efficacy. In the first case, anecdotal evidence is the norm, in the latter case it would be dismissed out of hand' (Mills & Bone 2000). Writing more than a decade after the shock announcement, the authors (2005) note that the list has had little impact on availability, but they do not speculate on the negative impact the call for withdrawal may have had on practitioner use. Bartram, however, is quick to suggest, writing in 1995, that the herb should be left to practitioner use only, that 'internal use today [is] discouraged in modern practice' and that excessive handling of the fresh plant may cause contact dermatitis.

The Commission E monograph for rue (dated 2 March 1989) (Blumenthal 1998) is one source from which the European Commission Committee for Proprietary Medicinal Products will have drawn. Here the dried leaf or dried aerial parts are linked with emmenogogic, antispasmodic, diuretic and antiinflammatory actions for use in menstrual disorders and discomforts; for loss of appetite and dyspepsia, circulatory disorders and arteriosclerosis, heart palpitations, nervousness and hysteria, fever, pleurisy and

©2009 Elsevier Ltd, Inc, BV
DOI: 10.1016/B978-0-443-10344-5.00032-X

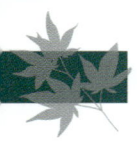

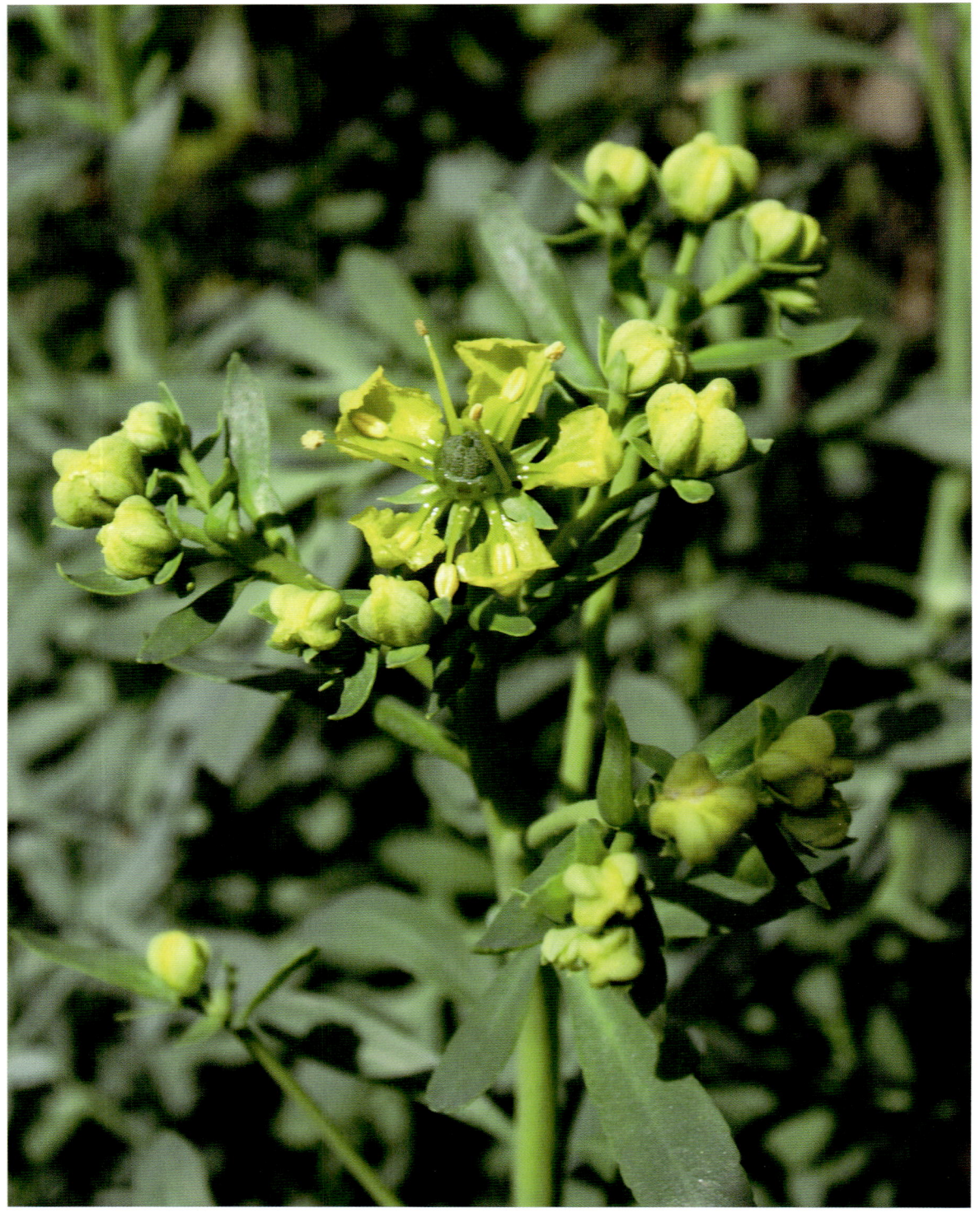

Figure 27.1 *Ruta graveolens,* rue (a garden in Somerset, August).

respiratory complaints, headache, neuralgic afflictions, toothache and weakness of the eyes. Both internally and externally, it is employed in arthritic complaints, dislocations, sprains, bone injuries and skin diseases. This represents quite a range of possible therapeutic actions but, according to the monograph, none of these applications has a verified effectiveness. Instead there is an unfavourable ratio of benefit to risk. The risks include contact dermatitis from the volatile oil component and phytophotodermatitis from the furocoumarins, while severe liver and kidney damage have been documented, and the deaths of pregnant women who used rue as an abortifacient reported. Therapeutic dosages can cause side-effects of melancholic moods, sleep disorders, tiredness, dizziness and spasms. The juice of the plant, particularly a fresh plant preparation, has been associated with painful irritations of the stomach and intestines, fainting, sleepiness, low pulse, abortion, swelling of the tongue and clammy skin.

Understandably, no dosage for rue is stated in the monograph but high doses are to be avoided, as the following case shows (Seak & Lin 2007). A woman of 78 in Taiwan took a decoction prepared with 50 g of fresh aerial parts decocted in 1000 mL of water boiled down to 250 mL. The plant material was positively identified as rue on further investigation. She took two doses a day and over the next 3 days developed increasing dyspnoea, dizziness, nausea, weakness and decreased urination. On admission she had a pulse of 41, blood pressure of 78/50, atrial fibrillation and an abnormal electrocardiogram, an international normalized ratio of over 12, hyperkalaemia and acute kidney failure, which was treated with haemodialysis. She was in hospital for 5 days and was well at a checkup 3 months later. She was taking medications for a 5-year history of hypertrophic cardiomyopathy and on further investigation had some mitral regurgitation but her normal pulse had been 78. The authors give a medical history and review the case in detail, including the possibility of a drug–herb interaction, and conclude that high dosage was the most likely cause.

Rue is a known abortifacient and is one of the plants traditionally used an as antifertility agent (de Laszlo & Henshaw 1954, Mengue et al 1997, O'Dowd 2001, Maurya et al 2004). It is also recommended to 'promote delayed menstruation' in self-help books such as Parvati (1979). Wood suggests that it is 'probably the single most important remedy in Latin American folk medicine' and Riddle (1991) cites ethnobotanical evidence of traditional abortifacient use among Hispanic people in New Mexico. The following report brings into focus the dangers of rue in this regard: a retrospective review of cases where herbal infusions had been taken to procure abortion found 86 cases (ages 14–47) from 1986 to 1999 which were reported to the Poison Centre in Montevideo, Uruguay. Twenty-six women took rue (*Ruta graveolens* or *Ruta chalepensis*), which was the most common herb used. Seventeen had abdominal pain and vomiting, 3 had jaundice, 11 had genital haemorrhage, 9 had abortion and 4 women died. One woman who died had also suffered a self-inflicted instrumental attempt at abortion (Ciganda & Laborde 2003). Gutiérrez-Pajares et al (2003) carried out a study on mice to determine whether rue affects preimplantation or embryo development, using aqueous extracts of the herb on the basis of a report from Chile that 500 mg twice a day is used by women there to prevent pregnancy.

Both this last study and another by de Freitas (2005) provide evidence that rue affects embryo development, producing abnormalities which lead to death of the embryo, while Al Mahmoud et al (2003), in a review of other studies where a range of preparations were used, found that implantation occurred but there was a higher rate of deaths of embryos. If embryo death leads to a sufficiently early spontaneous miscarriage, does this provide a modern explanation for the historical use of rue as an antifertility agent? Riddle, in reviewing this historical usage (1991), discusses both abortifacient and antifertility actions and explains how the extremely hot and particularly drying qualities of rue provide the Hippocratic rationale for the herb's power to dry up the male sperm or female seed, and both curb sexual desire and block conception if intercourse nevertheless takes place. This effect is enshrined in the Greek name for rue: peganon, from pegas meaning a congealed thing. Since the quality of moisture is required for fertility in Hippocratic and Galenic medical theory, a drying out and congealing of seed renders it unable to perform its role in conception. Riddle points out that rue is still used to control fertility today, but its employment in Western medicine came to an end by the19th century.

Use of rue as an abortifacient or antifertility agent requires knowledge of the correct dosage. Gutiérrez-Pajares et al (2003) found a significant and dose dependent increase in abnormal embryos in their study. Riddle (1991) cites Gargilius Martialis, a 3rd century AD retired soldier and land-owner, on concerns for the employment of rue by women, deeming foolish those who declare its power to inhibit and debilitate the generative seed and to kill embryos in the womb without consideration of the strength and dosage of the preparation, nor the circumstances in which it is taken. Rue must be taken in moderation 'so that it may not become a poison, rather than a remedy'. These studies support the recommendation that Rue should not be used in pregnancy or in women who intend to become pregnant.

A moderate dosage for rue will be required when treating other indications. In order to utilize its rutin content, which he says will be superior to rutin in isolated form, Weiss proposes a tea made with 1–2 tablespoons of dried rue to a cup of boiling water infused for 10–15 minutes. This is surely a large dose? If rutin in a complex is required for the treatment of circulatory disorders such as arteriosclerosis and capillary fragility, then the other herb he discusses in this regard, buckwheat *Fagopyrum esculentum*, must be preferable, and can be enjoyed as an item of the diet rather than as a medicine. Elsewhere in his text, Weiss proposes equal parts of dried rue leaf, hedge hyssop *Gratiola officinalis* and senna *Senna alexandrina* along with its corrective fennel seed *Foeniculum vulgare* as an effective emmenogogue. The inclusion of a laxative herb is very important, he says. The dose is 1 tablespoon (15 g) of herb to 500 mL of boiling water infused for 20 minutes. It is taken once daily, in the mornings within 1 hour of rising, on an empty stomach. Those among our modern authors who discuss rue (Bartram, Chevallier, Menzies-Trull, Williamson and Hoffmann) repeat the emmenogogue and spasmolytic actions listed in the *British Herbal Pharmacopoeia* – both due to the quinoline alkaloid arborinine according to Tyler (1993) – its indication in amenorrhoea, prohibition in pregnancy and the *British Herbal Pharmacopoeia* dose of 500 mg–1 g of dried herb three times a day. Hoffmann proposes a larger dose of 1–4 mL tincture 1:5 40% and 1–2 teaspoons dried herb to a cup of boiling water as an infusion. Wood takes a different approach. He provides the same contraindication and warning about contact but generally provides a homoeopathic description of the uses of rue and gives a dosage of 1–3 drops of the tincture. It is hard to agree with

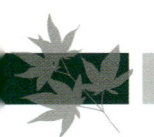

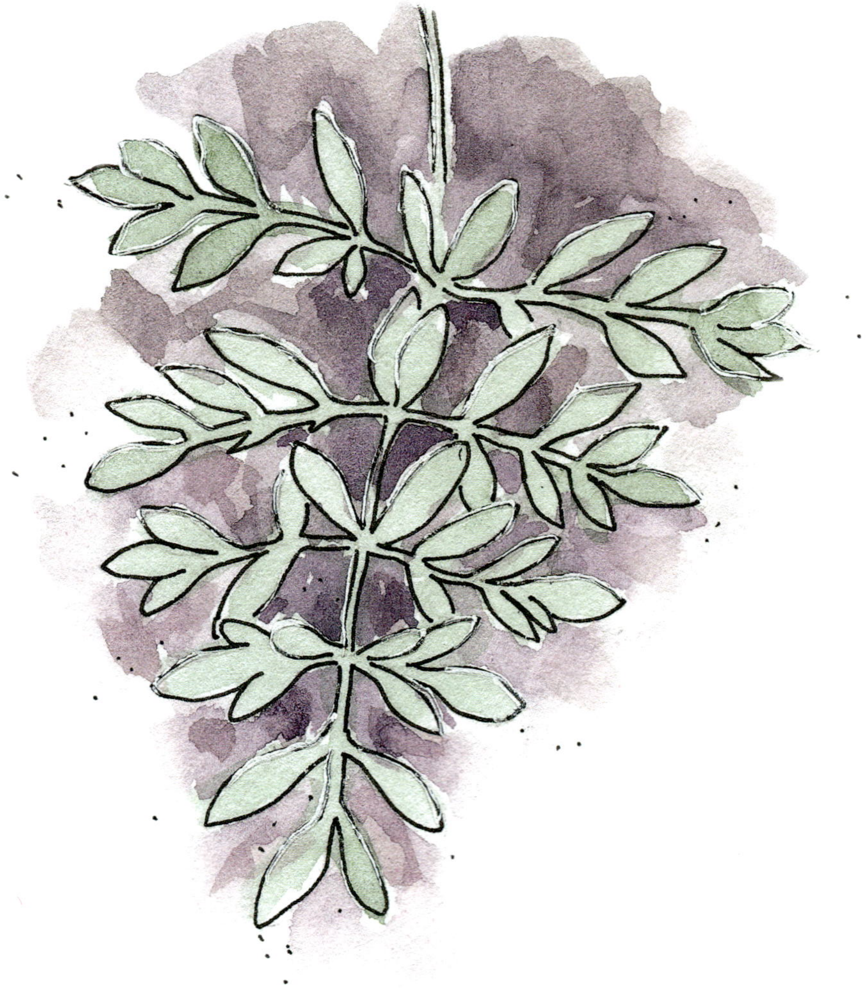

**Figure 27.2** *Ruta graveolens*, rue.

him that the vulnerary power of rue was unknown before Hahnemann's proving of the remedy to include strains, sprains, bruises and blows, when so many external applications are stated in the texts of the herbal tradition.

## RUE IN CLASSICAL MEDICINE

Dioscorides lists over a dozen external uses of rue. The herb infused into olive oil by cooking and applied to the abdomen helps inflations of the colon downwards and of the uterus, while the herb ground up with honey and applied to the perineum, 'from the genitalia to the anus', relieves uterine suffocation. A similar application is made to joints to relieve pain, while mixed with figs it disperses oedema. As a plaster with barley groats, it assuages severe eye pains and in combination with rose ointment and vinegar it is rubbed onto the head in cases of headache. Ground and inserted into the nostrils, it can stop nosebleeds; plastered on with the leaves of sweet bay, it helps inflammation of the testicles or with a cerate (wax) of myrtle it remedies their pustules. Rubbed on with salt and pepper, it treats dull-white leprosy, which is either vitiligo or psoriasis, and both raised and flat warts. Applied with honey and alum it is good for lichen-like eruptions of the skin. The fresh juice, warmed in a pomegranate shell and instilled, combats earache or mixed with the juice of fennel and honey then smeared on is a remedy for dim-sightedness. Another mixture with vinegar, white lead and rose ointment treats erysipelas, shingles and scurf. When a fresh leaf or two are chewed, it stops the smell and pungency of garlic and onions.

Pliny too records the majority of these uses, in some cases with the same ingredients, suggesting a common source. The herbal of pseudo-Apuleius, in a substantial entry for rue, reproduces fewer than half of them. For dimness of sight Pliny proposes the milk of a woman who has just borne a male child as an alternative ingredient to honey for the application of rue, or simply touching the corners of the eyes with a little of the juice. Engravers and painters, he adds, eat rue with bread or cress to preserve their sight. Rue with barley treats inflamed eyes, and with bay inflammation of the testicles. Apuleius requires the leaves and flowers of rue mixed with wine and applied to the eyes for mistiness and ulceration while restating Pliny's poultice with barley for inflammations, for which the pounded root may also be used. The fresh herb cooked in oil and mixed with wax as a cerate 'for the groin' copies the advice of Dioscorides for inflammation and swelling of the testicles but without the addition of myrtle. Pliny replaces the rose ointment in Dioscorides' mixture for headaches with rose oil, but if the headaches are chronic, he continues, barley flour should be used instead of rose oil. The juice of rue in vinegar is poured over the head in cases of phrenitis, or with the addition of wild thyme and bay, the liquid is rubbed into the head and neck. Apuleius requires the herb to be mixed with vinegar and rose oil and poured on the head for all head pains. Pliny states that injections of rue decocted in wine with hyssop *Hyssopus officinalis* are made for nosebleeds, and of the juice for earache. Honey and wine, or oil of rose or bay are added for hardness of hearing and tinnitus. Apuleius wants the herb itself inserted into the nose for bleeding but gives no treatment for ear pains. Applications to the abdomen for heartburn and severe colic are taken from Diocles, a physician of the 4th century BC, and involve mixing rue, vinegar and honey into barley meal, and for the latter pains boiling it in oil and applying the liquid on pieces of fleece. The simpler solution of Apuleius is to hold the herb in position on the skin over the organ. Treatment of skin eruptions and erysipelas in Pliny are the same as in Dioscorides, while that for vitiligo/psoriasis, warts, scrofula and the like require the addition of nightshade (undefined), lard and beef suet. Only the 'sacred fire' or erysipelas is mentioned in Apuleius, for which rue mixed with oil and vinegar is rubbed on.

Pliny offers other mixtures for external uses not mentioned by Dioscorides: the leaves boiled in oil for frostbite; carbuncles resolved by rue in vinegar, also cited in Apuleius; the mixture for nosebleeds as a mouthwash; a decoction of the plant applied to swollen breasts; an ointment of wild rue amazingly to resolve hernias; broken limbs healed by a wax plaster of rue seed; the root applied to bloodshot eyes and to heal scars and clear spots; finally, and despite it being a very heating herb which may be expected to open the pores of the skin, a bunch of rue boiled in rose oil with 1 oz of aloes checks the perspiration of those who have rubbed themselves with it. This formula is recommended for heartburn in Apuleius. The Myddfai physicians support Pliny's contention by recommending pounded rue rubbed into the skin as 'excellent for those hectic perspirations which so weaken a man'.

These external uses are handed down, in total or in part, through the Renaissance authors. They are partially reported in Ibn Sina, who adds baldness to the list of indications. Serapio only quotes Dioscorides. The medieval authors only report a few of the classical uses, but notably those for dim-sightedness and inflammation of the eyes. The *Old English Herbarium* reproduces fairly exactly the formulae for topical use in Apuleius for nosebleeds, eye pain and swelling and headache, but omits external applications for abdominal swelling. The *Red Book* of the Myddfai physicians lists thigh pains and bites of vipers, and the later 18th century prescriptions for topical use covers parasites in the skin, carbuncles, whitlows, cancer, arthritis and other aches, eye pain, sore throat with fever, a painful mouth and snake bites. The Salernitan herbal suggests heating rue and sage *Salvia officinalis* on a tile then apply to contusions while Dodoens describes bruising among the indications. Bauhin advises the distilled water of rue for nasal polyps and to purge the head. Macer and the Arabic authors include external applications for headache, repeated many centuries later by Dr Fernie (1897), from whom Grieve obtained the substantial part of her entry for rue. Robinson (1868) cites Professor Herman Boerhaave (1668–1738), a physician famed for his clinical teaching, on rue mixed with wine and salt to stop gangrene, restore vitality to a part, prevent suppuration and heal wounds. Fernie also transmits the benefit of rue for the eyes, reminding us that the visual nerve of Adam was purged by Milton's angel with 'Euphrasy [eyebright *Euphrasia officinalis*] and Rue'. He cites an old rhyme: 'Noble is Rue! It makes the sight of eyes both sharp and clear. With help of Rue, oh blear-eyed man! Thou shalt see far and near'. Bauhin reproduces the full Latin saying: 'nobilis est ruta qui alumina reddit acuta: auxilio rutae, vir lippe vedebis acute'. In addition to eye problems, Fernie proposes another external use, of compresses saturated with a strong decoction of the plant applied to the chest beneficially for chronic bronchitis.

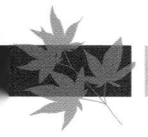

We have seen weakness of the eyes listed among the unverified indications of rue in the Commission E monograph. Bartram also includes this indication, while Juliette de Bairacli Levy (1966) offers seemingly her own preparation 'for eye ailments, including treatment of cataract': infuse a tablespoon of rue flowers for 3 days in a cup of water to which is added a teaspoon of white wine, the preparation to sit in a shallow dish in sunlight, or slowly heated in an oven with the door open if no sunshine is available. The eyes are then bathed several times daily with this water. A similarly gentle extraction is mentioned in Apuleius, where morning dew is collected from the plant in a small vessel and mixed with vinegar for bathing the eyes. Levy is well aware of the potency of rue and advises small doses. For internal use she suggests the ratio of a small teaspoon to a glass of water, as a 'standard brew' with a dose of only 2 tablespoons of the liquid twice daily. On the other hand, she seems familiar with the need for a substantially larger dose as an antidote to snake bite 'suck out the poison or cut out with the point of a sharp knife, in the usual way. Infuse 2 oz of fresh rue in a pint of beer, drink this and apply some frequently to the bitten area'. This dose is similar to that in the case of poisoning in the elderly Taiwanese woman but Levy's preparation is an infusion not a decoction and certainly not intended to be given to a person with cardiac hypertrophy and on medication for the problem.

It is apparent from the external applications, old and new, that fresh rue is used. Pliny specified that rue juice is extracted by pounding the plant with a sprinkling of water and the juice must be kept in a copper box. Are the levels of essential oil obtained sufficient to preserve the juice in this way? Conversely, aqueous infusions of the fresh plant will not extract as efficiently these same oils, thus rendering the resulting liquid for internal administration milder and potentially less toxic. The specification of the Commission E monograph for the dried leaves of rue has the same intention, since the quantity of volatile oils will be reduced in the drying process, but it is not the case that the Ancients did not appreciate the dangers of rue. We have already heard the opinion of Gargilius Martialis, and earlier Pliny too affirmed the risks to pregnant women of consuming rue in their diet, 'for I find that the foetus is killed by it'. It seems that the Romans, much more than the Greeks, used rue as a condiment. Fresh and dried rue were employed in the form of a bouquet garni or a sprig used to stir a sauce in the recipes of Apicius, while bunches of rue were pickled in brine for use at the table. 'It is prudent to assume that in his recipes rue was meant to be used invariably with moderation, even when this was not specifically recommended' (Andrews 1948).

Dioscorides does not warn that pregnant women should not eat rue, but states that it is emmenogogue. This action has passed down to the present day, in statements such as Fuch's 'if a pregnant woman drinks the juice, she will abort' and Turner's citing of Seth 'the juice of this herb is evil for women with child'. It is the only action listed in the *British Herbal Pharmacopoeia* to yield an indication (atonic amenorrhoea). According to Dioscorides the seed of rue quells the organ of generation, and this linked effect is discussed in herbals down to the 17th century, as, for instance, Pliny's 'for spermatorrhoea and frequent amorous dreams', Galen's 'inhibiting the appetite of Venus', 'for the flowing of semen' in Apuleius, Ibn Sina's 'dries up the seed, checks its flow and kills lust', Gerard's 'quencheth and drieth up the naturall seed of generation' and Culpeper's (1669) 'consumes the seed, and is an enemie to generation…is nought for women with child'. Hildegard tells us that lack of sexual release is also harmful. She advises that 'if a man is sometimes stirred up in delight, so that his sperm arrives at the point of emission but has in some way been retained within his body and he has begun to be ill from it', that he should take a preparation of rue and wormwood *Artemesia absinthium* in sugar, honey and wine in order to help the body void the 'noxious mucus' via urine and stool. Applicable to both sexes is Bauhin's observation that those who have devoted themselves and are sworn to chastity are greatly helped by a daily dose of 1 oz of the seeds in drink. Riddle (1991) interprets the statements in Soranus' Gynaecology, another 1st century AD text, on the use of rue as a vaginal suppository to imply an *antifertility* effect through contraceptive and abortifacient means. Both he and Mills & Bone (2000) identify the use of euphemistic language: Riddle says that Pliny's citation from Hippocrates that rue removes 'the foetus that has died before delivery' is a common circumlocution for abortion, while Mills & Bone argue that emmenogogues were used to 'bring on the menses' when they were delayed by pregnancy. Thus Dioscorides' words may provide sufficient warning to women of rue's power in this respect.

Dioscorides is more specific on other aspects of rue's potential toxicity. Both garden and wild varieties burn and ulcerate. He points out that 'the rue that grows on mountains and the wild is harsher than the cultivated and unfit to eat', that 'eating much wild rue is fatal: gathered for pickling when in bloom, it does redden and puff up the skin with itching and with a violent rash. People must thus harvest it after they have anointed their face and hands'. So, here is evidence of ancient knowledge of rue's ability to cause a contact dermatitis, and since rue flowers in the summer months and in sunny climates, it would have been difficult in former times to distinguish this from a phototoxic dermatitis. Furthermore, for internal consumption, the question of dosage is again crucial. Dioscorides balances his statement that eating much wild rue is fatal with the notion, of which he is sceptical, that ingestion of any amount is immediately followed by death 'They say...that the rue that grows in Macedonia by the river Haliacmon is fatal when eaten; this place is mountainous and full of vipers'. Pliny states that an overdose of the juice, which is normally taken in wine in doses of one acetabulum (around 60 mL), is poisonous, especially from the Macedonian rue specified by Dioscorides. 'Strangely enough, it is neutralized by the juice of hemlock; so there are actually poisons of poisons, and hemlock juice is good for the hands and face of those who gather rue'.

Pelikan gives us a modern take on rue's ability to combat poisons and infectious diseases. He contrasts abnormal astral forces operating in plants to render them poisonous, with rue's ability to assimilate these forces through the dominance of a cosmic 'I'-like nature. This is apparent in its formation of volatile oils and expression of a warmth principle, as also seen among the healing aromatic plants of the Labiate family. However, this warmth principle and expression through volatile oil production is particularly strong in rue. In order for rue to be tolerated, the human 'I'-impulses within the patient must also be strong. In this way rue protects the person from outside influences like infectious disease and poison. The strong fire and light forces within rue link both to its ability to treat the eyes and its power to cause blistering of the skin on contact.

## RUE, HARMALA AND POISON

It will be useful now to clarify here the difference between cultivated and wild rue, for there is some confusion in the later tradition. Dioscorides writes of the cultivated or garden rue and the wild rue that grows on mountains together as 'peganon'. He has a separate entry for the wild rue 'peganon agrion' called 'harmala', by the Syrians 'bessara' and by the Cappodocians 'moly'. It is sometimes called 'Syrian rue' but is the white-flowered harmal *Peganum harmala* from the Zygophyllaceae (USDA 2010). The fact that these plants of different families are both called wild rue sets up a confusion. For Dioscorides' peganon agrion or harmal is also used for dim-sightedness but there is no internal use mentioned for either the seed or root. Galen accords with Dioscorides in pointing out that the wild form of rue and harmala are both called 'wild rue' but differentiates garden and wild forms by attributing heating and especially drying qualities in the fourth degree to wild rue (a category reserved for agents which can inflame and blister the skin) and in the third degree to garden rue. Mattioli tells us that harmala is also deemed hot and dry in the third degree by Galen, and therefore it cuts thick humours, provokes diuresis and menstruation, and purges phlegm. Is this simply Galenic pharmacological theory or was harmal used internally in this way? It may be good for shoulder pain, according to Galen, but this could perhaps be achieved through topical application. Our later French edition of Mattioli as well as providing a description of harmala, states that the seed of wild rue (i.e. harmal) prepared and mixed with honey and sesame or almond oil is remarkable in purging melancholy by vomit and also treats epilepsy. It is added that the Arabs regard the seed as intoxicating and makes those who take it sleep long. Modern research has identified that one of the plant's alkaloids, harmaline, has a monoamine oxidase inhibitory effect, that as an entheogen (a substance that facilitates communion with the supernatural) it has been likened to the South American ayahuasca (which also causes vomiting) and that animal studies show it is an abortifacient and can reduce spermatogenesis. In modern Turkey, the seeds of harmal are hung in a house to protect from the 'evil eye' and in Iran an old Zoroastrian ritual is still occasionally carried out in restaurants where diners are exposed to the gaze of strangers whereby the seed capsules and other ingredients are placed on hot charcoals whereupon the seeds explode, releasing a fragrant smoke which is wafted about the diners' heads as protection.

Latin texts name garden rue 'ruta sativa' and wild rue 'ruta agrestis' or 'ruta sylvestris'. Mattioli correctly reads Dioscorides and comments that ruta sylvestris practically covers mount Salvatinus, demonstrating again that the wild peganon is found in mountainous areas. Gerard even includes the hills of Lancashire and Yorkshire as locations in which to find ruta sylvestris, though it is a native of southern Europe, but Parkinson is doubtful of the claim, sure that rue would not survive winter in the Pennines (the fact that Fernie (1897) and Grieve repeat the claim shows that they have read Gerard but not Parkinson on the matter). Mattioli admits that he has not yet seen (in 1554) the plant harmal, although it reportedly grows in the botanic gardens in Padua. He chastises Fuchs in his work called Paradoxes for misreading Ibn Sina on wild rue by assuming that Ibn Sina was discussing harmal when in fact he was following Dioscorides on the wild form of rue. Equally, Mattioli reckons that when the Mauritanians (Arabs of North Africa) speak of 'armala' (i.e. an unaspirated form of harmala) they mean the wild form of rue and if Italian apothecaries are following any of their prescriptions, they should prepare wild rue when 'armala is required. Mattioli makes no comment on the advice of Dioscorides not to use wild rue internally. Dodoens has a separate section for harmal but tells us that the wild form of rue is called 'harmel' in the apothecaries' shops. Turner regards the seeds of wild rue as safe to ingest but unhelpfully calls its root 'moly of the mountains' while Gerard falls prey to Fuch's misunderstanding by suggesting that 'Harmala', 'Harmel' and 'Besara' are simply alternative names for wild rue among the Arabic writers. In the 18th century Miller names the white-flowered harmal 'wild rue'. Location helps to distinguish the species, although this is unhelpful if the only examples are seen in botanical gardens. Cultivated or garden rue, according to Pliny, loves to grow in open, dry places, especially on clay and needs to be dressed with ashes, but it hates dampness, winter and manure. The wild form is found in mountainous areas, while harmal is a plant of desert regions. Harmal has become an invasive weed since being planted in New Mexico in the late 1920s and has since spread across the salt-desert shrub lands of the western USA, successfully competing with native species because of its drought tolerance (Moore 1989).

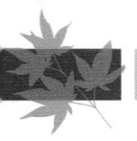

Despite the confusions over wild rue, Dioscorides' warnings that eating too much of this wild form can be fatal and handling it can blister the skin are passed down the tradition, from the Arabic writers to the Renaissance authors. Gerard, for instance, affirms that wild rue 'scorcheth the face of him that looketh upon it, raising up blisters, wheals, venometh the hands that touch it, and will also infect the face if it be touched before they are clean washed; therefore, it is not to be admitted to meat, or medicine'. Fernie (1897) later quotes the same statement and warns of inflammation of the skin but Grieve omits it and styles rue a topical rubefacient agent without this caution). Bauhin informs us that Guillaume Rondelais (1507–66), physician and botanist at the medical school in Montpellier, used to tell a story about meeting a man on pilgrimage to that city who came across rue on his journey and, having heard that Montpellier was beset by the plague, gathered the herb, placed it in his nostrils and held it in his hand for some time, whence the parts in contact with rue became greatly inflamed.

Rue is 'among our chief medicinal plants' says Pliny, and its extensive uses by ingestion are consistently passed down as far as Culpeper. We have heard of its emmenogogue action, to which is linked by Galenic pharmacology a diuretic one, although the indication was given by Hippocrates. Pliny, who tells us this and reckons the herb good for the kidneys, then marvels at how some use rue for incontinence of urine, while treatment of strangury is made by the usual internal administration or the application of an oil of rue over the bladder area. Mention has also been made of its ability to antidote the poison of a snake bite. Dioscorides includes not only reptile poisons but all deadly poisons, requiring a dose of one oxybaphon (a volume measurement of nearly 70 mL) of the seed taken in wine. Pliny regards the pounded leaves of any sort of rue in wine a powerful antidote, especially against aconite, mistletoe, poisonous fungi, snake bites, rabid dogs and scorpion and other stings. Apuleius advises the powdered seed drunk in wine and laid on for scorpion stings. Seth cited in Fuchs adds opium to the list of poisons rue antidotes. Pliny notes that weasels about to fight with snakes first protect themselves by eating rue. It is also good for fevers with rigors.

Serapio calls rue 'the ultimate medicine against the evil of poisons' and Dodoens, Gerard, Bauhin, Parkinson and Culpeper want it as a remedy against the plague. It was, after all, one of the ingredients of the 'vinegar of the four thieves' who robbed the houses of plague victims under the protection of their aromatic repellent. Quincy, Miller and Hill consider it an alexipharmic remedy against the plague or epidemic infections and fevers. Drury (1992) comments that the English courtrooms of today no longer have to contend with the threat of gaol fever (typhus) or the plague from defendants in the dock or from members of the public in the gallery, for which rue was used as a strewing herb as proof against these contagions of the Renaissance and early modern periods. A belief in rue's ability to combat poison thus has a long history and strong recommendation, since it is a constituent of the famous antidote of Mithridates, King of Pontus. Parkinson informs us that each morning the king, to protect himself against poisoning, would take 20 rue leaves mixed with a little salt, two walnuts and two figs, the whole beaten to a mass and ingested as a daily dose. We know this because, as Fernie (1897) relates, the Roman general Pompey found the formula in the satchel of the conquered king. The formula turns up in the Red Book of the physicians of Myddfai. Culpeper offers particular praise to Mithridates for his researches in physic, dismisses arguments that protection against cold poisons do not afford immunity against hot poisons but recommends instead that Mithridates' formula, to which Culpeper adds 20 juniper berries, taken in the quantity of a hazel nut, will preserve admirably the health of the body. This is because rue is a herb of the sun in Leo, an alexipharmic like juniper, which by fortifying the heart strengthens resistance to all disease. The herbs must be gathered, however, at the astrologically propitious hour.

## ANTHELMINTIC AND SPASMOLYTIC

Another traditional use for rue is as an anthelmintic. Dioscorides wants it boiled in olive oil and drunk to remove intestinal worms. This indication passes down through the Arabic and Renaissance sources, then is rarely mentioned, although Cullen recommends a strong decoction as an enema for ascarides in the rectum. Williamson states that the herb is reportedly anthelmintic and recent ethnobotanic research shows that rue is a popular traditional medicine in rural parts of Italy for worms and externally against head lice and parasites (Guarrera 1999). Despite being a non-indigenous herb, it is also in much demand by the people of the Bredasdorp/Elim area of South Africa not only for worms but also for bladder and kidney problems, convulsions, diabetes, fever, headache, stomach complaints and sinus problems, in doses of 1 teaspoon of the herb to a cup of boiling water (Thring & Weitz 2006). An anthelmintic action is derived from the volatile oils and bitterness of rue and leads us to consider the plant's actions in the digestive tract. Dioscorides notes that eaten or drunk it stops diarrhoea and, taken with dried dill *Anethum graveolens*, abdominal colic. Pliny says that the pounded leaves in wine with cheese are given to patients with dysentery. Rue soon relieves indigestion, flatulence and chronic stomach pains, and should be decocted with hyssop *Hyssopus officinalis* and taken in wine for colic and internal haemorrhage, and can be used externally on the abdomen and over the heart, as discussed above. Decocted with figs in wine, and the liquid reduced by half then drunk, it treats dropsy. Pliny wants rue for liver problems generally and the Arabic writers mention the spleen. Indications for diarrhoea, flatulence and colic have passed down the tradition to the present day. Hoffmann emphasizes the spasmolytic action of rue, easing griping and bowel tension by relaxing smooth muscle. When Fernie (1897) suggests that rue remedies the nervous indigestion and flatulence from which the Greeks suffered when eating before strangers and later mentions that it sometimes causes vomiting or purging, we wonder if he is a victim of the confusion between wild rue and harmal. Grieve too, following the *National Botanic Pharmacopoeia*, warns of taking rue after food 'on account of its emetic tendencies', whereas Bauhin proposes half a drachm (2 g) of the powdered herb in warm wine to comfort the stomachs of children weakened by frequent vomiting.

Rue has also been recommended for lung problems and its spasmolytic action offers a rational therapeutic for respiratory complaints. Only pleurisy is included in the unverified uses of the Commission E monograph, which disease fits the report of Dioscorides that the herb is 'good for pains on the side and chest, dyspnoea, cough, inflammation of the lungs'. Pliny mentions asthma but the *British Herbal Pharmacopoeia* restricts itself to an antitussive action without indications and the *National Botanic Pharmacopoeia* lists only croupy affections. Hoffmann suggests spasmodic coughs. Indeed little has been made of rue for lung problems since Culpeper's day, when rue may also have been given for purulent expectoration and the spitting of blood, using for the latter three sprigs of rue boiled in wine. Rather, the spasmolytic action combined with a stimulating effect has been thought useful for nervous complaints. The old herbals mention more serious neurological problems: Pliny proposes a decoction of the juice for epilepsy and Fernie (1897) writes that the Neapolitan physician Piperno commended rue in 1625 as a specific for epilepsy and vertigo. We may recall the Commission E noting dizziness as an adverse effect; Fernie mentions an unsteadiness of gait in regard to excessive doses, for a leaf or two chewed is sufficient in his opinion to relieve nervous headache, giddiness, hysterical spasm or palpitation (the praecordial pain in Apuleius for which the herb in wine is drunk before the patient lies down), and Grieve and Hoffmann repeat this advice. Quincy reckons that rue is good in all convulsive cases and thinks the best way to take it is to eat the fresh leaves with bread and butter. Cullen too is prepared to consider rue, 'a plant of several peculiarities' in the treatment of epilepsy, for which the inspissated juice or other extract may be used. Ibn Sina advocates rue internally and externally for paralysis and sciatica, for which latter Fernie suggests that the leaves should be bruised and applied. Macer recommends the bruised herb with cumin powder applied to an ache in any part. Indeed, an external liniment of rue is used topically for pain in present-day Mexico (Waldstein 2006). For lethargy, Turner's 'the forgetful disease', rue may be taken internally, as an enema or the vinegar of the fresh plant smelled. In Apuleius rue in vinegar is poured onto the head and in the *Old English Herbarium* it is sprinkled onto the temples. For instance, some recent research records application of a homoeopathic combination of rue and calcium phosphate in the treatment of neurocysticercosis which has neurological symptoms as the cysts are in the brain tissues (Banerji & Banerji 2001). Thirty-six patients were assessed with computerized tomography scans and treated for between 3 and 65 months, and 25 subjects became symptom-free.

The indication of paralysis is not continued, although Gerard writes of oil of rue warming and chafing all cold members that are rubbed with it. Instead Quincy naturally places rue among the hysterics, with cephalic qualities, and good for all nervous complaints in women which originate from the womb. Miller, Hill, Cullen, the *National Botanic Pharmacopoeia* and the *British Pharmaceutical Codex* (1934) follow suit. In the last case a dose of 0.12–0.3 mL of the oil should be taken on sugar or in hot water. The essential oil of rue is no longer recommended and indeed Wren prefers anyway an infusion of 1 oz to 1 pint (25 g to 500 mL), to be taken in cupful doses for hysteria and amenorrhoea. He warns that large doses are liable to produce inflammation and nerve derangements.

The Commission E monograph lists several adverse effects of rue on the nervous system: melancholic moods, sleep disorders, tiredness, dizziness and spasms. Just as we have seen with dizziness above, these anecdotal reports are likely to be linked with excessive dosage. It is not news to practising herbalists that a certain action of a herb obtained with a therapeutic dose can be paradoxically reversed with a different dose, usually a much larger one but also with micro-doses. Melancholy, poor sleep, tiredness and spasms may appear in the same disease, and may be provoked by inappropriately large doses of a stimulant medicine such as rue. On the other hand, there are two reports in the literature we have consulted about the generation of melancholy. Turner cites Simeon Seth (although this same statement does not appear in Fuch's citation) on the need for those of a choleric temperament suffering from an imbalance of the yellow bile humour to abstain from rue, since it will heat their blood too much, driving off the thinner part of it and leaving it melancholic in quality. Fernie (1897), not being attached to Galenic theory, mentions dullness and weight of mind as products of excessive dosage of rue. It is important with this herb, as we have heard several times, to establish a correct dosage for the indication.

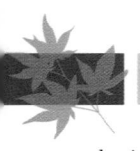

A final set of indications listed by Dioscorides for internal use of rue is pains of the hip joints and of the joints, and internal swellings and oedema. These passed down through the Arabic and Renaissance writers before being neglected. Treatment of the joints may be carried out by internal medicine and by external applications, as we have seen. A piece of recent research hints at some credence to the advice in the old herbals. An extract of rue was found to have an antiinflammatory action in vitro in a model which measures nitric oxide production and showed that this was related to inhibition of nitric oxide synthase. The authors found that although it was much more effective than pure rutin, the action was also related to concentration of rutin (Raghav et al 2006). Williamson mentions the antioedema effect of rutin and cites other research on the antiinflammatory action of rue. There are other plants which are safer sources of rutin, as we have already stated, but the unusual constituents of rue – aliphatic ketones, furocoumarins and alkaloids – may have specific actions of their own to complement this antiinflammatory effect.

We have seen a range of dosages employed in the above uses of rue, from the dew shaken from the flowers for an eye bath and a couple of fresh leaved chewed for nervous headache, palpitation and giddiness, to 2 oz of the fresh herb infused in a pint of beer for snake bite. This last use is unlikely to be repeated by herbal practitioners in a primary care setting, so we should instead consider the typical doses advocated. Again these have been as small as 2 tablespoons twice daily of an infusion made with a small teaspoon of rue to a glass of water, and as large as Weiss' infusion to obtain the benefits of rutin from rue, where 1–2 tablespoons of dried herb per cup of boiling water is used and the infusion taken three times daily. The *British Herbal Pharmacopoeia* states 0.5–1 g of the dried herb, as infusion, or 0.5–1 mL of the liquid extract 1:1 25% alcohol, three times daily. Grieve proposes 15–30 grains (1–2 g) of the powdered herb and 0.5–1 drachm (1.7–3.5 mL) of the liquid extract. Hoffmann offers a tincture dosage of 1–4 mL of tincture 1:5 40% alcohol. Wren states 1 oz of dried herb infused in 1 pint of boiling water, the infusion taken in cupful doses.

Bauhin writes that he must limit his comments on rue to what he himself has experienced of its efficacy, since it is virtually impossible to investigate the many claims made for rue by other authors. He provides instructions on how to prepare a distilled water, a conserve, a vinegar and an oil. For the latter, chopped and crushed fresh rue is infused in oil for 15 days in the sun or in a warm place, then decocted in a bain marie. The oil is strained and the process repeated twice more. As far as dosage is concerned, he proposes 1 drachm (4 g) of the powdered herb in warm wine for headaches due to cold. A handful of the (fresh?) herb decocted in wine until reduced by one third then strained, and with 4 oz sugar added, forms a drink for chest pain due to cold, to be taken morning and evening. In addition, 4 oz of the juice mixed with 1 drachm (4 g) of asafoetida seed *Ferula assafoetida* taken in a warm drink is helpful for epilepsy.

## RECOMMENDATIONS

Since rue is according to Galenic pharmacology very heating and drying, it is appropriate as an internal remedy for cold and phlegmatic presentations. These imbalances are much more likely in older people, whereas rue may be too stimulating and heating for younger people.

Rue should be considered for internal administration in:

- Obstructive lung diseases: asthma, chronic bronchitis, croup and spasmodic coughs. It may be considered for those convalescing from pleurisy and other inflammatory diseases of the lungs.
- As a carminative and antispasmodic it may be used for dyspepsia, colic and some cases of irritable bowel syndrome and diarrhoea.
- In nervous affections, including headache, spasms, light-headedness and functional palpitations. In small doses as a stimulant in lethargic states.
- Secondary amenorrhoea not linked to underlying disease. Weiss' formula above should be considered for use.
- Rue may have a role in premenstrual syndrome.
- To sharpen vision.
- Arthritis and rheumatism.
- For external use (with the need to protect the area treated from exposure to sunlight):
- Neuralgic pain, including shingles; arthritic pain of all kinds
- Scabies and other infestations, insect bites and stings

- Skin diseases where a stimulation of the affected skin is required to improve healing, or an anti-microbial effect is needed.
- As a rub for chest conditions such as bronchitis
- Research should be considered for the use of rue in epilepsy, mild cases of frostbite, vitiligo, lichen skin conditions and as a topical treatment in eye problems.

Dosage: the *British Herbal Pharmacopoeia* recommends 500 mg–1 g three times a day of dried herb. Equivalent dosage in liquid extract or tincture forms may be considered. Infusions of the fresh herb and specific tinctures should be used more cautiously in lower doses at first. A suitable fixed oil of rue and a derived ointment could be prepared for external use.

## CONSTITUENTS

Reviews: Williamson (2003), Stashenko et al (2000).

### Alkaloids

Furoquinolines, quinolines (Stashenko et al 2000).
Quinoline: graveoline, furoquinoline: kokusagenine; quinoline (fresh leaves, cultivated, USA) (Oliva et al 2003).
Quinoline: graveoline and eight analogues; furoquinoline: kokusagenine, skimmianine (cultivated, Bulgaria) (Kostova et al 1999).
Acridones, unique to Rutacea, mainly in roots and slightly in leaf base (Junghanns et al 1998).

### Volatile oil

Total 0.74% (38 compounds), linear ketones: 2-undecanone 47%, 2-nonanone 19%; monoterpenes 11%: alpha-pinene, limonene; oxygenated monoterpenes: 1,8-cineole, methyl salicylate 4% (aerial parts, Italy) (De Feo et a 2002).
(37 compounds), linear ketones: 2-nonanone 45.3%, 2-undecanone 31.1%; oxygenated monoterpenes (leaves, cultivated, Columbia) (Stashenko et al 1995).
Undecanone is responsible for the characteristic smell and insect repellant action and is used in sprays to repel dogs and cats.

### Furocoumarins

Total 0.4% (mean): psoralen 0.14%, bergapten (5-methoxypsoralen) 0.16%, xanthotoxin (8-methoxypsoralen) 0.1%, isoopimpinellin (5,8-methoxypsoralen) (leaves, cultivated, 19 plants, France). Total concentration was highest in fruits and leaves and similar in all 19 accessions (Milesi et al 2001).
Total 0.5% (mean): psoralen, xanthotoxin, bergapten. Total concentration was highest in leaves higher during fruiting, and did not vary between sites (cultivation, France) (Poutaraud et al 2000).
Rutamarin, bergapten, xanthotoxin, chalepin, rutaretin (Kostova et al 1999).
Chalepin, chalepensis, bergapten, psoralen, xanthotoxin, isopimpinellin (leaves, cultivated, Colombia) (Stashenko et al 2000).

### Flavonoids

Rutin 4% (Raghav et al 2006).

## RECOMMENDATIONS ON SAFETY

1. **Do not use in children.**
   Given the safety concerns discussed above, rue should not be used in children under any circumstances.
2. **Use caution in dosage.**
   The dosage of this plant is discussed above.
3. **Do not use where the patient may be pregnant or could become pregnant.**
   The authors and other sources discussed above indicate that rue can be an abortifacient.
4. **Do not apply to the skin without first conducting a small patch test.** Avoid exposing the treated part to the sun. Use gloves when gathering the plant as contact can cause an unpleasant, phototoxic skin reaction.
   Phytophotodermatitis is a light-sensitive contact dermatitis where skin which is exposed to sunlight comes into contact with an irritant substance and a red, oedematous rash, sometimes with blisters, develops, usually 1–2 days after exposure (Deleo 2004). The furocoumarins are linear

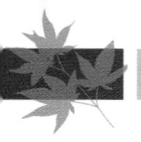

coumarins, containing a lactone group and the main ones are psoralen, bergapten and xanthotoxin (Eisenbrand 2007). A group of four adults and seven children applied fresh rue as an insect repellant and spent the afternoon outdoors. After 24 hours they developed reddish-purple rashes with blistering, which continued to erupt up to 12 days after the initial exposure. The rashes tended to be linear where the plant had been rubbed on the skin and people who had spent less time in the sun were less affected (Eickhorst et al 2007). A 2-year-old child suffered acute blistering on the hands and was poorly after touching the plant (Furniss & Adams 2007). A woman developed a painful rash after applying a decoction of dried rue the day before visiting a suntan parlour and again the rash was present where the rue extract had been applied (Wessner et al 1999).

# REFERENCES

Al Mahmoud MS, Elbetieha A, Al Muhur RA 2003 Anticonceptive and antifertility activities of various *Ruta graveolens* extracts in female rats. Acta Pharmaceutica Turcica 45:203–212.

Andrews AC 1948 The use of rue as a spice by the Greeks and Romans. The Classical Journal 3:371–373.

Banerji P, Banerji P 2001 Intracranial cysticercosis: an effective treatment with alternative medicines. In Vivo 15:181–184.

Blumenthal M (ed.) 1998 The complete German Commission E monographs. American Botanical Council.

Ciganda C, Laborde A 2003 Herbal infusions used for induced abortion. Journal of Toxicology Clinical Toxicology 41:235–239.

Culpeper N 1669 Pharmacopoeia londinensis or, the London dispensatory. London.

Davis PH (ed.) 1967 Flora of Turkey, vol 2. Edinburgh University Press, Edinburgh.

De Bairacli Levy J 1966 Herbal handbook for everyone. Faber & Faber, London.

De Feo V, De Simone F, Senatore F 2002 Potential allelochemicals from the essential oil of *Ruta graveolens*. Phytochemistry 61:573–578.

De Freitas TG, Augusto PM, Montanari T 2005 Effect of *Ruta graveolens* L. on pregnant mice. Contraception 71:74–77.

De Laszlo H, Henshaw PS 1954 Plant materials used by primitive peoples to affect fertility. Science 119:626–631.

Deleo VA 2004 Photocontact dermatitis. Dermatologic Therapy 17:279–288.

Drury S 1992 Plants and pest control in England circa 1400–1700: a preliminary study. Folklore 103:103–106.

Eickhorst K, DeLeo V, Csaposs J 2007 Rue the herb: Ruta graveolens – associated phytophototoxicity. Dermatitis 18:52–55. Online. Available: http://www.medscape.com/viewarticle/559986.

Eisenbrand G 2007 Toxicological assessment of furocoumarins in foodstuffs. Molecular Nutrition & Food Research 51:367–373.

Fernie WT 1897 Herbal simples approved for modern uses of cure. Boericke & Tafel, Philadelphia. Online. Available: http://www.gutenberg.org.

Furniss D, Adams T 2007 Herb of grace: an unusual cause of phytophotodermatitis mimicking burn injury. Journal of Burn Care Research 28:767–769.

Guarrera PM 1999 Traditional antihelmintic, antiparasitic and repellent uses of plants in Central Italy. Journal of Ethnopharmacology 68:183–192.

Gutiérrez-Pajares JL, Zúñiga L, Pino J 2003 *Ruta graveolens* aqueous extract retards mouse preimplantation embryo development. Reproductive Toxicology 17:667–672.

Junghanns KT, Kneusel RE, Gröger D, et al 1998 Differential regulation and distribution of acridone synthase in *Ruta graveolens*. Phytochemistry 49:403–411.

Kostova I, Ivanova A, Mikhova B, et al 1999 Alkaloids and coumarins from *Ruta graveolens*. Monatshefte für Chemie 130:703–707.

Maurya R, Srivastava S, Kulshreshta DK, et al 2004 Traditional remedies for fertility regulation. Current Medicinal Chemistry 11:1431–1450.

Mengue SS, Schenkel EP, Mentz LA, et al 1997 Plants used by pregnant women to induce menstruation (an inquiry to 6109 women in seven Brazilian cities). Acta Farmaceutica Bonaerense 16:251–258.

Milesi S, Massot B, Gontier E, et al 2001 *Ruta graveolens* L.: a promising species for the production of furanocoumarins. Plant Science 161:189–199.

Mills S, Bone K 2000 The principles & practice of phytotherapy. Churchill Livingstone, Edinburgh.

Moore M 1989 Medicinal plants of the desert and canyon west. Museum of New Mexico Press, Santa Fe.

O'Dowd MJ 2001 A history of medications for women. Parthenon, London.

Oliva A, Meepagal KM, Wedge DE, et al 2003 Natural fungicides from *Ruta graveolens* L. leaves, including a new quinolone alkaloid. Journal of Agricultural and Food Chemistry 51:890–896.

Parvati J 1979 Hygieia a woman's herbal. Wildwood House, London.

Poutaraud A, Bourgaud F, Girardin P, et al 2000 Cultivation of rue (*Ruta graveolens* L., Rutaceae) for the production of furanocoumarins of therapeutic value. Canadian Journal of Botany 78:1326–1335.

Raghav SK, Gupta B, Agrawal C, et al 2006 Anti-inflammatory effect of *Ruta graveolens* L. in murine macrophage cells. Journal of Ethnopharmacology 104:234–239.

Riddle JM 1991 Oral contraceptives and early-term abortifacients during classical antiquity and the Middle Ages. Past and Present 132:3–32.

Robinson M 1868 The new family herbal. W Nicholson, London.

Seak CJ, Lin CC 2007 *Ruta Graveolens* intoxication. Clinical Toxicology 45:173–175.

Stashenko EE, Villa HS, Combariza MY 1995 Comparative study of Colombian rue oils by high resolution gas chromatography using different detection systems. Journal of Microcolumn Separations 7:117–122.

Stashenko EE, Acosta R, Martinez JR 2000 High-resolution gas-chromatographic analysis of the secondary metabolites obtained by subcritical-fluid extraction from Colombian rue (*Ruta graveolens* L.). Journal of Biochemical and Biophysical Methods 43:379–390.

Thring TSA, Weitz FM 2006 Medicinal plant use in the Bredasdorp/Elim region of the Southern Overberg in the Western Cape Province of South Africa. Journal of Ethnopharmacology 103:261–275.

Tutin TG, Heywood VH, Burges NA, et al 1968 Flora Europaea, vol 2. Cambridge University Press, Cambridge.

Tyler V 1993 The honest herbal: a sensible guide to the use of herbs and related remedies. Pharmaceutical Products Press, New York.

USDA 2010 Plants profile for *Peganum harmala*. Online. Available: http://plants.usda.gov/java/profile?symbol=PEHA.

Waldstein A 2006 Mexican migrant ethnopharmacology: Pharmacopoeia, classification of medicines and explanations of efficacy. Journal of Ethnopharmacology 108:299–310.

Wessner D, Hofmann H, Ring J 1999 Phytophotodermatitis due to *Ruta graveolens* applied as protection against evil spells. Contact Dermatitis 41:232

Williamson E 2003 Potter's Herbal Cyclopaedia. CW Daniel, Saffron Walden.

# CHAPTER 28
# *Scrophularia nodosa*, figwort

## DESCRIPTION

**Family: Scrophulariaceae**      **Part used: aerial parts, root**

The genus contains over 200 species, which are mainly perennials. The erect stems are usually square with opposite leaves and bear lobed flowers, so can be confused with members of the Lamiaceae family. Distinguishing features of *Scrophularia* species are the terminal branched flowerheads and the characteristic staminodes (enlarged non-fertile stamens) and seed cases. The *Flora of Turkey* (Davis 1978) gives 56 *Scrophularia* species, including *Scrophularia nodosa*.

*Scrophularia nodosa* L. is a native, herbaceous perennial found in damp places. It is widespread in Europe. Smooth, erect, four-sided stems (50–120 cm) with acute stem-angles, bear serrate, opposite leaves with short petioles without stipules. Stalked clusters of small, tubular, five-lobed, greenish purple-brown flowers with a large upper lip occur in July. Under the upper lip is a tongue-shaped staminode (Makbul et al 2006). It is pollinated by wasps and the seeds are enclosed in small clusters of hard, brown, egg-shaped capsules. The root is white and tuberous.

**Other species used:** Water figwort *Scrophularia auriculata* L. is a similar plant that is found in wetter places. The stems are taller and more stout with more prominent wings on the stem angles. The roots are brown and stringy. A former synonym was *Scrophularia aquatica* but this has been discontinued (Ortega-Olivencia & Devesa 2002). *Scrophularia marilandica* is widespread in North America (USDA 2009) and is very similar to *Scrophularia nodosa* but has a more branching flowerheads. The sample which we grew had white nodules on the roots. *Scrophularia ningpoensis* is used in China (WHO 1989).

### Quality

Where the root is specified then only *Scrophularia nodosa* should be used.

## 'THE BROWN WORT' – BUT WHAT IS IT?

The descriptions given by the authors include much discussion of the identity of the plant under consideration. Earlier writers may be referring to a figwort or to a deadnettle. Dioscorides describes galeobdolon and the debate on the identity of this plant is explored in the chapter on *Lamium* species. As discussed later, some *Lamium* and *Scrophularia* species are not easily distinguished. They are listed consecutively by Gerard and Parkinson, although Parkinson also describes 'great figwort without knobbed roots', which could be *Scrophularia auriculata*. Alongside figwort is water betony or water figwort *Scrophularia auriculata*. Another reason for the confusion is that some of the actions are comparable. For example, Mattioli debates the differentiation of species and, after making recommendations for use of the leaves of stinking deadnettle for 'bruises, injuries, burns, strumas, tumours/swellings, gouts and wounds', he goes on to recommend external use of figwort root 'by which the aforesaid diseases are most usefully healed'. Before discussing figwort in more detail, what we can say is that the descriptions from the Renaissance are of figwort *Scrophularia nodosa* so that while there is uncertainty about the other plants, it is certain that figwort was used.

Many earlier recommendations are for external usage of the root. External use of the leaves is suggested combined with internal use of the leaves to heal wounds, places where the blood is congealed in the body and swellings of every sort, more especially haemorrhoids and swollen lymph nodes in the neck. The alterative usage which is most common today develops more clearly after the 13th century.

Dioscorides (IV 94) describes 'the brown wort: but some call it galepsis and others galeobdolon' as having delicate purple flowers and the 'entire little shrub' resembling the nettle (IV 93) in shape, leaf and stem, but the leaves are smoother and 'rather foul smelling when ground'. Beck gives *Scrophularia peregrina* nettle-leaved figwort, which fits

©2009 Elsevier Ltd, Inc, BV
DOI: 10.1016/B978-0-443-10344-5.00033-1

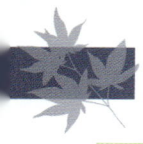

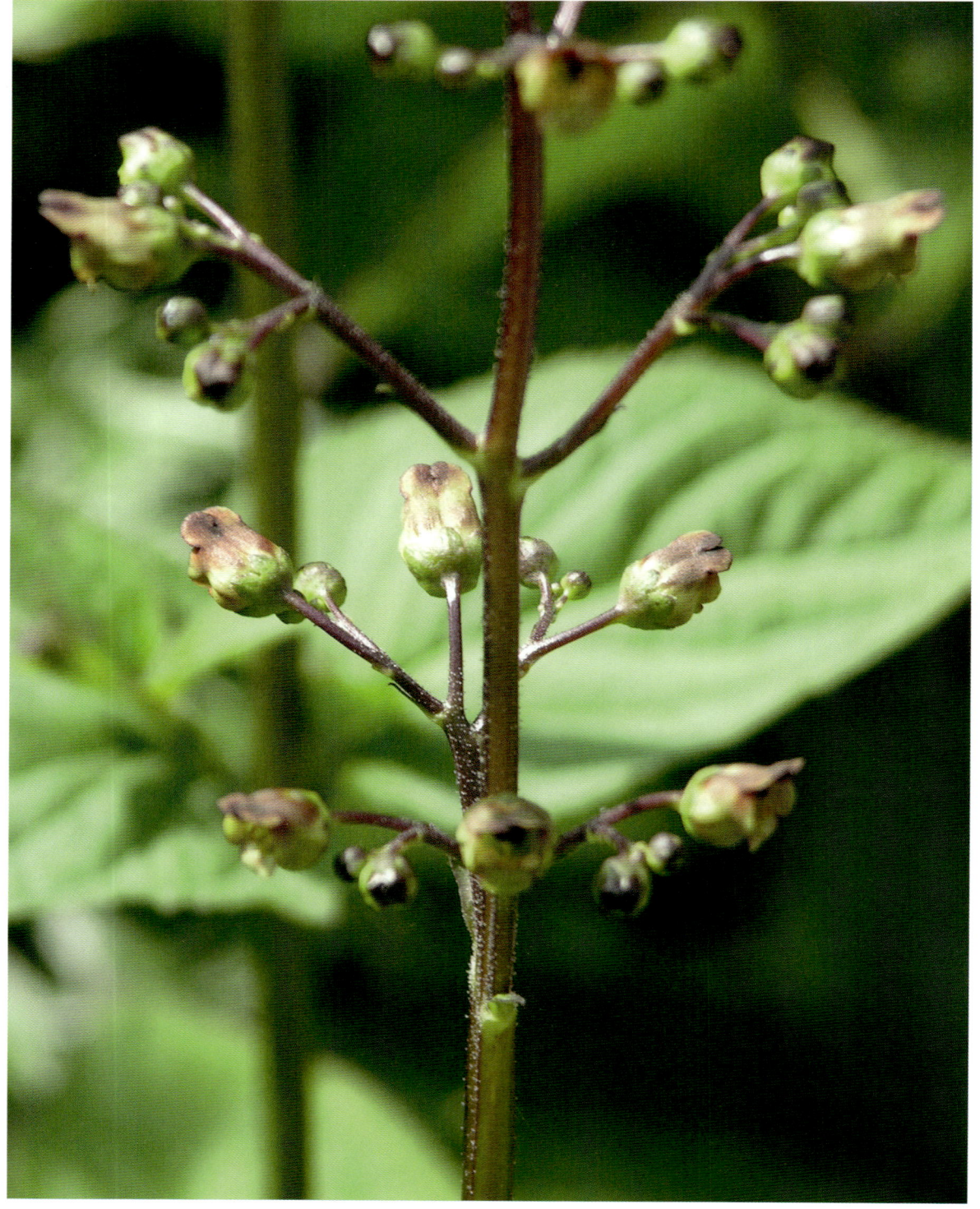

Figure 28.1 *Scrophularia nodosa*, figwort (a garden in Yorkshire, June).

the description given by Dioscorides (Polunin & Huxley 1978). Dioscorides refers to it as growing on fences, roadsides and 'building lots' (Beck) or 'house courtyards' (Fuchs), which would not describe *Scrophularia nodosa* as it is found in more moist sites. Mattioli also makes this point in his argument that figwort is not the galiopsis of Dioscorides. Makbul et al (2006) describe *Scrophularia nodosa* growing in Turkey so, apart from the habitat given, this could be the plant described by Dioscorides. *Scrophularia* species do have an unpleasant smell and the flowers can be described as reddish-purple or maroon. The indications given are plausible for figwort but the description is not conclusive.

The Renaissance authors give descriptions and I will start with Dodoens, who says the plant is called Scrophularia major in the shops and brownwort and wood betony in English. He describes two figworts with hollow stems as growing plentifully in the borders of fields, under hedges and on the edge of lakes and ditches. Dodoens notes an important distinguishing feature between *Scrophularia nodosa* and *Scrophularia auriculata*: the root of *Scrophularia nodosa* is solid, white and knobbly and the root of *Scrophularia auriculata* is stringy. Having confirmed this from plants in my garden, I have to agree with Dodoens that 'those that do not take heed to the difference in the roots, do gather the one for the other'. This suggests that the recommendations for use of the root must refer to the use of *Scrophularia nodosa*, but that use of the aerial parts may refer to either species. This proposal is supported by research into the constituents (see below), and the evidence that many species of *Scrophularia* are used worldwide.

The illustrations from Fuchs' text were published as a separate document in 1545 and a facsimile produced (Fuchs 1980). This lists galeopsis minor, small Braunwurz (brownwort) and the picture could be *Scrophularia nodosa*. Mattioli and Bauhin both decry Fuchs over the question of whether figwort smells as badly as stinking deadnettle but the picture given is plausibly *Scrophularia nodosa*. In contrast, Gerard and Parkinson use the same print, which could be figwort, but is not clear enough to be distinguishable. Parkinson gives a full description of figwort *Scrophularia nodosa* and Culpeper follows Parkinson in his description of 'common great figwort' as 3–4 feet high, growing in moist, shady places, in woods and lower parts of fields and meadows. Gerard gives three entries under great figwort and the first could be *Scrophularia nodosa*. The third, the yellow-flowered, flowers in May and is pictured with a hairy stem. This is a *Lamium*, as already confirmed by De l'Ecluse (Clusius). Parkinson calls figwort 'the great figwort', as does Gerard and refers to the white roots. Bauhin gives a picture which looks right for *Scrophularia nodosa* and is clear on the point that he does not consider figwort to be the galeopsis of Dioscorides. Bauhin claims that Fuchs has lost his sense of smell if he thinks this plant is the galeopsis of Dioscorides as it does not have a strong smell. This depends how the word 'strong' is used. The scent of figwort could be called strong as it is somewhat penetrating and lingering and has something of the unpleasant smell of woundwort *Stachys sylvatica*. Parkinson argues that the galeopsis of Dioscorides could be stinking deadnettle or hedge woundwort *Stachys sylvatica*. Miller describes the smell as like elder *Sambucus nigra* with which I would concur. It is interesting to trace the development of the nomenclature as Quincy gives Scrophularia major vulgaris of Parkinson and Scophularia nodosa foetida of Caspar Bauhin.

There are two further points on the identity of the plant used as figwort. Water betony is described by Gerard and Parkinson, who both use the same illustration, and Culpeper gives the description from Parkinson. The description of the seeds is of *Scrophularia auriculata* but the picture is of a Lamiaceae, possibly a *Stachys*. Finally, as Gerard notes, Scrophularia minor was used for lesser celandine *Ranunculus ficaria* as it has a knobbly root and is used to treat haemorrhoids which were called figs, so Scrophularia major means the larger of the plants used to treat haemorrhoids.

The text in Turner is unclear and it appears that he was not referring to the same entry in Dioscorides. The illustrations for 'clymenum or water betony' look like figworts with the characteristic seed pods. However, the text refers to plants with a four-squared stem like the bean stalk, leaves like plantain and little seed cases 'not unlike unto the claspers of the fish called polypus' which the translators give as octopus. Turner describes the herb given by Pliny as clymenos with a branched, hollow, jointed stem which is compared to an ivy with ivy-like leaves and seeds and the actions given are those of an astringent herb.

Although there are similar actions, figworts and *Lamium* species are, as Pelikan reveals, very different plants. Pelikan suggests that while at first glance some *Scrophularia* species resemble the Labiates, they have none of their powerful warmth nature and make no etheric oils; they rather take after the nightshades. Figwort itself is associated with shady streams and riverbanks, undergrowth and forest ditches. He observes the strong rootstock with tubers arising from nodes, and how, though the panicle rises and separates from the banked pairs of nettle-like leaves – these nettle-like leaves plus the throaty flowers suggesting strongly the Lamiaceae – it does not lead to the light, but to a dull brown olive-green gullet 'smelling as gloomy as nightshade' and speaking of the forces of the dark working in them. Pelikan points to its use not only for scrofula and tuberculous and glandular problems in children, as the name suggests, but further to its application for ulcers/boils, eczema in the head area, and even for goitre, as found in other plants with dammed energy around the roots, witnessed by knobbly swellings there. The relationship between figwort and the scrofulous process, he says, is signalled by the plant's overcoming of the swelling damp, the fight with the lack of light to achieve

**299**

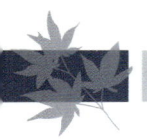

a transformation of the leaf buds into a successful and determined flowering, i.e. astralising, process; and he notes the appropriate nature of this process to affect a swollen organism lacking in etheric form which cannot manage sufficient light and astral suffusion. My impression gained from using figwort is that it is very different in action from any Lamiaceae and is an alterative which travels deeply into the tissues of the body.

## EXTERNAL USE FOR SWELLINGS OF ALL SORTS

The common thread throughout the authors is the use of figwort for swellings, in particular enlarged cervical glands, and externally for swollen haemorrhoids. The

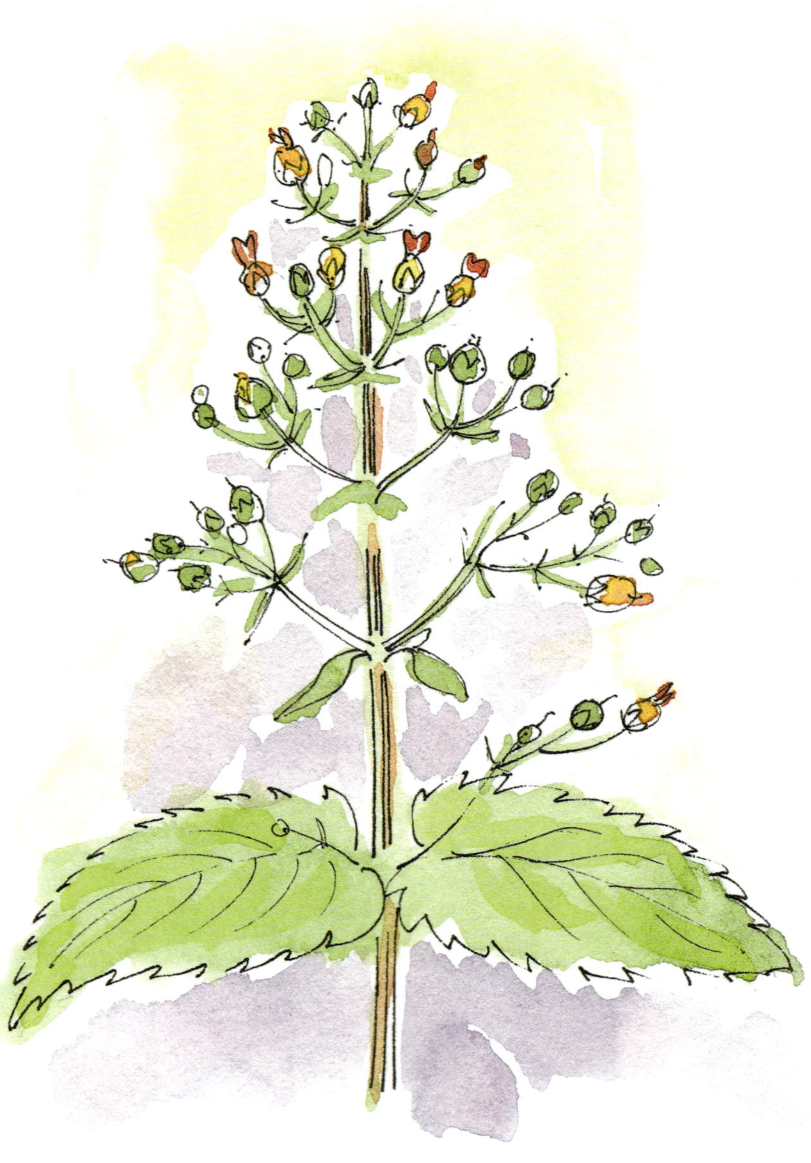

**Figure 28.2** *Scrophularia* sp., figwort.

recommendations of Dioscorides (IV 94) are only for external usage. He advises use of the leaves and stems to dissolve indurations (hardenings), tumours, scrofulous swellings of the glands, swellings of the glands and tumours of parotid glands. He gives an application as a plaster with vinegar twice daily, or the decoction as a rinse, and a plaster with salt for spreading ulcers, gangrenes and putrid humours. Translations vary and the term 'induration', hardening of the skin, could be linked with swollen glands under the skin, chronic inflammatory skin disease, abscesses or boils. Similar recommendations for external use as a plaster with vinegar are given by Fuchs and Mattioli, with reference back to Pliny, who states that it disperses lymph swellings, scrofula and parotid swellings. Mattioli gives the reference but it is not clear whether this does refer to an entry on figwort as we were not able to confirm this in the edition we used. Fuchs quotes Paul of Aegina as recommending figwort to soften and disperse hard swellings and use of a cataplasm (plaster) for corroding sores. Fuchs was able to use a new Greek version of this text published in Venice in 1528 and revised again for publication in Cologne in 1534 and Basel in 1538 (Meyer et al 1999).

Dodoens recommends leaves, stalks, seeds, root and juice to 'waste and dissolve all kinds of tumours, swellings and hardness, if it be pound with vinegar, and laid thereupon 2 or 3 times a day'. He then recommends the leaves of either species stamped and laid to 'old, rotten, corrupt, spreading and fretting ulcers and consuming sores'. He also gives the same recommendation of Dioscorides for a plaster with salt. He suggests external use of the fresh root and eating the fresh root to dry up and heal haemorrhoids. Bauhin gives the root as the main part to be used and lists scrofula, scabies, ulcers and cancers. Gerard recommends the leaves of water betony (water figwort) as of scouring and cleansing quality to 'mundify' foul and stinking ulcers, especially the juice boiled in honey'. Bauhin gives the same recommendation and adds a reference to use of the leaves dried in the oven and powdered. Mundify means to rebuild the tissues, and use of the terms 'scouring' and 'cleaning' suggests a use to cleanse wounds and remove dead tissue, before the use of demulcents to rebuild the tissue.

The authors give similar but varying suggestions for use of figwort as a face wash. Dodoens recommends washing the face with the juice of figwort to take away redness. This could be a more cautious rendition of the entry in Fuchs, who records other practitioners of the time as using 'the juice for a deformity of the face resembling elephantiasis'. Fuchs also records use in healing suppurating ulcers and piles and Turner writes 'The common herbaries write that scrophularia healeth rotting sores and the swelling sores of the fundament called figs of some writers. The juice is also good for the deformity of the face much like unto a lazar's sickness'. The plant is included in Volume 1 of Turner, which was published in 1551, and this reads like a translation of Fuchs, which was published in Latin in 1542. The editors of Turner give the plant as *Scrophularia auriculata*, but this could refer, as discussed above, to just these last three lines of the entry. Gerard states that 'it is reported' that use of the juice to wash the face takes away redness and deformity. Parkinson, in his entry for figwort, gives the distilled water of the whole plant as good for 'any foul deformity that is inveterate and the leprosy likewise'. This text could refer back to the original recommendation of Dioscorides for use of the plant in 'spreading ulcers' and we must remember that the identity of that plant is not clear. The recommendation for use on the face is ascribed to figwort by one author and to water betony by another and, in contrast to some herbs in this book, Parkinson does not shed much light here. Bauhin keeps to advising the distilled water of the root for redness of the face. The recommendations for use on the face are given by Grieve for water figwort, as 'the juice or distilled water of the leaves is good for bruises, whether inward or outward, as also to bathe the face and hands spotted or blemished or discoloured by sun burning'.

The herb is not given in Apuleius or Macer, but appears in the Salernital herbal, where it is recommended for scrofula and hard glands as an electuary, a preparation of the powder in honey, to be taken in the morning on an empty stomach with no food to be taken for 3 hours. It might also be prepared in pancakes followed by some pure white wine. It is not mentioned by Hildegard or by the Myddfai but has a brief mention in the Trotula (Green 2001) as a preparation of the root in honey, useful for 'thickness of the lips'.

## EXTERNAL USE OF THE BULBOUS WHITE ROOT

Most recommendations for use of the root are for external usage. Mattioli gives a recipe: the root is collected in autumn, cleaned, pounded with fresh butter and put in a moist place in a covered earthen pot. It is to be left for 15 days and then the butter gradually melted on a slow fire, strained, and applied to bruises, injuries, burns, strumas, tumours and painful joints. This same recipe is given by Bauhin, Gerard and Parkinson. Gerard specifies use in 'hard kernels' and 'haemorrhoid veins, or piles which are in the fundament'. Bauhin further recommends an application of the powdered root to haemorrhoids. Miller gives the same recommendation but no preparation. Parkinson gives a second ointment which he advises for scabs and lepra (the word lepra means a scaly condition of the skin in Greek). It is made using boiled roots or leaves with oil and wax. The term 'axungia' is used, which can be a soft animal fat, such as goose fat or the fat around the kidneys, which suggests that in current practice we would use a cream base rather than an ointment. Faivre (2007) gives a similar recipe from Quebec, Canada using 10 g leaves dried to a powder stirred into 10 g suet or beef fat melted with 20 g lard or pig fat and cooled.

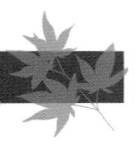

Later texts give external usages. Cook does not specify the part but recommends use of an ointment in lard for burns, inflammation, sore nipples, ringworm, eczema and piles. Wren gives usage internally and externally of the leaf and a poultice of leaves for all cutaneous eruptions including 'so called' scrofula, abscesses and wounds. The *National Botanic Pharmacopoeia* repeats the external usage for scrofulous sores, abscesses and gangrene. Use of a fomentation is advised for sprains, swellings, inflammations, wounds and diseased parts. Priest & Priest include external use on haemorrhoids. An ethnobotanical survey of 88 people in villages in the northwest Pyrenees, Spain found that the whole plant of *Scrophularia auriculata* is used externally as an antiseptic and for inflammation (Akerreta et al 2007).

## ALTERATIVES AND 'SCROFULA'

Figwort is mainly used now internally but Renaissance authors describe external and internal use together. Bauhin recommends a preparation from the root for hard tumours of the glands described as scrofula, since figwort helps by softening a tubercle caused by freezing cold humours. Parkinson recommends the decoction of figwort taken and the bruised herb applied to dissolve congealed, clotted blood after wounds, both internal and external, the kings evil and other 'knobs and kernels'. Gerard, Parkinson and Miller recommend figwort for scrofula in any part of the body, swellings and painful swelling of haemorrhoids if used inwardly or outwardly, as also cancerous stubborn ulcers. Bauhin gives the advice of 1 drachm (4 g) of root in a drink for worms in the belly but this is not repeated by other authors.

Before moving on to a discussion of usage as an alterative, it is worth looking at the description of the qualities of figwort given by the authors and the interpretation of the term scrofula. Fuchs states that figwort dries, thins and disperses, and the bitterness of taste indicates that it is of thin parts. Dodoens describes figwort as hot and dry in the third degree and of subtle parts, and Gerard repeats it as hot and dry. Bauhin described it as hot and dry, bitter and of subtle parts so that it thins and disperses. Looking at the use of words here, it is possible that it was described as hot and dry by virtue of its actions in that it was used for swellings which were considered to be caused by the agglomeration of cold humours.

The term 'scrofula' is used by the authors but interpretation of this term is difficult. Scrofula refers to the large swellings in the cervical glands caused by tuberculosis but Kiple (1997) argues that this would primarily have been bovine tuberculosis caught from drinking contaminated milk. A relevant modern study in Nepal of 155 adults aged 8–71 with cervical lymphadenitis found that 54% had tubercular lymphadenitis, 33% had reactive lymphadenitis and 11% had metastatic neck nodes (Maharjan et al 2009). French (1993) argues that scrofula was used by Renaissance authors in place of the term 'struma' from the Latin struo, 'to build up', which refers to a swelling or tumour. It would thus have been used to describe enlarged lymph nodes in any part of the body. Finally, Cullen describes four categories of scrofula, including scrofula vulgaris, of which the symptom was an itchy rash (Kiple 1997). Interpretation of the term scrofula becomes even more difficult because of its association in England and France with 'the king's evil'. Even the radical Culpeper uses the term 'the king's evil' although the Stuart kings used the effectiveness of the royal touch in curing this condition as evidence for the divine right of kings (Kiple 1997). French (2003) argues that no conclusion can be reached on its meaning partly because of the association with monarchies, pointing out that it was not used in Holland, which had no monarchy. As an example, he notes that when a new doctor arrived from Leiden in the late 18th century, the diagnosis of scrofula disappeared from the record book of the Aberdeen Infirmary. To conclude, it does seem possible that figwort was used in the treatment of lymphadenitis, ulceration and skin infections. It could therefore be recommended for infected eczema and other skin infections but also any condition where infection has led to enlarged lymph nodes.

In the 18th century, Quincy lists figwort as a detergent in Class 4 of the balsamics but says it is very little used. Hill refers to figwort merely as *Scrophularia* but describes *Scrophularia nodosa*. Hill repeats the recommendation for use of the fresh roots bruised and applied 'for the evil' and as a cooling poultice for piles. He recommends juice of the fresh root as an 'excellent sweetener of the blood' if taken in small doses for a long time. It is noteworthy that he gives the root whereas current practice is to use the aerial parts, but he is the first author to describe figwort as an alterative in the wider sense.

Cook recommends the use of a figwort *Scrophularia marilandica*, which grows in North America. He describes it as chiefly alterative, 'soothing and leaving behind a fair tonic impression'. He recommends it for 'irritable forms of scrofula' and for scaly and irritable skin affections, with yellow dock root *Rumex crispus* and *Stillingia sylvatica*. He claims 'an unusually excellent influence on kidneys which relieves torpor', moderate increase in flow of urine and describes figwort as 'amongst the most soothing tonics for irregular and painful menstruation'. The word tonic is used where the action of a herb is considered to improve the function of an organ, and this recommendation could reflect an antiinflammatory action as discussed below. The dose given is 2 fl oz three to four times a day of the decoction of 2 oz in 1 pint water, strained with force.

Scudder (1870) describes figwort as an alterative of which not too much must be expected but makes use of it in scrofula, secondary syphilis, 'chronic inflammation with exudation of material of low vitality' and chronic skin disease. Felter & Lloyd (1898) describe figwort as a pronounced but slow alterative and add use in dropsy and as a general deobstruent to the glandular system to the indications given by Scudder. The root in decoction 'is said' to relieve period pains. They recommend a fomentation or ointment in bruises, mammary inflammation, ringworm, piles, painful swelling, itch and skin eruptions 'of a vesicular character'. The dose of the infusion, or syrup, is given as 2–4 fl oz whereas the dose of a strong tincture (76% alcohol) is given as only 10–40 drops. They state that Goss valued it highly in conditions where the skin condition is poor so that ulceration arises from wounds, abrasions or bruising. Ellingwood gives some specific recommendations by Goss for use in 'enlarged lymphatics with perverted nutrition', ulcerations around the eyes, ears, nose, or face, full lips with a pink and white countenance and puffiness of the nostrils, and lastly, epiphyseal thickening and fullness of the joints. This list reflects the late 19th century interest in giving specific herbs for specific indications.

## CURRENT USE AS AN ALTERATIVE

Wren, followed by the *National Botanic Pharmacopoeia*, gives the actions of alterative, diuretic and anodyne. Figwort is considered not 'of paramount importance as an internal remedy'. Priest & Priest repeat Cook's description as a gently stimulating and relaxing alterative with lower abdominal and pelvic emphasis, but emphasize the deobstruent action on enlarged and engorged lymph glands, for mammary tumours and nodosities and enlarged glands, and externally for haemorrhoids. Deobstruent is a term used to describe the action of removing obstructions to flow, and they suggest the addition of hepatics and more stimulating diuretics. In more recent years, figwort is used as a more general alterative for all skin conditions. The *British Herbal Pharmacopoeia* recommends it for chronic skin disease, eczema, psoriasis and pruritus.

Although I have used this plant for 20 years, I had not previously grown it and was unaware of the tuberous roots until reading Dodoens. Going outside, digging a plant and finding the root was quite a shock. In addition, although suggested by recent authors, I have not used it externally. For example, Chevallier recommends external usage in healing wounds, burns, haemorrhoids and ulcers, and Bartram emphasizes the use of figwort in exudative skin eruptions and to encourage discharge and thus cleansing of abscesses, boils and infected wounds. In contrast, I have used it consistently internally as an alterative in chronic skin disease, in eczema, acne or psoriasis, and when looking for an alterative with some 'bite'. It has proved useful in itching. I had a very elderly patient who had recovered from cirrhosis of the liver and continued to take liver remedies, but who periodically suffered from intense itching, especially on the shoulders in the evening. Alternation of various herbs in the medicine showed that it was the figwort which most effectively controlled this symptom. Hoffmann perceives figwort as acting in a broad way to improve body function and bring about a state of inner cleanliness which he ascribes partly to diuretic and mild laxative actions. Chevallier describes it as a herb that supports detoxification of the body and advises it in any skin condition with itching and irritation. Hoffmann and Chevallier both recommend figwort in eczema and psoriasis. This is how I have used it over the years but the recommendations given by the authors suggest a usage in more deep-seated problems.

## USE IN ARTHRITIS?

Recent research has led to recommendations for increased use in inflammatory disease, especially in arthritis. This recommendation relies on the iridoid glycoside content. Iridoids are found in many *Scrophularia* species (Galíndez et al 2002) and an iridoid of special interest in *Scrophularia* species is harpagoside. This is amongst the active constituents of devil's claw *Harpagophytum procumbens*, widely used in arthritis to reduce pain and inflammation (Brien et al 2006, Qi et al 2006, Grant et al 2007). The use of *Harpagophytum procumbens* is of conservation concern because it is collected in the wild in the Namibian desert (Hachfeld & Schippmann 2000). Sesterhenn et al (2007) propose that *Scrophularia nodosa* could be a useful substitute as they found that the concentration of harpagoside in the leaves is similar to that in tubers of *Harpagophytum procumbens*. Faivre (2007) argues that the high concentration of harpagoside in a standardized fluid extract prepared from fresh plant material alongside the aucubin found in *Scrophularia* species but not in *Harpagophytum procumbens*, and the associated phenolic acids such as verbascoside, make *Scrophularia nodosa* a significant herb in the treatment of functional and arthritic joint disease. Faivre (2007) claims that it is very well tolerated and particularly useful in exacerbations of painful joint pain in, for example, the shoulder. This suggests that it could be particularly useful in psoriatic arthritis and thus of use as an alterative alongside other herbs in treatment of this condition. Patients with this condition often take disease-modifying antirheumatic drugs so that extra caution is needed in the choice of appropriate and supportive treatment (Gordon & Ruderman 2006). Harpagoside has been identified in other *Scrophularia* species such as *Scrophularia scorodonia*, where levels were highest in the leaves in July (Galíndez et al 2002) and *Scrophularia ningpoensis* (Tong et al 2006). Extraction of iridoid glycosides is most efficient in hot water (Suomi et al 2000).

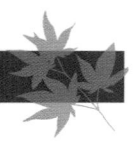

## RECOMMENDATIONS

- The *British Herbal Pharmacopoeia* recommends figwort in chronic skin disease, eczema, psoriasis and pruritus, and this agrees with the consistent recommendations by the authors for skin conditions. In addition, there is a consistent recommendation from the authors for use in wounds and ulcers that are or might become infected. External and internal usage together is often recommended. Figwort could be particularly useful in patients who are vulnerable to exacerbations of eczema caused by bacterial infections, and in patients with diabetes who are subject to poor wound healing and chronic skin infections.
- Figwort could be the alterative of choice in a prescription for psoriasis and in psoriatic arthritis.
- Usage for chronic infection with lymphadenitis must be recommended as long as the diagnosis is clear. Figwort could be the alterative of choice alongside available orthodox treatment where the patient has either primary or secondary tumours in the lymph nodes.
- The authors consistently recommend use of the root, mainly externally, for swollen and inflamed haemorrhoids.
- Dosage: the *British Herbal Pharmacopoeia* recommends 2–8 g three times a day of dried herb.

## CONSTITUENTS

Reviews: Barnes et al (2007), Williamson (2003).

### Iridoid glycosides

Harpagoside 1.05% (leaves), aucubin 0.43% (leaves), catalpol (trace) (root and aerial part, wild, Germany) (Sesterhenn et al 2007).
Harpagide, aucubin, catalpol (commercial, Germany) (Weinges & von der Eltz 1978).
Scrophuloside A2-A8 (Dinda et al 2007).
Eighteen acylated iridoid glycosides: aucubin, harpagide, catalpol glycosides and 8 new (Miyase & Mimatsu 1999).
Seeds, catapol-type glycosides: scopolioside A, scrophuloside A4, scrovalentinoside (wild, Ireland) (Stevenson et al 2002).
*Scrophularia auriculata* L. subsp. *pseudoauriculata*, iridoid glycosides: scrovalentinoside, scopolioside A; saponins: verbascosaponin A, verbascosaponin; phenylethanoid glycoside: verbascoside (wild, Spain) (Giner et al 1998).

### Phenylpropanoids

Phenylethanoid glycosides: seven known and two new (Miyase & Mimatsu 1999).

### Flavonoids

Diosmin, acacetin rhamnoside (Barnes et al 2007).

## RECOMMENDATIONS ON SAFETY

- Do not use figwort alongside digitalis or when the patient has a pacemaker or when there is tachycardia or an unstable heart rate.

The *British Herbal Pharmacopoeia* states that figwort contains cardioactive glycosides, increases myocardial contraction and therefore is to be avoided in ventricular tachycardia. Bartram gives the contraindication in tachycardia. Chevallier gives a contraindication if suffering from a heart condition, which is completely appropriate as he is writing for lay usage.

We have been unable to verify the presence of cardioactive glycosides, although they are referred to by Faivre (2007). Cardioactive glycosides or cardenolides are found in *Digitalis* species, which are either placed in the Scrophulariaceae family or in the Plantaginaceae (Taskova et al 2005). Triterpene glycosides are found in other *Scrophularia* such as *Scrophularia ningpoensis* (Li et al 2009). The uncertainty could reflect the lack of recent investigation into constituents other than the iridoid glycosides or could result from less exact methods of chromatography used in the past. There were two relevant references in older texts. Ellingwood (1919) states that 'according to Professor Lloyd a yellow powder has been obtained from the extract which has some of the properties of digitalis'. *The American Dispensatory* (Remington et al 1918) refers to a statement made in 1896 that the seeds are toxic, belonging to the digitalis group.

The lack of firm evidence supports the above recommendation but otherwise there appear to be no contraindications. Equally figwort cannot be expected to support cardiac function.

## REFERENCES

Akerreta S, Cavero RY, Calvo MI 2007 First comprehensive contribution to medical ethnobotany of western pyrenees. Journal of Ethnobiology and Ethnomedicine 3:26. Online. Available: http://www.pubmedcentral.nih.gov.

Barnes J, Anderson LA, Phillipson JD 2007 Herbal medicines, 3rd edn. Pharmaceutical Press, London.

Brien S, Lewith GT, McGregor G 2006 Devil's claw (Harpagophytum procumbens) as a treatment for osteoarthritis: a review of efficacy and safety. Journal of Alternative and Complementary Medicine 12:981–993.

Davis PH (ed.) 1978 Flora of Turkey, vol 6. Edinburgh University Press, Edinburgh.

Dinda B, Debnath S, Harigaya Y 2007 Naturally occurring iridoids: a review, part 1. Chemical and Pharmaceutical Bulletin 55:159–222.

Ellingwood F 1919 The American materia medica, therapeutics and pharmacognosy. Online. Available: http://www.henriettesherbal.com.

Felter HW, Lloyd JU 1898 King's American dispensatory. Online. Available: http://www.henriettesherbal.com 20 August 2009.

French RK 1993 Scrofula (scrophula). In: Kiple K F (ed.) The Cambridge world history of human disease. Cambridge University Press, Cambridge.

French RK 2003 Medicine before science. Cambridge University Press, Cambridge.

Faivre C 2007 Scrofularia nodosa. Phytothérapie 5: 154–158.

Fuchs L 1980 Holzschnitte, Die historischen Taschenbücher. Konrad Kölbl, Grünwald bei München.

Galíndez J de S, Diaz-Lanza AM, Matellano LF 2002 Biologically active substances from the genus Scrophularia. Pharmaceutical Biology 40:45–59.

Giner RM, Villalba ML, Recio MC, et al 1998 A new iridoid from Scrophularia auriculata ssp. pseudoauriculata. Journal of Natural Products 61:1162–1163.

Gordon KB, Ruderman EM 2006 The treatment of psoriasis and psoriatic arthritis: an interdisciplinary approach. Journal of the American Academy of Dermatology 54:S85–S91.

Grant L, McBean DE, Fyfe L, et al 2007 A review of the biological and potential therapeutic actions of Harpagophytum procumbens. Phytotherapy Research 21:199–209.

Green MH (ed.) 2001 The Trotula. University of Pennsylvania Press, Philadelphia.

Hachfeld B, Schippmann U 2000 Conservation data sheet 2: exploitation, trade and population status of Harpagophytum procumbens in southern Africa. Medicinal Plant Conservation 6:4–9. Online. Available: http://cmsdata.iucn.org.

Kiple KF 1997 Scrofula: the king's evil and struma africana. In: Kiple KF (ed.) Plague, pox & pestilence. Weidenfeld & Nicholson, London.

Li J, Huang X, Du X, et al 2009 Study of chemical composition and antimicrobial activity of leaves and roots of Scrophularia ningpoensis. Natural Product Research 23:775–780

Maharjan M, Hirachan S, Kafle PK, et al 2009 Incidence of tuberculosis in enlarged neck nodes, our experience. Kathmandu University Medical Journal 7:54–58.

Makbul S, Coşkunçelebi K, Türkmen Z, et al 2006 Morphology and anatomy of Scrophularia L. (Scrophulariaceae) taxa from NE Anatolia. Acta Botanica Cracoviensia Series Botanica 48:33–43.

Meyer FG, Trueblood EE, Heller JL 1999 The great herbal of Leonard Fuchs, vol 1. Stanford University Press, California.

Miyase T, Mimatsu A 1999 Acylated iridoid and phenylethanoid glycosides from the aerial parts of Scrophularia nodosa. Journal of Natural Products 62:1079–1084.

Ortega-Olivencia A, Devesa JA 2002 Proposal to conserve the name Scrophularia auriculata (scrophulariaceae) with a conserved type. Taxon 51:201–202.

Polunin O, Huxley A 1978 Flowers of the Mediterranean. Chatto and Windus, London.

Qi J, Chen JJ, Cheng ZH, et al 2006 Iridoid glycosides from Harpagophytum procumbens D.C. (devil's claw). Phytochemistry 67:1372–1377.

Remington JP, Wood HC et al 1918 The dispensatory of the United States of America. Online. Available: http://www.henriettesherbal.com.

Scudder MD 1870 Specific medication and specific medicines. Online. Available: http://www.henriettesherbal.com 18 Aug 2009.

Sesterhenn K, Distl M, Wink M 2007 Occurrence of iridoid glycosides in in vitro cultures and intact plants of Scrophularia nodosa L. Plant Cell Reports 26: 365–371.

Stevenson PC, Simmonds MSJ, Sampson J, et al 2002 Wound healing activity of acylated iridoid glycosides from Scrophularia nodosa. Phytotherapy Research 16:33–35.

Suomi J, Sirén H, Hartonen K, et al 2000 Extraction of iridoid glycosides and their determination by micellar electrokinetic capillary chromatography. Journal of Chromatography A868:73–83.

Taskova RM, Gotfredsen CH, Jensen SR 2005 Chemotaxonomic markers in Digitalideae (Plantaginaceae). Phytochemistry 66:1440–1447.

Tong S, Yan J, Lou J 2006 Preparative isolation and purification of harpagoside from Scrophularia ningpoensis hemsley by high-speed counter-current chromatography. Phytochemical Analysis 17: 406–408.

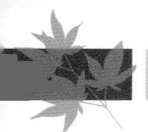

USDA 2009 National resources conservation service plants profile *Scrophularia* L. Online. Available: http://plants.usda.gov.

Weinges K, von der Eltz H 1978 Iridoid glycosides from *Scrophularia nodosa* L. Justus Liebigs Annalen der Chemie 12:1968–1973.

Williamson E 2003 Potter's herbal cyclopaedia. CW Daniel, Saffron Walden.

WHO 1989 Medicinal plants in China. World Health Organization, Manila.

# CHAPTER 29
# *Stachys officinalis*, wood betony

## DESCRIPTION

### Family: Lamiaceae

### Part used: aerial parts

The genus contains over 270 species (Conforti et al 2009) and is divided into sections. Recently *Stachys officinalis* (L.) Trevis. was placed in section Betonica of subgenus Betonica with *Stachys alopecuros* (Marin et al 2004). The genus has been revised more than once and *Stachys betonica* L. and *Betonica officinalis* are synonyms for *Stachys officinalis*. *Stachys officinalis* is a hardy perennial and found throughout Europe on open grassland and woodland.

Erect, straight, unbranched square stems (15–40 cm) bear narrow stem leaves. The stalked basal leaves are oval and bluntly toothed with a heart-shaped base. Dense, terminal, cylindrical spikes of reddish-purple magenta flowers occur in summer. The cylindrical flowerheads distinguish it from woundworts. The flowers are tubular with five lobes, the lower three lobes are bent back, and there are axillary flowers with a characteristic pair of leafy bracts below each whorl of flowers. The fruit is composed of four small nutlets hidden in the persistent, smooth five-toothed calyx.

**Other species used**: The woundworts such as hedge woundwort *Stachys sylvatica* are traditionally used for healing wounds but cannot be substituted for *Stachys officinalis*. *Stachys sylvatica* grows in more shady areas and spreads from a creeping rhizome. Erect hairy stems (to 90 cm) bear opposite, nettle-shaped leaves. The flower is claret red with white markings. It has a characteristic unpleasant smell. Marsh woundwort *Stachys palustris* grows in ditches, river margins and wet land and spreads from a creeping rhizome. It is distinguishable from *Stachys officinalis* as the flower heads are less solid and the pinkish-purple flowers have white markings (Akeroyd 2003). It readily hybridizes with *Stachys sylvatica* to form large clumps of *Stachys* x *ambigua*.

### Quality

Other *Stachys* are used as medicinal plants (Kartsev et al 1994, Vundać et al 2006, Conforti et al 2009) and it is possible that plant material collected in the wild is not all *Stachys officinalis*.

In *The Honest Herbal: A Sensible Guide to the Use of Herbs and Related Remedies* (Tyler 1993) the pharmacognocist Dr Varro Tyler writes: 'Betony or wood betony is one of those medicinal plants once believed to be good for practically everything whose use in folk medicine decreased over the years until it is now thought to be of relatively little value'. He indicates the plant's past reputation by citing Grieve on two old sayings: the Italian 'sell your coat and buy betony' and the Spanish 'he has as many virtues as betony' (Bauhin states that both of these are Italian sayings). He sees no need to list the 47 diseases it was thought to cure in Roman times because 'any one you can think of was probably included'. This former panacea, he concludes, is effective in treating diarrhoea and irritations of mucous membranes on account of its tannin content, and the flavonoids have been reported from Russia to lower blood pressure.

Wood betony has been included in our monographs because it is in very common use amongst herbalists in the UK, the authors included, primarily as a nerve tonic with special reference to the head, and thus a reliever of headaches. Clearly this action cannot be directly linked to its tannin content, except in cases of headache from sinusitis and head colds, as mentioned by Bartram, Chevalier and Wood. Actually there is no evidence, in what exists for this under-researched plant, that it contains any tannins. The putative hypotensive action linked to its flavonoid content seems more relevant to its use as a nervine agent but this action is only mentioned by several of our authors published after Tyler's *Honest Herbal*. There is no entry at all for wood betony in the *Complete Commission E Monographs* (Blumenthal 1998). In order to trace the origin of betony as a remedy for the head, we need to explore our earlier writers and to look as far back as

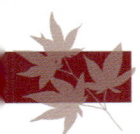

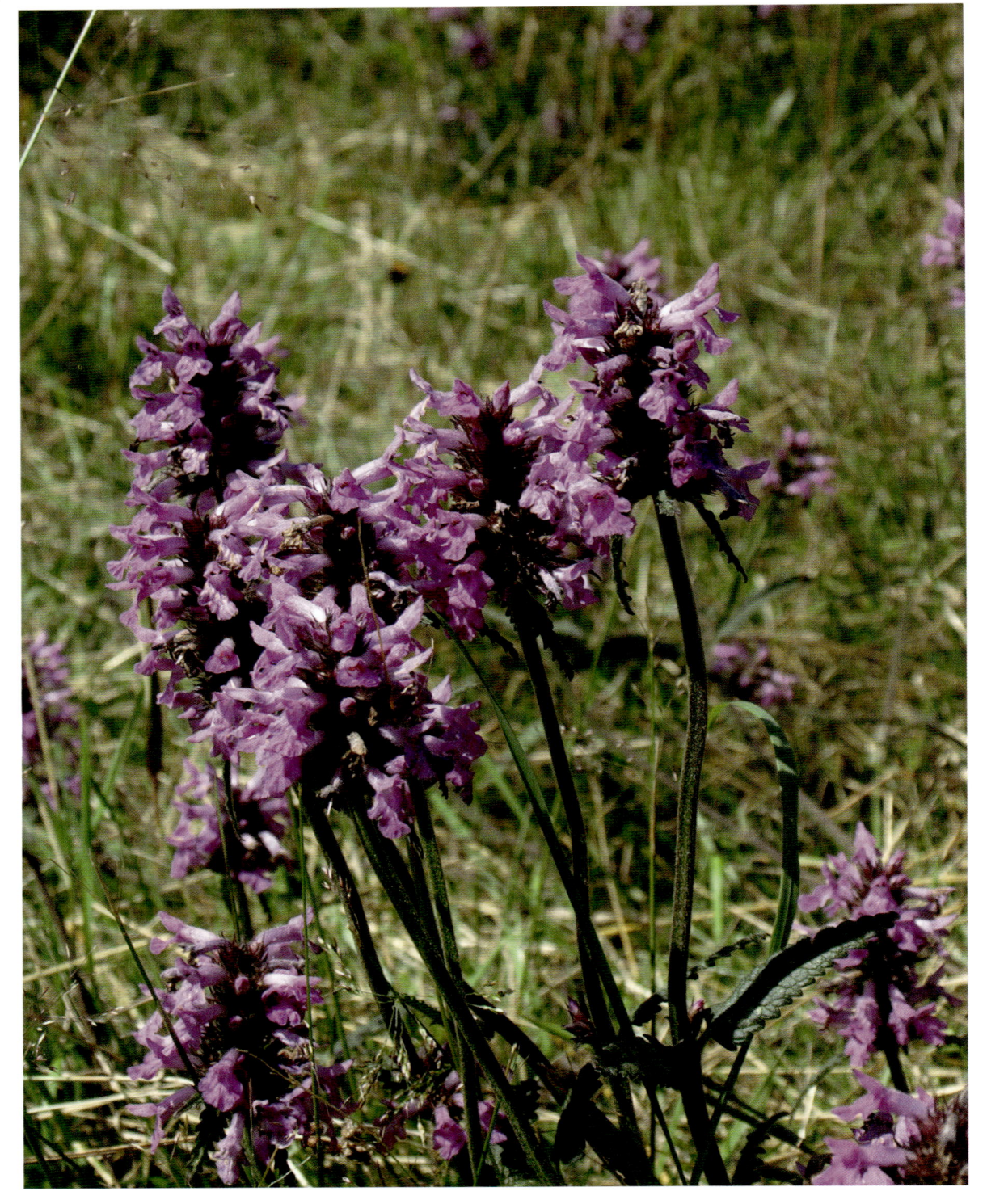

Figure 29.1 *Stachys officinalis,* wood betony (Farnley reservoir, Yorkshire, July).

Roman times in order to recount the history of this former panacea.

Antonius Musa, the physician to Emperor Augustus (63 BC to 14 AD), wrote an essay on betony and its power to cure 47 diseases. He is mentioned by name in our version of the Salernitan Herbal, where 39 separate conditions can be identified, and by Bauhin, Parkinson and Culpeper. Bauhin's list, directly cited from Musa, seems to consist of 44 uses. The large entry on Betony in the *Herbal of Apuleius Platonicus*, and in the *Old English Herbarium*, where there are 29 indications, are largely, although not wholly, based on Musa's writings. Separately, Dioscorides writes a not insubstantial entry on betony, in notable distinction to Pliny, who has very little to say. Let us explore the uses of betony cited from Musa by Bauhin, one by one but in an order suiting the modern practitioner, and to follow their transmission through to present-day authors in order to map out what remains of the knowledge of this panacea among the herbal practitioners and writers of today.

Dioscorides' (IV 1) name for betony is 'kestron', also 'psychrotrophon' because it is found in very cold places. Bauhin informs us that the name 'kestron' refers to betony's sharp spike of flowers. Dioscorides further states that it is called 'bettonica' or 'rosmarina' by the Romans and in the *Old English Herbarium* the former name is given, alongside the Old English 'biscopwyrt'. In later herbals the title 'betonica' is consistently used and there seems to be certainty about the identification of kestron.

Bauhin and the *Old English Herbarium* commence their list of the uses of betony with a protective influence, keeping safe men's bodies and souls, especially after dark, when nightmares and terrifying visions may arise. The plant protects holy places and sepulchres from such fearful sights. Only Dalechamps cites Musa by name on this aspect of betony, concluding that 'it is holy'. Our other authors, including Dioscorides and Pliny, do not mention the claim, except Grieve, who cites 'Apelius'. As a remedy for nightmares, it pops up later in Bartram and again in Menzies-Trull.

## BETONY FOR DIGESTION

Otherwise Dalechamps and Bauhin are consistent with each other in citing Musa. Concerning the organs of digestion, 4 drachms (16 g) of the leaves eaten daily for 3 days or taken in 4 cyathi (180 mL) of cooled water soothe pains of the stomach, and of the liver and intestines if taken in hot water, while in wine they heal defects of the spleen and allay inflammation of the colon. If the pain in the intestines is due not to 'crude juices' but to constipation, this dose taken in double the quantity of water, this time honeyed, will comfortably move the bowels. A lesser amount of herb, 3 drachms or 12 g, in goat's milk drunk for 3 days allays the vomiting of blood. Betony taken frequently in wine treats jaundice, and generally prevents drunkenness, removes a loathing for food and corrects dyspepsia. Musa's recommendations place much weight on the volumes of liquid in which the herb is taken and whether it is hot or cold. Dioscorides insists that the dried, powdered herb, kept in a clay pot, is the correct preparation of the herb, suggesting that the powder is simply stirred into the liquids which Musa proposes. Furthermore, Dalechamps and Bauhin emphasize how different the powers of the leaves and flowers are from those of the root: the root is unpleasant in the mouth and stomach, causing nausea, rumbling and vomiting, whereas the leaves are aromatic with a graceful, strengthening smell, and as food and medicine it is a friend of nature. Dioscorides concurs: the root of betony, drunk with honey water, provokes emesis and is employed only to void phlegm from the stomach. The *Old English Herbarium*, on the other hand, wants the whole of this 'very wholesome' herb, roots and all, to be gathered and powdered. Betony is to be plucked from the ground in August without using a tool of iron and cleaned, then dried and powdered. The Myddfai physicians are not specific, requiring simply a handful and a half of betony in warm water, or betony boiled in honey, for vomiting and sighing.

Dioscorides, perhaps drawing on Musa, also gives indications of stomach, liver and spleen problems, differentiating between water and wine as vehicles for betony in cases of liver disease and jaundice respectively. His dose for the latter is 1 holce (3.4 g), which is roughly a drachm. The same quantity in an oxymel replaces Musa's 14 g in wine for spleen ailments, but Musa's measure in honey water as a laxative is repeated, with only the volume of water increased to 10 cyathi (450 mL). Dioscorides includes heartburn under stomach pains. The herb promotes digestion in the dyspeptic if it is mixed into a little cooked honey. A dose the size of a bean is chewed and swallowed after food, then washed down with diluted wine for such stomach problems. Pliny's only internal use of betony is for the stomach.

Nearly a millennium later in the *Old English Herbarium*, the dose of betony is expressed as the weight of two or more coins, the plant is gently decocted more often than not and there is no mention of separate internal organs save the stomach. Otherwise, the indications of stomach pains, constipation, vomiting blood, nausea, vomiting and dyspepsia, abdominal pains and as an aid to digestion are repeated. The purgative power of betony is cited also by Macer and by Serapio and the Renaissance authors as far as Culpeper before disappearing. Likewise its effects on the organs of digestion and their deficiencies are to a greater or lesser extent repeated again as far as Culpeper. In the 18th century Miller describes it as a hepatic remedy. Perhaps he has read Galen, who states that betony is

THE WESTERN HERBAL TRADITION

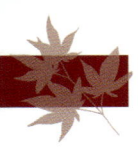

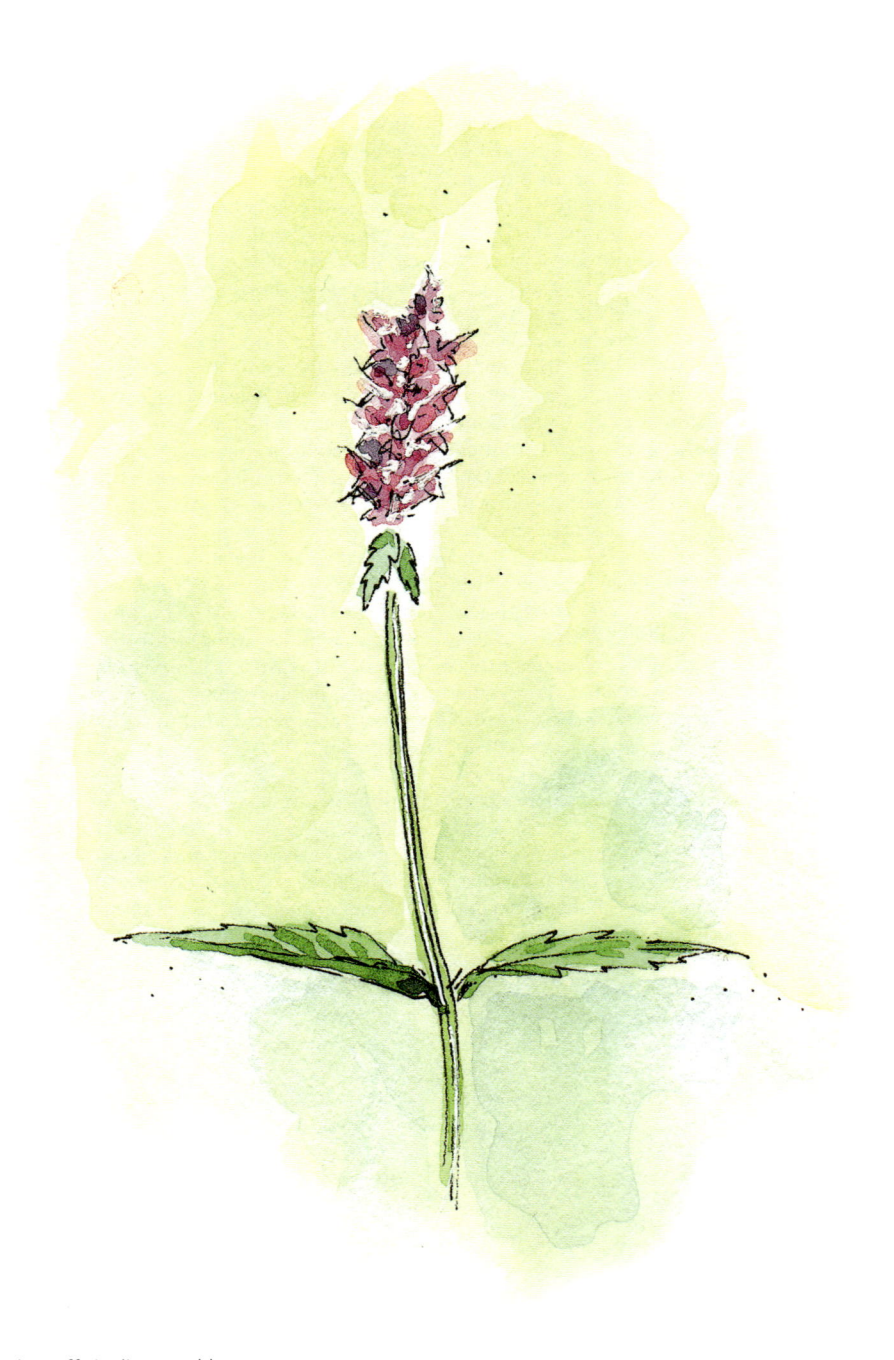

**Figure 29.2** *Stachys officinalis,* wood betony.

somewhat bitter and sharp, conferring the power to purge and cleanse the liver and so help acid eructations. Gerard adds obstructions of the gall to the list of indications. Later Cullen, in an age of energetic remedies, is more interested in the acrid, emetic root than in the aerial parts. Betony has been lavishly praised, he says, but 'very little virtue is found in it'. The American authors, during the Victorian revival of herbal medicines, do not report on it. Only Hool speaks up for 'one of the best known herbs in the vegetable kingdom' by naming it a stomachic for heartburn, stomach cramps, biliousness and colic. Grieve simply cites Gerard extensively, commenting otherwise that betony's carminative, astringent and alterative properties make it useful as a tonic in dyspepsia. It is also classed in Priest & Priest as a general tonic with stomachic action suitable for stomach pains and dyspepsia. Chevallier notes its slight bitterness by which it stimulates digestion and the liver and confers an overall tonic effect on the body. Menzies-Trull is more specific, suggesting a tonic action on stomach and intestines and as a treatment for nausea, dyspepsia, colic and, presumably following the link with tannins that Tyler made, diarrhoea, despite the old use of betony for constipation. Finally, Wood states that betony has a significant influence on the stomach and strengthens and regularizes functioning of the gastrointestinal tract by improving autonomic innervation. It is indicated in weak digestion, especially involving the gall-bladder, where wind, bloating, colic and either diarrhoea or constipation may be present.

## GENITO-URINARY USES

Other abdominal pains for which betony may be used relate to the urinary system and reproductive organs. Honey is required in the vehicle for kidney problems. Dalechamps and Bauhin report Musa advising 2 drachms (8 g) of herb mixed with honey for defects of the kidneys and double this dose in 4 cyathi of water (180 mL) to break stones. With the addition of 27 peppercorns and no honey, the herb is good for pains in the sides, which may refer to ureteric pain. Since the recommendation for dropsy follows that for stones, this may indicate oedema of renal origin, although ascites cannot be ruled out. Certainly Dioscorides specifies oedemata after kidney problems and bladder pain, for which 2 drachms (8 g) in honey water is the dose. He claims betony is diuretic, as does Galen, who confirms its use in kidney stones. On the other hand, Macer speaks of dropsy and this is how Dioscorides' oedemata is interpreted by Fuchs and the other Renaissance writers. The *Old English Herbarium* also offers recipes for both pains in the side and pains in the loins. In both cases betony is taken with peppercorns, 27 in the former recipe and 17 in the latter, the herbs being powdered and gently boiled in aged wine. Three cupfuls are taken warm at night on an empty stomach. Another recipe for sore loins with aching of the thighs requires less betony with no added peppercorns to be decocted in beer, or in warm water but definitely not beer, if the patient is feverish. The physicians of Myddfai give a different indication for betony juice mixed with a little wine, honey and nine peppercorns: it is to be drunk morning and evening for 9 days for headache. The uses in kidney and bladder problems, including stones, pass down more or less again as far as Culpeper. The Salernitan herbal recommends betony for pain in the penis also, and Gerard mentions bloody urine, both of which are possible symptoms of urinary stones. Quincy mentions its diuretic action. Betony's usefulness for urinary problems is then quite lost until Menzies-Trull and Wood list without comment enuresis, and in the latter text only, weak expulsion of urine. Clearly, the old indications for betony in relation to kidney and bladder have not been explored for centuries.

Musa affirms emmenogogic as well as diuretic actions for betony. The herb stimulates menstruation, brings a speedy delivery in childbirth and, at a dose of 2 drachms (8 g) in hot water or honey water, eases womb pains due to cold. Dioscorides and Galen also consider betony to stimulate menstruation. Dioscorides offers a dose of 1 drachm (4 g) in water with or without honey for uterine pains and uterine suffocation. Bauhin explains that this action is due to the sharpness and heat of betony. However, the texts he has sourced seem to have additional interpolated material. For instance, he claims that Pliny also lists the herb as an emmenogogue – an action missing from the augmented list of Pliny's cited in Fuchs and Dalechamps, suggesting numerous corruptions of Pliny's *Natural History* then in circulation. Bauhin claims too that Galen's assessment of betony as hot in the third degree is the reason why it not only stimulates menstruation and expels the afterbirth at the end of labour, but is also an abortifacient. The Salernitan herbal advises 2 drachms (8 g) of betony for women who have great difficulty in giving birth, alone with hot water if they have a fever, or with mirabolans if fever is absent. Equally a pessary of the decocted herb inserted while a syrup of the herb with honey is ingested will cleanse the womb and promote conception. These treatments are not recorded by Serapio, and no entry at all for betony is found in Ibn Sina, nor are they repeated by the other writers of the Medieval period, save Macer's partial restatement of Dioscorides. Hildegard proposes that a woman takes betony in wine often for heavy menstruation 'at the wrong time'. It is also a remedy, she continues, to counter a magical spell which incites a man to fall madly in love with a woman, or vice versa, or generally to banish foolishness in a person, for 'at times the deceit of the devil extends his shadow over it, and over similar herbs'. In these cases the herb is applied externally because the eating of betony 'harms his understanding and intellect, and makes him nearly mad'.

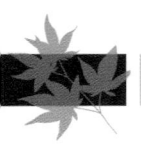

Uterine pain, suffocation and labour reappear as indications based on the emmenogogic action of betony from Fuchs onwards, when Dioscorides is being closely studied. The English writers Gerard and Parkinson speak of 'cleansing of the mother' and the 'falling down of pains of the mother' respectively. Neither mention suffocation, but it is the related indication of hysteria which appears after more than two and a half centuries in the *National Botanic Pharmacopoeia*. The other uterine uses, and betony's emmenogogic action, are not mentioned after Culpeper. Only Chevallier among the modern writers warns against taking betony during pregnancy. Where Quincy recommends a decoction *after* a hard labour, he is referring to the herb's tonic effect.

## BETONY AND THE NERVOUS SYSTEM

When Musa includes three treatments with betony for the nervous system, one concerns trauma and probably both the other two bear some relation to indications contemplated by modern practitioners. Firstly, the leaves powdered and applied heal severed nerves. Other traumas appearing elsewhere in Musa's list of conditions are ruptures, and in those who have tumbled down from a high place, for which 3 drachms (12 g) in old wine is used. It is not clear whether internal or external administration is meant here, but the former is presumed, since The *Old English Herbarium* specifies internal ruptures and Dioscorides mentions ruptures with spasms, uterine problems and suffocations, for which cases he advises 1 drachm of the powdered leaves in water or honey water. We have already noted, too, when discussing mugwort, that uterine suffocations are renamed hysterical affections in the later tradition. To this supposed nervous state we can add Musa's 'unnerved' or enfeebled condition (Bauhin's 'resolutos'), unless another traumatic injury such as the wrenching of a joint is meant. The Salernitan herbal, however, advises betony for those in a weakened state, where 1 drachm (4 g) in 3 cyathi (135 mL) of good wine taken daily for 5 days will be curative. The same dose in vinegar and honey water to miraculously restore the strength of those who have made a long journey is Musa's third indication. The *Old English Herbarium* wants a coin's weight of betony decocted in sweet wine as a pick-me-up 'if a person becomes tired from much riding or much walking'. Dioscorides makes no mention of weakness or fatigue but recommends betony for epileptics and the insane. Galen mentions epilepsy also, together with ruptures and spasms.

These indications are passed down to some extent through our authors. While Serapio describes wounds of the nerves and convalescence and the Salernitans repeat severed nerves and fatigue without acknowledging Musa's authorship as Dalechamps and Bauhin do, others are silent on these uses because Dioscorides does not mention them. Parkinson suggests 'any vein or sinew that is cut' and in a separate statement lists palsy alongside epilepsy. Others mix ruptures with cramps, spasms, internal pains and colic. Fuchs, Turner, Dodoens, Gerard and Mattioli presumably, if he had written more on this herb, follow Dioscorides in giving epilepsy and madness as conditions treatable but do not mention Musa's fatigue. Since Parkinson (and Culpeper, because he has copied Parkinson's entry) does mention fatigue, we once again assume that he has enjoyed the benefit of Bauhin's herbal. On the other hand, Parkinson omits madness as an indication, but includes epilepsy and also continual pains in the head which may be severe enough to produce a frenzy. This last is a use for betony that has persisted in texts to the present day.

We find an earlier recording of head pain in Serapio alongside scalp laceration, trauma to the cranium and inflamed eyes. Powdered betony is to be applied topically to join the wound together and even to draw out shards of broken bone but the plaster must be renewed often, every third day according to Musa from whose essay these uses are taken. The *Old English Herbarium* suggests drinking betony in beer for a shattered skull and its editor rightly questions this radical departure from the Latin text of its source and from Dioscorides. She wonders whether the Old English text is referring to migraine, which can feel as if the skull is broken, but this seems fanciful since we have no reason to believe this does not refer to the healing of head wounds. More than 200 years later and from the then dominant culture, Serapio proposes to relieve pain in the head by placing the powdered root or herb on the forehead, while in the Salernitan herbal, itself influenced by Arabic writings, a decoction in wine is made for ingestion in cases of headache due to vapours rising from the stomach, or a gargle made from betony and poisonous stavesacre decocted in vinegar for headache due to cold. The 18th century writers first emphasize the head as the main target for medicinal effects. Quincy describes betony as 'accounted by all a very good cephalick' and proposes its inclusion in a herbal tobacco, the smoking of which corrects rheums in the head. He too cites Musa on wounds to the head and reports that a plaster of betony is official in the London dispensatory but little used. Miller confirms the plaster, as well as a conserve of the flowers, as official preparations and lists head pains, convulsions, nervine affections, vertigo and sore eyes as indications. Smoking betony in a mix with tobacco cures headaches, but Hill deems this a more uncertain method of treatment. The herb gathered when just coming into flower, Hill writes, and given presumably as a tea, treats disorders of the head and all nervous complaints. Cullen countenances the use of betony as a mild sternutatory for symptoms in the head but dismisses the suggestions of Bartholin and Pauli that the herb is hypnotic and anodyne. It is tempting to conclude that the later indication of headache derives from the earlier one for head trauma, in which headache would be inevitable.

Betony is not among Coffin's botanic remedies and is not mentioned by the American writers. Fox writes that it is excellent for those distracted by pain in the head, and the herb will cure dizziness and all nervous complaints in the head, including 'softening of the brain'. Hool denotes it as nervine and tonic, treating headache, pains in head and face, neuralgia and delirium, for which he recommends betony 1 oz, rosemary *Rosmarinus officinalis* ½ oz, and English scullcap, *Scutellaria galericulata*, ½ oz infused in 2 pints of boiling water, steeped for 20 minutes, strained and taken in wineglassful doses three or four times a day. As a daily tea, for Grieve tells us that the weak infusion has somewhat the taste of tea and is used extensively as a substitute for tea, or in fevers and insensibility Hool proposes 1 oz each of betony, greater burnet *Sanguisorba officinalis*, raspberry leaf *Rubus idaeus*, agrimony *Agrimonia eupatoria*, meadowsweet *Filipendula ulmaria* and wood avens *Geum urbanum*, ¼ oz of the mixture to be infused for 10 minutes in a pint of boiling water and drunk sweetened in place of tea or coffee. The *National Botanic Pharmacopoeia* adds palpitations to the indications for the herb, confirms that it is usually used in combination with other herbs and assures that it may be used with the utmost safety and benefit in all cases of cerebral affections. Grieve's contributions to the history of betony involve a citation from the *Medicina Britannica* of 1666 concerning the curing of very obstinate headaches with a daily decoction of betony in new milk and support for Cullen's evaluation of the sternutatory action of the plant: 'a pinch of the powdered herb will provoke violent sneezing. The dried leaves formed an ingredient in Rowley's British herb snuff, which was at one time quite famous for headaches'.

The modern focus is on a cephalic action. Priest & Priest consider betony 'especially indicated for neuralgic and ischaemic conditions affecting the head', including forgetfulness and lack of concentration. The *British Herbal Pharmacopoeia* styles it sedative and bitter, and lists headache, specifically that in neurasthenia, a now outdated term which may include today's chronic fatigue syndrome, anxiety states, neuralgia, vertigo (Bartram has dizziness) and hysteria. It proposes a use in combination with skullcap *Scutellaria lateriflora* and states a dose of 2–4 g dried herb by infusion, 2–4 mL of the liquid extract and 2–6 mL of tincture 1:5 45%. Chevallier adds 'frayed nerves' and pre-menstrual syndrome, like hysteria an echo of the old classification as a herb for treating the womb, and Menzies-Trull includes chorea, nervous eye disorders, amnesia, menopausal depression, panic attacks and cerebral atrophy. He too proposes combinations of herbs: betony with skullcap *Scutellaria lateriflora* or valerian *Valeriana officinalis* for nervous headaches, with elder flower *Sambucus nigra* for headache from a cold or chill, with milk thistle *Silybum marianum* for memory loss, and Hool's mix with skullcap and rosemary for neuralgia or ischaemia of the head. Menzies-Trull, Hoffmann and Wood list hypertension among the indications. Wood suggests betony for Parkinson's disease, stroke and as a restorative after concussion, as well as for insomnia. The herb is suited to tall, thin intellectuals dissociated from their body, he says, or for elderly people disconnected from their surroundings. We may recall the magical uses we have heard of from Musa and Hildegard, when we read Wood extending the traditional European use for demon possession to cover unwanted alien abduction experiences. Who says that betony is now of little value?

## OTHER APPLICATIONS

Wood alone among the modern authors also mentions a lower respiratory condition treatable with betony, namely bronchitis. The respiratory tract is in fact another body system for which betony is recorded as having uses. Dalechamps and Bauhin state Musa's recommendation of the herb in warm water as beneficial to those sighing and breathing with difficulty; while the leaves in honey help consumptives, especially those who cough up purulent matter. Betony in an eclegma, or thick syrup made from honey, sometimes conveyed to the mouth on a root of liquorice which is licked clean, and taken for 9 days eases a cough. Dioscorides also mentions betony with honey for tuberculosis and for internal abscesses, while 3 obols (1.7 g) of the powdered herb in 1 cyathos (45 mL) of tepid and diluted wine helps those that spit blood (haemoptysis). Galen states that betony cleanses the lungs and Serapio repeats this, adding a strengthening action None of these points is listed in the *Old English Herbarium*. The Salernitan herbal repeats Musa and Dioscorides, but with different dosages or length of administration of the remedy. Macer mentions cough only. These indications are once again passed down in full or in part through the Renaissance writers as far as Culpeper before disappearing.

Musa proposes betony for the treatment of intermittent malarial fevers and continual fevers, but Dioscorides makes no such proposal nor that of the plant bruised with salt and placed in the nostrils for nosebleed. It appears only in those authors drawing from Musa, here Dalechamps, Bauhin, the *Old English Herbarium*, the Salernitan herbal and Parkinson, who sources Bauhin. These same authors cite another use from Musa, of a decoction of the roots and powdered herb applied externally to a painful, gouty joint. This time Serapio repeats the use as well as does Miller in the 18th century alongside rheumatism, for which conditions a diet drink of betony, wood sage (the hepatotoxic *Teucrium scorodonia*) and ground-pine *Ajuga chamaepitys* was recommended The other strand to betony's former reputation for joint problems commences

313

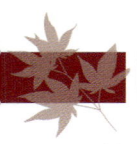

with the treatment by internal administration for hip pains in Dioscorides and Galen, which are duly transmitted, sometimes as sciatica, by the Renaissance herbalists (see the discussion of hip pain under ground ivy, Chapter 18). Grieve also lists rheumatism, attributing an alterative action to betony, and her indication is repeated by Priest & Priest, Bartram, Menzies-Trull and Wood. For this condition, Menzies-Trull wants it prescribed with skullcap *Scutellaria lateriflora* and black cohosh *Cimicifuga racemosa*.

Finally, there is a range of external uses to which betony has been put. Musa reports that a decoction of the roots in water, reduced to a third, then fomented or the powdered leaf applied heals pains of the eyes. The expressed juice of the leaves or the pounded leaves macerated in water eases pains in the ears if inserted lukewarm after being mixed with rose-oil. Internally, 1 drachm (4 g) of the leaves infused in 4 cyathi (180 mL) of hot water draws down through the lower organs that blood whose vapours rise back to pour into the eyes while the leaves of this herb eaten will sharpen the sight. These may have some relevance to the differential diagnosis and treatment of head pain and sinusitis. The decoction in old wine or vinegar stops toothache, if the mouth is regularly washed with it. Mixed with sheep fat to form an ointment, the herb heals carbuncles. It counters poison and the bites of snakes or any poisonous or rabid animal, when not only taken internally but also applied externally on a plaster. Applied with salt, it can heal sinuous and burrowing ulcers.

Dioscorides too notes the use of betony for bites of wild animals, as does Galen, but the former also countenances the herb neutralizing deadly poisons. For this last misfortune, 1 holce (3.5 g) of the powdered herb is taken in wine. Indeed, if this is drunk beforehand, it will protect against harm from ingesting a deadly poison. On the other hand, the *Old English Herbarium* advises that betony is effective by causing a vomiting up of the poison taken if the herb and root to the weight of three coins is decocted in 4 cups of wine and drunk down. In the same text appear an ointment for boils on the face and a poultice for neck and throat problems, while the herb taken beforehand prevents drunkenness. Macer proposes the herb for all recent wounds and Miller adds the drawing of splinters to wound healing. Gerard recommends it for worms. Again these uses are variously transmitted down the centuries, until the external applications disappear by the 18th century.

In conclusion, we can agree with Tyler that betony has been proposed for virtually any disease conceived of, certainly up to Culpeper's time. It has been advocated for gastrointestinal, urinary, gynaecological, respiratory, musculoskeletal and skin problems. It treats the organs of special sense and has had a limited use in problems of the nervous system, before becoming a special cephalic remedy for a variety of nervous problems. Only the cardiovascular system is not mentioned, but this could be related to the lack of understanding of diseases of the heart and circulation before the mid 18th century.

There is little research available to support this. What does exist usually features other species of betony. Eighty-three patients with chronic cholecystitis and cholangitis received stachyglen (total flavonoids from the herb *Stachys neglecta*) for 3–4 weeks and it was found that stachyglen exerts a choleretic effect (Peleshchuk et al 1974).

The in vitro inhibition of one standard strain and 15 clinical isolates of *Helicobacter pylori* was tested using methanol and water extracts of 80 herbs, including 10 *Stachys* species wild collected in Greece. *Stachys alopecuros* was included in the 13 most useful herbs alongside three species of *Origanum* but the position of *Stachys officinalis* was not given (Stamatis et al 2003).

The volatile oils of eight species of *Stachys* growing in Greece were tested against six bacteria and five fungi, and *Stachys scardica* was the most effective, but, as in many studies, no oil inhibited growth of *Pseudomonas aeruginosa* (Skaltsa et al 2003). Studies have shown antioxidant activity in a range of *Stachys* species and found a correlation with the concentration of polyphenols (Háznagy-Radnai et al 2006, Matkowski & Piotrowska 2006, Khanavi et al 2009) although Vundać et al (2007) argue that only the scavenging of free radicals is significant. Matkowski & Piotrowska (2006) included *Stachys officinalis* in their research into the antioxidant activity of several medicinal herbs. Betony, along with white horehound *Marrubium vulgare*, showed itself the strongest of the plants tested in inhibiting lipid oxidation.

Until further research is forthcoming, this former panacea is probably better considered in practice as a tonic, not only of the nervous system but of the digestive system also, owing to its bitter, aromatic and spasmolytic qualities. It should not be forgotten as a herb for respiratory catarrh, while its virtue as a diuretic and urinary herb and with regard to hypertension, prohibition in pregnancy, or its true effects on the bowel should be subject to further testing, including, where ethical, clinical trials.

## RECOMMENDATIONS

- Headache, anxiety, depression, and symptoms of nervous origin; neuralgia, chronic fatigue syndrome, debility and convalescence.
- Dyspepsia and weak digestion, nausea, heartburn, colic, irritable bowel syndrome.
- Upper and lower respiratory catarrh, sinusitis.
- Topically on wounds.

Dosage: the *British Herbal Pharmacopoeia* recommends 2–4 g three times a day of dried herb. This dosage range for the dried herb seems to match that of Dioscorides, who advises the powdered herb be taken in wine or another vehicle. Betony in tablet form could be used today. Other authors propose a dose of as much as 8 g with honey to remedy genito-urinary problems, without indication of length of treatment, and to 12 g or even 16 g in acute conditions. This last dose is said to induce a laxative effect. These larger doses are likely to have been used for short periods only.

## RECOMMENDATIONS ON SAFETY

- No safety concerns are documented.

## CONSTITUENTS

Reviews: Williamson (2003).

### Volatile oils

Monoterpenes 0–5%; oxygenated monoterpenes 0.4–1.4%; sesquiterpenes 62–71%; oxygenated sesquiterpenes 4–11% (Radulović et al 2007).
Total 0.04%, monoterpenes 0.6%; sesquiterpenes 71%: germacrene D 42.8%, gamma-cadinene 6.3%, delta-cadinene 5%, alpha-amorphene 3.9%, alpha-cadinol 2.3%, alpha-bergamotene 1.2%, beta-bourbonene 1.9% (wild, Serbia) (Grujic-Jovanovic et al 2004).
Total 0.5%, sesquiterpenes: isocaryophyllene 22.9%, beta-caryophyllene (Chalchat et al 2001).
Total 0.02%, germacrene D 20.1%, beta-caryophyllene 14.6%, caryophyllene oxide 7.9%, beta-humulene 6.7% (wild, Croatia) (Vundać et al 2006).
*Stachys sylvatica*, sesquiterpenes: germacrene D, beta farnesene, mint sulphide; alkane: n-tetracosane (wild, Italy) (Tirillini et al 2004).

### Phenylpropanoids

Total polyphenols 6.75%, phenolic acids 2.7%, flavonoids 0.15% (Vundać et al 2007).

### Phenolic acids

Caffeic acid 3.8% (cultivated, Hungary) (Háznagy-Radnai et al 2006).

### Phenylethanoid glycosides

Acetoside, betonyosides A-F, campneosides II, forsythoside B, leucosceptoside B (cultivated, Japan) (Miyase et al 1996).

### Flavonoids

Flavone glycosides: tricin glycosides, luteolin glycoside and C-glycoside, apigenin diglycoside and apigenin coumaroylglucoside (Marin et al 2004).
Apigenin glycosides and C-glycosides, quercetin glycosides (Háznagy-Radnai et al 2006).

### Tannins

Total 5.6% calculated as gallic acid 6% (Háznagy-Radnai et al 2006).

## REFERENCES

Akeroyd J 2003 The encyclopaedia of wild flowers. Parragon, Bath.

Blumenthal M (ed.) 1998 The complete German Commission E monographs: therapeutic guide to herbal medicines. American Botanical Council, Austin, Texas.

Chalchat JC, Petrovic SD, Maksimovic ZA, et al 2001 Essential oil of *Stachys officinalis* (L.) Trevis, Lamiaceae from Montenegro. Journal of Essential Oil Research 13:286–287.

Conforti F, Menichini F, Formisano C, et al 2009 Comparative chemical composition, free radical-scavenging and cytotoxic properties of essential oils of six *Stachys* species from different regions of the Mediterrane'an area. Food Chemistry 116:898–905.

Grujic-Jovanovic S, Skaltsa HD, Marin P, et al 2004 Composition and antibacterial activity of the essential oil of six *Stachys* species from Serbia. Flavour and Fragrance Journal 19:139–144.

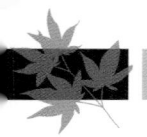

Háznagy-Radnai E, Czigle S, Zupkó I, et al 2006 Comparison of antioxidant activity in enzyme-independent system of six *Stachys* species. Fitoterapia 77:521–524.

Kartsev VG, Stepanichenko NN, Auelbekov SA 1994 Chemical composition and pharmacological properties of plants of the genus *Stachys*. Chemistry of Natural Compounds 30:645–654.

Khanavi M, Hajimahmoodi M, Cheraghi-Niroomand M 2009 Comparison of the antioxidant activity and total phenolic contents in some *Stachys* species. African Journal of Biotechnology 8:1143–1147.

Marin PD, Grayer RJ, Grujic-Jovanovic S, et al 2004 Glycosides of tricetin methyl ethers as chemosystematic markers in *Stachys* subgenus Betonica. Phytochemistry 65:1247–1253.

Matkowski A, Piotrowska M 2006 Antioxidant and free radical scavenging activities of some medicinal plants from the Lamiaceae. Fitoterapia 77:346–353.

Miyase T, Yamamoto R, Ueno A 1996 Phenylethanoid glycosides from *Stachys officinalis*. Phytochemistry 43:475–479.

Peleshchuk AP, Kravchenko AI, Pavlenko KA, et al 1974 Stachyglen treatment of patients with chronic cholecystitis and cholangitis. Vrachebnoe delo 1:65–69 (abstract).

Radulović N, Lazarević J, Ristić N, et al 2007 Chemotaxonomic significance of the volatiles in the genus *Stachys* (Lamiaceae): essential oil composition of four Balkan *Stachys* species. Biochemical Systematics and Ecology 35:196–208.

Skaltsa HD, Demetzos C, Lazari D, et al 2003 Essential oil analysis and antimicrobial activity of eight *Stachys* species from Greece. Phytochemistry 64:743–752.

Stamatis G, Kyriazopoulos P, Golegou S, et al 2003 In vitro anti-*Helicobacter pylori* activity of Greek herbal medicines. Journal of Ethnopharmacology 88:175–179.

Tirillini B, Pellegrino R, Bini LM 2004 Essential oil composition of *Stachys sylvatica* L. from Italy. Flavour and Fragrance Journal 19:330–332.

Tyler V 1993 The honest herbal: a sensible guide to the use of herbs and related remedies. Pharmaceutical Products Press, London.

Vundać VB, Pfeifhofer HW, Brantner AH, et al 2006 Essential oils of seven *Stachys* taxa from Croatia. Biochemical Systematics and Ecology 34: 875–881.

Vundać VB, Brantner AH, Plazibat M 2007 Content of polyphenolic constituents and antioxidant activity of some *Stachys* taxa. Food Chemistry 104:1277–1281.

Williamson E 2003 Potter's Herbal Cyclopaedia. CW Daniel, Saffron Walden.

# CHAPTER 30
# *Tussilago farfara*, coltsfoot

## DESCRIPTION

### Family: Asteraceae
### Part used: leaf, flower

*Tussilago farfara* L. is found throughout Eurasia and is established in North America. It is a pioneer plant and can grow on very alkaline soils. It is low growing and spreads vegetatively by rhizomes. The *Flora of Turkey* (Davis 1975) gives 1 *Tussilago* species: *Tussilago farfara*.

Erect, scaly woolly stems (to 15 cm) bear single terminal yellow flowers with yellow disc and ray florets. The flowers precede the leaves and appear early in the year, in March to April in Britain. The large, round, heart-shaped leaves arise directly from the rootstock and have radial veins and crinkly, slightly toothed edges. They have a thick white downy covering underneath. The 'clock' of seeds is composed of achenes, which are viable for only a few months (Myerscough & Whitehead 1966).

### Quality

Coltsfoot colonizes waste land such as former open-cast mining sites and should not be collected where the soil is polluted by industrial waste.

Adverse events have resulted from collection of the wrong plant such as butterbur *Petasites hybridus*. The leaves of butterbur also appear after the flowers which are pinkish white spikes, but the leaves are much larger and coarser. The plants are clearly distinguishable with a field guide (Akeroyd 2003). Substitution of *Petasites* species can occur with dried leaf material as they are difficult to distinguish.

The concentration of pyrrolizidine alkaloids in coltsfoot varies widely (Lebada et al 2000) and cultivation of a pyrrolizidine alkaloid-free variety is being developed in Austria.

## NAMES AND ASSOCIATIONS

The shape of the coltsfoot leaf has inspired many of its names – bull's hoof, foalswort, folefoot, horsehoof, ungula caballina; it also carries the practical name cough-wort. Dioscorides has several terms for the plant – bechion, pithion, pechion and petronion. Mattioli cites Galen that it is called bechium because it is thought to heal 'buchas', cough, shortness of breath, asthma. Hence we find a Greek precedent for tussilago, itself from tussis meaning cough. Perhaps the strangest name for the plant is filius ante patrem, the son before the father, which describes the exceptional appearance, fruiting and dying back of the flowers before any leaves appear. Such an unusual rhythm has drawn remark from a number of authors. Dioscorides (III 112) says some suppose it has neither stems nor flowers. It apparently led Pliny to believe this was the case, which Mattioli suggests is not unreasonable, the flowers with their short-lived appearance often only recognized by experts or those who come upon their path by fortune. Quincy obviously does not care for the name, occasioned, he says, by 'some persons of conceit'. Simonis (1983) expresses the strange rhythm more poetically 'the plant breathes out first and then in'. He remarks too how it is the first of the Asteraceae family to appear in the year, and very early compared to the majority of his family, which, as the most advanced in the plant world, usually 'adorn the height of the year'. The leaves can then flourish unparalyzed by the usual subsequent flowering process, while the next year's flower buds are prepared underground through the late summer. Simonis relates this and other rhythms within the plant to an interpenetrating of sun and moon forces in a 'mercurial equilibrium' and links this nature to Steiner's consideration of the lung/liver relationship, but detailed examination of these ideas is beyond the remit of this text.

Many authors, including Dodoens, Bauhin and Gerard, write of coltsfoot's relationship with water; how it likes to grow on moist ground or near water, and Mattioli even relates how water seekers search out the plant because they

©2009 Elsevier Ltd, Inc, BV
DOI: 10.1016/B978-0-443-10344-5.00035-5

THE WESTERN HERBAL TRADITION

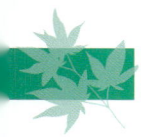

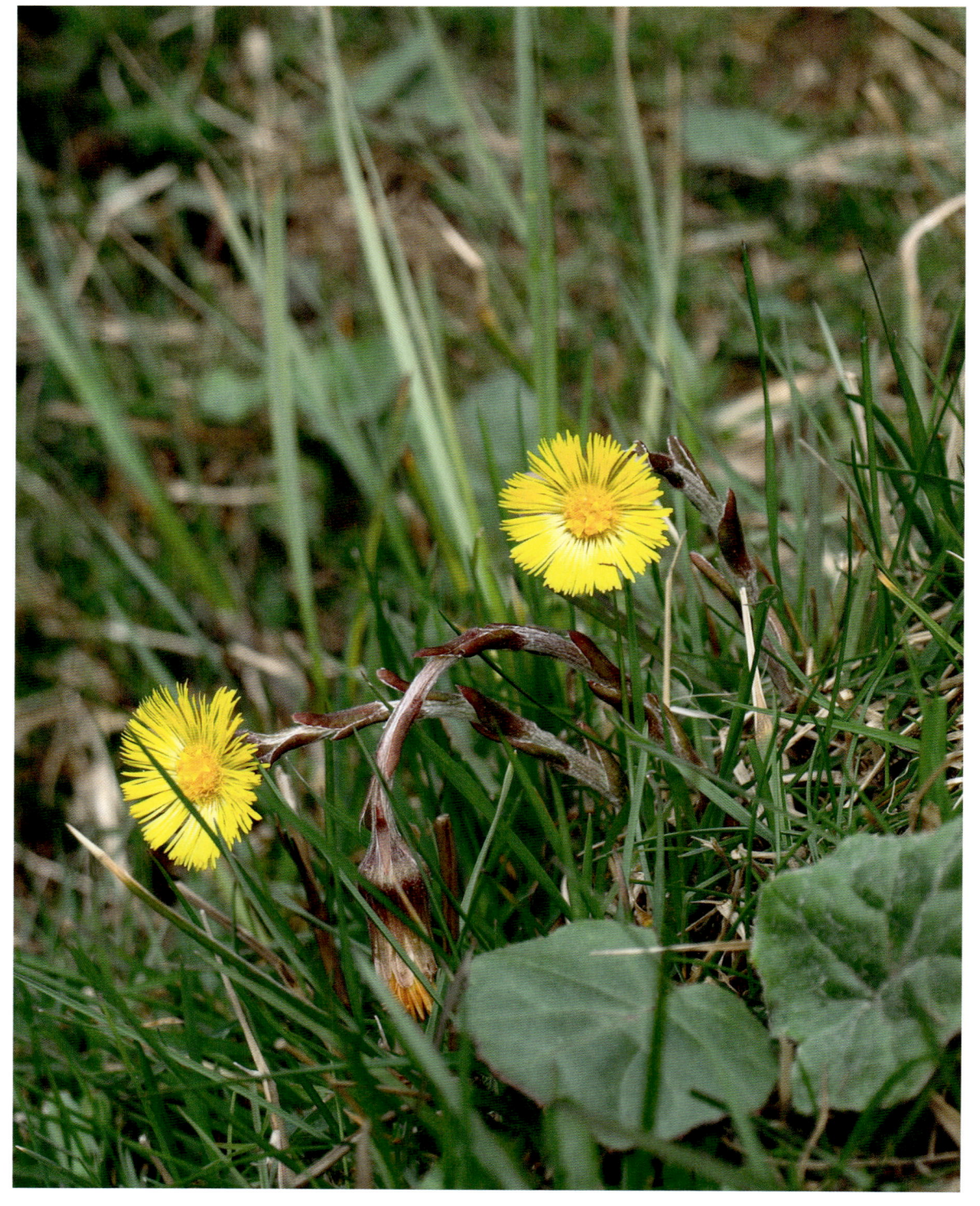

Figure 30.1 *Tussilago farfara*, coltsfoot (Wharfedale, Yorkshire, April).

know its presence indicates a water source. Yet Simonis (1983) says it likes to grow on rubble in waste places and Culpeper says it grows as well in wet grounds as in drier places. In a different element, Mattioli observes how this plant also provides the best tinder. The whitish down which grows on the roots, collected, wrapped in linen cloths and decocted with lye for a while, then with a little saltpeter added and dried in the sun 'is the best tinder of all to create a fire struck from flintstone for it is so greedy of fire that it is lit immediately on the first striking of the steel'.

## OUTSTANDING LUNG HERB

Medicinally there is considerable accord on the virtues of coltsfoot. It appears to be well regarded by all except a few later authors concerned about the pyrrolizidine alkaloid content (see later discussion). Grieve says it has been termed 'nature's best herb for the lungs and her most eminent thoracic'; Fox says it 'cures where other medicines fail'; Weiss labels it the remedy of choice in chronic cases of cough; Hill dubs it 'of excellent virtues'; and Quincy says 'it is by all received as an excellent pectoral'. Its central theme is as a cough herb, with a small number of other faculties added to this core, mainly in relation to liver and skin. Only Hildegard, of all our authors, omits the cough action. It is hot, she says and is used in a mixture for a liver injured and hardened by immoderate intake of many foods. The recipe reads 'he should make incisions in coltsfoot, and twice as much plantain root, and insert the mush from mistletoe from a pear tree (the same amount as the coltsfoot').

## INTERNAL USE? THE OLDER PERSPECTIVE

Dioscorides has only one use for internal consumption of coltsfoot – the root, boiled in hydromel, expels a dead embryo/foetus. This use is rarely repeated in later texts. Other preparations in Dioscorides are for external use only or taken in via the lungs as smoke. He begins with external application of the leaves ground up with honey to treat erysipelas and all inflammations. The dried leaves are burned and the fumes inhaled through a funnel to treat dry cough and orthopnoea (see under hyssop, Chapter 19). He adds that it will break abscesses of the chest too, but the 'it' is ambiguous, whether the inhaled fumes or the plant as a whole, and how taken is not clear and other authors have interpreted this variously.

Neither Pliny nor Galen necessarily advocate internal use. They both suggest the herb is burnt and the fumes inhaled, Pliny says through a pipe. Galen is equally as ambiguous as Dioscorides. It is slightly sharp, moderately bitter, he says, and so will break abscesses of the chest without harm, but again no mode of application is clear. The young leaves, Galen continues, applied externally, help parts blocked by harsh inflammation because of the admixture of a watery substance in which all fresh, green and tender things share, to a greater or lesser degree. The dried leaves are more bitter.

The *Old English Herbarium*, Ibn Sina, Serapio and the Salernitan herbal carry no entry for the herb.

## INTERNAL USE – LATER IDEAS

Later authors introduce internal use for cough, some expand application of the bitter principle, and some consider its qualities, while most repeat the Ancients' recommendations too. Dodoens and Turner simply repeat Dioscorides. Culpeper assigns the herb to Venus. Parkinson, followed by Culpeper, includes the burnt herb use but takes up Galen that fresh coltsfoot is cooling and drying, but when dried and the moisture evaporated it becomes hotter and dry, and hence good against thin rheums that are causing the cough, thickening and drying it; while the fresh leaves or juice, or their syrup, are good for a hot dry cough, wheezings and shortness of breath. He suggests the distilled water alone or in a mixture with elder *Sambucus nigra* and nightshade *Solanum nigrum* for hot agues, both drunk, 2 oz at a time, and applied on cloths to the head and stomach. This mix can also be applied to any hot swellings and other inflammations, including St Anthony's fire (possibly erysipelas or herpes zoster, for which coltsfoot could be effective, or ergotism, for which topical treatment is almost certainly useless), burns, 'wheales' and pustules from heat, and burning piles. This mixture possibly originates from Bock – Simonis cites the same recipe from this source. Gerard adds the fresh green leaves, being cold, are good for ulcers in inflammation, otherwise he reads as Galen and Dioscorides, interpreting the breaking of abscesses (impostumes) of the breast/chest as relieved by inhaling the fumes, not as drunk in internal use.

The herb was clearly taken internally in the 18th century. Miller says the leaves and flowers are frequently put into 'pectoral apozems'; Quincy confirms this, telling us that as an excellent pectoral it enters many shop compositions of that intention as well as appearing frequently in extemporaneous prescriptions. It makes a decoction smooth and healing, he says. Quincy notes that it might be used in stronger form 'But Dr Fuller, in his *Medicina Gymnastica*, thinks such preparations of it are not enough charged with the herb; and is for having the decoctions made with it boil'd to the consistence almost of a syrup; which he recommends for a wonderful restorative, in wastings of the

319

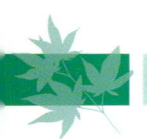

lungs and consumptions'. He does not actually specify internal use, but in the absence of other instruction, this mode might be assumed, since too he next writes of its healing qualities smoked a tobacco and how many account it a good cooler and healer outwardly used 'and Etmuller says he knew a woman who cured ulcers of the breast with it'. Quincy sites this herb in Class 2 of the Balsamics, the Restoratives. They are very like the Emollients of Class 1, which are 'such things as sheathe and soften the asperity of the humours and relax and supply the solids at the same time'. The restoratives have a peculiar quality, he says, 'they are of a more subtile and adhesive nature, whereby they pass the finest strainers or secretions, and enter into the nourishment of the remotest parts. All under this class are rather nutrimental than medicinal; and are more administered to repair the wastes of the constitution, than

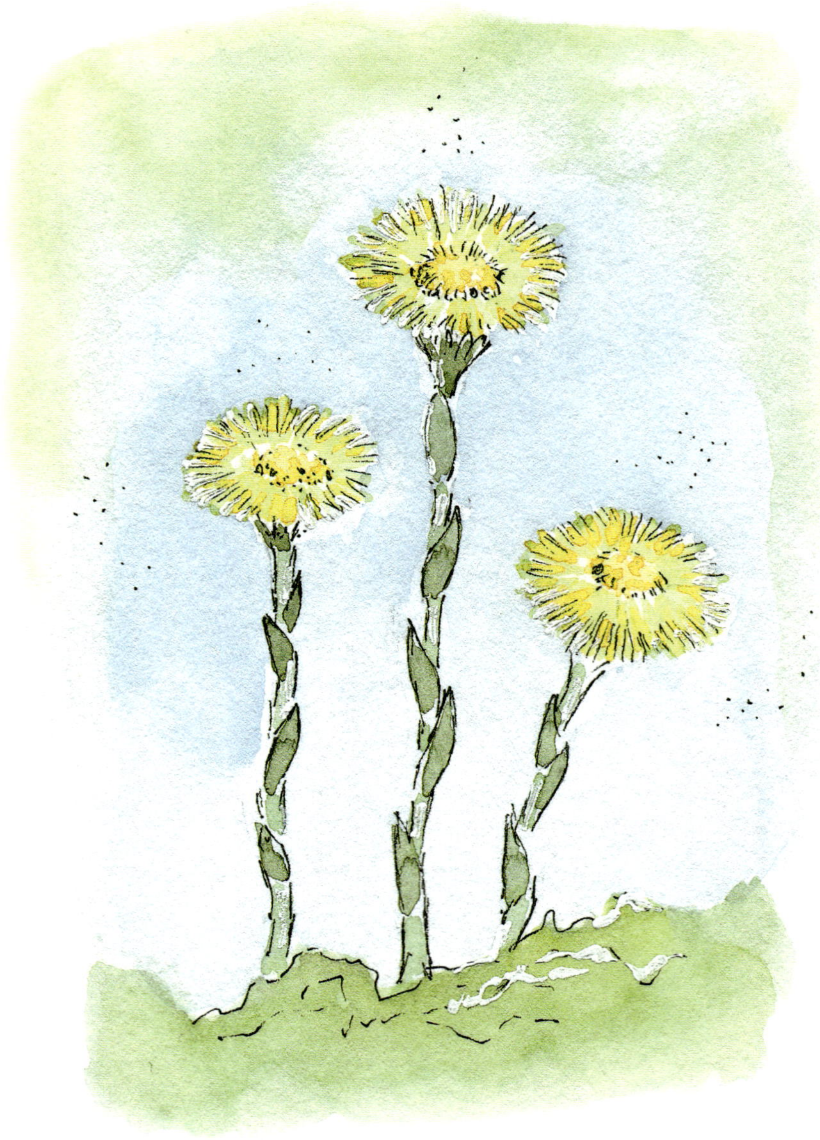

**Figure 30.2** *Tussilago farfara*, coltsfoot.

to alter and rectify its disorders. Whatsoever can answer this end, must be both endu'd with a disposition to enter into and mix with the most subtle of the animal fluids and to fall into and adhere with such interstices of the solids as have been wore away by action and stand in need of recruit'. Coltsfoot's tonic as well as mucilage properties might be recognized here.

Ellingwood has no entry for coltsfoot. Cook, writing in the USA, confirms earlier uses to some extent and adds some new dimensions. He speaks only of the roots, however, which are stimulant and relaxant, of agreeable and warming taste, with some demulcent properties. 'Its warm infusion promotes outward circulation, increases expectoration, and leaves a warm and slightly tonic impression'. Its principal use, he says, is for debilitated coughs, whooping cough and humid forms of asthma. He suggests combining it with cherry *Prunus virginiana* or boneset *Eupatorium perfoliatum*, although he adds, unlike most others, 'its virtues have probably been overrated'. Use for chronic catarrh is then introduced, as a snuff; and then as a liver herb, though via another voice 'Professor SE Carey tells me that this agent will prove fairly depurative to the liver in doses of half a drachm (2 g) three times a day; and that it is a good hepatic tonic of the moderately stimulating grade in scrofulous cases'. Thus we have a link made between the bitter nature of coltsfoot and its old external application for the skin. Is this a use from practical experience or a 'Chinese whispers' misinterpretation of the Ancients' texts.

## RECIPES

Fox tells us the herb was well known and gathered freely by the women of Yorkshire and Lancashire for coltsfoot wine, but despite being most excellent for pulmonary disorders, it was probably not valued enough because of its abundance. For colds and severe coughs, he says, take 2 oz of the dried plant, boil in 3 gills water, leave 15 minutes, sweeten with honeyed or candied sugar, take a wineglass full four times a day; half the amount for children. Hool praises coltsfoot's virtue, taken 'at all times when there is disease of the lungs', its influence more apparent when inflammation is present. He offers a recipe too; coltsfoot 1 oz, marshmallow leaf *Althaea officinalis* ½ oz, elecampane *Inula helenium* ¼ oz, capsicum *Capsicum annuum* ½ teaspoon, in one quart boiling water until cool, then strain and add ½ oz antispasmodic tincture; take 2 tablespoonfuls every 4 hours.

Simonis (1983) cites other authors as praising coltsfoot leaves for the scrofulous constitution of loose form with pale skin, skin ulcers, glandular swellings and the beginnings of lung and glandular tuberculosis. Mattausch, he says, claims the leaves were indicated in convulsive and chesty coughs and they work particularly well in patients who have an 'irritable constitution'. He suggests a recipe from Marzell, who says that in some regions a syrup is made from coltfoot leaves by taking an earthenware pot and filling it alternately with layers of coltsfoot leaves and sugar; the pot is then sealed well and buried for a long time in the earth where the leaves should undergo a kind of fermentation. This syrup, when ready, is taken by the spoonful.

## TOBACCO

Grieve summarizes the uses from the Ancients. We can see from the entry that coltsfoot was a popular herb in Grieve's day. 'One of the most popular cough remedies', she terms it, usually given with horehound *Marrubium vulgare*, marshmallow *Althaea officinalis* and ground ivy *Glechoma hederacea*. She gives a recipe for British Herbal Tobacco in which coltsfoot in the main ingredient, together with buckbean *Menyanthes trifoliata*, eyebright *Euphrasia officinalis*, betony *Stachys officinalis*, rosemary *Rosmarinus officinalis*, thyme *Thymus vulgaris*, lavender *Lavandula angustifolia* and chamomile flowers *Matricaria recutita*, which relieves asthma and old bronchitis, catarrh and other lung troubles, having none of the disadvantages of normal tobacco, she assures us. She gives quantities for the decoction of 1 oz leaves in a quart of water boiled down to 1 pint, sweetened with honey or liquorice, taken in teacupful doses frequently, for colds and asthma. She also remarks on a stronger decoction sounding rather like that of Dr Fuller from Quincy, so strong as to be sweet and glutinous, which 'has proved of great service in scrofulous cases, and with wormwood [*Artemisia absinthium*] has been found efficacious in calculus complaints'. Again one assumes it is drunk, but there is no specific instruction to that purpose.

## MODERN RECOMMENDATIONS – INTRODUCING THE PYRROLIZIDINE ALKALOID QUESTION

Weiss addresses the question of carcinogenic compounds in the herb and the experiments done to establish their nature, but concludes 'investigations of this kind may be of scientific interest but have no relevance whatsoever when it comes to practical therapy … all this has no bearing on the genuine value of the coltsfoot … The amount of the potentially carcinogenic pyrrolizidine alkaloids found in the dried plant drug was so small that it may be disregarded'. Weiss values the distinctive combination of mucilage and bitter, making coltsfoot a good tonic as well as a cough herb. He calls it the remedy of choice in chronic cases, especially for chronic emphysema and silicosis, diseases included in Priest & Priest's specific indications. The leaves and flowers are used. He suggests a relief for the enduringly irritating morning cough for sufferers of these complaints by making a flask of coltsfoot tea, sweetened with honey, at night and keeping it by the bedside for use the following morning before rising, thus avoiding the unpleasant coughing spasms otherwise regularly appearing at the beginning of the day.

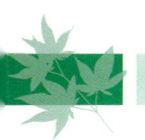

The *British Herbal Pharmacopoeia* notes the actions of coltsfoot as expectorant, antitussive, demulcent and anticatarrhal; indicated for bronchitis, laryngitis, pertussis and asthma, with specific indications for chronic spasmodic bronchial cough, and may be combined with horehound *Marrubium vulgare* and mullein V*erbascum thapsus* in irritating cough. There is no recording of pyrrolizidine alkaloids here. Priest & Priest similarly carry no mention of the alkaloids and they designate it a diffusive expectorant, sedative and demulcent, with stimulant and relaxant auxiliary properties for debilitating and chronic conditions, especially with tubercular diathesis, specific for chronic emphysema and silicosis, pertussis and asthma. They recommend combining with elecampane or mullein for persistent cough. There are no references to smoking the herb, nor to external application of any kind, for skin inflammations nor for pectoral use.

Modern authors are more cautious about using coltsfoot, with reference to the pyrrolizidine alkaloids. Bartram rehearses its uses, yet adds a note that thyme and elecampane are preferable for internal use, nor should the herb be taken in pregnancy and lactation. There does, however, appear to be lingering appreciation of the herb. Williamson notes, as well as the list of pulmonary diseases addressed, how the polysaccharides are antiinflammatory and immunostimulant, as well as demulcent, and how the flavonoids have antiinflammatory and antispasmodic action, hence useful for coughs and colds. She argues the pyrrolizidine alkaloids have not caused problems in rats on low dose regimes and 'appear not to cause damage to human chromosomes in vitro'. She suggests, however, that significant quantities should not be used. Chevallier argues the pyrrolizidine alkaloids are largely destroyed when the parts are boiled to make a decoction, but this is not supported by the evidence on safety (see below). He limits use though to the leaves, and for no more than 3–4 weeks at a time, and not in pregnancy and lactation, nor for children under 6 years old. Hoffman writes similarly though he cites Commission E's more generous allowance of 4–6 weeks. Menzies-Trull records no caution among his comprehensive list of uses which reprise traditional applications including external use for chest and skin. He describes it as a favourite remedy in cough prescriptions. Wood suggests its use for liver and gallbladder, together with respiratory and other conditions. However, its main indication is as a lung herb and safety considerations preclude its use primarily for the liver.

## RECOMMENDATIONS

- Our recommendations err on the side of caution since the scientific evidence offers confusing, often conflicting information. Pending more firm evidence we suggest use within cautious limits. The herb should only be used as infusion and should not be used for children or in pregnancy and lactation. There appears to be no contraindication to external application.
- In cough prescription for up to 6 weeks' use, particularly for stubborn, old cough.
- Particularly for emphysema and silicosis.
- External application for lung problems, as a poultice.
- External application for inflammations of the skin.

Dosage: the *British Herbal Pharmacopoeia* recommends 600 mg–2 g three times a day of dried aerial parts. However, given the safety concerns discussed below, the lowest effective dose should be sought.

## CONSTITUENTS

Reviews: Barnes et al (2007), Williamson (2003).

### Pyrrolizidine alkaloids

(1 ppm = 1 microgram per gram)

### Leaf

Unsaturated pyrrolizidine alkaloids: senkirkine 0.5–46.6 ppm (mean 17.9), senecionine 0–0.9 ppm present in only four samples (10 samples, cultivated, Austria) (Lebada et al 2000).
Senkirkine 0.45 ppm, senecionine not detected (1:40 decoction for 15 minutes, commercial, Poland) (Mroczek et al 2002).
Senkirkine 0.52–73.5 ppm (mean 39.6 ppm) (11 preparations from five samples, decoction for 15 minutes, commercial, Eastern Europe) (Bartkowski et al 1997).
Saturated pyrrolizidine alkaloids: tussilagine, isotussilagine and isomers (Passreiter 1992).

### Flower buds

Senkirkine 19.5–46.6 ppm, senicionine 0 to under 1 ppm (commercial powder, Singapore) (Jiang et al 2009).
Senkirkine 0.45 ppm, senecionine not detected (flowers, commercial, Poland) (Mroczek et al 2002).

### Mucilage

Leaf: total 7–8%, unspecified (Barnes et al 2007).

### Sesquiterpenes

Oplopane-type: tussilagone (Liu et al 2008), five new sesquiterpenes (flower buds, commercial, Japan) (Yaoita et al 1999).
Bisabolane-type: cryptomerion, two new sesquiterpenes; oplopane-type; aromadendrane-type: spathulenol; hydroxytremetone (flower buds, commercial, Japan) (Yaoita et al 2001).
Notonipetranone-type six (Kikuchi & Suzuki 1992).

### Triterpenes

Bauerenol and isobauereno (flower buds) (Yaoita & Kikuchi 1998).

### Chromones

Two chromones (flower buds, wild, China) (Wu et al 2008).

### Flavonoids

Quercetin glycosides (flower buds, semi-wild, South Korea) (Kim et al 2006).

### Tannins

Up to 17% unspecified (Barnes et al 2000).

## RECOMMENDATIONS ON SAFETY

1. Use caution in dosage and duration of usage and consider using other expectorants before using coltsfoot.

To evaluate the safety of any medicine, the effectiveness must be considered. Coltsfoot has been considered effective because of its mucilage content but there are other useful demulcent plants such as marshmallow (see Chapter 8). It has been shown to have an antioxidant action (Kim et al 2006) and an antiseptic action (Barnes et al 2007), but an in vitro study of the antibacterial qualities of Siberian medicinal plants found that the results for coltsfoot were similar to those for yarrow *Achillea millefolium*, another member of the Asteraceae family (Kokoska et al 2002). Elecampane (see Chapter 20) is an Asteraceae, which is an effective expectorant and contains sesquiterpenes and may be fully equivalent to coltsfoot immature flower buds, which are widely used in China (Chan et al 2006).

2. Coltsfoot should not be used in children under the age of 18 or in pregnancy and lactation.

Coltsfoot contains pyrrolizidine alkaloids (PAs), which are widespread plant toxins and their incidence in medicinal plants has been reviewed extensively (Roeder 1995, Stegelmeier et al 1999). The compounds are not part of the medicinal benefit of a plant but are toxins whose ingestion should be avoided. Hepatotoxicity of medicinal plants is of concern for regulators (Willett et al 2004) but in this case it is a known and thus predictable mechanism rather than an idiosyncratic response.

The structure of different PAs varies and the most toxic compounds are unsaturated PAs, in particular diesters with a macrocyclic ring. The main PAs in coltsfoot are of this type: senkirkine, which is an otonecine-type PA, and senecionine, which is a retronecine-type PA. It also contains saturated PAs, such as tussilagine, which are safe. Senecionine is perhaps the most researched PA as it is found in *Senecio* species where usage has been linked to deaths. Young children are particularly susceptible (Steenkamp et al 2000) and use of *Senecio* species has been banned in Britain (MHRA 2008), therefore despite its long usage, there are serious concerns about the use of coltsfoot as a medicinal plant.

These concerns are based on studies of the metabolism of PAs. Metabolism of PAs in the liver is primarily by carboxylesterases, which hydrolyze the alkaloids into the corresponding necine base and necic acid. As with all detoxification in the liver, the aim is to produce water-soluble compounds but the rate of metabolism varies widely between individuals. Where PAs are not fully metabolized by carboxylesterases, another phase I reaction

323

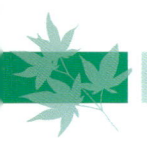

occurs, which is metabolism by cytochrome p450 3A4. This leads to an activated product, a pyrrole, which is then detoxified if it conjugates with glutathione. This reaction is catalyzed by glutathione S-transferases. If this step does not occur and the pyrrole is not detoxified, it forms adducts with DNA and RNA which leads to cell death. Cell death also occurs because of crosslinks made between pyrroles and proteins in the cytoskeleton (Coulombe et al 1999). This leads to characteristic hepatic injury and veno-occlusive liver disease, which was first described in Jamaica (Stuart & Bras 1957). A review summarizes research (Fu et al 2004). Other comprehensive reviews are Bertram et al (2001) Prakash et al (1999), Chojkier (2003) and a short summary is given by Denham (1996). Chou & Fu (2006) were able to isolate DNA adducts derived from dehydropyrrolizidines in the livers of female rats one day after they had been fed coltsfoot flowers for 3 days. The rats were given 10 times the recommended dose but the importance of this study is that it shows that these adducts can occur with coltsfoot. Bone (1990) argues that, as senecionine is either not present in coltsfoot or found at very low concentrations, then it is relatively safer than *Petasites* species. However, it has since been shown that otonecine-type and retronecine-type PAs have been found to form the same type of dehydropyrrolizidine-derived DNA adducts (Fu et al 2004).

Guidance on the safe limits for content of pyrrolizidine alkaloids in dried herb material was set in Germany in 1992. The limits are 1 microgram daily for up to 6 weeks where there is a positive Commission E monograph and 0.1 microgram daily where there is no supporting monograph. An exception was made for coltsfoot teas, where the limit was set at 10 micrograms daily (Bundesanzeiger 1992). The limits continue to be used and referred to by other sources (Lebada et al 2000).

The limit of 10 micrograms for coltsfoot teas or infusions is based on the argument that the level of extraction into teas is low and thus the full content of pyrrolizidine alkaloids will not be available. This may reflect methods of analysis in 1992, not the actual rate of extraction. It has actually been argued that otonecine-type PAs such as senkirkine may be more soluble in water than other PAs as they exist in an ionized form as well as the usual non-ionized form (Fu et al 2004). This is supported by a study referred to by Westerdorf (1992), where up to 80% of the senkirkine in a tea from young shoots of coltsfoot was extracted into the aqueous phase. One part per million (ppm) equals 1 microgram/gram so we can compare the concentrations given above with the dose recommended by Commission E. Bartkowski et al (1997) decocted 11 samples of coltsfoot leaf in water for 15 minutes and the mean concentration of senkirkine was 40 ppm, i.e. 40 micrograms per gram. This means that the total daily dose of coltsfoot leaves as a tea would have to be 250 mg to be within the limits. Lebada et al (2000) found a mean concentration of 18 micrograms/gram, which would give a dose of 500 mg to be within the limits. Extraction is lower at room temperature: a study of extracts from one sample of coltsfoot leaf found that there were 2.9 ppm of senkirkine in a sample stirred in water at room temperature for 30 minutes and 9.3 ppm in a sample refluxed in water for 15 minutes (Lebada et al 2000).

The recommendation of teas makes another assumption that has since been questioned. Part of the total concentration of PAs in plant material is present as the corresponding N-oxide. These are water soluble and thus may be excreted via the bowel without being absorbed. However, this assumes that the water soluble N-oxides of senecionine found in the plant material are not reduced to PAs in the acid conditions in the stomach. There is some evidence from an animal study that N-oxides can be absorbed and reduced to pyrroles in the liver (Wang et al 2005). PAs are difficult to analyze and it has been argued that determination of the total content, including N-oxides, is important in any evaluation of safety (Cao et al 2008). To conclude, teas and infusions will be safer than more concentrated extracts but there may not be the margin of safety that has been assumed.

3. Coltsfoot should be used short term unless there are overriding reasons for continuing its use in a particular patient.

Many commentators consider that although there is a dose below which there is no frank liver disease, there is no safe dose as genotoxicity and thus changes leading to cancer may be occurring without any symptoms.

The only feeding study published is now over 30 years old and is discussed by Bone (1990). Four groups of ten rats were fed different doses of coltsfoot flower buds. A dose-dependent incidence of hemangioendothelial sarcoma in the liver was found and the group fed the lowest dose did not develop tumours. Bone (1990) discusses the relevance of feeding studies on animals and argues that they are generally not relevant as the doses are not equivalent. However, there have been more recent studies of the mechanisms of carcinogenicity for PAs (Fu et al 2004, Wang et al 2005). It is outside the remit of this book to take this discussion further as there is a strong argument that there are many other carcinogenic factors in life and that orthodox drugs are used which are known to be carcinogenic. It can equally be argued that a low daily dose of coltsfoot is completely safe as the liver would be able to metabolize any PA.

4. Coltsfoot should not be taken alongside *Hypericum perforatum* or any medications for the treatment of epilepsy.

*Hypericum perforatum* has been shown to induce cytochrome p450 3A4. Induction of cytochrome p450 3A4 has been found to increase the rate of metabolism of pyrrolizidine alkaloids to dehydropyrroles, which are the active toxins (Chojkier 2003, Fu et al 2004). Coltsfoot should not be taken alongside any medications for the treatment

of epilepsy because some epilepsy medications induce cytochrome p450s (Perucca 2006).
5. Positive identification of the plant material must be carried out.

We found two adverse event reports putatively involving coltsfoot. In 1988 a case was reported of a baby who died at 38 days who was suffering from veno-occlusive disease. Analysis of the tea which his mother had drunk throughout pregnancy identified both *Tussilago farfara* and root of *Petasites hybridus* (Westerdorf 1992). The main pyrrolizidine alkaloid in butterbur *Petasites hybridus* is senecionine with its isomer integerrimine (Langer et al 1996). The concentration varies widely between different samples but is highest in the rhizome (Chizolla et al 2000).

A boy of 18 months from southern Tyrol was admitted with vomiting, diarrhoea, subfebrile temperature, distended abdomen and abdominal pain. On examination the liver was enlarged, 3 cm below the costal margin. Biopsy showed haemorrhagic congestion of zones II and III of the acinus. Fortunately, after 6 weeks of therapy there was remission of the symptoms, no signs of portal hypertension and the child made a full recovery. Subsequent ultrasound evaluation was normal. Further investigation found that since he was 3 months old, the child had been consuming up to 500 mL daily of a tea. Collection and examination of the herb material showed that the herb had been collected in error. It was not coltsfoot but alpendost *Adenostyles alliariae*. It was found to contain a high concentration of seneciphylline and its corresponding N-oxide such that the authors estimate that the boy could have consumed 60 micrograms/kg of body weight per day (Sperl et al 1995).

## REFERENCES

Akeroyd J 2003 The encyclopaedia of wild flowers. Parragon, Bath.

Bartkowski JPB, Wiedenfeld H, Roeder E 1997 Quantitative photometric determination of senkirkine in farfarae folium. Phytochemical Analysis 8:1–4.

Barnes J, Anderson LA, Phillipson JD 2007 Herbal medicines, 3rd edn. Pharmaceutical Press, London.

Bertram B, Hemm I, Tang W 2001 Mutagenic and carcinogenic constituents of medicinal herbs used in Europe or in the USA. Pharmazie 56:99–120.

Bone K 1990 Coltsfoot – is it safe? British Journal of Phytotherapy 1:32–35.

Bundesanzeiger 1992 Protection against drug risks – Phase II German Medicines Act. Bundesanzeiger 17 June 1992.

Cao Y, Colegate SM, Edgar JA 2008 Safety assessment of food and herbal products containing hepatotoxic pyrrolizidine alkaloids: interlaboratory consistency and the importance of N-oxide determination. Phytochemical Analysis 19:526–533.

Chan C-K, Kuo M-L, Shen J-J, et al 2006 Ding Chuan Tang, a Chinese herb decoction, could improve airway hyper-responsiveness in stabilized asthmatic children: a randomized, double-blind clinical trial. Pediatric Allergy & Immunology 17:316–322.

Chizolla R, Ozelsburger S, Langer T 2000 Variability in chemical constituents in *Petasites hybridus* from Austria. Biochemical Systematics and Ecology 28:421–432.

Chojkier M 2003 Hepatic sinusoidal-obstruction syndrome: toxicity of pyrrolizidine alkaloids. Journal of Hepatology 39:437–446.

Chou MW, Fu PP 2006 Formation of DHP-derived DNA adducts in vivo from dietary supplements and Chinese herbal plant extracts containing carcinogenic pyrrolizidine alkaloids. Toxicology and Industrial Health 22:321–327.

Coulombe RA Jr, Drew GL, Stermitz FR 1999 Pyrrolizidine alkaloids crosslink DNA with actin. Toxicology and Applied Pharmacology 154:198–202.

Davis PH (ed.) 1975 Flora of Turkey, vol 5. Edinburgh University Press, Edinburgh.

Denham A 1996 Using herbs that contain pyrrolizidine alkaloids. European Journal of Herbal Medicine 2:27–3

Fu PP, Xia Q, Lin G, et al 2004 Pyrrolizidine alkaloids – genotoxicity, metabolism enzymes, metabolic activation, and mechanisms. Drug Metabolism Reviews 36:1–55.

Jiang Z, Liu F, Goh JJ, et al 2009 Determination of senkirkine and senecionine in *Tussilago farfara* using microwave-assisted extraction and pressurized hot water extraction with liquid chromatography tandem mass spectrometry. Talanta 79:539–546.

Kikuchi M, Suzuki N 1992 Studies on the constituents of *Tussilago farfara* L. II Structures of new sesquiterpenoids isolated from the flower buds. Chemical and Pharmaceutical Bulletin 40:2753–2755.

Kim MR, Lee JY, Lee HH 2006 Antioxidative effects of quercetin-glycosides isolated from the flower buds of *Tussilago farfara* L. Food and Chemical Toxicology 44:1299–1307.

Kokoska L, Polesny Z, Rada V, et al 2002 Screening of some Siberian medicinal plants for antimicrobial activity. Journal of Ethnopharmacology 82 51–53.

Langer T, Mostl E, Chizzola R, et al 1996 A competitive enzyme immunoassay for the pyrrolizidine alkaloids of the senecionine type. Planta-Medica 62:267–271.

Lebada R, Schreier A, Scherz S, et al 2000 Quantitative analysis of the pyrrolizidine alkaloids senkirkine and senecionine in *Tussilago farfara* L. by capillary electrophoresis. Phytochemical Analysis 11:366–369.

Liu Y-F, Yang X-W, Lu W, et al 2008 Determination and pharmacokinetic study of tussilagone in rat plasma by RP-HPLC method. Biomedical Chromatography 22:1194–1200.

MHRA 2008 Prohibited and restricted herbal medicines. Online. Available. http://www.mhra.gov.uk Howweregulate/Medicines/Herbalmedicines/ Prohibitedorrestrictedherbalingredients/index.htm.

Mroczek T, Glowniak K, Wlaszczyk A 2002 Simultaneous determination of N-oxides and free bases of pyrrolizidine alkaloids by cation-exchange solid-phase extraction and ion-pair high-performance liquid chromatography. Journal of Chromatography A 949:249–262.

Myerscough PJ, Whitehead F 1966 Comparative biology of *Tussilago farfara* L., *Chamaenerion angustifolium* (L.) Scop., *Epilobium adenocaulon* Hausskn. 1 General biology and germination. New Phytologist 65:192–210.

Passreiter CM 1992 Co-occurrence of 2-pyrrolidineacetic acid with four isomeric tussilaginic acids in *Arnica* species and *Tussilago farfara*. Planta Medica 58(Suppl 1):A694–A695.

Perucca E 2006 Clinically relevant drug interactions with antiepileptic drugs. British Journal of Clinical Pharmacology 61:246–255.

Prakash AS, Pereira TN, Reilly PE, et al 1999 Pyrrolizidine alkaloids in human diet. Mutation Research 443:53–67.

Roeder E 1995 Medicinal plants in Europe containing pyrrolizidine alkaloids. Pharmazie 50:83–98.

Sperl W, Stuppner H, Gassne I, et al 1995 Reversible hepatic veno-occlusive disease in an infant after consumption of pyrrolizidine-containing herbal tea. European Journal of Pediatrics 154:112–116.

Simonis WC 1983 Medizinisch-botanische Wesensdarstellungen einzelner heilpflanzen, Band 3, Mysterienpflanzen. Novalis, Berlin.

Steenkamp V, Stewart MJ, Zuckerman M 2000 Clinical and analytical aspects of pyrrolizidine poisoning caused by South African traditional medicines. Therapeutic Drug Monitoring 22:302–306.

Stegelmeier BL, Edgar JA, Colegate SM, et al 1999 Pyrrolizidine alkaloid plants, metabolism and toxicity. Journal of Natural Toxins 8:95–116.

Stuart KL, Bras G 1957 Veno-occlusive disease of the liver. Quarterly Journal of Medicine 26:291–315.

Wang YP, Yan J, Fu PP, et al 2005 Human liver microsomal reduction of pyrrolizidine alkaloid N-oxides to form the corresponding carcinogenic parent alkaloid. Toxicology Letters 155:411–420.

Westerdorf J 1992 Pyrrolizidine alkaloids – *Tussilago farfara*. In De Smet PAGM (ed.) Adverse effects to herbal drugs. vol 1. Springer Verlag, Stuttgart.

Willett KL, Roth RA, Walker L 2004 Workshop overview: hepatotoxicity assessment for botanical dietary supplements. Toxicological Sciences 79:4–9.

Williamson E 2003 Potter's herbal cyclopaedia. CW Daniel, Saffron Walden.

Wu D, Zhang M, Zhang C, et al 2008 Chromones from the flower buds of *Tussilago farfara*. Biochemical Systematics and Ecology 36:219–222.

Yaoita Y, Kikuchi M 1998 Triterpenoids from flower buds of *Tussilago farfara* L. Natural Medicines 52:273–275.

Yaoita Y, Kamazawa H, Kikuchi M 1999 Structures of new oplopane-type sesquiterpenoids from the flower buds of *Tussilago farfara* L. Chemical and Pharmaceutical Bulletin 47:705–707.

Yaoita Y, Suzuki N, Kikuchi M 2001 Structures of new sesquiterpenoids from farfarae flos. Chemical and Pharmaceutical Bulletin 49:645–648.

# CHAPTER 31
# *Verbena officinalis*, vervain

## DESCRIPTION

### Family: Verbenaceae                                   Part used: aerial parts

*Verbena officinalis* L. is a hardy, herbaceous perennial found in Eurasia, North and South America. It is found on rough grassland on dry soils. The *Flora of Turkey* (Davis 1982) gives two *Verbena* species, including *Verbena officinalis*.

It forms an evergreen rosette which overwinters. Erect, hairy, woody, square stems (to 70 cm) bear opposite leaves with the lower leaves deeply lobed with serrated edges. Clusters of small pinkish lilac flowers with a two-lipped, five lobed tubular corolla occur on slender branched spikes in June to September. The calyx is long and tubular and the fruit contains four nutlets.

A study carried out on waste ground the UK over 13 years found that population density depended on winter temperature in that plants died below −17°C, and summer temperature as seed germination required a temperature of above 19°C (Woodward 1997).

**Other species used:** *Verbena hastata* is a taller North American species that is easy to cultivate. It has bright green, larger, toothed leaves, a dark stem and branching flowerheads of blue flowers. It is discussed in American texts (Henriette's Herbal Homepage 2009). Lemon verbena *Aloysia triphylla* (syn. *Lippia citriodora*) is a half-hardy lemon scented member of the Verbenaceae that is native to South America (Bown 1995). It is cultivated in Europe and flourishes in a warm climate.

### Quality

In a study in Spain where aerial parts were collected every week in June and July, the concentration of the iridoid glycoside verbenalin was highest just before flowering (Calvo et al 2000).

Historical sources suggest a range of harvesting times. The herb is gathered in midsummer and the 'dog days' until the plant has gone to seed (Bryce 1987). To obtain the juice, collection early in the season is necessary since the stems later become long and woody.

---

Vervain is an example of an ancient medicine which has fallen out of, and back into, favour in our history of its 2000 years of use. It was one of the sacred herbs of the European tradition and according to Pliny no plant was more highly revered by the Romans than this. But our Arabic writers do not mention it, and the medieval sources emphasize its external usage, medicinal as well as magical. The latter uses were predictably condemned by Renaissance writers such as Gerard. Quincy notes in the early 18th century that vervain is little taken internally compared to its external use. Yet the first mention of the plant as a nerve tonic, its major action for herbal practitioners today, is proposed by Parkinson nearly 80 years before Quincy. This does not prevent vervain from disappearing from conventional medicine, for Cullen does not mention it in his *Lectures on Materia Medica*. Then another seven decades pass before vervain is written about again, this time by the Americans Coffin and Cook concerning their native species *Verbena hastata*, for which they propose only internal administration. Wren reckons the European and American species are synonymous as medicinal herbs and from this assertion a modern set of indications in herbal medicine is constructed. This parity is attested by the value placed on a bitterness and an opening action on the liver shared by both species: Dioscorides recommends 1 drachm (4 g) of 'Hiera Botane' or sacred herb *Verbena officinalis* mixed with half as much frankincense in 1 cotyle (274 mL) of aged wine, taken warm on an empty stomach for 4 days in cases of jaundice; Cook writes of blue vervain *Verbena hastata* that a 'free use of a concentrated decoction many times will open and sustain the liver and gall-ducts so effectually as to cure intermittents'. In other respects, however, the American indications for blue vervain have dominated those few applications that have managed to pass down through the European tradition. We have used vervain *Verbena officinalis* on very many occasions as a nerve tonic with thymoleptic qualities for cases of depression, anxiety and insomnia, in convalescence and for chronic fatigue syndrome, cases of restless legs and headache and sometimes for abdominal pains.

©2009 Elsevier Ltd, Inc, BV
DOI: 10.1016/B978-0-443-10344-5.00036-7

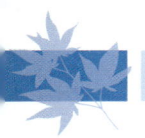

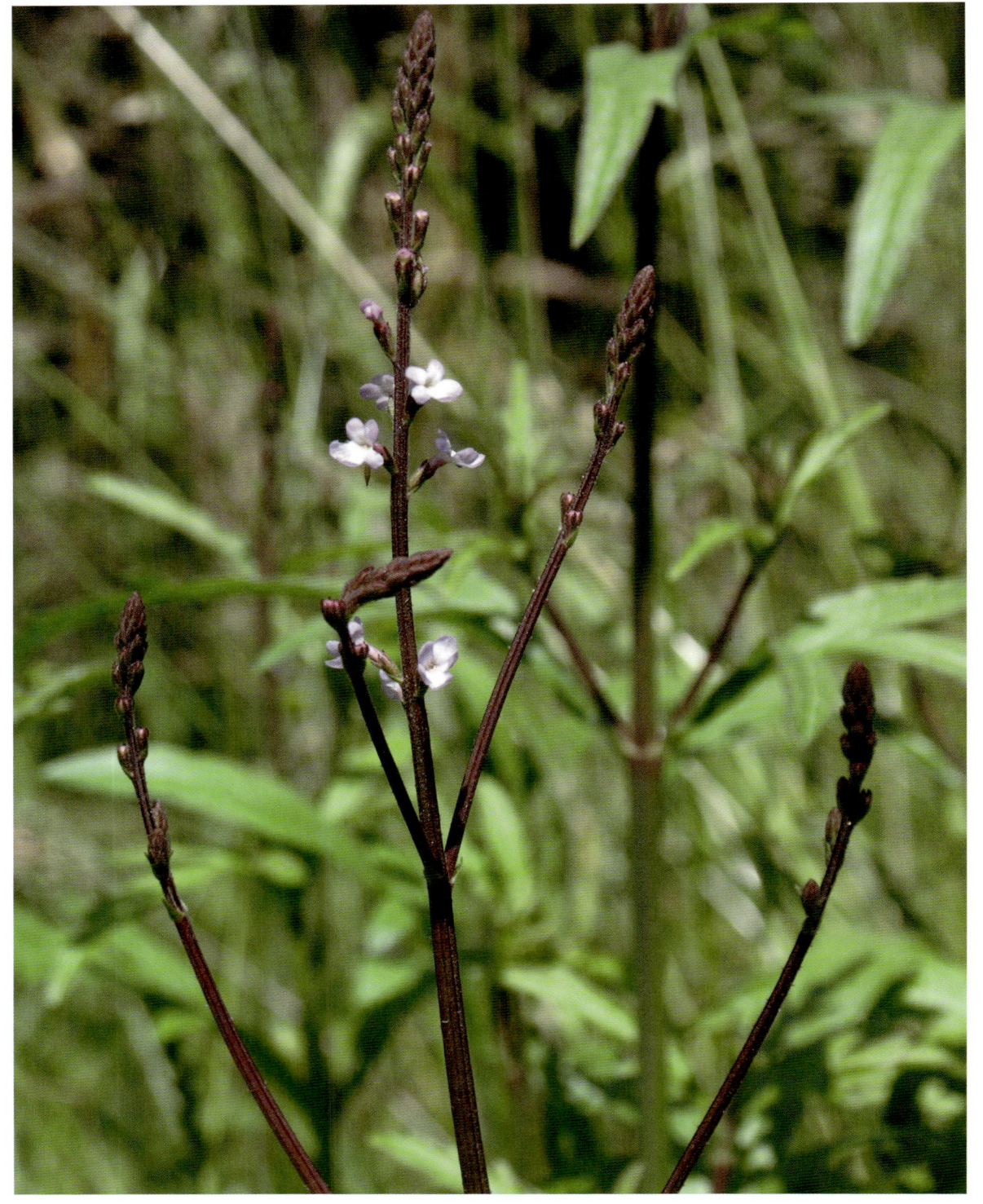

Figure 31.1 *Verbena officinalis*, vervain (Hardwick Hall, Derbyshire, August).

Dioscorides (IV 60) presents us with two possible herbs named 'peristerion' which Beck names as separate species: the first peristerion, so-called because doves delight to be near it, 'generally found with a single stem and a single root' whose leaves are 'split and whitish growing from the stem' is identified as *Lycopus europaeus*, today called gypsywort; the second the holy vervain, 'hiera botane' *Verbena officinalis*, which 'some called … peristerion. It sends out shoots … angular and knobby, surrounded at intervals by leaves resembling oak leaves except they are narrower, less indented at the periphery and grayish'. At the same time Pliny also records that there are two kinds of 'hiera botane', one of which has many leaves and thought to be a female plant, while the other male plant has fewer leaves, although he adds that some authorities see only one plant in the two forms, for they both have the same properties. These two contemporaneous opinions thus set up a continuing confusion concerning the identity of vervain. Later writers group the two plants together but distinguish them by form, name and powers, according to Bauhin: between the upright peristerion or verbena recta, and the sprawling hiera botane or verbena supina. As to form, writers such as Fuchs claim that it was Dioscorides who discriminated between upright and sprawling kinds, although his actual words quoted above fail to support this notion. Mattioli and Turner seem to take the plant named hiera botane as vervain and speculate on the true identity of the other peristerion. As to medicinal powers, Dioscorides writes of peristerion that its leaves applied in a pessary with rose ointment or fresh pig fat stop uterine pains, while as a poultice with vinegar it checks erysipelas and with honey it controls putrid humours and resolves and cicatrises wounds. Galen's peristerion has a drying power enabling it to close up wounds. Where Dodoens makes an attempt to separate out the uses of peristerion from those of hiera botane, he attributes a Dioscoridean indication to the wrong one. Mostly he lists the indications without differentiation, noting that both kinds are of a drying power. Gerard makes no attempt at distinguishing separate indications, but reckons the temperature of both plants as very dry, binding and also cooling with a list of virtues in common.

It is the hiera botane of Dioscorides that treats jaundice as well as ague, its leaves applied in a plaster to the bites of reptiles, chronic swellings and inflammations and to clean filthy sores, and a decoction of the entire plant as a gargle to remove scabs from the tonsils and heal spreading mouth ulcers. It is a sacred herb because it is used in amulets during purificatory offerings. Also noted by Dioscorides is that the sprinkling around of an infusion of the plant at drinking parties seems to make the guests merrier, while the harvesting of specifically the third joint of the stem from the ground with its surrounding leaves is necessary to treat a tertian ague, and the fourth joint in a quartan ague. Pliny records only the treatment of snake bite by the herb crushed in wine but relates much more concerning sacred and magical uses. He too notes its benefit at parties, but only later, in the *Grete Herbal* of 1526, is a quantity specified: four leaves and four roots of vervain, to be steeped in wine and sprinkled about the house where the guests will be (Brooke 1992). Pliny notes that the altar of Zeus is cleansed by it, that it is carried by Rome's envoys to her enemies, that the Gauls employ it in fortune-telling and sooth-saying and the Persian Magi 'madly' imagine that those who have been rubbed with the plant win friends and obtain their wishes, banish fevers and cure all diseases.

## PURIFICATION, PEACE AND LOVE MAGIC

Purification of sacred places has formed a key use of the sprigs of this sacred herb. The Romans used them to cleanse the altars and temples dedicated to Jupiter. In Egypt the herb was dedicated to Isis and played an important role in religious ceremonies. The Druids held a sprig of vervain during the act of soothsaying or speaking divine prophecies, having first made offerings to Mother Earth in grand ceremonies surrounding the gathering of the plant (De Cleene & Lejeune 2002). In medieval Europe, vervain was considered one of the magical midsummer plants, but there were rules for its gathering. It had to be collected at midsummer, during the solstice of the Sun. People in Germany cast their posies of vervain and mugwort *Artemisia vulgaris* onto the St John's day fire on 24 June. Pliny writes of the Magi that they required vervain to be gathered at the rising of the constellation of Sirius the Dog Star, when neither Sun nor Moon was shining. A circle had first to be drawn around the plant with iron, and after gathering, some wax and honey was given back to the Earth in its place. Culpeper mocks similar instructions in the London Dispensatory for the gathering of scuills, questioning how anyone might know which astronomical rising of the star the physicians of the College meant, for instance the heliacal rising of Sirius before dawn, or its acronycal rising after sunset (Culpeper 1669). De Cleene & Lejeune (2002) suggest that no exact astronomical event was specified, merely the gathering of the herb before dawn during the dog days, roughly 3 July to 11 August, when Sirius would be bright in the eastern sky.

In ancient Rome, priests of the College of the Fetiales were garlanded with flowering sprigs of vervain in the course of their duties, which were to examine the causes of conflicts between Rome and other peoples and to establish whether Rome was within her rights. If so, and the opponents did not pay the damages claimed by the priests, then war would be declared on that people. If not, then a pig would be slaughtered and the priests would send their envoys, called 'verbenarii', with sprigs of vervain in their hands to negotiate peace. This practice is said to date back

THE WESTERN HERBAL TRADITION

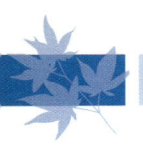

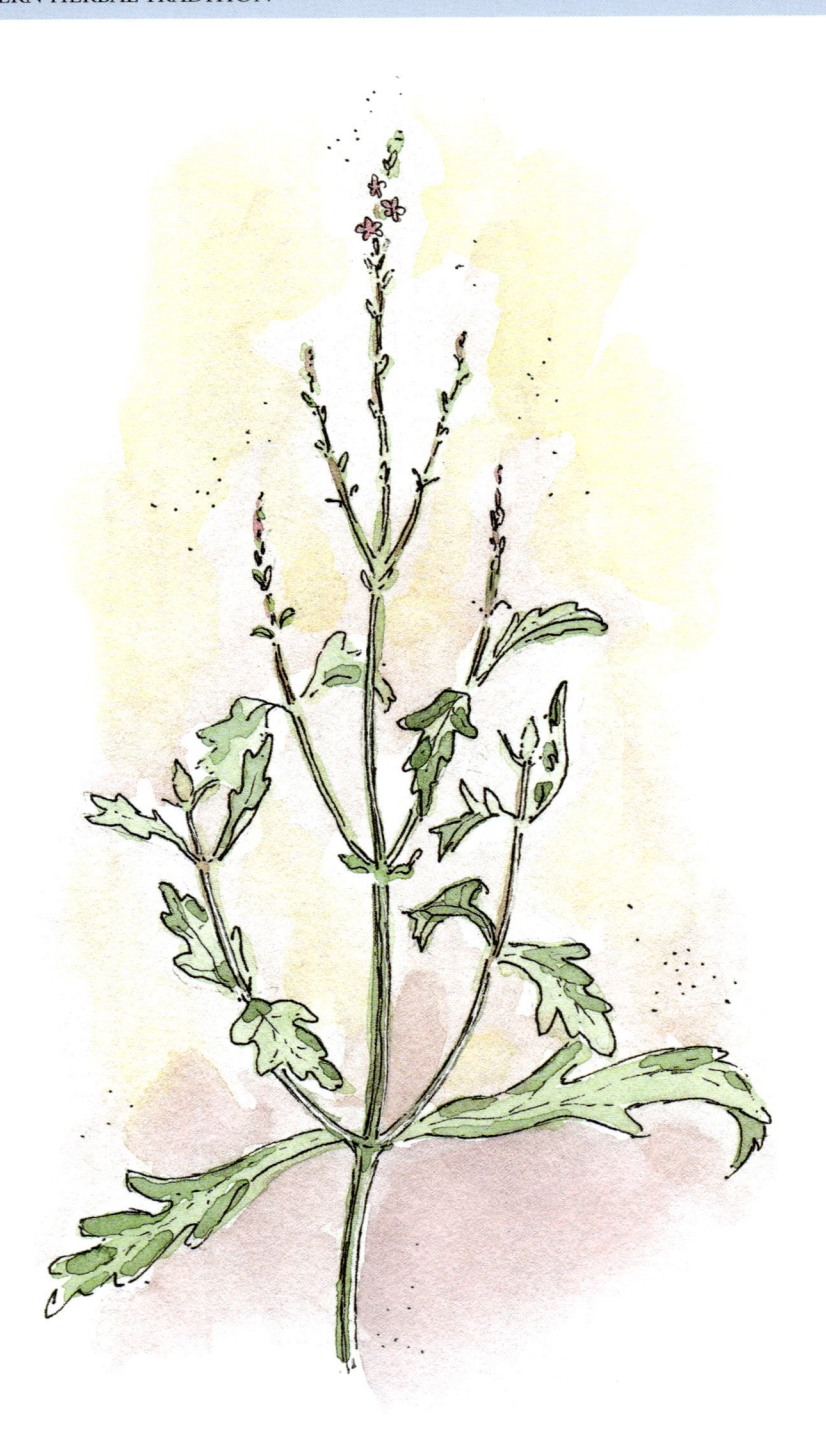

**Figure 31.2** *Verbena officinalis*, vervain.

to the very founding of Rome itself and seems to have been followed also by the Magi of Persia and later among Germanic peoples (De Cleene & Lejeune 2002). It is likely that vervain was not the sole plant used in these rituals, for 'verbenae' refers to a number of cooling herbs such as myrtle, olive and laurel (Lewis & Short 1890).

Vervain is also said to have been dedicated by the Romans to Venus since, as Virgil testifies, it was used in love magic and the preparation of love potions (De Cleene & Lejeune 2002). This enchantment is reflected in vervain's epithet of 'you tempt me' in the language of flowers (De Latour 1819). To counter the spell, this same 'Enchanter's Weed' or 'Herbe aux Sorcieres' was used to drive away evil and undesirable people. It was said that 'Vervain and Dill hinder witches from their will' (De Cleene & Lejeune 2002). Vervain was hung on stable doors in Greece to protect and bring luck; guns were rubbed with the plant so that they would never miss, and armour also, so that it might remain impervious to arrows and other weapons (De Cleene & Lejeune 2002). He who carries vervain about his person, says the Salernitan herbal, will be protected against all serpent bites (or dogs in Apuleius and the *Old English Herbarium* under peristerion), while Macer wants the bruised herb applied to the bite. It was used in a more magical way also by being hung round the neck rather than ingested, as Turner and Culpeper suggest, for garlands of this herb as a crown for the head are recommended in the Salernitan herbal to treat a headache. Gerard tells us that this method comes from Archigenes, but another method cited by Fuchs from Aetius becomes the approved treatment in the London Dispensatory: an oil of vervain is used to anoint the head. Culpeper adds a proviso that the headache must not be accompanied by inflammation or fever, presumably because, like Parkinson, he regarded the herb as hot and dry in quality. For Culpeper, vervain is 'an herb of Venus, and an excellent herb for the womb, to strengthen it, and remedy all the cold griefs of it, as Plantain doth the hot'. The fact of vervain's bitterness adds credence to the assessment of a heating power, but Galen himself only states the plant's drying action and several authors go no further than this. However, the Salernitan herbal repeats the Roman classification of the plant as cold and dry, and Hildegard writes that it is more cold than hot, while Macer has hot and dry in the second degree, like Parkinson and Culpeper. Eighteenth century recommendations of the herb for diseases of cold and phlegm suggest the acceptance of vervain as heating and drying.

## EUROPEAN MEDICINAL USES

Now that we have returned to medicinal virtues of vervain, let us look at the medieval sources. The Old English Herbarium lists one internal use of the powdered herb peristerion, taken in drink to disperse poison, and indications for vermenaca. These include liver pain, headache, wounds of various kinds including the bites of snakes, spiders and mad dogs, 'for those who have clogged veins so that blood cannot get to the genitals', an indication recalling the employment of vervain in love magic, and for those who cannot keep their food down. Two new uses are mentioned: for bladder stones and for swollen glands. Grieve tells us that the name verva n comes from the Celtic 'fer' and 'faen' meaning 'to drive away the stone'. The Salernitan herbal specifies the root in mead or bladder stones, Macer wants equal parts of vervain betony *Stachys officinalis* and saxifrage in white wine and Fuchs cites Aetius of Amida and Simeon Seth on the herb taken in drink with honey for unspecified stones. Parkinson and Culpeper after him state that vervain cleanses the kidneys and bladder of humours which engender stones, and helps to break stones and expel gravel. Quincy comments more generally on indurations and obstructions of the liver, spleen, kidneys and mesentery, Coffin lists diuretic and anti-scorbutic actions and both Priest & Priest and Bartram refer to vervain's influence on hepatic and renal function. Stainton (1900) makes it a kidney tonic and Chevallier suggests a use in gall-stones. It is reasonable to identify a herbal diuretic action (Bisset & Wichtl 2001) and there is also some evidence that vervain can be useful in cases of urinary stones (Mills & Bone 2000).

As for swollen glands, this is named scrofula by the Myddfai physicians and vervain as a simple is recommended to be inwardly taken and externally applied, using the whole plant, until the swelling is dispersed. Hildegard describes topical compresses for swellings of the throat and corroding ulcers. The juice of vervain boiled in wine with honey is proposed by the teachers of Salerno for any swelling, growth or abscess of the throat which hinders swallowing. This may include seats of the tonsils and takes us back to Dioscorides, but the recommendation for scrofula is not passed down into Renaissance herbals. There is a surprise re-appearance, however, in Victorian England, when Fernie (1897) writes that 'the vervain has fallen of late years into disfavour as a British Herbal Simple, though a pamphlet has recently appeared, written by a Mr Morley, who strongly advises the revived use of the herb for benefiting scrofulous diseases. Therein it is ordered that the root of vervain shall be tied with a yard of white satin ribband round the neck of the patient until he recovers. Also an infusion and ointment are to be prepared from the leaves of the plant'. A prescription for scrofula is also recorded by John Skelton in *The Science and Practice of Medicine*, published by the National Association of Medical Herbalists of Great Britain in 1904 but with an introduction by the author from 1870. A decoction of vervain, coltsfoot *Tussilago farfara* and the poisonous dog's mercury *Mercurialis perennis* and spurge laurel *Daphne laureola*, with added poke root *Phytolacca americana* and Spanish juice (liquorice *Glycyrrhiza glabra*) is prescribed for internal administration, while the enlarged glands are covered with flannel during the day and treated with hot wormwood compress at night. A poultice of white pond lily *Nymphaea alba* is used instead if the glands appear ripe for suppuration. The detail of Skelton's treatment suggests actual use but for reasons of likely toxicity could no longer be repeated today.

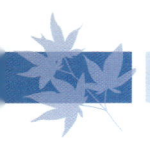

Another medieval topical use for vervain involves applying the fresh juice to the chest while the herb is available, or the dried and powdered herb with honey in winter, for chest complaints. The Myddfai physicians recommend this to counter the effects of scrofula on the lungs, while the Salernitan herbal insists the plants used must be gathered when the sun is at its highest point, presumably mid-summer rather than noon. Macer accounts the herb generally good for stomach, liver and lungs and Fuchs reads the same in his copy of Pliny, the interpolation emphasizing the benefits of vervain for consumption.

The Byzantine sources Aetius of Amida and Simeon Seth cited by Fuchs, and Paul of Aegina cited by Dalechamps, provide yet more external uses: hair loss, toothache and loose teeth, mouth ulcers and fistulae. To these are added abdominal colic, elephantiasis, epilepsy, common or quotidian fevers, gout and hip pains by internal medicine. These citations appear where we might have expected comments in Renaissance herbals on new uses of vervain among contemporary doctors. The plant's common name 'simpler's joy' might suggest an enthusiastic usage outside trained medical practice, especially given the extent of vervain's reputation in magic, and the popular tendency to deploy elaborate rituals in the use of medicinal plants (Webster 2008). Could a superstitious reverence of the plant have diminished its standing among more qualified and professionally aware practitioners? Some writers want to distance themselves from such practices. Gerard chooses Dioscorides' recommendation of vervain in agues to reprimand improper practice:

> It is reported to be of singular force against the tertian and quartaine fevers: but you must observe mother Bumbies rules to take just so many knots or sprigs and no more, least it fall out so that it do you no good, if you catch no harme by it. Many odde olde wives fables are written of vervaine tending to witchcraft and sorcerie, which you may reade else where, for I am not willing to trouble your eares with reporting such trifles, as honest eares abhorre to heare … Most of the later physitions do give the juice or decoction hereof to them that have the plague: but these men are deceived, not only in that they looke for some truth from the father of falsehood and leasings, but also because in stead of a good and sure remedy they minister no remedy at all: for it is reported that the Divell did reveale it as a secret and divine medicine.

Quincy cites a magical use of vervain from Marcellus Empiricus, a Gallic physician of the 5th century AD and author of a book on medicines (De Medicamentis), before complaining that 'many country people pretend to do great feats with it in agues, by applying it to the wrist in the form of a cataplasm, and also to cure gouty pains and swellings being use in the same manner'. Miller and Hill describe only physical applications: Miller recommends vervain for diseases of cold and phlegm, for clearing obstructions of the liver and spleen including jaundice, for gout and watery, inflamed eyes already mentioned by Parkinson, and as a vulnerary; Hill comments only on its ability to warm the stomach, open the liver and spleen and, with continued use, to remove nervous conditions. This last indication may stem from Parkinson's opinion that the herb is good for those who are frantic and is the earliest mention we have found of vervain's primary indication today.

Parkinson also establishes other indications, which will have been read more often in Culpeper's rendering of the same virtues of vervain. He emphasizes benefits for defects of the stomach, liver, spleen, kidneys and also the lungs, treating cough, wheezing and breathlessness, and generally for all inward pains. It will cause a good colour in the face and body. Vervain kills worms in the belly and its distilled water, dropped into the eyes for films and mists 'wonderfully comforteth the optick veins'. Among the external uses are ointments for pain and swelling in the groin and for haemorrhoids, the juice or bruised herb to cleanse pustules, freckles and morphew (possibly a type of psoriasis). He lists gout and fistulas, which we have already seen mentioned in Byzantine sources.

## VERVAIN OF THE AMERICAS

Where later writers have included any of the older indications, they are likely to have come from Culpeper. This includes Dioscorides' indication for jaundice in the *British Herbal Pharmacopoeia*, and references to lung conditions (Robinson 1868, Brooke 1992), but these are negligible compared to the importance of the descriptions by Coffin and Cook of the American *Verbena hastata*. Take vervain's use in gynaecology: Cook discusses vervain as a relaxant tonic with mild laxative effects indicated in recent obstructions of the menses, from which is derived an emmenogogue action and an indication of amenorrhoea (Priest & Priest, Bartram, Hoffmann), which has nothing to do with Culpeper's original assertion, that vervain is a sympathetic remedy for the womb correcting all cold diseases of that organ. The relaxant effect becomes an antispasmodic action, useful in gall-bladder inflammation (*British Herbal Pharmacopoeia*, Hoffmann), acute spasms of bronchitis and pertussis as well as dysmenorrhoea (Priest & Priest), seizures (Hoffmann) muscle spasm, neuritis and ear neuralgia (Menzies-Trull) and labour pains (Coffin). None of these writers mentions abdominal colic cited by the old Byzantine writers, or repeats Parkinson's 'all inward pains'. Both Coffin and Cook note vervain also as a treatment for worms, with an action similar to that of balmony *Chelone glabra*. Coffin highlights vervain's diaphoretic action 'one of the strongest sweating medicines in nature. It is good for colds, coughs and pains in the head, and some years ago was highly esteemed as a remedy for consumption'. The *National Botanic Pharmacopoeia* advocates its use in some forms of fevers only and it remains a mild diaphoretic for coughs and colds in the *British Herbal Pharmacopoeia*, to be taken as a simple infusion of 1 oz of herb to 1 pint of water according to Wren and only for the early stages of fever for Hoffmann. Coffin is also full of praise for vervain's emetic action 'It ranks next to lobelia … As an emetic it supercedes the use of antimony and ipecacuanha … I generally give a teaspoon of the pulverized herb every half hour in a tea of pennyroyal (*Mentha pulegium*) or raspberry leaves (*Rubus idaeus*) until it operates, taking great care to keep the patient warm in bed, with a hot brick or stone to the feet, and use freely of cayenne or ginger tea, taken as hot as convenient during its operation'. Cook too relates that a warm infusion of vervain proves emetic if used freely. Chevallier thinks that the bitter terpenoid verbenalin may be responsible for the effect. Yet this action goes without mention or caution in Priest & Priest, Grieve, whose entry for vervain is short as if she could not be bothered with it, Bartram and the *British Herbal Pharmacopoeia*. Perhaps Cook's conclusion that 'this article is nearly overlooked by the profession, but deserves decided attention' is just as true today. So, a recent survey by researchers looking at 16th and 17th century herbals for citations of herbs indicated for rheumatic disorders, which included vervain in that number (Adams et al 2009), is most welcome. The uses mentioned in the herbals of Bock, Fuchs and Tabernaemontanus, of vervain decocted in wine for topical application to painful parts, including gout of the feet, is linked by the authors to ethnobotanical field studies in Italy and Serbia which report knowledge of vervain's analgesic and antiphlogistic properties and topical use in rheumatic disorders, and to in vitro and in vivo evidence which may explain these effects.

Recent research identifies four types of constituents in vervain which have been shown to be antiinflammatory: iridoid glycosides, phenylpropanoid glycosides, flavonoids and triterpenoids, which has led to recommendations that the plant merits further research for use particularly as a tea (Deepak & Handa 2000a, Bilia et al 2008).

Use of vervain is reported in recent ethnographic surveys for many disorders. Vervain is used in traditional Chinese medicine and is described as cold, bitter, anticoagulant, detoxifying and diuretic and used for amenorrhea, traumatic injuries; hepatitis, mastitis; liver cirrhosis and ascites, nephritic oedema and urinary tract infections (Revolutionary Health Committee of Hunan Province 1978). A study of medicinal plant knowledge amongst the Bai people, in the Himalayan foothills in southwest China documented use of 176 plants. The whole plant of vervain is used, as a decoction or poultice, as an anthelmintic, to treat injuries and, eaten raw, to 'strengthen bones and tendons'. The authors note the continuing influence of the herbal manuals distributed in the 1970s to improve rural healthcare (Weckerle et al 2009). A survey of markets in Yunnan, southwest China documented use of 216 plants. Aerial parts of verbena are collected in the wild and used for cold-fever, hepatitis and enteritis (Lee et al 2008). A European survey in rural northern Portugal documented use of 88 plants and found that verbena is used for depression, nervousness, stress and insomnia (Neves et al 2009). Another survey in the Italian Alps documenting the use of 58 species found that the whole plant of vervain is collected and used for coughs and asthma. The dose given is 3 cups of tea daily for several weeks (Vitalini et al 2009). A third survey in central Italy documented use of 96 plants. Aerial parts of vervain are used as a plaster to stop bleeding and aid in wound healing and for rheumatic pains in the knees and elbows. Aerial parts are used too as a poultice for thyroid problems. The herb is chopped together with *Thymus longicaulis* subsp. *longicaulis* and *Parietaria diffusa*, added to bean flour and beaten egg white and applied with a cloth to the neck for 4–5 hours or preferably overnight. It is applied for 3 days, stopped for 3 days and the cycle is repeated three times (Guarrera et al 2005).

Western herbalists writing about vervain feature its relaxant tonic action on the nervous system. Perhaps more readily available in the shops is Lemon verbena *Verbena triphylla*, which makes a refreshing tea possessing nervine properties also. It is used in traditional medicine in South America for depression and to calm the nerves (Carnat et al 1999, Ceuterick et al 2008). It has similar constituents to vervain (Bilia et al 2008), including the iridoid glycoside verbenalin and the phenylpropanoid glycoside verbascoside. The concentration of verbascoside

# THE WESTERN HERBAL TRADITION

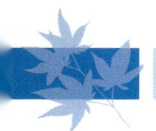

is substantially higher in lemon verbena (Bilia et al 2008). It is more aromatic with a lemony aroma as the volatile oil contains geranial, neral and limonene (Carnat et al 1999, Svoboda & Greenaway 2003) which renders the tea more pleasant to take.

However, our medicinal herb is *Verbena officinalis* and the writers variously describe its principal indications as a nervine agent: as a sedative and anxiolytic for nervous disorders and breakdowns, irritability, over-sensitivity, withdrawal from tranquillizers or mood-altering drugs, paranoid tendency, hysteria, agoraphobia, generalized seizures, fits and convulsions; as a thymoleptic in depression and melancholia, and specifically for the depression and debility of convalescence after fevers such as influenza, in recovery from chronic illness or in post-natal or post-operative depression; as a nerve tonic in chronic fatigue syndrome, nervous exhaustion and insomnia, for which last it is often prescribed as an infusion with other relaxant herbs in Mességué's (1981) 'tea of happiness': 2 parts vervain, chamomile *Matricaria recutita* and lime flowers *Tilia* x *vulgaris*; 1 part peppermint *Mentha piperita* and (additional to Mességué's four herbs) lavender *Lavandula angustifolia*.

## RECOMMENDATIONS

- Nervous disorders: stress, anxiety and depression, withdrawal from tranquillizers or mood-altering drugs, agoraphobia, chronic fatigue syndrome, nervous exhaustion and insomnia; sexual neurosis; headache; restless leg syndrome.
- Convalescence: depression and debility after fevers such as influenza or in recovery from chronic illness; post-natal or post-operative depression.
- Digestion: abdominal colic, jaundice, gall-bladder inflammation, intestinal worms.
- Respiratory: colds and fevers, tightness of the chest, bronchitis, asthma, pertussis, sinusitis.
- Urinary: urinary stones, urinary tract infections.
- Reproductive: dysmenorrhoea.
- Topical: wounds, bites, oral and throat inflammation, muscle spasms and rheumatic conditions.

Daily dosage: the *British Herbal Pharmacopoeia* recommends 2–4 g three times a day of dried herb.

## CONSTITUENTS

Barnes et al (2007), Bisset & Wichtl (2001), Bradley (2006), Williamson (2003).

### Iridoid glycosides

Verbenalin 0.34%, hastatoside 0.3% (tender parts, wild, India) (Deepak & Handa 2000b); dihydrocornin, aucubin (Bradley 2006).
Verbenalin, hastatoside (decoction, tea, ethanol tincture, wild, Italy) (Bilia et al 2008).
Verbenalin 1.49–2.73%, hastatoside 0.5% (six samples, commercial, Switzerland) (Müller et al 2004).
Verbenalin was the most abundant constituent (cultivated, Spain) (Calvo et al 1997).

### Triterpenes

Beta-sitosterol, ursolic acid, oleanolic acid (Deepak & Handa 1998); ursolic acid, two new triterpenes (collected, India) (Deepak & Handa 2000a).

### Phenylpropanoids

Phenylpropanoid glycosides: verbascoside (acteoside) 0.24% (tender parts, wild, India) (Deepak & Handa 2000b).
Verbascoside, isoverbascoside, eukovoside (wild, Italy) (Bilia et al 2008). Concentration was higher in the ethanolic tincture than in the infusion or decoction.

### Flavonoids

Flavone glycosides: luteolin 7-diglucuronide, apigenin 7-diglucuronide (Müller et al 2004).
Apigenin 7-glucoside, luteolin glycosides, diosmetin glycosides, chrysoeriol galactoside (wild, Egypt) (Kawashty et al 2000).
Luteolin 7-diglucuronide, apigenin 7-diglucuronide (decoction, wild, Italy) (Bilia et al 2008). In this study the flavone glycosides were extracted into the tea but not into the ethanol tincture, whereas Calvo et al (1997) found the flavonoids were extracted into a methanolic tincture.
Luteolin and glycoside, 6-hydroxyluteolin and glycoside, apigenin and glycoside, 6-hydroxyapigenin and glycoside (Calvo et al 1997).

## RECOMMENDATIONS ON SAFETY

1. Do not use in pregnancy.
   Several sources suggest that this herb should not be used in pregnancy (Bradley 2006, Brooke 1992) and it has been investigated in China as a possible herb to terminate early pregnancy (Zhang et al 2004).
2. Vervain should not be drunk with meals by vegetarians and vegans.
   Mills & Bone (2000) state that phenylpropanoids interfere with non-haem iron absorption and include vervain in the list of herbs where this may be of concern. A study in Morocco using an in vitro model of digestion found that non-haem iron absorption was decreased by vervain, although vervain had one third of the level of polyphenols in tea (Zaida et al 2006). This was an in vitro study designed to estimate the effect of drinking tea, vervain or mint teas on women weaning their babies and so would require further confirmation.

## REFERENCES

Adams M, Berset C, Kessler M, et al 2009 Medicinal herbs for the treatment of rheumatic disorders – a survey of European herbals from the 16th and 17th century. Journal of Ethnopharmacology 121:343–359.

Barnes J, Anderson LA, Phillipson JD 2007 Herbal medicines, 3rd edn. Pharmaceutical Press, London.

Bilia AR, Giomi M, Innocenti M, et al 2008 HPLC-DAD-ESI-MS analysis of the constituents of aqueous preparations of verbena and lemon verbena and evaluation of the antioxidant. Journal of Pharmaceutical and Biomedical Analysis 46:463–470.

Bisset NG, Wichtl M (eds) 2001 Herbal Drugs and Phytopharmaceuticals, 2nd edn. Medpharm, Stuttgart.

Bown D 1995 Encyclopedia of herbs. Dorling Kindersley, London.

Bradley PR 2006 British herbal compendium, vol 2. British Herbal Medicine Association, Bournemouth.

Brooke E 1992 A woman's book of herbs. The Women's Press, London.

Bryce D (ed.) 1987 The herbal remedies of the physicians of Myddfai. Llanerch Enterprises, Lampeter.

Calvo MI, San Julian A, Fernandez M 1997 Identification of the major compounds in extracts of *Verbena officinalis* L. (Verbenaceae) by HPLC with post-column derivatization. Chromatographia 46:241–244.

Calvo MI, Crespo A, Fernandez M 2000 Seasonal variations of the iridoids, flavonoids and verbascoside content from *Verbena officinalis* L. Acta Horticulturae 516:169–174.

Carnat A, Carnat AP, Fraisse D 1999 The aromatic and polyphenolic composition of lemon verbena tea. Fitoterapia 70:44–49.

Ceuterick M, Vandebroek I, Torry B, et al 2008 Cross-cultural adaptation in urban ethnobotany: the Colombian folk pharmacopoeia in London. Journal of Ethnopharmacology 120:342–359.

Culpeper N 1669 Pharmacopoeia Londinensis. London: George Sawbridge.

Davis PH (ed.) 1982 Flora of Turkey, vol. 7. Edinburgh University Press, Edinburgh.

De Cleene M, Lejeune MC 2002 Compendium of symbolic and ritual plants in Europe. Man & Culture Publishers, Ghent.

Deepak M, Handa SS 1998 3alpha,24-dihydroxy-urs-12-en-28-oic acid from *Verbena officinalis*. Phytochemistry 49:269–271.

Deepak M, Handa SS 2000a Antiinflammatory activity and chemical composition of extracts of *Verbena officinalis*. Phytotherapy Research 14:463–465.

Deepak M, Handa SS 2000b Quantitative determination of the major constituents of *Verbena officinalis* using high performance thin layer chromatography and high pressure liquid chromatography. Phytochemical Analysis 11:351–355.

De Latour C 1819 Le langage des fleurs. A Pihan Delaforest, Paris.

Fernie WT 1897 Herbal simples approved for modern uses of cure. Boericke & Tafel, Philadelphia. Online. Available: http://www.gutenberg.org.

Guarrera PM, Forti G, Marignoli S 2005 Ethnobotanical and ethnomedicinal uses of plants in the district of Acquapendente (Latium, Central Italy). Journal of Ethnopharmacology 96:429–444.

Henriette's Herbal Homepage 2009 *Verbena hastata*. Online. Available: http://www.henriettesherbal.com/plants/verbena/hastata.html.

Kawashty SA, El-Garf IA 2000 The flavonoid chemosystematics of Egyptian *Verbena* species. Biochemical Systematics and Ecology 28:919–921.

Lee S, Xiao C, Pei S 2008 Ethnobotanical survey of medicinal plants at periodic markets of Honghe Prefecture in Yunnan Province, SW China. Journal of Ethnopharmacology 117:362–377.

Lewis C, Short C 1890 A Latin dictionary. Clarendon Press, Oxford.

Mességué M 1981 Health secrets of plants and herbs. Pan books, London.

Mills S, Bone K 2000 The principles and practice of phytotherapy. Churchill Livingstone, Edinburgh.

Müller A, Ganzera M, Stuppner H 2004 Analysis of the aerial parts of *Verbena officinalis* L. by micellar electrokinetic capillary chromatography. Chromatographia 60:193–197.

Neves JM, Matos C, Moutinho C, et al 2009 Ethnopharmacological notes about ancient uses of medicinal plants in Trás-os-Montes (northern of Portugal). Journal of Ethnopharmacology 124: 270–283.

Revolutionary Health Committee of Hunan Province 1978 Barefoot doctor's manual. Routledge Kegan Paul, London.

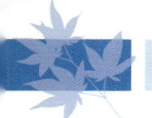

Robinson M 1868 The new family herbal. W Nicholson, London.

Stainton R 1990 *Verbena officinalis* in perspective. British Journal of Phytotherapy 1:34–46.

Svoboda KP, Greenaway RI 2003 Lemon scented plants. International Journal of Aromatherapy 13:23–32.

Vitalini S, Tomè F, Fico G 2009 Traditional uses of medicinal plants in Valvestino (Italy). Journal of Ethnopharmacology 121:106–116.

Webster C 2008 Medicine, magic and mission at the end of time. Yale University Press, New Haven.

Weckerle CS, Ineichen R, Huber FK, et al 2009 Mao's heritage: medicinal plant knowledge among the Bai in Shaxi, China, at a crossroads between distinct local and common widespread practice. Journal of Ethnopharmacology 123:213–228.

Williamson E 2003 Potter's herbal cyclopaedia. CW Daniel, Saffron Walden.

Woodward FI 1997 Life at the edge: a 14-year study of a *Verbena officinalis* population's interactions with climate. The Journal of Ecology 85:899–906.

Zaida F, Bureau F, Guyot S, et al 2006 Iron availability and consumption of tea, vervain and mint during weaning in Morocco. Ann Nutr Metab 50:237–241.

Zhang SX, Wang HQ, Ou N 2004 Studies on the effect of *Verbena officinalis* extract on decidual stromal cells of early pregnancy in vitro. Chinese Journal of Natural Medicines 2:242–246 (Chinese, English abstract only).

# CHAPTER 32
# *Viola odorata*, sweet violet; *Viola tricolor*, heartsease

## DESCRIPTION

### Family: Violaceae                                                      Part used: aerial parts

There are over 90 *Viola* species in Europe. The *Flora of Turkey* (Davis 1965) gives 20 *Viola* species, including *Viola odorata* and *Viola tricolor*.

*Viola odorata* L. is a low-growing perennial with a stout rootstock found in hedgerows, rough land and margins of woodlands. It is native to Europe south of the Alps and west into France, but has naturalized in more northern areas because of widespread cultivation (Marcussen 2006).

The stalked leaves arise in a rosette from the sturdy rootstock and are heart-shaped and hairy with an oval stipule. The fragrant, five-petalled dark violet or white flowers occur in spring and it may flower again in early autumn. The leafless flower stalks curve sharply so that the flower hangs down. The lowest petal has a prominent nectar-filled spur and the five sepals have basal appendages. The small seeds form in a three-valved capsule and it also spreads by long creeping stolons.

**Other species used**: Parma violets are cultivated for cut flowers and for their fragrance. The leaves are shiny green and the flowers are double. A study of six specimens cultivated in France and 31 wild *Viola* species found that Parma violets are cultivars of *Viola alba* (Malécot et al 2007). Parma violets are tender and flower from autumn to spring depending on the variety. They are considered to have been introduced to Europe, certainly by the early 19th century as they were grown alongside many other violets in the gardens of the Empress Josephine at Malmaison (Coombs 1981). The violet became a symbol of the House of Bonaparte. In the 19th century, cultivation of numerous varieties in market gardens and orchards, for cut flowers and button holes was an enormous trade in northern and southern France and England, especially in Middlesex (Coombs 1981).

*Viola yedoensis* is a perennial and is used in China in the treatment of acute skin infections (WHO 1989, Zhou et al 2009).

Other common species of violet are scented or faintly scented and are not used. White violet *Viola alba* is white with non-rooting runners. Hairy violet *Viola hirta* is similar to *Viola odorata* but hairy with no runners and usually found on chalk or limestone. *Viola × scabra* is the cross between *Viola hirta* and *Viola odorata* (Stace 1991). Early dog-violet *Viola reichenbachiana* and common dog-violet *Viola riviniana* have veined throats, more pointed leaves, and flowers and leaves arise from the same stems (Grey-Wilson 1994). Marsh violet *Viola palustris* has veined pale violet flowers and rounded leaves (Akeroyd 2003). Field pansy *Viola arvensis* is similar to *Viola tricolor* with creamy yellow flowers and longer sepals (Grey-Wilson 1994) and the two species form crosses which are difficult to distinguish (Rimkiene et al 2003). *Viola* species are illustrated in Gibbons & Brough (1996).

### Quality

Given the similarity between species, it is hard to believe that only the leaves of *Viola odorata* are collected. The French Pharmacopoeia includes *Viola lutea* and *Viola calcarata* (Bradley 2006). Leaves of the many aromatic cultivars could be collected as they are cultivars rather than hybrids.

### Family: Violaceae

*Viola tricolor* L. is annual, biennial or perennial with a short or absent rhizome. Stems (up to 30 cm) bear alternate oval toothed leaves with a rounded base and conspicuous deeply lobed, pinnate leaf-like stipules. Flowers 1–2.5 cm) across occur in summer, vary in colour and contain white, yellow and violet of varying tones. The petals are longer than the sepals which is a distinguishing feature. It has a weak fragrance.

*Viola tricolor* subsp. *tricolor* is an annual weed of cultivated soil. *Viola tricolor* subsp. *curtisii* is a perennial with rhizomes and mainly found in coastal dunes and heathland.

### Quality

Heartsease is vulnerable to drying out in early summer as it has small roots so is vulnerable to changes of land use which introduce more aggressive plants (Rimkiene et al 2003). The garden pansy *Viola × wittrockiana* Hams is not used. The pansy was bred from *Viola tricolor* by nurserymen working in Britain in the early 19th century, and then crossed with other *Viola* species in Scotland to develop the show pansy (Genders 1958). Pansies contain similar flavonoids to *Viola tricolor*, which have been shown to be antioxidant (Vukics et al 2008a), but further research would be needed to confer any advantage, and as they are hybrids, there may be as yet unknown disadvantages.

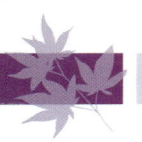

## *Viola odorata*, sweet violet

### A COOLING HERB

The current uses of viola appear to be somewhat metamorphosed within its broad ancient themes, referring to a diverse and sporadic tradition in some degree, with some expansions and one or two additions. Chevallier and Hoffman record its main use now as a cough remedy, for coughs, colds and catarrh. Hoffman expands on its alterative and antiinflammatory properties, useful in skin conditions, urinary tract infections and rheumatism. Both authors cite recent application for cancer. The *British Herbal Pharmacopoeia* specifies it expectorant and antineoplastic.

Violet nature, according to tradition, is cooling. It belongs to a smaller group of plants, cold and moist in nature, which treat either symptoms of heat or dryness. This cooling property is employed, according to Dioscorides (IV 121), to ease heartburn, eye inflammations and prolapse of the anus, as external application of the leaves as a plaster. The purple flower helps in sore throats and in epilepsy in children, the infusion taken internally. Pliny expands on this. He records purple, white and yellow varieties. The purple, as Dioscorides but with no distinction as to leaves or flowers, is applied for stomach inflammation, to the forehead when the head burns, for watering eyes, anal and uterine prolapse, and he adds its use for abscesses. Moreover, violets are placed on the head to disperse the after effects of drinking and its headaches; then follows use in water for quinsies and for epilepsy in children, again as Dioscorides. Its seed neutralizes

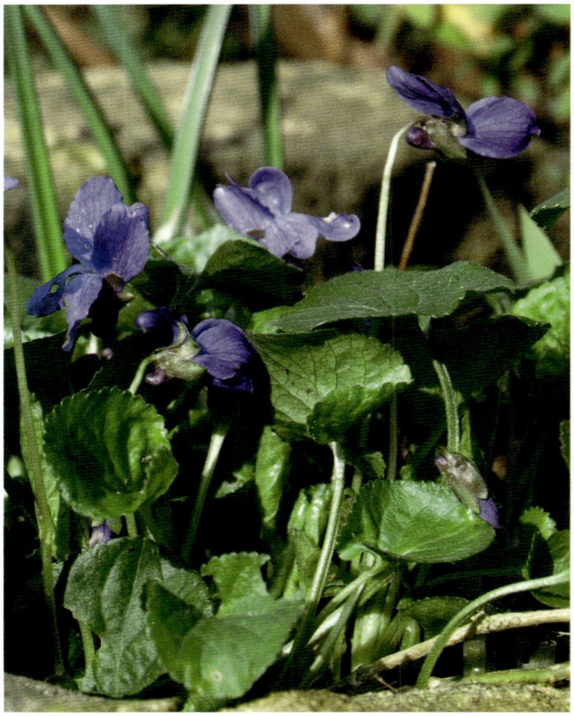

**Figure 32.1** *Viola odorata*, sweet violet (a garden in Yorkshire, March).

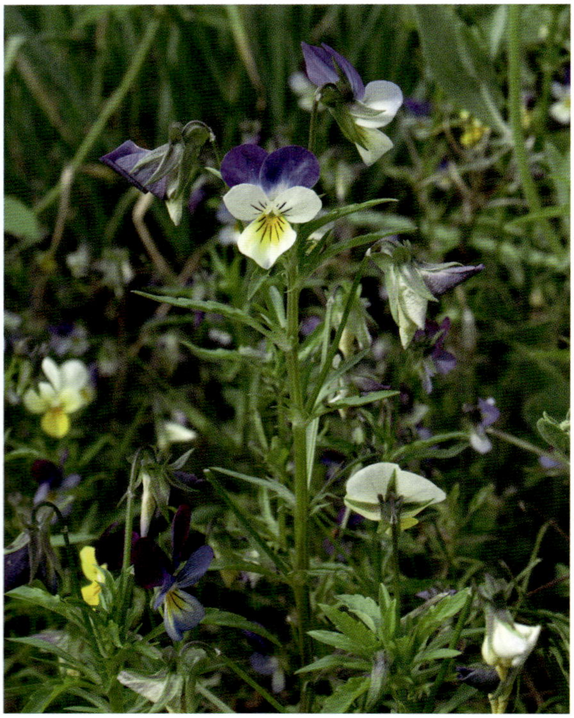

**Figure 32.2** *Viola tricolor*, heartsease (Hardwick Hall, Derbyshire, August).

scorpion stings. The white and yellow violets, to be used dried and over 1 year old to increase their potency, are diuretic, reduce menstrual discharge; the white disperse abscesses, while the yellow, half a cyathus (22 mL) in 3 cyathi of water (135 mL), promotes menstruation. Its roots, presumably the yellow variety, although he does not specify, with vinegar as liniment, soothe the spleen and gout, while for eye inflammations myrrh *Commiphora molmol* and saffron *Crocus sativus* are added. With wax ointment they, again presumably the yellow, heal cracks in the anus and other moist parts of the body; in vinegar they heal abscesses. Galen ascribes the virtues of violets to their cool, watery nature. Topically with polenta they are good for hot inflammations, a burning mouth of the stomach and the eyes. So with some few additions from Pliny, our three ancient sources mainly converge. So far, there is no mention specifically of use for cough, though quinsy is at least heading in that direction.

## ECHOES, CHANGES AND ADDITIONS

With the medieval herbals there are echoes, changes and additions. Macer writes of 'vyolet' as cold in the first degree, moist in the second; how it is good for sore, swollen or 'blasted' eyes, the root being stamped with myrrh and saffron – no distinction here between the purple and the yellow; for head wounds a plaster of the leaves stamped with honey and vinegar – is this a version of 'when the head burns'?; and as a foot bath and a binding for the temples for poor sleep due to sickness, 'and ye shall sleep well by the Grace of God'. The *Old English Herbarium* carries two uses: for fresh or old wounds (not just the head this time), swellings and calluses, the leaves are applied with lard. Then violet's use for constipation is introduced; take the flowers mixed with honey and soaked in very good wine to relieve the constipation. Hildegard records a number of uses. She begins with use of the oil for the eyes, against fogginess of the eyes. She gives a recipe for this oil 'take good oil and make it boil in a new pot, either in the sun or over a fire. When it boils, put violets in so that it becomes thickened. Put this in a glass vessel and save it. At night put this unguent around the eyelids and eyes. Although it shan't touch the inside of the eyes, it will expel the fogginess'. She continues that if the eyes are inflamed, foggy and painful, then violet, rose juice and fennel juice are mixed in the ratio of 3:6:2 parts, respectively, add a little wine and again rub round the external parts of the eyes. To anointing for heaviness in the head, Hildegard adds use for kidneys or 'any other place fatigued by palsy' by application of the juice of violets added to goat tallow and half as much old fat. Head pain is relieved by violet juice with olive oil and goat tallow, and this mixture will also rid crabs (lice or scabies) from the body. Tertian fevers, presumably due to violet's cooling properties, are helped by 3 parts violet with 1 part plantain and 2 parts savory, frequently eaten with vinegar or roasted salt. An early reference to use for lungs then follows, but a use linked directly with melancholy 'anyone oppressed by melancholy with a discontented mind, which then harms his lungs, should cook violets in pure wine. He should strain this through a cloth, add a bit of galingale, and as much licorice as he wants, and so make spiced wine. When he drinks it, it will check the melancholy, make him happy and heal his lungs. This presumably hails from the phthisical diathesis delineated in the *Hippocratic Corpus*, where tendency to cerebral and lung diseases is the dominant diathesis.

*The Trotula* (Green 2001) applies violet's cooling nature; juice of violets for excessive flux of the menses through 'too much bile'; the herb along with marshmallow, roses and root of rush for pain in the womb from heat 'made hot from the use of Venus'; the oil, made in the same way as rose oil, anointed on the liver, pulse points, temples, palms of the hand and soles of the feet, to extinguish heat in acute diseases; and in various treatments, together with rose and marshmallow, for women with a hot constitution, determined by insertion of a diagnostic pessary prepared as described under mugwort.

The Salernitan herbal reads much like the Ancients: it is cold in the first degree, moist in the second, is moistening, sweetening, softening, cooling and loosening; the oil for an overheated liver, head pain caused by heat, the bruised, cooked plant applied to 'inflamed apostemes' in the early stages; bathing the feet and forehead in a hot decoction induces sleep in acute fevers. Two recipes are offered; violet syrup, which has more virtue made with fresh flowers, is prepared thus; place violets in water overnight, then cook, strain and add sugar; violet sugar, which will keep for 3 years is made by taking 1 lb flowers to 3–4 lb sugar; chop the violets and mix with the sugar in a glass container; place in the sun for 3 days, stirring every day.

The source of these mediaeval recommendations is no doubt via the Arabic writers, who wrote widely on violet, and here too we find hearty recommendations for use for the lungs, along with applications from the Ancients, plus additions. Ibn Sina tells us violets are cold and moist in the first degree, they balance the blood. The leaves with barley flour as bandage calm hot swellings. The oil is good for skin eruptions. To smell violets or apply their oil calms headache due to blood humour. For hot inflammations of the eyes the oil is applied or the infusion drunk. Inflammations of the stomach are eased too. The syrup 'softens nature' and helps rectal prolapse. Thus far he follows the Ancients. But then he diversifies: for a hot cough, violets boiled with sugar lenify the chest; syrup of violets is useful for pleuritis and inflammation of the lungs; the syrup is also diuretic and helps illnesses of the kidneys, and dried violets purge bile. Compare here Hildegard and the Trotula. Simeon Seth, cited in Fuchs, says with the gastrointestinal tract and offers cautions; violets are useful for

339

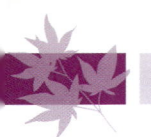

pains of the intestines but offend the heart; smelled or drunk they ease pains of the head due to yellow bile; they induce sleep; they moisten a dry head and cool a hot one, but will render moist heads liable to defluxion. Bauhin and Mattioli cite Mesue, and Bauhin adds that Mesue describes viola's powers more accurately than others. Fresh violets are cold and moist in the first degree, says Mesue, although when dry they cool and moisten less. Bauhin's version of Mesue continues: for in a fresh preparation an excrementitious moisture is purgative by a lubricating action and it dampens heat, then breaks it by drying and its bitter taste purges the heat by a drawing action. Mattioli writes of the same ideas in Mesue: so being dried they have more heat and less humidity; so dried, their faculties are more ejective not because they soften but because they dissolve. Fresh violets thus cool, easing hot pains in the manner of narcotics, extinguish all inflammations, soothe the trachea and lungs, purge yellow bile and extinguish its heat, and ease headache from a hot cause; they bring sleep. Violets carry off inflammations of the throat, pleurisy and other hot swellings of the lungs; dried they greatly help liver inflammation, dry obstruction there and help jaundice; they counter inflammatory fevers. They allay thirst but provoke a runny nose. The juice and syrup soothe.

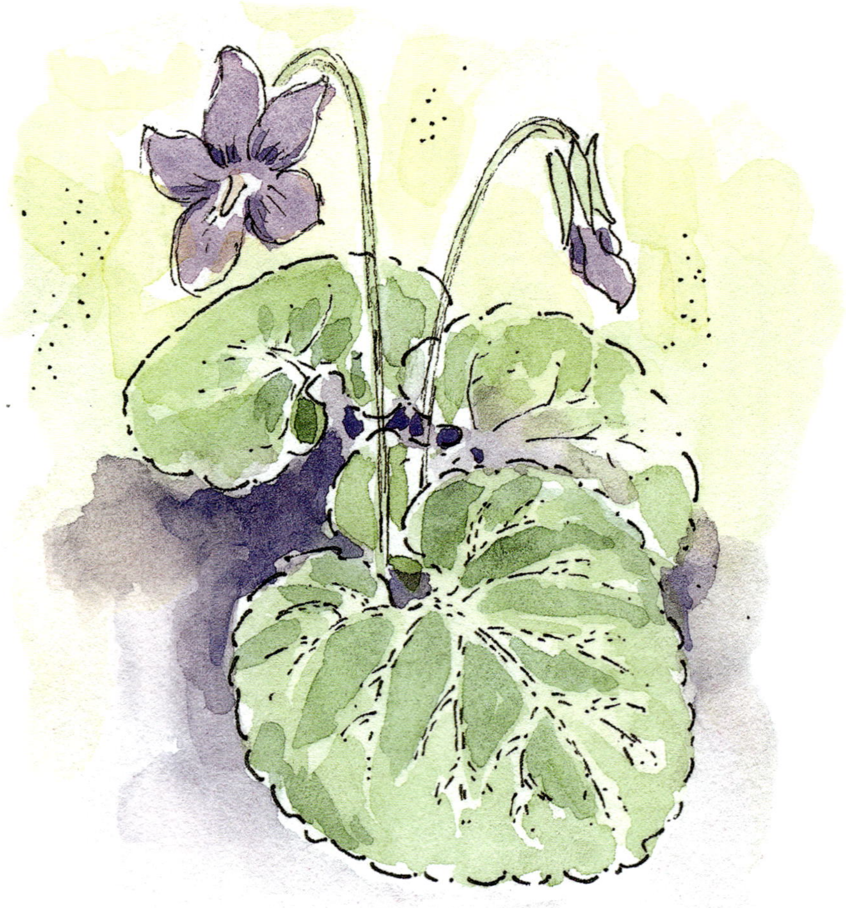

Figure 32.3 *Viola odorata*, sweet violet.

*Viola odorata*, sweet violet; *Viola tricolor*, heartsease

Honey of violets is more cleansing and less cooling; sugar of violets works the other way round. The dose of the syrup, Mesue says, is 2–4 oz; the dose of the juice, which does not tolerate much preparation, is 1–2 oz; the vinegar, which reduces fever wonderfully, 4–8 oz; the preserve 1½–3 oz. Dalechamps, citing Mesue, adds that since violets purge weakly, some add half its quantity of turbith or scammony (this is poisonous) and make troches (lozenges), for violets and oil of violets retard the violence of medicines and are added to them for that purpose.

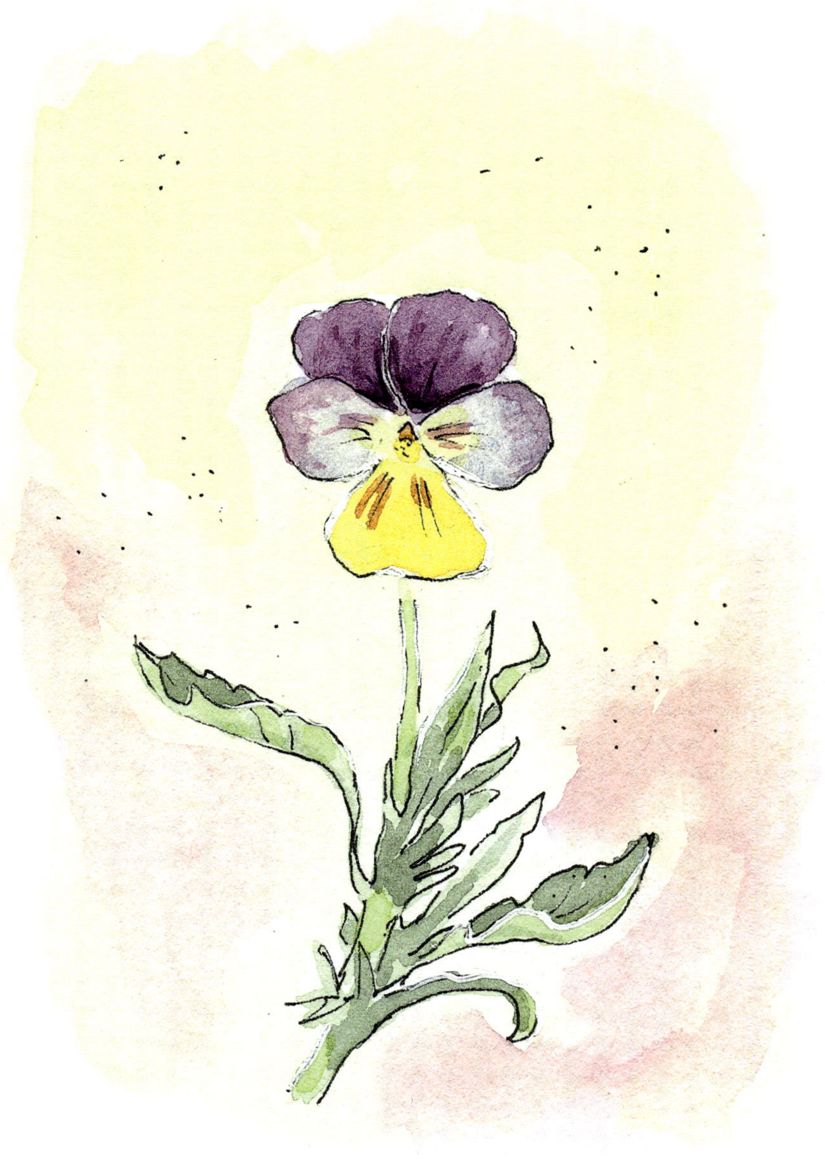

**Figure 32.4** *Viola tricolor*, heartsease.

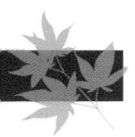

## RENAISSANCE USE

The Renaissance writers rehearse the themes. A number, for example Gerard, Parkinson and Dodoens, relate the origin of the Greek name for violet, 'Ion'. How either, according to Nicander, it was named after the nymphs of Ionia, who first gave the flower to Jupiter; or rather after the 'young damosell, Io' (Gerard), 'that sweete girle or pleasant damosell' (Dodoens) whom Jupiter courted and then, 'after that he had got her with child' (Dodoens) turned her into a cow, or 'trim heiffer' according to Dodoens, to protect her from the jealous eyes of Hera. Jupiter then caused the flowers to grow as fragrant food for his erstwhile mistress. The Latin term 'viola' is then proffered to come from 'vitula' meaning heifer. De Cleene & Lejeune (2003) add that the violet is dedicated to Persephone, goddess of fertility and queen of the underworld; it is often associated with death, particularly of a young person. In Christian legend the violet hangs its head because the shadow of the cross fell on the flower.

Gerard is comprehensive in his coverage of violets. He begins with a more 'moral' influence through their beauty; violets '… have a great prerogative above others, not only because the minde conceiveth a certain pleasure and recreation by smelling and handling of those most odoriferous of flours, but also for that very many by these violets receive ornament and comely grace … yea gardens themselves receive by these the greatest ornament of all, chiefest beauty and most gallant grace; and the recreation of the minde which is taken hereby, cannot be but very good and honest'. He lists seven sorts: purple garden, white garden, double garden, white double, yellow, wild, field and one found in Germany. The virtues cover the Ancients, Arabic writers and 'later phisitians'. He lists by mode of application. The flowers are good for all inflammations, especially the lungs; they take away hoarseness of the chest, ruggedness of the windpipe and jaws, allay heat of the liver, kidneys and bladder, ease the heat of burning agues, temper sharpness of choler and take away thirst. The oil, made from fresh, moist violets, put on the testicles (this is the only reference I found to this part of the body) counters hot and dry distempers to allow sleep; mixed with egg yolk it eases pain of the fundament and haemorrhoids; also in enemas and poultices to cool and ease pain. Dried violets are mixed with medicines, according to 'later physitians', says Gerard, to comfort and strengthen the heart. The leaves taken internally cool, moisten and make the belly soluble. Externally they cool hot inflammations by themselves or with barley flour, and, after Galen and Dioscorides, this same mixture thus cools a burning stomach and eyes and can be applied to the 'fundament that is fallen out'. He cites Pliny's use as garlands for surfeiting, heaviness of the head, squinancie (quinsy) or inward swellings of the throat, the falling sickness, especially in young children, and the seed against scorpion stings. Three or four ounces of the syrup softens the belly and purges choler. He offers a recipe:

*First make of clarified sugar by boyling a simple syrryup of a good consistence or meane thicknesse, whereunto put the floures cleane picked from all manner of filth, as also the white ends nipped away, a quantitie according to the quantitie of the syrup, to your owne discretion, wherein let them infuse or steepe foure and twenty houres, and set upon a few warm embers; then strain it, and put more violets in to the same syrup; thus do three or foure times, the oftner the better; then set them upon a gentle fire to simper, but not to boyle in any wise; so have you it simply made of a most perfect purple colour, and of the smell of the floures themselves. Some do adde thereto a little of the juice of the floures in the boyling, which maketh it of better force and virtue. Likewise some do put a little quantitie of the juice of lymons in the boyling, which doth greatly encrease the beauty thereof, but nothing at all the vertue.*

The decoction is taken for hot fever, inflamed liver and other organs, and the juice, syrup or conserve can be used similarly. The syrup is used too for inflammation of the lungs and breast, pleurisy and cough, fever and agues in young children, for burning fevers, pestilent diseases, inflammation of the throat, mouth and uvula, quinsy and epilepsy in children. Sugar violet heals inflammations and sore throat, comforts the heart, eases headache and promotes sleep. The leaves are used with other plants such as 'Mercurie' (dog's mercury which is poisonous) and mallows in plasters, oils, cataplasms, poultices and enemas.

Fuchs, Dodoens and Dalechamps all write similarly, citing Dioscorides, Pliny, Galen, Mesue and others. Dodoens and Mattioli both point out it is clear Galen and the Greeks had not discovered the laxative property of violets. Mattioli stresses the gentleness of the remedy in this respect; it can be used without harm. Culpeper too remarks on its mildness and ascribes the herb to Venus. He otherwise follows Parkinson almost word for word, covering the same areas as Gerard and the rest. Bauhin's coverage is thorough, as usual. On reading his text, his frequent mention of the general recommendation for epilepsy in children, e.g. citing Bayrum 'for epilepsy in children, especially when the fever is acute', presents the suggestion that the epilepsy referred to might be simply the convulsions occurring in children with a high fever, rather than epilepsy itself. Is this perhaps what Dioscorides meant? Violets' cooling properties would suggest a more obvious and effective use here.

## 18TH CENTURY DISCREPANCY

Quincy in the 18th century refers only to the opening qualities of violets. He ranks them among the cathartics, not the cordials, despite Miller's designation of them as one of the four cordial flowers. They are 'in everyone's acquaintance for their use in medicine'. Although the syrup is the only preparation, and used less often than formerly, he says, 'although among the nurses it still remains in its wonted esteem, for a safe and gentle purger of young children'. He suggests a dose of $\frac{1}{4}$–1 oz. It is too gentle, however, for purging adults: 'no dose is sufficient to make it a proper purge to them'. This heralds Cullen's later estimation of the purgative virtue as little to be depended upon. Quincy's discussion of the actions of cathartics, however, makes interesting reading. He says 'The peristaltic or vermicular motion of the guts, is such as continually propels forward their contents, from the pylorus down to the rectum. Now every irritation either quickens that motion in its natural order, or occasions some little inversions of it. In both, what but slightly adhered to the coats or inner membranes, will be loosen'd and shook off and carried forward with their contents; and they will also be more agitated, and thus render'd more fluid. By this only is it manifest, how a cathartic hastens and increases the discharges by stool. But the same manner of operation also carries its effects much further in proportion to the force of the stimulus. For where it is great, all the appendices of the bowels and even all the viscera in the abdomen, will by a consent of their parts, that is, a communication of nerves, be pulled or twitched, so as to affect their respective juices in the same manner as the intestines themselves affect their contents. The consequence of which must be, that a great deal will be drained back into the intestines, and made a part of what they discharge. And when we consider the vast number of glands in the intestines, with the outlets of those viscera opening there into, and particularly of the pancreas and liver; it will be no wonder what vast quantities, especially in full constitutions, may be carried off by one small purge'.

Miller suggests broader actions for violets and designates them one of the four cordial flowers. (Culpeper has five cordial flowers: rose *Rosa* species, viola, borage *Borago officinalis*, bugloss *Echium vulgare* and lemon balm *Melissa officinalis*). They are cooling, moistening and laxative, good in affections of the breast and lungs, helping coughs and pleuritic pains. He records purging in children 'to open and cool their bodies'. He mentions use in enemas and ointments against inflammations. The seed is reckoned good for the stone and gravel, he says. He concords with Quincy that the only official preparation is the syrupus violarum. Hill offers a recipe for the syrup of violets; boiling water is to be poured upon the flowers, just enough to cover them, and it is to stand all night. It is then strained and sugar added at the rate of 2 lb to each pint, and then melted over a fire. He, like Quincy, accounts it mainly a gentle purge for children, although he adds the use of the dried leaves in decoction for enemas and the infusion works by urine.

## MORE MODERN APPLICATION AND CANCER

The plant does not appear in Cook or Ellingwood in the USA. The *National Botanic Pharmacopoeia* summarizes the view in the early part of the 20th century. Inflammation of the eyes, sleeplessness, pleurisy, jaundice and quinsy 'are but a few of the ailments for which it was held potent'. The general assessment in this herbal is not encouraging; 'it is still found in the pharmacopoeias though many of the virtues ascribed to it in the Middle Ages have not stood the test of time and greater experience'. This might be a rather severe judgement, particularly given the narrow range of application mode and lack of emphasis or perhaps sufficient appreciation of its broader cooling properties within its earlier context. Its reputation as an anti cancer herb is explored in Potter's Bulletin of May 1902, cited by the *National Botanic Pharmacopoeia*, recording the case of a 67-year-old lady whose malignant throat tumour was cleared in 14 days on use of this herb. They suggest a handful of fresh green violet leaves infused in 1 pint of boiling water covered for 12 hours; this is strained and warmed; then a piece of lint, soaked in this infusion, is placed 'where the malady is', covered with oilskin or flannel and changed when dry or cold.

Grieve writes expansively on violets, covering various traditions and more modern use, this latter being mainly as a colouring agent and perfume and as source of the medicinally employed syrup of violets. She records Macer's use against 'wykked sperytis', their association with death of the young and Napoleon's adoption of them as his emblem. She gives detailed advice on their cultivation. The chemical constituents are introduced: the odorous principle and the blue colouring, the glycoside viola-quecitin, and salicylic acid. The laxative properties are covered, syrup of violets being found in the *British Herbal Pharmacopoeia* for infants in doses of $\frac{1}{2}$–1 teaspoon or more with equal quantities of oil of almonds. Older uses are summarized. Grieve also reports on the action of the underground stems or rhizomes as strongly emetic and purgative, sometimes used as adulterant to ipecacuanha. 40 to 50 grains (2600–3250 mg), she says, of the powdered root is said to 'act violently, inciting nausea and great vomiting and nervous affection, due to the pronounced emetic qualities of the alkaloid contained'. The seeds are recorded as purgative and diuretic in urinary complaints, particularly for gravel. She then introduces its more recent use as cancer treatment, internal and external, especially for cancer of the throat and tongue. Later she mentions cancer of the colon in the context of the great quantity of fresh leaf supply needed for such treatment. She gives a recipe and a resounding commendation for an ointment; 'place 2 oz of the best lard in a jar in the oven till it becomes quite clear. Then add about 36 fresh violet leaves. Stew them in the lard for about an hour till the leaves are the consistency of cooked cabbage. Strain and when cold put into a covered pot for use. This is a good old-fashioned Herbal remedy which has been allowed to fall into disuse. It is good as an application for superficial tubercles in the glands of the neck, Violet Leaves Tea being drunk at the same time'.

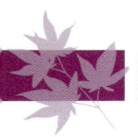

Weiss refers to its reputation as a 'native cough remedy'. Although the flowers are gathered to make the syrup, their use, he says, is for colouring other remedies rather than as a cough remedy. Unlike Grieve, Weiss tells us the most valuable part is the root containing saponin, glycoside, anthocyan and small amount of emetine-like alkaloid. While the alkaloid does not occur in sufficient amounts to compare with ipecacuanha, the saponin offers a useful expectorant prescribed in chronic bronchitis. The British Herbal Pharmacopoeia makes no mention of the root. The dried leaves and flowers are expectorant and antineoplastic, indicated for malignant disease both internally and externally, bronchitis and chronic naso-pharyngeal catarrh.

So quite a journey from Dioscorides and Galen – heartburn, eyes, prolapse, sore throat, inflammations and epilepsy to a sometime laxative, cough remedy and latterly anticancer application. Some more recent writers still seem to deem the herb worthy of inclusion and presumably, hence, use. Chevallier and Hoffman we have seen recommend its use for coughs, colds, catarrh and wider applications. Menzies Trull, categorizing its primary action as demulcent expectorant, gives the many traditional uses and introduces application in malignant conditions. Wood tells us the leaves and flowers are used together; he notes an affinity to the lymphatic system and thus an indication in lymphatic stagnation and swollen glands together with dry skin and constipation. He notes too its use in cancer of the breast, lymphatics, lungs and skin, citing Hall's recommendation in changes in components of the blood that may foreshadow cancer.

Bartram records the plant's actions as mild antiseptic, soothing expectorant, used in bronchitis, children's chest complaints and persistent cough; also for mouth ulcers, cystitis with hot acid urine, urethritis, vaginal trichomonas, and fibroids as a douche to ease pain. It is internally and externally antineoplastic, he says, used in cancer of the lungs, alimentary canal and breast. He makes the same reference as Potter's Bulletin to the lady with throat cancer. Williamson too has a broad enough coverage; 'it has been used in syrups for coughs and colds, bronchitis and catarrh; and externally for skin inflammation. Antiinflammatory and diuretic effects have been reported for a leaf extract. It is reputed to be expectorant and anti-microbial due to saponin content'.

## RECOMMENDATIONS

- Syrup of flowers for coughs, colds and catarrh.
- Syrup as laxative for children.
- Leaves as antiinflammatory in fevers and rheumatism.
- A cooling demulcent for urinary conditions.
- A cooling liver herb for bile/bilious conditions.
- For indications of heat – heartburn, anger.

Dosage: the *British Herbal Pharmacopoeia* recommends 2–4 g three times a day of dried herb but the history of use of violets indicates fresh leaf preparations, mainly the syrup for children in Quincy's dose of $\frac{1}{4}$–1 fl oz (7–30 mL) and as a vehicle for stronger lung remedies for adults.

Since herbalists today are just as likely to prescribe another Viola species, namely *Viola tricolor*, we have included a discussion of this herb for completeness.

## Viola tricolor

### A LATER DISCOVERY

This violet does not appear in Dioscorides, Galen nor Pliny. It first appears among our authors in the 1500s. Parkinson tags 'Pansyes' or 'Hearts ease' to the end of the entry for garden violets, denoting them somewhat hotter and drier, yet very temperate. Their viscous or glutinous juice mollifies, though less so than mallows; like violets it is good for hot diseases of the lungs and chest, agues, convulsions and the falling sickness in children; the decoction is used to bathe those troubled with the itch or scabs; the juice or distilled water helps old sores; and it has a reputation for healing green wounds too, he says. Culpeper, under a separate entry from violets, says heart'sease is really saturnine (yet under the sign of Cancer) 'something cold, viscous and slimy'; a strong decoction of the herbs and flowers, or syrup if preferred, is an excellent cure for venereal disease, the 'French pox', since the herb is 'a gallant antivenereal'. It is the spirit of it, he says, which is good for convulsions in children, and the falling sickness, as well as a remedy for inflammations of the lungs and breasts, 'pleurisy, scabs, itch, etc.'.

Dodoens and Fuchs differ little from Parkinson and Culpeper in designation of use, but diverge somewhat in their rationale. Fuchs names *Viola tricolor* a herb of Jupiter, warm and dry, in taste sticky and a little sharp or biting, little different from the temperament of comfrey. It has a certain cutting power, he says, so that 'nowadays' they teach its use for asthmatics and inflammation of the chest. It can purge pus collected in the thorax and chest. Consequently, he adds, it is used to help epilepsy in children. It aids pruritus and eczema and all imperfections of the skin through its moderate sharpness and astringency; and because of its stickiness it heals ulcers. Dodoens agrees it is dry and temperate in cold and heat. It is again tempting to wonder, as in sweet violet, whether the falling sickness in children, referred to by the Renaissance authors here, might not be simply convulsions resulting from high temperature, but Dodoens on this matter is more specific; he says, 'These floures boyled and drunken, do cure and stay the beginnings of the falling evill, or the disease of young children that fome and cast up froth (wherefore it is called in high Dutch Freyscham) [presumably frei Schaum, literally free foam]'. He continues, as others, with the whole herb to cleanse the lungs and breast, as very good for fevers and inward inflammations or heats. The final paragraph, referring to external and internal use of the powder in wine for healing wounds, is still in Latin in our copy, so whether an addition or translation omission is not clear.

Dodoens offers a number of names for the plant – in Greek flox and flogion, Latin Viola flammea, Flamma, 'at this time' Viola tricolor, herba trinitatis, iacea and herba clavellata, indicating some past tradition, but its source is obscure. In English he says the plant is called Pances, Love in idleness and Harts-ease, in French Pensee and Pensee menue. Gerard offers us four types of the plant: heartsease *Viola tricolor*; upright heartsease 'Viola assurgens tricolor'; wilde pansies 'Viola tricolor sylvestris'; and stony heartsease 'Viola tricolor petraea'. If the attribution is correct, he perhaps solves the Greek source for us, saying 'it seemeth to be the viola flammea, which Theophrastus calleth floga, which is also called flogion', though it was clearly little repeated by other writers. Gerard adds other names, herba trinitatis, pensees in French, paunsies in English, live in idleness, cull me to you and three faces in a hood. For Gerard the herb is 'obscurely cold, but more evidently moist, of tough and slimy juice, like mallow, hence it moistens and softens though to a lesser extent'. He repeats the familiar uses 'as the later physitions write: for ague especially in children to combat 'convulsions' and fits of the falling sicknesse it is thought to cure'. Use for lungs, skin and ulcers follows; for the French disease too, attributed to a report of Costaeus: 'it doth wonderfully ease the paines … and cureth the same'.

Bauhin reprises the above uses. He includes in addition the distilled water for inflammations and pains of the belly in children, and its use for angina, which is here angina of the throat, tonsillitis. He cites Camerarius on distillation of the leaves, stems and flowers to be drunk for 9 days or more by those with venereal disease, since it brings on a sweat. He cites Mattioli too who recommends similarly the distilled water to induce sweating, the herb being hot and dry. Bauhin adds how Mattioli says he has much experience of its use. In the 1554 text, Mattioli describes the herb, expresses doubt whether this iacea, 'as it is called by some' is that which some modern writers praise for ruptures of the intestines, as comfrey; and how some say it brings considerable help for those with breathing afflictions and inflammation of the lungs, and to heal itch and other blemishes of the skin. He makes no claims here regarding his own experience. Could this then perhaps date at least Mattioli's exploration of the plant's virtues, so that in a later manuscript he could claim wide experience in its use?

In the 18th century Miller has only a bare record; the leaves only are used 'but seldom'. It is accounted mucilaginous and vulnerary, good to take off the gripes in children and to prevent fits arising from thence. I cannot find the plant in Quincy, Hill nor later Cullen. It does not appear in Cook nor Ellingwood.

## MODERN APPLICATIONS

Grieve offers many more names for this plant, among them: love lies bleeding, love idol, Jack-jump-up-and-kiss-me, Kit run in the fields, stepmother, pink-eyed John, bouncing Bet. Discussing the names, she tells how the plant was prized for its potency as a love charm 'in ancient days', hence perhaps its name heartsease. Along with the uses familiar from the Renaissance authors, Grieve records the flowers were formerly considered cordial and good in diseases of the heart, attributing to this use a further possible origin of the name heartsease. Grieve offers no source for use of the plant as cordial. There is no obvious mention of this in our authors up to this point. Perhaps it stems more from a folk tradition, or perhaps even from a misinterpretation somewhere of the word angina. Leyel (1949) accords the herb cordial properties. She cites the past uses as in our authors, adds 'a good herb in disorders of the blood', and mentions its use in moist cutaneous eruptions in children', particularly crusta lactea and tinea capitis. Then she continues 'it has derived the name heartsease partly from its early use as a heart tonic and it can be taken quite safely to relieve palpitation of the heart and to soothe a tired and irritable heart. Since Leyel edited Grieve's book, we should not be too surprised at a similar entry, but it does not take us nearer to a source for the 'early use' in this context.

Wren's edition of 1932 records on diaphoretic and diuretic actions, used in blood disorders and catarrhal infections, with chief use for moist cutaneous eruptions in children, and then a reference to our earlier use for convulsions – it 'is said to prevent convulsions', and here the convulsions covered are those in both epilepsy *and* asthma.

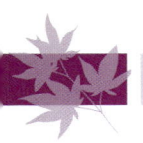

Weiss carries no reference to the heart. It is a saponin drug, he says, with adequate literature to commend it for skin conditions. He cites its successful use by paediatricians for eczema in infants, milk crust and other chronic skin conditions, used as a tea internally, added to feeds or mixed with milk, and externally as compress. It can be useful for eczema in adults too, though taken over a long time. Adults may use it in powder form. In this context, it is interesting that an in-vitro study showed that the infusion, decoction and ethanolic extract of aerial parts of heartsease showed antimicrobial activity against seven bacteria and *Candida albicans*. These extracts were more effective than extracts with solvents which selected for particular types of compound (Witkowska-Banaszczak et al 2005). This included moderate activity against *Pseudomonas aeruginosa*, which is an unusual finding. Weiss adds French sources reporting efficacy in tuberculous skin conditions.

The *British Herbal Pharmacopoeia* is a little broader. It records actions as expectorant, diuretic, antirheumatic, antiinflammatory and laxative; with indications for pertussis, acute bronchitis, cystitis, polyuria and dysuria, capillary fragility and cutaneous affections, specifically for eczema and skin eruptions with serous exudate particularly associated with rheumatic symptoms. It is noteworthy that there is no diaphoretic action mentioned here, given this designation in Wren and its earlier reputation in bringing on sweats in venereal disease. Such diaphoresis may represent a key action in remedying skin conditions.

Modern authors tend to stay close to the *British Herbal Pharmacopoeia* and the older tradition and omit any cordial reference. Chevallier and Hoffman cover the familiar ground of skin conditions, chest complaints, diuresis and rheumatism. Hoffman explains 'Both the salicylates and the rutin contained in heartsease are anti-inflammatory. This action helps explain the traditional use of the herb for arthritis. The saponins account for its expectorant action, while the mucilage it contains soothes the chest'. He adds that the high rutin concentration will help counter capillary fragility, hence its benefit for bruising, broken capillaries and oedema; use in atherosclerosis, hence against high blood pressure, and a laxative action are included too. Wood suggests the name heartsease stems from the French pensees, since the heart is associated with thoughts and how the original use was to reduce excessive and unwanted thoughts. He suggests the use for eczema originated in homeopathy, though use in, for example, Parkinson, for itch, scabs and old sores demonstrates an older tradition. Bartram adds alterative, depurative, antiallergic and anti-acne actions to the British Herbal Pharmacopoeia list, noting the herb as rich in zinc. We find here too a recent reprise of the indication for venereal disease with Bartram citing 'some success reported by Dr Schlegel, Moscow, for STDs generally, with ulceration'. He adds too its use for milk crust and ringworm, for prevention of capillary haemorrhage in steroid therapy and that it is still taken as daily in Russia 'by those with a tendency to TB and scrofula'.

## RECOMMENDATIONS

- Acute and chronic skin conditions, internal and external.
- Eczema and other exudative complaints – internal and external.
- Urinary conditions.
- Arthritic and rheumatic conditions.
- For avoiding convulsions in children with a high temperature.

Dosage: the *British Herbal Pharmacopoeia* recommends 2–4 g three times a day of dried herb.

## VIOLA ODORATA CONSTITUENTS

Reviews: Bradley (2006), Williamson (2003).

### Polysaccharides

Mucilage 18% (flowers, wild, France) (Lamaison et al 1991).
Mucilage, mainly galactose, glucose and galacturonic acid (leaves, wild, Russia) (Drozdova & Bubenchikov 2005).

### Volatile oils

var. Parma, total 0.02%, characteristic aliphatic aldehydes: nona-2,6-dienal; aliphatic alcohols (leaf, cultivated, France) (Cu et al 1992).
Flowers, total 0.003% diethylphthalate 26%, alpha-curcumene 18%, zingiberene 17%, dihydro-beta-ionone 10% (Bradley 2006); trans-alpha-ionone gives the characteristic fragrance (Werkhoff et al 1991).

### Phenylpropanoids

Anthocyanins 4%, total flavonoids 1.1%: flavonol glycosides (flowers, wild, France) (Lamaison et al 1991).
Leaf, flower, methyl salicylate (Bradley 2006).

### Macrocycylic peptides

Leaf, macrocyclic peptides with 28–37 amino acids, which are very stable because of a unique knot formed of three disulfide bonds in a cysteine knot. They are common in Violaceae such as *Viola odorata* and may have a cytotoxic action through disruption of membranes (Herrmann et al 2008).

## VIOLA TRICOLOR CONSTITUENTS

Reviews: Bisset & Wichtl (2001), Bradley (2006), Williamson (2003).

### Polysaccharides

Total 10%, highest during flowering (Bradley 2006).

### Saponins

Recent studies have not confirmed the presence of triterpene saponins in violet and heartsease (Bradley 2006).

### Carotenoids

Violaxanthins (Molnar et al 1986).

### Phenolic acids

Total 0.3% (mean of 11 samples, repeated over 7 years, cultivated, Lithuania) (Rimkiene et al 2003).

### Flavonoids

Up to 2%, mainly rutin, higher in flowers (Bradley 2006).

### Flavonol diglycosides

Quercetin diglycosides, kaempferol diglycoside, isorhamnetin diglycoside (commercial, Hungary) (Vukics et al 2003b).
Quercetin and glycosides (wild, Hungary) (Papp et al 2004).

### Flavone glycosides

Apigenin-C-diglycosides, luteolin-C-diglycosides, chryosoeriol-C-glycoside; apigenin-C,O-glycosides (commercial, Hungary) (Vukics et al 2008b).
Luteolin glycoside (wild, Hungary) (Papp et al 2004).

### Tannins

Total 3% (11 samples, mean of 8 years, cultivated, Lithuania) (Rimkiene et al 2003).

### Macrocyclic peptides

(Svangård et al 2004), found in all *Viola* species so far investigated (wild, Sweden) (Göransson et al 2003), see *Viola odorata*.

## RECOMMENDATIONS ON SAFETY

- Do not use in people with glucose-6-phosphate dehydrogenase (G6PD) deficiency.

G6PD deficiency is an inherited disorder which makes the person vulnerable to haemolytic anaemia in response to triggers such as certain drugs. It is most common in people of Mediterranean and African ancestry. An infant of 9 months was given half a cup of tea of heartsease. The child became ill within an hour and moderate haemolysis was treated in hospital and the child was well after 24 hours (Behmanesh & Abdollahi 2002). Reading undertaken in the course of preparing this book suggests that in some countries herbal teas are given to infants with less caution than would be normal in Britain.

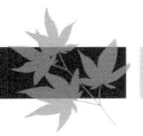

A study on the dried whole plant, including roots, of *Viola yedoensis* isolated two dicoumarins, dimeresculetin and euphobetin, and the coumarin esculetin (Zhou et al 2009). The in vitro study found that all three compounds showed anticoagulant activity using models which represent the intrinsic coagulation pathway, the extrinsic pathway and the transformation of fibrinogen into fibrin. This in vitro study was designed in the search for new pharmaceuticals. Whether the compounds are absorbed or absorbed at adequate concentration to have the same effect in vivo is not known.

## REFERENCES

Akeroyd J 2003 The encyclopaedia of wild flowers. Parragon, Bath.

Behmanesh Y, Abdollahi M 2002 Haemolysis after consumption of *Viola tricolor*. WHO Drug Information 16:15–16.

Bisset NG, Wichtl M (eds) 2001 Herbal drugs and phytopharmaceuticals, 2nd edn. Medpharm, Stuttgart.

Bradley PR 2006 British herbal compendium, vol 2. British Herbal Medicine Association, Bournemouth.

Coombs RE 1981 Violets. Croom Helm, London.

Cu JQ, Perineau F, Gaset A 1992 Volatile components of violet leaves. Phytochemistry 31:571–573.

Davis PH (ed.) 1965 Flora of Turkey, vol 1. Edinburgh University Press, Edinburgh.

De Cleene M, Lejeune MC 2003 Compendium of symbolic and ritual plants in Europe. Man and Culture Publishers, Ghent.

Drozdova IL, Bubenchikov RA 2005 Composition and antiinflammatory activity of polysaccharide complexes extracted from sweet violet and low mallow. Pharmaceutical Chemistry Journal 39:197–200.

Genders R 1958 Pansies, violas and violets. Garden Book Club, London.

Gibbons B, Brough P 1996 Wild flowers of Britain & Northern Europe. Chancellor Press, London.

Göransson U, Broussalis AM, Claeson P 2003 Expression of *Viola cyclotides* by liquid chromatography-mass spectrometry and tandem mass spectrometry sequencing of intercysteine loops after introduction of charges and cleavage sites by aminoethylation. Analytical Biochemistry 318:107–117.

Green MH (ed.) 2001 The Trotula. University of Pennsylvania Press, Philadelphia.

Grey-Wilson C 1994 Wild flowers of Britain and Northwest Europe. Dorling Kindersley, London.

Herrmann A, Burman R, Mylne JS 2008 The alpine violet, *Viola biflora*, is a rich source of cyclotides with potent cytotoxicity. Phytochemistry 69:939–952.

Lamaison JL, Petitjean-Freytet C, Carnat A 1991 Comparative study of *Viola lutea* Huds., *V. calcarata* L. and *V. odorata* L. Plantes Medicinales et Phytotherapie 25:79–88.

Leyel H 1949 Hearts-ease: herbs for the heart. Faber and Faber, London.

Malécot V, Marcussen T, Munzinger J, et al 2007 On the origin of the sweet-smelling Parma violet cultivars (Violaceae): wide intraspecific hybridization, sterility, and sexual reproduction. American Journal of Botany 94:29–41.

Marcussen T 2006 Allozymic variation in the widespread and cultivated *Viola odorata* (Violaceae) in western Eurasia. Botanical Journal of the Linnean Society 151:563–571.

Papp I, Apati P, Andrasek V, et al 2004 LC-MS analysis of antioxidant plant phenoloids. Chromatographia 60:S93–S100.

Molnar P, Szabolcs J, Radics L 1986 Naturally occurring di-cis-violaxanthins from *Viola tricolor*: isolation and identification by 1HNMR spectroscopy of four di-cis-isomers. Phytochemistry 25:195–199.

Rimkiene S, Ragazinskiene O, Savickiene N 2003 The cumulation of wild pansy (*Viola tricolor* L.) accessions: the possibility of species preservation and usage in medicine. Medicina (Kaunas, Lithuania) 39:411–416.

Stace C 1991 New flora of the British Isles. Cambridge University Press, Cambridge.

Svangård E, Göransson U, Hocaoglu Z 2004 Cytotoxic cyclotides from *Viola tricolor*. Journal of Natural Products 67:144–147.

Vukics V, Kery A, Guttman A 2008a Analysis of polar antioxidants in heartsease (*Viola tricolor* L.) and Garden pansy (*Viola x wittrockiana* Gams.). Journal of Chromatographic Science 46:823–827.

Vukics V, Ringer T, Kery A, et al 2008b Analysis of heartsease (*Viola tricolor* L.) flavonoid glycosides by micro-liquid chromatography coupled to multistage mass spectrometry. Journal of Chromatography A 1206:11–20.

Werkhoff P, Bretschneider W, Güntert M, et al 1991 Chirospecific analysis in flavor and essential oil chemistry. B, Direct enantiomer resolution of trans-α-ionone and trans-α-damascone by inclusion gas chromatography. Zeitschrift für Lebensmittel-Untersuchung und –Forschung 192:111–115.

Williamson E 2003 Potter's herbal cyclopaedia. CW Daniel, Saffron Walden.

WHO 1989 Medicinal plants in China. World Health Organization, Manila.

Witkowska-Banaszczak E, Bylka W, Matlawska I, et al 2005 Antimicrobial activity of *Viola tricolor* herb. Fitoterapia 76:458–461.

Zhou HY, Hong JL, Shu P, et al 2009 A new dicoumarin and anticoagulant activity from *Viola yedoensis* Makino. Fitoterapia 80:283–285.

# Index

Abdominal pain, *Stachys officinalis* (wood betony), 311
Abortions
   *Apium graveolens* (wild celery), 84
   *Daucus carota* (wild carrot), 149–150
   *Ocimum basilicum* (basil), 223–224
   *Ruta graveolens* (rue), 283–285
Abscesses
   *Galium aparine* (goosegrass), 175
   *Rosa damascene* (damask rose), 259
   *Tussilago farfara* (coltsfoot), 319
Absinthe, safety, 118
*Achillea millefolium* (yarrow), 187, 204–205, 217, 246
Achlorhydria, *Artemisia absinthium* (wormwood), 116
*Adiantum capillus-veneris* (maidenhair fern), 175
*Aesculus hippocastanum* (horse-chestnut), 246
*Agrimonia eupatoria* (agrimony), 47–55, 48f, 50f
   Coffin, 51
   constituents, 54b
      antioxidants, 53
      condensed tannins, 54
      flavone glycosides, 54
      flavonoids, 54
      flavonol glycosides, 54
      hydrolyzable tannins, 54
      isoflavonoids, 54
      phenolic acids, 54
      polyphenols, 53
      silica content, 53
      tannins, 54
      triterpenes, 54
      volatile oil, 54
   Cook, 52
   Cullen, 51
   Culpeper, 49–50
   Dioscorides, 47
   dosage, 54
   Ellingwood, 52
   Fuchs, 47–49
   Galen, 47
   Green, 51
   Grieve, 47–49
   Herbal of Pseudo-Apuleius, 49
   Hildegard of Bingen, 49
   Hill, 51
   Hool, 51

   National Botanic Pharmacopoeia, 51
   Parkinson, 47–49
   parts used, 47
   Pelikan, 53
   quality, 47
   Quincy, 51
   recommendations, 53–54
      astringent, 52–53
      combination therapies, 129, 277, 313
      diabetes mellitus, 54
      diarrhoea, 52–54
      dysmenorrhoea, 54
      exanthemas, 54
      jaundice, 51
      leucorrhoea, 54
      liver disease, 52, 54
      menorrhagia, 54
      non-mainstream uses, 51–52
      spring tonic, 52
      tonic, 52
      topical uses, 50–51
      urinary tract infections, 54
      wounds, 53–54
   Renaissance, 47–49
*Agrimonia odorata*, 47–49
Agrimony *see Agrimonia eupatoria* (agrimony)
*Ajuga chaemapitys* (ground pine), 139, 313–314
*Alcea rosea* (hollyhock), 67–78
   combination therapies, 264–265
   description, 67
   *see also Althaea officinalis* (marshmallow)
*Alchemilla vulgaris* (lady's mantle), 57–65, 58f, 60f
   Apuleius, 59
   British Herbal Pharmacopoeia, 62
   constituents, 64b
      flavonoids, 62, 64
      hydrolyzable tannins, 64
      tannins, 62, 64
      triterpenes, 64
   Culpeper, 59–60
   Dalechamps, 57–59, 61
   description, 57
   Dodoens, 59–60
   dosage, 63
   Fuchs, 59
   Grieve, 62
   Hill, 61–62
   Mattioli, 59

   *The National Botanic Pharmacopoeia*, 62
   nomenclature/identification, 57–59
   Parkinson, 59, 61
   parts used, 57
   Pelikan, 63
   Pliny, 57–59
   quality, 57
   Quincy, 61
   recommendations, 63
      antioxidant, 62–63
      astringency, 62
      breast laxity, 61, 63
      conception problems, 61
      diarrhoea, 63
      gastrointestinal system, 62
      heavy periods, 63
      leucorrhoea, 61, 63
      menorrhagia, 63
      miscarriages, 61
      skin ageing, 63
      vomiting, 63
      'women's herb', 59–61
      wounds, 59–61, 63
   research, 62–63
   safety, 63–64
   Salernitan school, 59
   Tragus, 59
   Treben, Maria, 62
   Williamson, 62
Alexipharmic panacea, *Centaurium erythraea* (centuary), 141–142
Alkaloids
   *Galium aparine* (goosegrass), 179
   *Glechoma hederacea* (ground ivy), 188
   *Ruta graveolens* (rue), 293
Allergic contact dermatitis
   *Arctium lappa* (burdock), 102
   *Inula helenium* (elecampene), 207
Allergies
   *Apium graveolens* (wild celery), 87
   *Artemisia vulgaris* (mugwort), 133
   *Aloysia triphylla* (lemon verbena), 264–265, 333–334
   *Alpinia galanga* (galangal), 248
*Althaea officinalis* (marshmallow), 67–78, 68f, 70f
   British Herbal Pharmacopoeia, 75
   Coffin, 73
   constituents, 76b–77b
      coumarins, 76
      flavonoids, 77

# INDEX

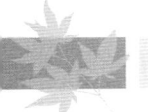

high molecular weight polysaccharides, 74
phenolic acids, 76
polysaccharides, 76
Culp, 73
Dalechamps, 72
description, 67–71
Dioscorides, 67, 71
Dodoens, 69, 72
dosage, 76
18th century, 73–76
*On the Faculties of Foods*, 70
Fernie, 74
Fuchs, 71
Galen, 69–71
Gerard, 72
Hill, 73
Hippocrates, 67–69
Ibn Sina, 67, 71
Mattioli, 69–72
Myddfai, physicians of, 71
*National Botanic Pharmacopoeia*, 74
19th Century, 73–76
nomenclature problems, 70–71
Parkinson, 72–73
Pelikan, 75–76
*Pharmacopoeia Londinensis*, 73
Pliny, 69, 71–72
Priest, 75
Quincy, 73
recommendations, 76–77
  astringents, 69–70, 72
  bronchitis, 74
  combinations, 75
  combination therapies, 127–128, 177, 205, 248, 277, 321
  cough, 71, 74–75
  dandruff, 67
  diarrhoea and vomiting, 69–70
  diuretics, 69
  dysentery, 69–70
  emollients, 73
  gastrointestinal tract, 76
  gynaecological problems, 69
  haemorrhages, 67–69
  lachrymal fistulas/abscesses, 67
  mixed remedies, 72
  neuralgic pain, 74
  respiratory system, 76
  swellings, 69
  topical uses, 76
  urinary problems, 76
  wounds, 69
Robinson, 74
safety, 77
  drug interactions, 77
Salernitan herbal, 71
Serapio, 71
temperament, controversy of, 71–73
Theophrastus, 67–69
Turner, 67, 71
Weiss, Rudolf, 75
Wood, 76
Wren, 74
Amenorrhoea, *Ruta graveolens* (rue), 292
*The American Dispensatory*, *Scrophularia nodosa* (figwort), 304
Ancient Greece, weights and measures, 42t
Ancient Rome, weights and measures, 42t
Ancients, *Rosa damascene* (damask rose), 257–258
Andreas Vesalius, *Ocimum basilicum* (basil), 224–225
Andrews, A C
  *Daucus carota* (wild carrot), 147, 150
  *Hyssopus officinalis* (hyssop), 193
Angina, *Hyssopus officinalis* (hyssop), 193–195
Anglo-Saxon sources, 2
Anorexia
  *Artemisia absinthium* (wormwood), 116
  *Centaurium erythraea* (centuary), 142
Anthelmintics
  *Artemisia absinthium* (wormwood), 112–113, 116
  *Centaurium erythraea* (centuary), 140
  *Hyssopus officinalis* (hyssop), 193–197
  *Ruta graveolens* (rue), 290–292
Anthocyanins, *Rosa damascene* (damask rose), 268
Anthroposophical medicine, 39
Antibacterals
  *Inula helenium* (elecampene), 207
  *Ocimum basilicum* (basil), 226
  *Viola tricolour* (heartsease), 346
Anticatarrhals
  *Glechoma hederacea* (ground ivy), 187–188
  *Ocimum basilicum* (basil), 227
Anticonvulsants, *Viola tricolour* (heartsease), 345–346
Antidepressants, *Ocimum basilicum* (basil), 225
Antiinflammatories
  *Arctium lappa* (burdock), 99
  *Glechoma hederacea* (ground ivy), 187
  *Tussilago farfara* (coltsfoot), 322
*Verbena officinalis* (vervain), 333
*Viola odorata* (sweet violet), 344
Antimicrobials, *Arctium lappa* (burdock), 98
Antioxidants
  *Agrimonia eupatoria* (agrimony), 53
  *Alchemilla vulgaris* (lady's mantle), 62–63
  *Apium graveolens* (wild celery), 85–86
  *Arctium lappa* (burdock), 99
  *Ocimum basilicum* (basil), 226
  *Rubus idaeus* (raspberry), 276
Antiperspirants, *Rosa damascene* (damask rose), 257–258
Antiseptics
  *Ocimum basilicum* (basil), 225
  *Viola odorata* (sweet violet), 344
Antispasmodics
  *Fumaria officinalis* (fumitory), 170
  *Paeonia officinalis* (paeony), 235
  *Ruta graveolens* (rue), 292
  *Tussilago farfara* (coltsfoot), 322
Antitussives, *Inula helenium* (elecampene), 207
Antonius Musa, *Stachys officinalis* (wood betony), 309
Anxiety, *Stachys officinalis* (wood betony), 314
Aphrodisiacs
  *Apium graveolens* (wild celery), 84
  *Daucus carota* (wild carrot), 149
*Apium graveolens* (wild celery), 79–89, 80f, 82f
  *British Herbal Pharmacopoeia*, 81
  Chevallier, 84
  constituents, 86b–87b
    flavonoids, 87
    furanocoumarins, 87
    phthalides, 87
    volatile oils, 86–87
  Cullen, 79
  Culpeper, 83–84
  Dalechamps, 79–81
  Dioscorides, 79, 81–83, 85
  Dodoens, 83–84
  dosage, 86–87
  folklore, 82–83
  Fuchs, 81, 83–84
  Galen, 81, 83
  Gerard, 83–84
  Grieve, 85
  Hildegard of Bingen, 81
  Hippocrates, 79
  hot and dry theme, 83–84
  Ibn Sina, 81, 83
  identification problems, 79–82
  Mattioli, 81–82
  Miller, 84–85

350

# INDEX

Myddfai texts, 85
Palladius, 79
Parkinson, 83–84
parts used, 79
Pelikan, 86
Pliny, 79, 81–82
quality, 79
Quincy, 84–85
recommendations, 86–87
    abortions, 84
    antioxidant, 85–86
    as aphrodisiac, 84
    arthritis, 85–86
    calmative, 86
    combination therapies, 83–86, 195
    contraception, 84
    diuretic, 86
    hormone effects, 84
    *see also specific effects*
    later uses, 84–85
    menses, 83, 86
    modern uses, 85–86
    as nervine, 85
    swollen breasts, 84
    topical use, 86
    urinary tract, 86
Renaissance, 79–81, 83–84
safety, 87–88
    allergy, 87
    furanocoumarin reactions, 88
    oral allergy syndrome (OAS), 87–88
    phytophotodermatitis, 88
    pregnancy, 87
    thyroxine supplements, 87
Sturtevant, 79
Theophrastus, 79
Turner, 81–82
Apothecaries' system, 43
Apuleius, 1, 6
    *Alchemilla vulgaris* (lady's mantle), 59
    *Arctium lappa* (burdock), 95–98
    *Artemisia vulgaris* (mugwort), 129
    *Centaurium erythraea* (centaury), 140
    *Daucus carota* (wild carrot), 149–150
    *Glechoma hederacea* (ground ivy), 183
    *Inula helenium* (elecampane), 206
    *Ocimum basilicum* (basil), 225
    *Paeonia officinalis* (paeony), 235–236
    *Potentilla erecta* (tomentil), 247–248
    *Ruta graveolens* (rue), 288, 291
    *see also The Herbal of Pseudo-Apuleius*

Arabic authors, 1
Arber, Ann R, 1
    *Herbals, their Origins and Evolution: A Chapter in the History of Botany 1470-1670*, 1, 26–27
*Arctium lappa* (burdock), 91–103, 92f
    Apuleius, 95–98
    Bartram, 91–93
    Bauhin, 96–97
    *The British Pharmaceutical Codex*, 91–93
    Chevallier, 93
    Coffin, 93–96
    constituents, 101b
        flavonoids, 101
        lignans, 100–101
        phenolic acids, 101
        polyacetylenes, 101
        polysaccharides, 101
        volatile oil, 101
    Cook, 93–95
    Culpeper, 91, 95–96
    Dalechamps, 96–97
    Dioscorides, 95–96
    dosage, 101
    early texts, 95–96
    Essiac, 98–100
        recipe, 98–99
    Fuchs, 96–97
    Galen, 96
    Gerard, 97
    Grieve, 91–93, 95
    Hoffman, 93
    Hool, 93–95
    Mattioli, 96
    Mill, 96
    Myddfai physicians, 95
    nomenclature problems, 95
    parts used, 91
    Pliny, 96
    quality, 91–95
    Quincy, 93–95
    recommendations, 98–101
        antiinflammatory, 99
        antimicrobial actions, 98
        as antioxidant, 99
        arthritis, 100
        breast cancer, 100
        cancer, 99–101
        combination therapies, 93–95, 98, 130, 169
        COX-2 inhibition, 99
        cystitis, 98
        depurative actions, 93
        diuretic, 91–93, 97, 100
        gastrointestinal system, 100
        inducible nitrogen oxide synthase (iNOS), 99–100
        leucorrhoea, 100

        miscarriage, 101
        osteoarthritis, 95
        skin disease, 93, 100–101
        topical uses, 101
        womb laxity, 100
    Renaissance, 95–96
    safety, 102
        allergic contact dermatitis, 102
    Salernitan texts, 97
    Turner, 96–97
    Williamson, 98
    Wren, 95
*Arctium minus* (lesser burdock), 91
*Aristolchia* (birthwort), 139
Aristophanes, *Drimia maritima* (squill), 159
Aristotle, *Rubus idaeus* (raspberry), 271–273
*Artemisia abrotanum* (southernwood), 128
*Artemisia absinthium* (wormwood), 105–121, 106f, 108f
    Barker, 114
    Bartram, 115
    Bauhin, 110, 113–114
    bitters, 111–112
    *British Herbal Pharmacopoeia*, 113, 116
    constituents, 117b
        flavonoids, 117
        phenolic acids, 117
        phenypropanoids, 117
        sesquiterpene lactones, 117
        volatile oils, 117
    Cook, 105, 110–111, 114
    Cullen, 111–115
    Culpeper, 105–107, 113
    Dalechamps, 110, 113–114
    Dioscorides, 107–109, 112, 115
    Dodoens, 110, 112
    dosage, 116–117
    Ellingwood, 110–111
    Fuchs, 105, 110
    Galen, 105–107, 109
    Gerard, 112
    Grieve, 105, 113–114
    Hildegard of Bingen, 105, 110, 114
    Hill, 110–111
    Ibn Sina, 105–107, 109–110, 112–113, 115
    identity, 107
    Menzies-Trull, 113–115
    Miller, 110, 112–115
    Mills, 111, 113
    *National Botanic Pharmacopoeia*, 114
    *Old English Herbarium*, 109, 115
    Parkinson, 107, 110
    parts used, 105

**351**

# INDEX

Pelikan, 116
Pliny, 109, 112–113, 115
quality, 105
Quincy, 110, 112–113, 115
recommendations, 116–117
    achlorhydria, 116
    anorexia, 116
    anthelmintic, 112–113, 116
    astringent properties, 107–109
    atonic dyspepsia, 116
    atonic vaginal discharge, 113
    bad breath, 116
    biliary disorders, 111–112
    combination therapies, 112–113, 288
    depression, 116
    digestion, 107–109
    emmenagogue action, 113
    eyes, 115
    gall bladder, 116
    gastrointestinal system, 109
    hormonal effects, 113
    jaundice, 110
    leucorrhoea, 113
    melancholy, 114
    mental health, 114
    nausea and vomiting, 116
    oedemata, 107–109
    rheumatic pain, 115
    sore throats, 115
    spleen disease, 107–109
    topical use, 115–116
safety, 118–119
    porphyria, 118
    pregnancy, 118
Salernitan herbal, 105–107, 113
Serapio, 109–110, 112–114
Steiner, Rudolf, 116
Turner, 110
*see also* Absinthe
*Artemisia vulgaris* (mugwort), 123–134, 124f, 126f
Apuleius, 129
Bauhin, 127–129
Brassavola, Antonio Musa, 125–127
constituents, 132b
    coumarins, 132
    flavones, 132
    flavonoids, 132
    monoterpenes, 132
    polyphenols, 132
    sesquiterpenes, 132
    volatile oils, 132
Cook, 130
Culpeper, 125, 127, 129–130
Dalechamps, 125–128
Dioscorides, 123–125, 129
Dodoens, 127, 129
dosage, 131

Falloppio, Gabrielle, 125–127
Fuchs, 125–127
Galen, 123–125
Gerard, 127, 129
Grieve, 123, 129–130
Hoffman, 130
Hool, 128
Ibn Sina, 130
Mabey, 130
Mattioli, 125–127
Menzies-Trull, 130
nomenclature problems, 123–125
*The Old English Herbarium*, 125, 129
Parkinson, 129
Pliny, 123, 129
quality, 123–127
Quincy, 130
recommendations, 131–132
    combination therapies, 127–130
    digestion, 129
    gout, 130–131
    gynaecological problems, 127–129
    joint problems, 129
    labour facilitation, 128
    menstrual problems, 131
    migraine, 130
    nervous affections, 130–131
    opium antidote, 130–131
    premature birth prevention, 128
    spirituality, 130–131
    suppressed menstruation, 128
    unexplained infertility, 131
    urinary problems, 129
    urinary stones, 129
Renaissance, 129
Ruellius, 125–127
safety, 133
    allergies, 133
    lactation, 133
    malaria therapy, 133
    pregnancy, 133
Salernitan herbal, 129–130
Salernitan Plateraius, 127–128
Stevens, John, 128–129
*Trotula*, 127–128, 130
Turner, 123–125
*Woman's Herbal Book of Health*, 130
Arteriosclerosis, *Ruta graveolens* (rue), 285–287
Arthritis
    *Apium graveolens* (wild celery), 85–86
    *Arctium lappa* (burdock), 100
    *Centaurium erythraea* (centaury), 142
    *Lamium album* (white deadnettle), 217

    *Potentilla erecta* (tomentil), 245–246, 250
    *Ruta graveolens* (rue), 292
    *Scrophularia nodosa* (figwort), 303–304
    *Viola tricolour* (heartsease), 346
*Articella* (Constantine the African), 8
Asthma
    *Hyssopus officinalis* (hyssop), 193
    *Rubus idaeus* (raspberry), 276
    *Ruta graveolens* (rue), 291
    *Tussilago farfara* (coltsfoot), 321
    *Viola tricolour* (heartsease), 345–346
Astringents
    *Agrimonia eupatoria* (agrimony), 52–53
    *Alchemilla vulgaris* (lady's mantle), 62
    *Althaea officinalis* (marshmallow), 69–70, 72
    *Artemisia absinthium* (wormwood), 107–109
    *Glechoma hederacea* (ground ivy), 187
    *Paeonia officinalis* (paeony), 233–235
    *Potentilla erecta* (tomentil), 241–246, 248
    *Rosa damascene* (damask rose), 263
    *Rosa damascene* (damask rose) recommendations, 263
    *Rubus idaeus* (raspberry), 271, 276–277
Atonic dyspepsia, *Artemisia absinthium* (wormwood), 116
Atonic vaginal discharge, *Artemisia absinthium* (wormwood), 113
Atopic dermatitis, *Lamium album* (white deadnettle), 217
*Atropa belladonna* (deadly nightshade), 248–249
Averoes, 7
Avicenna *see* Ibn Sina (Avicenna)
Avoirdupois system, 42–43

Bacterial infections, *Rubus idaeus* (raspberry), 276
Bad breath, *Artemisia absinthium* (wormwood), 116
Barker, J
    *Artemisia absinthium* (wormwood), 114
    *Hyssopus officinalis* (hyssop), 193, 197
    *Rosa damascene* (damask rose), 264
Bartram, Thomas, 3, 19
    *Arctium lappa* (burdock), 91–93
    *Artemisia absinthium* (wormwood), 115

# INDEX

*Daucus carota* (wild carrot), 149
*Encyclopedia of Herbal Medicine*, 19
*Ruta graveolens* (rue), 285–287
*Verbena officinalis* (vervain), 332–333
Basil *see Ocimum basilicum* (basil)
Bauhin, Johann, 2, 12–13
    *Arctium lappa* (burdock), 96–97
    *Artemisia absinthium* (wormwood), 110, 113–114
    *Artemisia vulgaris* (mugwort), 127–129
    *Centaurium erythraea* (centaury), 139–140
    *Drimia maritima* (squill), 160
    *Fumaria officinalis* (fumitory), 167
    *Glechoma hederacea* (ground ivy), 186
    *Historica plantarum universalis*, 12–13
    *Hyssopus officinalis* (hyssop), 196
    *Inula helenium* (elecampene), 203
    *Lamium album* (white deadnettle), 213, 215–216
    *Paeonia officinalis* (paeony), 235–236
    *Potentilla erecta* (tomentil), 243–245, 247
    *Rosa damascene* (damask rose), 257, 260
    *Rubus idaeus* (raspberry), 275
    *Ruta graveolens* (rue), 290, 292
    *Scrophularia nodosa* (figwort), 301–302
    *Stachys officinalis* (wood betony), 309, 311, 313–314
    *Tussilago farfara* (coltsfoot), 317–319
    *Verbena officinalis* (vervain), 329
    *Viola odorata* (sweet violet), 339–343
    *Viola tricolour* (heartsease), 345
Bayberry (*Myrica cerfera*), 248
Beach, Wooster, 32
Beauty, *Rosa damascene* (damask rose), 265
Beck, L Y
    *Daucus carota* (wild carrot), 145
    *Glechoma hederacea* (ground ivy), 183
    *Rosa damascene* (damask rose), 258
*Bellis perennis* (daisy), 185
Belly ache, *Paeonia officinalis* (paeony), 233–234
Betony *see Stachys officinalis* (wood betony)
*Bidens tripartita* (bur-marigold, water agrimony), 47–49
Bile cleansing, *Fumaria officinalis* (fumitory), 167

Biliary disorders, *Artemisia absinthium* (wormwood), 111–112
Bilious conditions
    *Potentilla erecta* (tomentil), 244
    *Stachys officinalis* (wood betony), 309–311
    *Viola odorata* (sweet violet), 344
Birth preparation, *Rubus idaeus* (raspberry), 280
*Birthwort* (*Aristolchia*), 139
Bistort (*Polygonium bistorta*), 127–128
Bites
    *Centaurium erythraea* (centaury), 142
    *Inula helenium* (elecampene), 205
Bitters, *Artemisia absinthium* (wormwood), 111–112
Black cohosh (*Cimicifuga racemosa*), 203, 313–314
Black eyes, *Hyssopus officinalis* (hyssop), 193
Bladder problems, *Stachys officinalis* (wood betony), 311
Bladder stones
    *Galium aparine* (goosegrass), 177–178
    *Verbena officinalis* (vervain), 331
Bloodletting, Thomson, Samuel, 29
Blood purification
    *Fumaria officinalis* (fumitory), 165–167
    *Galium aparine* (goosegrass), 173–175
Bock, Hieronymus *see* Tragus
Bogbean (*Menyanthes trifoliata*), 93–95, 321
Boils, *Galium aparine* (goosegrass), 175, 177
Bone, Kerry, 4, 19–22
Boneset (*Eupatorium perfoliatum*), 321
*The Botanic Guide to Health* (Coffin), 16–17
*Botanicum Officinale* (Miller), 15
Bradley, Peter, 3, 19
Bramble *see Rubus fruticosa* (bramble)
Brassavola, Antonio Musa, *Artemisia vulgaris* (mugwort), 125–127
Breast cancer, *Arctium lappa* (burdock), 100
Breast laxity, *Alchemilla vulgaris* (lady's mantle), 61, 63
Breathlessness, *Inula helenium* (elecampene), 203
*British Herbal* (Hill), 16
*British Herbal Compendium*, *Glechoma hederacea* (ground ivy), 181
*The British Herbal Pharmacopoeia*, 3, 19
    *Alchemilla vulgaris* (lady's mantle), 62
    *Apium graveolens* (wild celery), 81

*Artemisia absinthium* (wormwood), 113, 116
*Centaurium erythraea* (centaury), 141
*Daucus carota* (wild carrot), 151
*Drimia maritima* (squill), 162
*Fumaria officinalis* (fumitory), 165, 167, 170
*Galium aparine* (goosegrass), 178
*Glechoma hederacea* (ground ivy), 181
*Hyssopus officinalis* (hyssop), 197
*Inula helenium* (elecampene), 204–205
*Potentilla erecta* (tomentil), 248–249
*Rosa damascene* (damask rose), 264
*Rubus idaeus* (raspberry), 277
*Ruta graveolens* (rue), 285–288, 291
*Scrophularia nodosa* (figwort), 303–304
*Stachys officinalis* (wood betony), 313
*Tussilago farfara* (coltsfoot), 322
*Verbena officinalis* (vervain), 332–333
*Viola odorata* (sweet violet), 338
*Viola tricolour* (heartsease), 346
*The British Pharmaceutical Codex*
    *Arctium lappa* (burdock), 91–93
    *Ruta graveolens* (rue), 291
*British Pharmacopoeia*, 15
    *Rosa damascene* (damask rose), 264
Bronchitis
    *Althaea officinalis* (marshmallow), 74
    *Inula helenium* (elecampene), 203–205
    *Ruta graveolens* (rue), 293
    *Tussilago farfara* (coltsfoot), 321
    *Viola odorata* (sweet violet), 344
Brown, P S, 30
Bruises
    *Hyssopus officinalis* (hyssop), 195, 198
    *Scrophularia nodosa* (figwort), 301–302
Buchan, William, 32
    *Domestic Medicine (The Family Physician)* 32
Bufadienolides, *Drimia maritima* (squill), 161–162
Burdock *see Arctium lappa* (burdock)
Bur-marigold (*Bidens tripartita*) 47–49
Burns
    *Galium aparine* (goosegrass) 175
    *Scrophularia nodosa* (figwort), 301–303

# INDEX

*Calendula officinalis* (marigold), 165–167
Calmative, *Apium graveolens* (wild celery), 86
Cancer
   *Arctium lappa* (burdock), 99–101
   *Galium aparine* (goosegrass), 173–175
   *Scrophularia nodosa* (figwort), 301–302
   *Viola odorata* (sweet violet), 343–344
Canker, *Rubus idaeus* (raspberry), 277
*Capsella bursa-pastoris*, 246
*Capsicum annuum* (cayenne pepper)
   combination therapies, 93–95, 248, 276–278, 321
   Thomson, Samuel, 29
Carcinogens, *Ocimum basilicum* (basil), 228
Cardenolides, *Drimia maritima* (squill), 161, 163
Cardiac glycosides
   *Drimia maritima* (squill), 157, 161–162
   *Scrophularia nodosa* (figwort), 304
Carmichael, A G, *Potentilla erecta* (tomentil), 245
Carminatives
   *Inula helenium* (elecampene), 205–207
   *Ocimum basilicum* (basil), 226–227
Carotenoids, *Viola tricolour* (heartsease), 347
Carrot, wild *see Daucus carota* (wild carrot)
Catarrh
   *Hyssopus officinalis* (hyssop), 195, 198
   *Viola odorata* (sweet violet), 344
*Cautions Against the Immoderate Use of Snuff* (Hill), 16
Cayenne pepper *see Capsicum annuum* (cayenne pepper)
*Centaurium erythraea* (centaury), 135–144, 136f, 138f
   Apuleius, 140
   Bauhin, 139–140
   *British Herbal Pharmacopoeia*, 141
   Coffin, 137, 140
   constituents, 142b–143b
      coumarins, 143
      flavonoids, 143
      phenolic acids, 143
      secoiridoid glycosides, 142–143
      sterols, 143
      xanthones, 143
   Culpeper, 135–137, 139–141
   Dalechamps, 139–140
   Dioscorides, 135, 137, 139–140

Dodoens, 137, 139
dosage, 142
Fernie, 140
Fox, 140
Fuchs, 139–140
Galen, 137, 139–140, 142
Gerard, 137, 139
Grieve, 140
Hoffman, 140–141
Hool, 140
Ibn Sina, 137, 140
Mattioli, 139–140
Menzies-Trull, 140–141
Miller, 135–137, 140
Parkinson, 139–140
part used, 135
Pelikan, 140–141
Pliny, 137
quality, 135
Quincy, 139–141
recommendations, 142
   alexipharmic panacea, 141–142
   anorexia, 142
   anthelmintic, 140
   arthritis, 142
   bites, 142
   combination therapies, 93–95, 139, 141, 165–167, 169
   depression, 140
   dyspepsia, 142
   emmenagogue, 141
   eye conditions, 139
   fevers, 139–140
   gout, 139
   hip ailments, 139–140
   indigestion, 140
   irritable bowel syndrome, 142
   joint pain, 142
   muscular pain, 142
   musculoskeletal conditions, 139–140
   sciatica, 139
   stings, 142
   tendon diseases, 139
   topical uses, 142
   ulcers, 137
   viscous humours, 140–141
   wound healing, 137–139, 142
Riddle, 141
Robinson, 140
safety, 143
   pregnancy, 143
Serapio, 139–140
Turner, 139–140
Wood, 140
Centuary *see Centaurium erythraea* (centuary)
Cephalic action, *Stachys officinalis* (wood betony), 313

Chamomile *(Matricaria recutita)*, 129, 187, 248–249, 321, 334
Cherry *(Prunus virginiana)*, 321
Chevallier, Andrew, 3, 19
   *Apium graveolens* (wild celery), 84
   *Arctium lappa* (burdock), 93
   *Fumaria officinalis* (fumitory), 170
   *Hyssopus officinalis* (hyssop), 197
   *Inula helenium* (elecampene), 204–205
   *Lamium album* (white deadnettle), 217
   *Paeonia officinalis* (paeony), 235, 237
   *Potentilla erecta* (tomentil), 249
   *Rosa damascene* (damask rose), 264
   *Ruta graveolens* (rue), 285–287
   *Scrophularia nodosa* (figwort), 303
   *Stachys officinalis* (wood betony), 309–312
   *Verbena officinalis* (vervain), 331–333
   *Viola odorata* (sweet violet), 338, 344
   *Viola tricolour* (heartsease), 346
Cheyne, George, 32
Chickweed *(Stellaria media)*, 129
Children
   *Ruta graveolens* (rue), 293
   *Tussilago farfara* (coltsfoot), 323
Cholangitis, *Stachys officinalis* (wood betony), 314
Cholecystitis, *Stachys officinalis* (wood betony), 314
Chromones, *Tussilago farfara* (coltsfoot), 323
Chronic cholecystitis, *Stachys officinalis* (wood betony), 314
Chronic heart failure, *Drimia maritima* (squill), 162
*Cimicifuga racemosa* (black cohosh), 203, 313–314
*Cinnamomum zeylanicum* (cinnamon), 225
*Circa Instans* (Matthaeus Platearius), 9
Cloves *(Syzygium aromaticum)*, 225, 276
Clusius, *Lamium album* (white deadnettle), 213
Coffin, Albert Isaiah, 3, 16–17, 29, 31, 187
   *Agrimonia eupatoria* (agrimony), 51
   *Althaea officinalis* (marshmallow), 73
   *Arctium lappa* (burdock), 93–96
   *The Botanic Guide to Health*, 16–17
   *Centaurium erythraea* (centuary), 137, 140
   *The Diseases of Women and Children*, 16–17

*Galium aparine* (goosegrass), 175, 177
*Rubus idaeus* (raspberry), 277–278
*Skleton's Botanic Reader*, 16–17
*Stachys officinalis* (wood betony), 313
*A Treatise on Midwifery*, 16–17
*Verbena officinalis* (vervain), 331–333
Colds
   *Hyssopus officinalis* (hyssop), 195
   *Viola odorata* (sweet violet), 344
Colic, *Stachys officinalis* (wood betony), 309–311
Colitis, *Potentilla erecta* (tomentil), 249
Colouring agent, *Viola odorata* (sweet violet), 343–344
Combination therapies
   *Achillea millefolium* (yarrow), 187, 204–205, 217, 246
   *Adiantum capillus-veneris* (maidenhair fern), 175
   *Aesculus hippocastanum*, 246
   *Agrimonia eupatoria* (agrimony), 277, 313
   *Ajuga chaemapitys* (ground pine), 139, 313–314
   *Alcea rosea* (hollyhock), 264–265
   *Aloysia triphylla* (lemon verbena), 264–265
   *Alpinia galanga* (galangal), 248
   *Althaea officinalis* (marshmallow), 75, 177, 205, 248, 277, 321
   *Apium graveolens* (wild celery), 83–86, 195
   *Aristolchia* (birthwort), 139
   *Artemisia absinthium* (wormwood), 112–113, 288
   *Artemisia vulgaris* (mugwort), 127–130
   *Atropa belladonna*, 248–249
   *Bellis perennis* (daisy), 185
   *Capsella bursa-pastoris*, 246
   *Capsicum annuum* (cayenne pepper), 248, 276–278, 321
   *Centaurium erythraea* (centuary), 139, 141
   *Cimicifuga racemosa* (black cohosh), 203, 313–314
   *Cinnamomum zeylanicum* (cinnamon), 225
   *Commiphora molmol* (myrrh), 177, 338–339
   *Crocus sativus* (saffron), 338–339
   *Daphne laureola* (spurge laurel), 331–332
   *Echinacea augustifolia*, 203
   *Eleutherococcus senticoccus*, 217

*Eupatorium perfoliatum* (boneset), 321
*Euphrasia officinalis* (eyebright), 321
*Filipendula ulmaria* (meadowsweet), 313
*Foeniculum vulgare* (fennel), 285–287
*Fumaria officinalis* (fumitory), 165–167, 169
*Galium aparine* (goosegrass), 175, 177
*Gentiana lutea* (gentian), 139
*Geum urbanum* (wood avens), 277, 313
*Glechoma hederacea* (ground ivy), 185, 187, 321
*Glycyrrhiza glabra* (liquorice root), 187, 203–204, 233, 331–332
*Gratiola officinalis* (hedge hyssop), 285–287
*Hamamelis virginiana* (witch hazel), 247–248
*Harpagophytum procumbens* (devil's claw), 303–304
*Hermodactylus tuberosus*, 246–247
*Humulus lupulus* (hops), 248
*Hyssopus officinalis* (hyssop), 195, 197, 225, 287
*Inula helenium* (elecampene), 187, 203–205, 225, 321
*Juniperus communis* (juniper), 177–178
*Lamium album* (white deadnettle), 211, 217
*Lavandula angustifolia* (lavender), 321, 334
*Leonurus cardiaca* (motherwort), 225
*Linum usissitatum* (linseed), 177–178
*Lobelia inflata* (lobelia), 203, 248, 276–277
*Marrubium vulgare* (horehound), 321–322
*Matricaria recutita* (chamomile), 187, 248–249, 321, 334
*Melaleuca alternifolia* (tea tree oil), 177
*Melissa officinalis* (lemon balm), 248–249
*Mentha piperita* (peppermint), 248–249, 334
*Mentha pulegium* (pennyroyal), 332–333
*Menyanthes trifoliata* (bogbean), 321
*Mercuralis perennis* (dog's mercury), 331–332
*Myrica cerfera* (bayberry), 248
*Ocimum basilicum* (basil), 225
*Paeonia lactiflora* (paeony), 233

*Parietaria diffusa*, 333
*Peganum harmala* (white-flowered harmal), 289
*Petroselinon crispum* (parsley root), 177–178
*Phytoclacca americana* (poke root), 331–332
*Picrasma excelsa* (quassia), 177–178
*Potentilla erecta* (tomentil), 245–248
*Primula veris* (cowslip), 205
*Prunus virginiana* (cherry), 321
*Quercus rober* (oak), 277–278
*Rhus aromatica*, 177
*Rosa damascene* (damask rose), 264–265
*Rosmarinus officinalis* (rosemary), 313, 321
*Rubus idaeus* (raspberry), 141, 276–278, 313, 332–333
*Rumex crispus* (dock), 302
*Ruta graveolens* (rue), 285–289
*Sambuccus niger* (elderflower), 175, 313, 319
*Sanguisorba officinalis* (greater burnet), 313
*Scrophularia nodosa* (figwort), 302–304
*Scutellaria galericulata* (English skullcap), 313
*Scutellaria lateriflora*, 313–314
*Scutellaria lateriflora* (skullcap), 313
*Senna alexandrina* (senna), 285–287
*Silybum marianum* (milk thistle), 313
*Solanum nigrum* (nightshade), 319
*Stachys officinalis* (wood betony), 313, 321
*Stillingia sylvatica*, 302
*Symphyticum officinale* (comfrey), 203–204
*Syzygium aromaticum* (cloves), 225, 276
*Teucrium chamaedrys* (germander), 139
*Teucrium scordonia* (wood sage), 313–314
*Thymus longicaulis*, 333
*Thymus vulgaris* (thyme), 321
*Tilia* (lime), 334
*Tussilago farfara* (coltsfoot), 205, 319, 321–322, 331–332
*Urtica dioica* (stinging nettle), 85–86
*Valeriana officinalis*, 313
*Valeriana officinalis* (valerian), 277–278
*Verbascum thapsis* (mullein), 204–205, 322
*Verbena officinalis* (vervain), 331–333

# INDEX

*Verbena triphylla* (lemon verbena), 333–334
*Viola odorata* (sweet violet), 338–339
*Zingiber officinale* (ginger), 177–178, 246, 248
Comfrey *(Symphyticum officinale)*, 203–204
*Commiphora molmol* (myrrh), 127, 177, 338–339
Common dog-violet *(Viola riviniana)*, 337
Common mallow *see Malva sylvestris* (common mallow)
*Compleat English Dispensatory* (Quincy), 15
Compounds, The Salernitan herbal, 26
Conception aid
  *Alchemilla vulgaris* (lady's mantle), 61
  *Daucus carota* (wild carrot), 149
  *Ocimum basilicum* (basil), 223
Condensed tannins
  *Agrimonia eupatoria* (agrimony), 54
  *Potentilla erecta* (tomentil), 249–250
Constantine the African, 8
  *Articella*, 8
  *Pantegni*, 8
  *Viaticum*, 8
Constipation, *Rosa damascene* (damask rose), 267
Constituents, 41–42
  *see also individual species; specific constituents*
Contraception, *Apium graveolens* (wild celery), 84
Convalescence, *Verbena officinalis* (vervain), 334
Convulsions
  *Paeonia officinalis* (paeony), 235–237
  *Viola tricolour* (heartsease), 346
Cook, William, 3, 17, 32
  *Agrimonia eupatoria* (agrimony), 52
  *Arctium lappa* (burdock), 93–95
  *Artemisia absinthium* (wormwood), 105, 110–111, 114
  *Artemisia vulgaris* (mugwort), 130
  *Daucus carota* (wild carrot), 150–151
  *Galium aparine* (goosegrass), 177
  *Hyssopus officinalis* (hyssop), 196
  *Inula helenium* (elecampene), 203, 206
  *Paeonia officinalis* (paeony), 235
  *Rosa damascene* (damask rose), 263
  *Rubus idaeus* (raspberry), 277–278
  *Scrophularia nodosa* (figwort), 302

*Verbena officinalis* (vervain), 332–333
Cordial powders, *Rosa damascene* (damask rose), 262
*Coriandrum sativum* (coriander), 81
Coughs
  *Althaea officinalis* (marshmallow), 71, 74–75
  *Daucus carota* (wild carrot), 152
  *Glechoma hederacea* (ground ivy), 187–188
  *Hyssopus officinalis* (hyssop), 195, 198
  *Inula helenium* (elecampene), 203
  *Rosa damascene* (damask rose), 263
  *Rubus idaeus* (raspberry), 276
  *Tussilago farfara* (coltsfoot), 319, 321–322
  *Viola odorata* (sweet violet), 344
Coumarins
  *Althaea officinalis* (marshmallow), 76
  *Artemisia vulgaris* (mugwort), 132
  *Centaurium erythraea* (centuary), 143
  *Galium aparine* (goosegrass), 179
Cowslip *(Primula veris)*, 205
COX-2 inhibition, *Arctium lappa* (burdock), 99
Creeping cinquefoil *(Potentilla reptans)*, 241
*Crocus sativus* (saffron), 338–339
Crohn's disease, *Potentilla erecta* (tomentil), 249
Croup, *Rubus idaeus* (raspberry), 276
*Cruydeboek* (Dodoens), 12
Cullen, William, 3, 16
  *Agrimonia eupatoria* (agrimony), 51
  *Apium graveolens* (wild celery), 79
  *Artemisia absinthium* (wormwood), 111–115
  *Fumaria officinalis* (fumitory), 167, 169–170
  *Hyssopus officinalis* (hyssop), 196
  *Potentilla erecta* (tomentil), 248
  *Rosa damascene* (damask rose), 263
  *Rubus idaeus* (raspberry), 276
  *Ruta graveolens* (rue), 290–291
  *Stachys officinalis* (wood betony), 312–313
  *Verbena officinalis* (vervain), 327
  *Viola odorata* (sweet violet), 343
Culpeper, Nicholas, 2, 14–15
  *Agrimonia eupatoria* (agrimony), 49–50
  *Alchemilla vulgaris* (lady's mantle), 59–60
  *Althaea officinalis* (marshmallow), 73

*Apium graveolens* (wild celery), 83–84
*Arctium lappa* (burdock), 91, 95–96
*Artemisia absinthium* (wormwood), 105–107, 113
*Artemisia vulgaris* (mugwort), 125, 129–130
*Centaurium erythraea* (centuary), 135–137, 139–141
classification system, 24
*Daucus carota* (wild carrot), 149–150
*Drimia maritima* (squill), 157–161
*The English Physician* (Culpeper's Herbal), 14–15, 27
*Fumaria officinalis* (fumitory), 165, 167
*Galium aparine* (goosegrass), 178
*Glechoma hederacea* (ground ivy), 185–187
*Hyssopus officinalis* (hyssop), 196
*Inula helenium* (elecampene), 203, 205–207
*Key to Galen and Hippocrates, theor Method of Physick*, 15
*Lamium album* (white deadnettle), 216
*Ocimum basilicum* (basil), 221–223
*Paeonia officinalis* (paeony), 233–236
*A Physicall Directory (A Translation of the London Dispensatory)*, 14–15
*Potentilla erecta* (tomentil), 244–248
*Rosa damascene* (damask rose), 260–262
*Rubus fruticosa* (bramble), 275
*Ruta graveolens* (rue), 290–291
*Scrophularia nodosa* (figwort), 299, 302
*Stachys officinalis* (wood betony), 311–312
*Tussilago farfara* (coltsfoot), 317–319
*Verbena officinalis* (vervain), 331–332
*Viola odorata* (sweet violet), 342–343
*Viola tricolour* (heartsease), 344–345
Culpeper's Herbal *see The English Physician (Culpeper's Herbal)*
Curtis, Alva, 32
Cystitis
  *Arctium lappa* (burdock), 98
  *Galium aparine* (goosegrass), 177
  *Glechoma hederacea* (ground ivy), 187

Daily tonic, *Drimia maritima* (squill), 159

# INDEX

Daisy *(Bellis perennis)*, 185
Dalechamps, Jacques, 2
   *Alchemilla vulgaris* (lady's mantle), 57–59, 61
   *Althaea officinalis* (marshmallow), 72
   *Apium graveolens* (wild celery), 79–81
   *Arctium lappa* (burdock), 96–97
   *Artemisia absinthium* (wormwood), 110, 113–114
   *Artemisia vulgaris* (mugwort), 125–128
   *Centaurium erythraea* (centaury), 139–140
   *Fumaria officinalis* (fumitory), 167, 169
   *Galium aparine* (goosegrass), 177–178
   *Glechoma hederacea* (ground ivy), 185–186
   *Inula helenium* (elecampane), 203
   *Lamium album* (white deadnettle), 213, 215
   *Potentilla erecta* (tomentil), 243–248
   *Stachys officinalis* (wood betony), 309, 311–312
   *Verbena officinalis* (vervain), 332
   *Viola odorata* (sweet violet), 339–343
Damask rose *see Rosa damascene* (damask rose)
Dandelion *(Taraxacum officinale)*, 165–167
Dandruff, *Althaea officinalis* (marshmallow), 67
*Daphne laureola* (spurge laurel), 331–332
Daucine, *Daucus carota* (wild carrot), 151
*Daucus carota* (wild carrot), 145–154, 146f, 148f
   Andrews, 147, 150
   Apuleius, 149–150
   Bartram, 149
   Beck, 145
   *British Herbal Pharmacopoeia*, 151
   constituents, 153b
      daucine, 151
      flavonoids, 153
      furanocoumarins, 153
      porphyrins, 151
      volatile oils, 153
   Cook, 150–151
   Culpeper, 149–150
   Dioscorides, 145–151
   Dodoens, 147
   dosage, 152
   Galen, 145–150
   Gerard, 147, 149–150
   Grieve, 151
   Hippocrates, 149–150
   identity problems, 145–149
   Mattioli, 145–148
   Miller, 149
   Oribasius, 147
   Pelikan, 151
   Pliny, 145, 147, 149–150
   quality, 145
   Quincy, 150
   recommendations, 151–152
      abortifacient, 149–150
      aphrodisiac, 149
      conception aid, 149
      cough, 152
      gastrointestinal effects, 150, 152
      gout, 152
      gynaecology, 149–150
      reproduction, 149–150, 152
      rheumatic conditions, 152
      thread worms, 152
      topical uses, 152
      urinary problems, 149, 152
   Riddle, 149–150
   safety, 152
      pregnancy, 152
   Salernitan herbal, 149–150
   Serapio, 147
   Theophrastus, 147
   Turner, 149
   Weiss, 151
*Daucus gingidium*, 145
Deadly nightshade *(Atropa belladonna)*, 248–249
Debility, *Rosa damascene* (damask rose), 264
*De Historia Stirpium Commentarii* (Fuchs), 10–11
De l'Obel, Matthias, *Potentilla erecta* (tomentil), 247
*De Materia Medica* (Dioscorides), 1, 4, 23
Deodorants, *Rosa damascene* (damask rose), 257–258
Depression
   *Artemisia absinthium* (wormwood), 116
   *Centaurium erythraea* (centaury), 140
   *Ocimum basilicum* (basil), 225–226
   *Stachys officinalis* (wood betony), 314
Depurative actions, *Arctium lappa* (burdock), 93
Dermatitis, *Galium aparine* (goosegrass), 175
*De Simplicium Medicamentorum Temperamentis ac Facultatibus Libri Undecim* (Galen of Pergamon), 23
Devil's claw *(Harpagophytum procumbens)*, 303–304
*De Viribus Herbarum* (Macer's Herbal), 8
Dewberry *(Rubus caesius)* 271
Diabetes mellitus, *Agrimonia eupatoria* (agrimony), 54
Diaphoretics
   *Hyssopus officinalis* (hyssop), 197
   *Inula helenium* (elecampane), 206–207
Diarrhoea
   *Agrimonia eupatoria* (agrimony), 52–54
   *Alchemilla vulgaris* (lady's mantle), 63
   *Althaea officinalis* (marshmallow), 69–70
   *Potentilla erecta* (tomentil), 243–244, 249–250
   *Rosa damascene* (damask rose), 258, 264, 267
   *Rubus idaeus* (raspberry), 277, 280
Digestion
   *Artemisia absinthium* (wormwood), 107–109
   *Artemisia vulgaris* (mugwort), 129
   *Ocimum basilicum* (basil), 225
   *Verbena officinalis* (vervain), 334
Dioscorides, 1, 4–5
   *Agrimonia eupatoria* (agrimony), 47
   *Althaea officinalis* (marshmallow), 67, 71
   *Apium graveolens* (wild celery), 79, 81–83, 85
   *Arctium lappa* (burdock), 95
   *Artemisia absinthium* (wormwood), 107–109, 112, 115
   *Artemisia vulgaris* (mugwort), 123–125, 129
   *Centaurium erythraea* (centaury), 135, 137, 139–140
   *Daucus carota* (wild carrot), 145–151
   *De Materia Medica*, 1, 4, 23
   *Drimia maritima* (squill), 157, 159–160
   *Fumaria officinalis* (fumitory), 167, 170
   *Galium aparine* (goosegrass), 173
   *Hyssopus officinalis* (hyssop), 191, 193, 195–197
   *Inula helenium* (elecampane), 201, 205–206

**357**

# INDEX

*Lamium album* (white deadnettle), 213
*Leontice leontopetalum*, 57–59
*Ocimum basilicum* (basil), 221–225
*Paeonia officinalis* (paeony), 231, 233–236
*Potentilla erecta* (tomentil), 241–248
*Rosa damascene* (damask rose), 255, 257–259
*Rubus idaeus* (raspberry), 273–274
*Ruta graveolens* (rue), 287–292
*Scrophularia nodosa* (figwort), 297–301
*Stachys officinalis* (wood betony), 309, 311–314
translations of, Mattioli, 11
*Tussilago farfara* (coltsfoot), 319
*Verbena officinalis* (vervain), 327
*Viola odorata* (sweet violet), 338–339, 342–343
Diosmin, *Hyssopus officinalis* (hyssop), 197
Disease resistance, *Potentilla erecta* (tomentil), 245
*Diseases of Women* (Webb), 32–33
*The Diseases of Women and Children* (Coffin), 16–17
Diterpenes, *Glechoma hederacea* (ground ivy), 188
Diuretics
  *Althaea officinalis* (marshmallow), 69
  *Apium graveolens* (wild celery), 86
  *Arctium lappa* (burdock), 91–93, 97, 100
  *Drimia maritima* (squill), 157, 160
  *Fumaria officinalis* (fumitory), 171
  *Galium aparine* (goosegrass), 177–178
  *Glechoma hederacea* (ground ivy), 187
  *Hyssopus officinalis* (hyssop), 195–197
  *Inula helenium* (elecampene), 206
  *Ocimum basilicum* (basil), 224
  *Rosa damascene* (damask rose), 267
  *Stachys officinalis* (wood betony), 311
  *Viola tricolour* (heartsease), 346
Dock (*Rumex crispus*), 93–95, 169, 302
Dodoens, Rembert, 2, 12
  *Alchemilla vulgaris* (lady's mantle), 59–60
  *Althaea officinalis* (marshmallow), 69, 72
  *Apium graveolens* (wild celery), 83–84
  *Artemisia absinthium* (wormwood), 110, 112

*Artemisia vulgaris* (mugwort), 127, 129
*Centaurium erythraea* (centuary), 137, 139
*Cruydeboek*, 12
*Daucus carota* (wild carrot), 147
*Fumaria officinalis* (fumitory), 167
*Glechoma hederacea* (ground ivy), 183, 185
*Historie of Plantes*, 12
*Hyssopus officinalis* (hyssop), 191–195
*Inula helenium* (elecampene), 203, 205–207
*Lamium album* (white deadnettle), 213
*Ocimum basilicum* (basil), 225
*Paeonia officinalis* (paeony), 233, 235–236
*Potentilla erecta* (tomentil), 243–245, 247–248
*Rosa damascene* (damask rose), 255–257, 260–261
*Rubus fruticosa* (bramble), 275
*Rubus idaeus* (raspberry), 275
*Ruta graveolens* (rue), 290
*Scrophularia nodosa* (figwort), 299, 301–303
*Stachys officinalis* (wood betony), 312
*Stirpium historiae pentades sex sive librui XXX*, 12
*Tussilago farfara* (coltsfoot), 317–319
*Viola odorata* (sweet violet), 342–343
*Viola tricolour* (heartsease), 345
Dog's mercury (*Mercurialis perennis*), 331–332
*Domestic Medicine (The Family Physician)* (Buchan), 32
Dosages, 42–44
  parts to calculate proportions, 44
  pre-metric units, 42–44
  see also individual species
*Drimia maritima* (squill), 155–164, 156f, 158f
  Aristophanes, 159
  Bauhin, 160
  *British Herbal Pharmacopoeia*, 161
  constituents, 162b
    bufadienolides, 161–162
    cardenolides, 161, 163
    cardiac glycosides, 157, 161–162
    flavonoids, 162
    polysaccharides, 162
    proscillaridin, 161
    steroidal saponins, 161
  Culpeper, 157–161

Dioscorides, 157, 159–160
dosage, 160–162
  calculation, 161
Galen, 157–159
Hill, 160
Ibn Sina, 159
Mattioli, 157, 160
*The Old English Herbarium*, 159–160
part used, 155
Pliny, 157, 159–161
quality, 155–157
recommendations, 162
  chronic heart failure, 162
  daily tonic, 159
  diuretic, 157, 160
  dropsy, 160
  dyspnoea, 160
  expectorant, 157
  gastrointestinal problems, 157–159
  topical use, 157, 159
Robinson, 161
safety, 162–163
  drug interactions, 162
  hypertension, 162
  kidney disease, 162
  pregnancy, 163
Salernitan herbal, 159
Stannard, 159–160
Theophrastus, 157
Turner, 157–159
*Drimia sanguinea*, 155
Dropsy
  *Drimia maritima* (squill), 160
  *Galium aparine* (goosegrass), 173–175
Drug interactions
  *Althaea officinalis* (marshmallow), 77
  *Drimia maritima* (squill), 162
  *Tussilago farfara* (coltsfoot), 324
Dry conserve, *Rosa damascene* (damask rose), 262
Duration of use, *Tussilago farfara* (coltsfoot), 323–324
Dysentery
  *Althaea officinalis* (marshmallow), 69–70
  *Potentilla erecta* (tomentil), 243–245, 249
  *Rubus idaeus* (raspberry), 277
Dysmenorrhoea
  *Agrimonia eupatoria* (agrimony), 54
  *Verbena officinalis* (vervain), 334
Dyspepsia
  *Artemisia absinthium* (wormwood), 116
  *Centaurium erythraea* (centuary), 142

# INDEX

Stachys officinalis (wood betony), 314
Dyspnoea, *Drimia maritima* (squill), 160

Earache, *Galium aparine* (goosegrass), 177
Early dog-violet (*Viola reichenbachiana*), 337
Ear problems, *Hyssopus officinalis* (hyssop), 198
*Echinacea angustifolia*, 203
Eczema
    *Fumaria officinalis* (fumitory), 165–167, 171
    *Paeonia officinalis* (paeony), 237
    *Scrophularia nodosa* (figwort), 302, 304
    *Viola tricolour* (heartsease), 346
The Edinburgh New Dispensatory (Quincy), 15
18th Century, 2–3
    *Rosa damascene* (damask rose), 263–264
    *Viola odorata* (sweet violet), 343
Elderflower (*Sambuccus niger*), 175, 313, 319
Elecampene see *Inula helenium* (elecampene)
*Eleutherococcus senticoccus*, 217
Ellagitannins, *Rubus idaeus* (raspberry), 276
Ellingwood, Finley, 3, 17
    *Agrimonia eupatoria* (agrimony), 52
    *Artemisia absinthium* (wormwood), 110–111
    *Galium aparine* (goosegrass), 175, 177
    *Tussilago farfara* (coltsfoot), 321
Embryo development, *Ruta graveolens* (rue), 285
Emmenagogues
    *Artemisia absinthium* (wormwood), 113
    *Centaurium erythraea* (centuary), 141
    *Ocimum basilicum* (basil), 223–224, 228
    *Ruta graveolens* (rue), 285–288
    *Stachys officinalis* (wood betony), 311–312
    see also Menstrual problems
Emollients, *Althaea officinalis* (marshmallow), 73
Empedocles, 25
Emphysema, *Tussilago farfara* (coltsfoot), 322
Encyclopedia of Herbal Medicine (Bartram), 19

Endometriosis, *Paeonia officinalis* (paeony), 237
The English Physician (Culpeper's Herbal), 14–15, 27
English skullcap (*Scutellaria galericulata*), 313
Epilepsy
    *Hyssopus officinalis* (hyssop), 193–195, 197, 199
    *Paeonia officinalis* (paeony), 236, 238
    *Ruta graveolens* (rue), 291, 293
    *Stachys officinalis* (wood betony), 312
Errata Recentiorum Medicorum (Fuchs), 10–11
Erysipelas
    *Galium aparine* (goosegrass), 173–175
    *Rosa damascene* (damask rose), 261
Essiac see *Arctium lappa* (burdock)
*Eupatorium cannabinum* (hemp agrimony), 49
*Eupatorium perfoliatum* (boneset), 321
*Euphrasia officinalis* (eyebright), 321
Exanthemas, *Agrimonia eupatoria* (agrimony), 54
Expectorants
    *Drimia maritima* (squill), 157
    *Hyssopus officinalis* (hyssop), 196–197
    *Inula helenium* (elecampene), 207
    *Ocimum basilicum* (basil), 227
    *Viola odorata* (sweet violet), 344
External use see Topical uses
Eyebright (*Euphrasia officinalis*), 321
Eye conditions
    *Artemisia absinthium* (wormwood), 115
    *Centaurium erythraea* (centuary), 139
    *Fumaria officinalis* (fumitory), 170–171
    *Ocimum basilicum* (basil), 221–224
    *Ruta graveolens* (rue), 288
    *Stachys officinalis* (wood betony), 314
    *Viola odorata* (sweet violet), 338–339

Face wash, *Scrophularia nodosa* (figwort), 301
Falloppio, Gabrielle, *Artemisia vulgaris* (mugwort), 125–127
Fatigue, *Stachys officinalis* (wood betony), 312
Fennel (*Foeniculum vulgare*), 285–287
Fernie, W T
    *Althaea officinalis* (marshmallow), 74
    *Centaurium erythraea* (centuary), 140

*Glechoma hederacea* (ground ivy), 187
*Inula helenium* (elecampene), 206
Fevers
    *Centaurium erythraea* (centuary), 139–140
    *Galium aparine* (goosegrass), 179
    *Hyssopus officinalis* (hyssop), 196–197
    *Potentilla erecta* (tormentil), 245
    *Rosa damascene* (damask rose), 259, 267
    *Viola odorata* (sweet violet), 342
Figwort see *Scrophularia nodosa* (figwort)
*Filipendula ulmaria* (meadowsweet), 93–95, 313
Flatulence, *Ocimum basilicum* (basil), 224
Flavone(s), *Artemisia vulgaris* (mugwort), 132
Flavone glycosides, *Agrimonia eupatoria* (agrimony), 54
Flavonoid(s)
    *Agrimonia eupatoria* (agrimony), 54
    *Alchemilla vulgaris* (lady's mantle), 62, 64
    *Althaea officinalis* (marshmallow), 77
    *Apium graveolens* (wild celery), 87
    *Arctium lappa* (burdock), 101
    *Artemisia absinthium* (wormwood), 117
    *Artemisia vulgaris* (mugwort), 132
    *Centaurium erythraea* (centuary), 143
    *Daucus carota* (wild carrot), 153
    *Drimia maritima* (squill), 162
    *Galium aparine* (goosegrass), 179
    *Glechoma hederacea* (ground ivy), 188
    *Hyssopus officinalis* (hyssop), 198
    *Lamium album* (white deadnettle), 219
    *Rosa damascene* (damask rose), 268
    *Rubus idaeus* (raspberry), 280
    *Ruta graveolens* (rue), 293
    *Scrophularia nodosa* (figwort), 304
    *Stachys officinalis* (wood betony), 315
    *Tussilago farfara* (coltsfoot), 323
    *Verbena officinalis* (vervain), 333–334
    *Viola tricolour* (heartsease), 347
Flavonoid diglycosides, *Viola tricolour* (heartsease), 347
Flavonoid glycosides
    *Agrimonia eupatoria* (agrimony), 54
    *Hyssopus officinalis* (hyssop), 197
    *Rosa damascene* (damask rose), 268

**359**

# INDEX

*Rubus idaeus* (raspberry), 280
*Viola tricolour* (heartsease), 347
Fleabane *(Inula graveolens)*, 201
*Flora Britannica* (Hill), 16
*Flora Europaea*, 41
Fluxes of the blood, *Potentilla erecta* (tomentil), 248
*Foeniculum vulgare* (fennel), 285–287
Folklore, *Apium graveolens* (wild celery), 82–83
Fox, William, 3, 17
    *Centaurium erythraea* (centuary), 140
    *Galium aparine* (goosegrass), 177
    *Hyssopus officinalis* (hyssop), 196
    *Inula helenium* (elecampene), 203–204, 206
    *The Model Family Botanic Guide*, 17
    *Rubus idaeus* (raspberry), 277
    *Stachys officinalis* (wood betony), 313
    *Tussilago farfara* (coltsfoot), 319, 321
Fuchs, Leonard, 2, 10–11, 27
    *Agrimonia eupatoria* (agrimony), 47–49
    *Alchemilla vulgaris* (lady's mantle), 59
    *Althaea officinalis* (marshmallow), 71
    *Apium graveolens* (wild celery), 81, 83–84
    *Arctium lappa* (burdock), 96–97
    *Artemisia absinthium* (wormwood), 105, 110
    *Artemisia vulgaris* (mugwort), 125–127
    *Centaurium erythraea* (centuary), 139–140
    *De Historia Stirpium Commentarii*, 10–11
    *Errata Recentiorum Medicorum*, 10–11
    *Fumaria officinalis* (fumitory), 167
    *Galium aparine* (goosegrass), 173, 177–178
    *Glechoma hederacea* (ground ivy), 183, 185–186
    *Hyssopus officinalis* (hyssop), 191–193
    *Inula helenium* (elecampene), 203
    *Lamium album* (white deadnettle), 213–215
    *Paeonia officinalis* (paeony), 233–237
    *Potentilla erecta* (tomentil), 243–244
    *Rubus fruticosa* (bramble), 275
    *Scrophularia nodosa* (figwort), 299–301

*Stachys officinalis* (wood betony), 311–312
*Verbena officinalis* (vervain), 332
*Viola odorata* (sweet violet), 342–343
*Viola tricolour* (heartsease), 345
*Fumaria bastardii*, 165
*Fumaria capreolata*, 165
*Fumaria muralis*, 165
*Fumaria officinalis* (fumitory), 165–172
    Bauhin, 167
    *British Herbal Pharmacopoeia*, 165, 167, 170
    Chevallier, 170
    constituents, 171b
        isoquinoline alkaloids, 171
        phenylpropanoids, 171
    Cullen, 167, 169–170
    Culpeper, 165, 167
    Dalechamps, 167, 169
    Dioscorides, 167, 170
    Dodoens, 167
    dosage, 171
    Fuchs, 167
    Galen, 167
    Grieve, 169–170
    Hoffman, 169
    Ibn Sina, 167
    Knight, 169
    Macer, 167
    Menzies-Trull, 170
    Miller, 170
    Parkinson, 167
    parts used, 165
    Pelikan, 169
    quality, 165
    recommendations, 171
        antispasmodic, 170
        bile cleansing, 167
        blood cleansing, 165–167
        combination therapies, 93–95, 165–167, 169
        diuretic, 171
        eczema, 165–167, 171
        eyes, 170
        gastrointestinal system, 168–170
        laxative, 171
        lepra, 167–169
        melancholia, 169
        pernicious humours, 167–169
        psoriasis, 169
        skin disorders, 167–171
        topical use, 170–171
    Robinson, 169
    safety, 171
        eye conditions, 171
    Salernitan herbal, 167, 169–171
    Serapio, 167
    Weiss, 170

Fumitory *see Fumaria officinalis* (fumitory)
Furanocoumarins
    *Apium graveolens* (wild celery), 87–88
    *Daucus carota* (wild carrot), 153
Furocoumarins, *Ruta graveolens* (rue), 293

Gaius Plinius Secundus *see* Pliny the Elder
Galangal *(Alpinia galanga)*, 248
Galen of Pergamon, 1, 5–6, 23
    *Agrimonia eupatoria* (agrimony), 47
    *Althaea officinalis* (marshmallow), 69–71
    *Apium graveolens* (wild celery), 81, 83
    Arabic translations, 6
    *Arctium lappa* (burdock), 96
    *Artemisia absinthium* (wormwood), 105–107, 109
    *Artemisia vulgaris* (mugwort), 123–125
    categorization system, 24
    *Centaurium erythraea* (centuary), 137, 139–140, 142
    *Daucus carota* (wild carrot), 145–150
    *De Simplicium Medicamentorum Tempramentis ac Facultatibus Libri Undecim*, 23
    *Drimia maritima* (squill), 157–159
    dry *vs.* moist, 25
    *Fumaria officinalis* (fumitory), 167
    *Galium aparine* (goosegrass), 178
    *Glechoma hederacea* (ground ivy), 183
    heat *vs.* cold, 25
    *Hyssopus officinalis* (hyssop), 193, 195
    *Inula helenium* (elecampene), 203, 206
    *Ocimum basilicum* (basil), 221–223
    *Paeonia officinalis* (paeony), 234–237
    *Potentilla erecta* (tomentil), 245, 247–248
    purgatives, 24–25
    *Rosa damascene* (damask rose), 255, 258–259
    *Rubus fruticosa* (bramble), 275
    *Ruta graveolens* (rue), 289
    *Stachys officinalis* (wood betony), 311–312, 314
    *Tussilago farfara* (coltsfoot), 319
    *Verbena officinalis* (vervain), 329
    *Viola odorata* (sweet violet), 342–343

# INDEX

*Galeopsis tetrahit* (hemp-nettle), 211
*Galium aparine* (goosegrass), 165–167, 173–180, 174f, 176f
   *British Herbal Pharmacopoeia*, 178
   Coffin, 175, 177
   constituents, 179b
      alkaloids, 179
      coumarins, 179
      flavonoids, 179
      iridoid glycosides, 179
      polyphenolic acids, 179
      volatile oils, 179
   Cook, 177
   Culpeper, 178
   Dalechamps, 177–178
   Dioscorides, 173
   dosage, 179
   Ellingwood, 175, 177
   Fox, 177
   Fuchs, 173, 177–178
   Galen, 178
   Mattioli, 178
   Menzies-Trull, 178
   Myddfai physicians, 173–175, 177–178
   *National Botanic Pharmacopoeia*, 177–178
   part used, 173
   Pliny, 173, 177
   Priest, 175, 177
   quality, 173
   recommendations, 178–179
      abscesses, 175
      bladder stones, 177–178
      blood purification, 173–175
      boils, 175, 177
      burns, 175
      cancer, 173–175
      combination therapies, 175, 177
      cystitis, 177
      dermatitis, 175
      diuretic, 177–178
      dropsy, 173–175
      earache, 177
      erysipelas, 173–175
      fevers, 179
      as food, 178
      gout, 173–175
      jaundice, 178
      pneumonia, 173–175
      premenstrual sore breasts, 177
      rheumatism, 173–175
      ringworm, 175
      skin disease, 178–179
      swollen glands, 179
      topical use, 175, 177
      ulcers, 175
      urinary tract infections, 177, 179
      wounds, 175
   Renaissance texts, 178
   safety, 179
   Scudder, 177
*Galium spurium*, 173
Gall bladder
   *Artemisia absinthium* (wormwood), 116
   *Verbena officinalis* (vervain), 332–333
Gallotannins, *Paeonia officinalis* (paeony), 238
Gastrointestinal system
   *Alchemilla vulgaris* (lady's mantle), 62
   *Althaea officinalis* (marshmallow), 76
   *Arctium lappa* (burdock), 100
   *Artemisia absinthium* (wormwood), 109
   *Daucus carota* (wild carrot), 150, 152
   *Drimia maritima* (squill), 157–159
   *Fumaria officinalis* (fumitory), 168–170
   *Glechoma hederacea* (ground ivy), 181, 187
   *Hyssopus officinalis* (hyssop), 198
   *Paeonia officinalis* (paeony), 234
   *Rubus fruticosa* (bramble), 275
   *Rubus idaeus* (raspberry), 275–277
   *Viola odorata* (sweet violet), 339–341
*Genrall Historie of Plantes* (Gerard), 13
Gentian *(Gentiana lutea)*, 139
*Gentiana lutea* (gentian), 139
Gerard, John, 2, 13–14
   *Althaea officinalis* (marshmallow), 72
   *Apium graveolens* (wild celery), 83–84
   *Arctium lappa* (burdock), 97
   *Artemisia absinthium* (wormwood), 112
   *Artemisia vulgaris* (mugwort), 127, 129
   *Centaurium erythraea* (centuary), 137, 139
   *Daucus carota* (wild carrot), 147, 149–150
   *Genrall Historie of Plantes*, 13
   *Glechoma hederacea* (ground ivy), 185
   *Hyssopus officinalis* (hyssop), 193–195
   *Inula helenium* (elecampene), 203, 206–207
   *Lamium album* (white deadnettle), 215
   *Paeonia officinalis* (paeony), 233
   *Potentilla erecta* (tormentil), 245–246
   *Rosa damascene* (damask rose), 260–262
   *Rubus idaeus* (raspberry), 273, 275, 277–278
   *Ruta graveolens* (rue), 289–291
   *Scrophularia nodosa* (figwort), 297, 299, 301–302
   *Stachys officinalis* (wood betony), 312
   *Tussilago farfara* (coltsfoot), 317–319
   *Verbena officinalis* (vervain), 327, 329, 331
   *Viola odorata* (sweet violet), 342–343
   *Viola tricolor* (heartsease), 345
Germander *(Teucrium chamaedrys)*, 139
*Geum urbanum* (wood avens), 277, 313
Gill-Ale, *Glechoma hederacea* (ground ivy), 186–187
Gill-Tea, *Glechoma hederacea* (ground ivy), 186–187
Ginger *(Zingiber officinale)*, 98, 112–113, 177–178, 246, 248
Glass, Samuel, 32
*Glechoma hederacea* (ground ivy), 181–189, 182f, 184f
   Apuleius, 183
   Bauhin, 186
   Beck, 183
   *British Herbal Compendium*, 181
   *British Herbal Pharmacopoeia*, 181
   Coffin, 187
   constituents, 188b
      alkaloids, 188
      diterpenes, 188
      flavonoids, 188
      lectin, 188
      lignans, 188
      phenolic acids, 181, 188
      triterpenes, 181, 183, 188
      ursolic acid, 183
      volatile oils, 181, 188
   Culpeper, 185–187
   Dalechamps, 185–186
   Dodoens, 183, 185
   Fernie, 187
   Fuchs, 183, 185–186
   Galen, 183
   Gerard, 185
   Gill-Ale, 186–187
   Gill-Tea, 186–187
   Grieve, 187
   Hildegard of Bingen, 183–185
   *Historia Plantarum Universalis*, 186
   *London Dispensatory*, 185–186
   Mattioli, 183
   Myddfai physicians, 185

# INDEX

nomenclature, 185
Parkinson, 185–186
part used, 181
Pelikan, 181, 183
quality, 181–186
Quincy, 186–187
recommendations, 187–188
    anticatarrhal, 187–188
    antiinflammatory, 187
    astringent, 187
    combination therapies, 185, 187, 321
    cough, 187–188
    cystitis, 187
    digestive system, 181
    diuretics, 187
    gastrointestinal system, 187
    hip problems, 183, 185–186
    inflammed skin, 188
    jaundice, 185
    kidneys, 187
    menses, 185
    menstruation, 185–186
    tinnitus, 183–186
    topical use, 188
    urination, 185
Renaissance, 185
safety, 188
    lactation, 188
    pregnancy, 188
Salernitan herbal, 183–185
Wood, 187
*Glechoma longituba*, 181
Glucose-6-dehydrogenase deficiency, *Viola odorata* (sweet violet), 347
*Glycyrrhiza glabra* (liquorice root), 187, 203–204, 233, 331–332
Goddesses, *Rosa damascene* (damask rose), 265
Goethe, Johann Wolfgang von, 37–40
    leaf shapes, 38, 39f
    spirituality, 37–38
Golden seal *(Hydrastis candensis)*, 98
Goosegrass see *Galium aparine* (goosegrass)
Gout
    *Artemisia vulgaris* (mugwort), 130–131
    *Centaurium erythraea* (centaury), 139
    *Daucus carota* (wild carrot), 152
    *Galium aparine* (goosegrass), 173–175
    *Potentilla erecta* (tomentil), 246–247
    *Verbena officinalis* (vervain), 332
*Gratiola officinalis* (hedge hyssop), 285–287

Greater burnet *(Sanguisorba officinalis)*, 313
Greco-Roman authors, 1–4
Greece ancient, weights and measures, 42t
Green, M H, *Agrimonia eupatoria* (agrimony), 51
Grief, *Ocimum basilicum* (basil), 225–226
Grieve, Maud, 3, 18
    *Agrimonia eupatoria* (agrimony), 47–49
    *Alchemilla vulgaris* (lady's mantle), 62
    *Apium graveolens* (wild celery), 85
    *Arctium lappa* (burdock), 91–93, 95
    *Artemisia absinthium* (wormwood), 105, 113–114
    *Artemisia vulgaris* (mugwort), 123, 129–130
    *Centaurium erythraea* (centaury), 140
    *Daucus carota* (wild carrot), 151
    *Fumaria officinalis* (fumitory), 169–170
    *Glechoma hederacea* (ground ivy), 187
    *Hyssopus officinalis* (hyssop), 193, 197
    *Inula helenium* (elecampene), 205–206
    *Lamium album* (white deadnettle), 216
    *A Modern Herbal*, 18
    *Ocimum basilicum* (basil), 221
    *Potentilla erecta* (tomentil), 247–248
    *Rosa damascene* (damask rose), 264
    *Rubus idaeus* (raspberry), 276
    *Ruta graveolens* (rue), 287–291
    *Scrophularia nodosa* (figwort), 301
    *Tussilago farfara* (coltsfoot), 319, 321
    *Verbena officinalis* (vervain), 331–333
    *Viola odorata* (sweet violet), 343–344
    *Viola tricolour* (heartsease), 345
Grohman, G, *Rosa damascene* (damask rose), 265
Ground ivy see *Glechoma hederacea* (ground ivy)
Ground pine *(Ajuga chaemapitys)*, 139, 313–314
*Guaiacum officinale* (guaiacum), 128–129
Gynaecological conditions
    *Althaea officinalis* (marshmallow), 69

*Artemisia vulgaris* (mugwort), 127–129
*Daucus carota* (wild carrot), 149–150
*Ocimum basilicum* (basil), 226
*Paeonia officinalis* (paeony), 237

Haemorrhages, *Althaea officinalis* (marshmallow), 67–69
Haemorrhoids
    *Potentilla erecta* (tomentil), 247–248
    *Scrophularia nodosa* (figwort), 303
Haller, J S, 30
*Hamamelis virginiana* (witch hazel), 247–248
*Harpagophytum procumbens* (devil's claw), 303–304
Headaches
    *Inula helenium* (elecampene), 206
    *Rosa damascene* (damask rose), 259, 267
    *Stachys officinalis* (wood betony), 312–314
Head pain, *Viola odorata* (sweet violet), 339
*Healing Plants* (Pelikan), 18
Heartburn, *Stachys officinalis* (wood betony), 309–311
Heart disease, *Rosa damascene* (damask rose), 261, 267
Heart failure, *Drimia maritima* (squill), 162
Heartsease see *Viola tricolour* (heartsease)
Heat, importance of, Thomson, Samuel, 29
Hedge hyssop *(Gratiola officinalis)*, 285–287
Hedge woundwort *(Stachys sylvatica)*, 307
Hemp agrimony *(Eupatorium cannabinum)*, 49
Hemp-nettle *(Galeopsis tetrahit)*, 211
*The Herbal of Pseudo-Apuleius*, 1, 6, 25
    *Agrimonia eupatoria* (agrimony), 49
    *Malva sylvestris* (common mallow), 70–71
    *Ruta graveolens* (rue), 287
    *Stachys officinalis* (wood betony), 309
    translations, 8, 25–26
*Herbals, their Origins and Evolution: A Chapter in the History of Botany 1470-1670* (Arber), 1, 26–27
*Hermodactylus tuberosus*, 246–247
High molecular weight polysaccharides, *Althaea officinalis* (marshmallow), 74

Hildegard of Bingen, 2, 9, 26
    *Agrimonia eupatoria* (agrimony), 49
    *Apium graveolens* (wild celery), 81
    *Artemisia absinthium* (wormwood), 105, 110, 114
    *Glechoma hederacea* (ground ivy), 183–185
    *Hyssopus officinalis* (hyssop), 195–196
    *Inula helenium* (elecampene), 205–206
    *Lamium album* (white deadnettle), 215–216
    *Liber Simplicus Medicinae*, 9
    *Paeonia officinalis* (paeony), 233–234
    *Physica*, 1
    *Potentilla erecta* (tomentil), 245
    *Rosa damascene* (damask rose), 257–259
    *Rubus idaeus* (raspberry), 275–276
    *Ruta graveolens* (rue), 288
    *Scrivias (Know the Way)*, 9
    *Tussilago farfara* (coltsfoot), 319
    *Viola odorata* (sweet violet), 339
Hill, John, 3, 16
    *Agrimonia eupatoria* (agrimony), 51
    *Alchemilla vulgaris* (lady's mantle), 61–62
    *Althaea officinalis* (marshmallow), 73
    *Artemisia absinthium* (wormwood), 110–111
    *British Herbal*, 16
    *Cautions Against the Immoderate Use of Snuff*, 16
    *Drimia maritima* (squill), 160
    *Flora Britannica*, 16
    *Inula helenium* (elecampene), 203
    *Ocimum basilicum* (basil), 225
    *Rosa damascene* (damask rose), 263
    *Ruta graveolens* (rue), 291
    *Stachys officinalis* (wood betony), 312–313
    *Tussilago farfara* (coltsfoot), 319
    *The Useful Family Herbal*, 16
    *The Vegetable System*, 16
    *Verbena officinalis* (vervain), 332
Hip disease
    *Centaurium erythraea* (centaury), 139–140
    *Glechoma hederacea* (ground ivy), 183, 185–186
    *Inula helenium* (elecampene), 206
    *Potentilla erecta* (tomentil), 246
Hip pain, *Ruta graveolens* (rue), 292
Hippocrates
    *Althaea officinalis* (marshmallow), 67–69

*Apium graveolens* (wild celery), 79
*Daucus carota* (wild carrot), 149–150
Hippocratic Corpus, 30
    *Viola odorata* (sweet violet), 339
*Historia Plantarum Universalis*, *Glechoma hederacea* (ground ivy), 186
Historical sources, 1–22
    Anglo-Saxon, 2
    Arabic authors, 1
    18th Century, 2–3
    Greco-Roman authors, 1–4
    Medieval medicine, 8
    19th Century, 3, 16–22, 29–35
    Renaissance/Early Modern, 2
    20th Century, 3
    21st Century, 3–4
    see also specific titles; specific workers
*Historica plantarum universalis* (Bauhin), 12–13
*Historie of Plantes* (Dodoens), 12
Hoffman, David, 4, 19
    *Arctium lappa* (burdock), 93
    *Artemisia vulgaris* (mugwort), 130
    *Centaurium erythraea* (centaury), 140–141
    *Fumaria officinalis* (fumitory), 169
    *Hyssopus officinalis* (hyssop), 197
    *Rubus idaeus* (raspberry), 277
    *Ruta graveolens* (rue), 285–287, 290–291
    *Stachys officinalis* (wood betony), 313
    *Tussilago farfara* (coltsfoot), 322
    *Verbena officinalis* (vervain), 332–333
    *Viola odorata* (sweet violet), 338, 344
    *Viola tricolour* (heartsease), 346
Hollyhock see *Alcea rosea* (hollyhock)
Honey of roses, 261–262
Hool, Richard, 3, 18
    *Agrimonia eupatoria* (agrimony), 51
    *Arctium lappa* (burdock), 93–95
    *Artemisia vulgaris* (mugwort), 128
    *Centaurium erythraea* (centaury), 140
    *Hyssopus officinalis* (hyssop), 196–197
    *Stachys officinalis* (wood betony), 313
Hops (*Humulus lupulus*), 248
Horehound (*Marrubium vulgare*), 321–322
Hormone effects
    *Apium graveolens* (wild celery), 84
    *Artemisia absinthium* (wormwood), 113

Horse-chestnut (*Aesculus hippocastanum*), 246
Hot and dry theme, *Apium graveolens* (wild celery), 83–84
*Humulus lupulus* (hops), 248
*Hydrastis candensis* (golden seal), 98
Hydrolyzable tannins
    *Agrimonia eupatoria* (agrimony), 54
    *Alchemilla vulgaris* (lady's mantle), 64
    *Potentilla erecta* (tomentil), 250
    *Rubus idaeus* (raspberry), 280
Hypertension, *Drimia maritima* (squill), 162
*Hyssopus officinalis* (hyssop), 191–199, 192f, 194f
    Andrews, 193
    Barker, 193, 197
    Bauhin, 195
    *British Herbal Pharmacopoeia*, 197
    Chevallier, 197
    constituents, 198b
        diosmin, 197
        flavonoid glycosides, 197
        flavonoids, 198
        phenolic acids, 198
        volatile oils, 197–198
    Cook, 196
    Cullen, 195
    Culpeper, 196
    Dioscorides, 191, 193, 195–197
    Dodoens, 191–195
    dosage, 198
    Fox, 196
    Fuchs, 191–193
    Galen, 193, 195
    Gerard, 193–195
    Grieve, 193, 197
    Hildegard of Bingen, 195–196
    Hoffman, 197
    Hool, 196–197
    Ibn Sina, 193–195
    identity questions, 191–193
    limitation, 196
    Mattioli, 191–193
    Menzies-Trull, 197
    Miller, 196
    Myddfai physicians, 195
    Parkinson, 191–193, 195
    part used, 191
    Pelikan, 197–198
    Pliny, 195
    quality, 191
    Quincy, 196
    recommendations, 193–198
        angina, 193–195
        anthelmintic, 193–197
        asthma, 193
        black eyes, 195

# INDEX

bruises, 195, 198
catarrh, 195, 198
colds, 195
combination therapies, 195, 197, 225, 287
cough, 195, 198
diaphoretic, 197
digestive system, 198
diuretic, 195–197
ear problems, 198
epilepsy, 193–195, 197
expectorant, 196–197
fevers, 196–197
inflammation, 195
liver, 195–196
lungs, 196
nervous conditions, 198
respiratory system, 195–196, 198
sore throats, 193, 198
stomach, 195–196
topical use, 198
Robinson, 196–197
safety, 199
  epilepsy, 199
  ketone levels, 199
Salernitan herbal, 195
*Trotula*, 195
Weiss, 197
Wood, 197

Ibn Sina (Avicenna), 1, 6–7
  *Althaea officinalis* (marshmallow), 67, 71
  *Apium graveolens* (wild celery), 81, 83
  *Artemisia absinthium* (wormwood), 105–107, 109–110, 112–113, 115
  *Artemisia vulgaris* (mugwort), 130
  *Centaurium erythraea* (centaury), 137, 140
  *Drimia maritima* (squill), 159
  *Fumaria officinalis* (fumitory), 167
  *Hyssopus officinalis* (hyssop), 193–195
  *Inula helenium* (elecampene), 203, 206
  *Ocimum basilicum* (basil), 224–225
  *Paeonia officinalis* (paeony), 234–235
  *Qanun* (Canon of Medicine), 6–7
  *Rosa damascene* (damask rose), 259
  *Ruta graveolens* (rue), 287–290
  *Viola odorata* (sweet violet), 339–341
Ibn Wafid *see* Serapio the Younger (Ibn Wafid)
Identification problems
  *Daucus carota* (wild carrot), 145–149

*Hyssopus officinalis* (hyssop), 191–193
*Tussilago farfara* (coltsfoot), 317, 325
Indigestion, *Centaurium erythraea* (centaury), 140
Inducible nitrogen oxide synthase (iNOS), *Arctium lappa* (burdock), 99–100
Infections, *Potentilla erecta* (tomentil), 245
Infectious diseases, *Ruta graveolens* (rue), 289
Infertility, *Artemisia vulgaris* (mugwort), 131
Inflammations
  *Hyssopus officinalis* (hyssop), 195
  *Scrophularia nodosa* (figwort), 302
  *Tussilago farfara* (coltsfoot), 322
  *Viola odorata* (sweet violet), 342
Inflamed skin, *Glechoma hederacea* (ground ivy), 188
Infusion of roses, 262
Injuries, *Scrophularia nodosa* (figwort), 301–302
International Plants names, 41
*Inula britannica*, 201
*Inula conyza*, 201
*Inula graveolens* (fleabane), 201
*Inula helenium* (elecampene), 201–210, 202f, 204f
  Apuleius, 206
  Bauhin, 203
  British Herbal Pharmacopoeia, 204–205
  Chevallier, 204–205
  constituents, 207b
    polysaccharides, 207
    sesquiterpene lactones, 208
    volatile oils, 207
  Cook, 203, 206
  cordial preparations, 205–206
  Culpeper, 203, 205–207
  Dalechamps, 203
  Dioscorides, 201, 205–206
  Dodoens, 203, 205–207
  dosage, 207
  Fernie, 206
  Fox, 203–204, 206
  Fuchs, 203
  Galen, 203, 206
  Gerard, 203, 206–207
  Grieve, 205–206
  Hildegard of Bingen, 205–206
  Hill, 203
  Ibn Sina, 203, 206
  Mattioli, 203, 206
  Miller, 203, 206
  Myddfai physicians, 203, 206–207

Parkinson, 206
part used, 201
Pliny, 201, 203, 206
Priest, 203–204, 206
Quincy, 203
recommendations, 207
  antitussive, 207
  bactericidal agent, 207
  bites, 205
  breathlessness, 203
  bronchitis, 203–205
  carminative preparations, 205–207
  combination therapies, 187, 203–205, 225, 321
  cough, 203
  diaphoretic, 206–207
  diuretic, 206
  expectorant, 207
  headache, 206
  hip disease, 206
  itchy skin, 206
  lung disease, 204–205
  menstruation, 206
  mood alteration, 206
  respiratory system, 201–206
  scar formation, 207
  stomach problems, 205
  tonic, 205, 207
  topical use, 206–207
  tuberculosis, 203–204
  ulcers, 206–207
  urination, 206
safety, 207–209
  allergic contact dermatitis, 207
  lactation, 207
  pregnancy, 207
Salernitan herbal, 205–206
Serapio, 203, 206
Tragus, 203
Turner, 203, 205–206
*Inula japonica*, 201
*Inula racemosa*, 201
*Inula royleana*, 201
*Inula viscosa*, 201
Iridoid glycosides
  *Galium aparine* (goosegrass), 179
  *Lamium album* (white deadnettle), 218
  *Scrophularia nodosa* (figwort), 304
  *Verbena officinalis* (vervain), 333–334
Irritable bowel syndrome
  *Centaurium erythraea* (centaury), 142
  *Potentilla erecta* (tomentil), 249
Isoflavonoids, *Agrimonia eupatoria* (agrimony), 54

Isoquinoline alkaloids, *Fumaria officinalis* (fumitory), 171
Itchy skin, *Inula helenium* (elecampene), 206

Jaundice
  *Agrimonia eupatoria* (agrimony), 51
  *Artemisia absinthium* (wormwood), 110
  *Galium aparine* (goosegrass), 178
  *Glechoma hederacea* (ground ivy), 185
  *Potentilla erecta* (tomentil), 243–245
  *Verbena officinalis* (vervain), 332–333
Joint problems
  *Artemisia vulgaris* (mugwort), 129
  *Centaurium erythraea* (centuary), 142
  *Rosa damascene* (damask rose), 267
*Juniperus communis* (juniper), 177–178

Ketone levels, *Hyssopus officinalis* (hyssop), 199
*Key to Galen and Hippocrates, theor Method of Physick* (Culpeper), 15
Kidney disease
  *Drimia maritima* (squill), 162
  *Glechoma hederacea* (ground ivy), 187
  *Rosa damascene* (damask rose), 261
  *Ruta graveolens* (rue), 290
  *Scrophularia nodosa* (figwort), 302
  *Stachys officinalis* (wood betony), 311
Kidney stones, *Rubus idaeus* (raspberry), 275
Knight, C, *Fumaria officinalis* (fumitory), 169

Labour facilitation, *Artemisia vulgaris* (mugwort), 128
Lachrymal fistulas/abscesses, *Althaea officinalis* (marshmallow), 67
Lactation
  *Artemisia vulgaris* (mugwort), 133
  *Glechoma hederacea* (ground ivy), 188
  *Inula helenium* (elecampene), 207
  *Ocimum basilicum* (basil), 228
  *Tussilago farfara* (coltsfoot), 323
Lady's mantle *see Alchemilla vulgaris* (lady's mantle)
Lambertianin C, *Rubus idaeus* (raspberry), 276
*Lamium album* (white deadnettle), 211–220, 212f, 214f
  Bauhin, 213, 215–216
  Chevallier, 217
  Clusius, 213

constituents, 218b–219b
  flavonoids, 219
  iridoid glycosides, 218
  phenolic acids, 218
  phenylpropanoid glycosides, 219
  phenylpropanoids, 218–219
  phytoecdysteroids, 219
  tannins, 219
  triterpenes, 218
  volatile oil, 218
Culpeper, 216
Dalechamps, 213, 215
Dioscorides, 213
Dodoens, 213
dosage, 218
18th Century, 216
Fuchs, 213–215
Gerard, 213
Grieve, 216
Hildegard of Bingen, 215–216
identification problems, 213
Mattioli, 213
Menzies-Trull, 217
Miller, 216
Myddfai texts, 216
*National Botanic Pharmacopoeia*, 216
19th Century, 216
*The Old English Herbarium*, 215–216
Parkinson, 213, 215
parts used, 211
Pelikan, 217–218
Pliny, 213–215
quality, 211
Quartan, 215
Quincy, 216
recommendations, 211, 217–218
  arthritis, 217
  atopic dermatitis, 217
  combination therapies, 211, 217
  leucoma, 215–216
  leucorrhoea, 215, 218
  menorrhagia, 215–216, 218
  scabies, 216
  urtication, 217
  wounds, 218
Renaissance, 213–215
research applications, 217
safety, 218–219
Tragus, 213
Turner, 213–215
Weiss, 216–217
Wood, 217
*Lamium galeobdolon* (yellow deadnettle), 211, 213
*Lamium maculatum* (spotted deadnettle), 213
Laryngitis, *Rubus idaeus* (raspberry), 277

Lassitude, *Rosa damascene* (damask rose), 264
*Lavandula angustifolia* (lavender), 321, 334
Laxatives
  *Fumaria officinalis* (fumitory), 171
  *Ocimum basilicum* (basil), 224–225
  *Rosa damascene* (damask rose), 260, 263–264
  *Viola odorata* (sweet violet), 342–344
Leaf shapes, Goethe, Johann Wolfgang von, 38, 39f
Lectin, *Glechoma hederacea* (ground ivy), 188
Lemon balm (*Melissa officinalis*), 248–249
Lemon verbena (*Aloysia triphylla*), 264–265, 333–334
Leoniceno, Nicholaus, 23
*Leontice leontopetalum*, Dioscorides, 57–59
*Leonurus cardiaca* (motherwort), 225
Lepra, *Fumaria officinalis* (fumitory), 167–169
Lesser burdock (*Arctium minus*), 91
Leucoma, *Lamium album* (white deadnettle), 215–216
Leucorrhoea
  *Agrimonia eupatoria* (agrimony), 54
  *Alchemilla vulgaris* (lady's mantle), 61, 63
  *Arctium lappa* (burdock), 103
  *Artemisia absinthium* (wormwood), 113
  *Lamium album* (white deadnettle), 215, 218
  *Potentilla erecta* (tomentil), 247–248
  *Rosa damascene* (damask rose), 267
*Libellus de Re Herbaria* (Turner), 21
*Liber Aggregatus in Medicinus Simplicibus* (Serapio the Younger), 1, 7
*Liber Simplicus Medicinae* (Hildegard of Bingen), 9
Lignans
  *Arctium lappa* (burdock), 100–101
  *Glechoma hederacea* (ground ivy), 188
Lime (*Tilia*), 334
Linseed *see Linum usissitatum* (linseed)
*Linum usissitatum* (linseed)
  combination therapies, 177–178
  lignans, 100
Liquorice root (*Glycyrrhiza glabra*), 187, 203–204, 233, 331–332
Liver disease
  *Agrimonia eupatoria* (agrimony), 52, 54

**365**

# INDEX

*Hyssopus officinalis* (hyssop), 195–196
*Rosa damascene* (damask rose), 261, 267
*Stachys officinalis* (wood betony), 309
*Livre des Simples Medicines*, 9
*Lobelia inflata* (lobelia)
   combination therapies, 203, 248, 276–277
   Thomson, Samuel, 29
*The London Dispensatory*, 15
   *Glechoma hederacea* (ground ivy), 185–186
Loves, *Rosa damascene* (damask rose), 265
Lung conditions
   *Hyssopus officinalis* (hyssop), 196
   *Inula helenium* (elecampene), 204–205
   *Ruta graveolens* (rue), 291
   *Verbena officinalis* (vervain), 332–333
   see also Respiratory system
Lymphadenitis, *Scrophularia nodosa* (figwort), 304

Mabey, R, *Artemisia vulgaris* (mugwort), 130
Macer, 2
   *Fumaria officinalis* (fumitory), 167
   *Ruta graveolens* (rue), 291
   *Verbena officinalis* (vervain), 331
   *Viola odorata* (sweet violet), 339
Macrocyclic peptides
   *Viola odorata* (sweet violet), 347
   *Viola tricolour* (heartsease), 347
Magical uses, *Verbena officinalis* (vervain), 332
Maidenhair fern *(Adiantum capillus-veneris)*, 175
Malaria
   *Artemisia vulgaris* (mugwort), 133
   *Stachys officinalis* (wood betony), 313–314
Male paeony *(Paeonia mascula)*, 231, 232f
*Malva sylvestris* (common mallow), 67–78
   description, 67
   Herbal of Apuleius, 70–71
   recommendations, 74
   see also *Althaea officinalis* (marshmallow)
Marigold *(Calendula officinalis)*, 165–167
Marlow, John, 32–33
*Marrubium vulgare* (horehound), 321–322
Marsh violet *(Viola palustris)*, 337

Marsh woundwort *(Stachys palustris)*, 307
*Matricaria recutita* (chamomile), 129, 187, 248–249, 321, 334
Matthaeus Platearius, *Circa Instans*, 9
Mattioli, Pietro Andrea Gregorio, 2, 11, 27
   *Alchemilla vulgaris* (lady's mantle), 59
   *Althaea officinalis* (marshmallow), 69–72
   *Apium graveolens* (wild celery), 81–82
   *Arctium lappa* (burdock), 96
   *Artemisia vulgaris* (mugwort), 125–127
   *Centaurium erythraea* (centuary), 139–140
   *Daucus carota* (wild carrot), 145–148
   *Drimia maritima* (squill), 157, 160
   *Galium aparine* (goosegrass), 178
   *Glechoma hederacea* (ground ivy), 183
   *Hyssopus officinalis* (hyssop), 191–193
   *Inula helenium* (elecampene), 203, 206
   *Lamium album* (white deadnettle), 213
   *Ocimum basilicum* (basil), 225
   *Paeonia officinalis* (paeony), 233, 235–237
   *Potentilla erecta* (tomentil), 243
   *Rosa damascene* (damask rose), 255, 257, 260
   *Rubus fruticosa* (bramble), 275
   *Rubus idaeus* (raspberry), 273, 275
   *Ruta graveolens* (rue), 289–290
   *Scrophularia nodosa* (figwort), 300–302
   *Stachys officinalis* (wood betony), 312
   translations of Dioscorides, 11
   *Viola odorata* (sweet violet), 339–341
   *Viola tricolour* (heartsease), 345
Meadowsweet *(Filipendula ulmaria)*, 93–95, 313
*Medical Inquiries and Observations* (Rush), 30
Medieval age, 8
   *Rosa damascene* (damask rose), 258–259
   *Viola odorata* (sweet violet), 339
*Melaleuca alternifolia* (tea tree oil), 177
Melancholia
   *Artemisia absinthium* (wormwood), 114

*Fumaria officinalis* (fumitory), 169
*Rosa damascene* (damask rose), 267
*Melissa officinalis* (lemon balm), 248–249
Memory loss, *Stachys officinalis* (wood betony), 313
Menopause or Change of Life in Women (Webb), 32–33
Menopause, *Paeonia officinalis* (paeony), 237
Menorrhagia
   *Agrimonia eupatoria* (agrimony), 54
   *Alchemilla vulgaris* (lady's mantle), 63
   *Lamium album* (white deadnettle), 215–216, 218
   *Potentilla erecta* (tomentil), 245–246
   *Rosa damascene* (damask rose), 267
Menstrual problems
   *Alchemilla vulgaris* (lady's mantle), 63
   *Apium graveolens* (wild celery), 83, 86
   *Artemisia vulgaris* (mugwort), 128, 131
   *Glechoma hederacea* (ground ivy), 185–186
   *Inula helenium* (elecampene), 206
   *Paeonia officinalis* (paeony), 235, 237
   *Potentilla erecta* (tomentil), 246, 250
   *Rosa damascene* (damask rose), 263
   *Rubus idaeus* (raspberry), 278
   *Scrophularia nodosa* (figwort), 302
   *Stachys officinalis* (wood betony), 311–312
   *Viola odorata* (sweet violet), 338–339
   see also Emmenagogues
Mental health, *Artemisia absinthium* (wormwood), 114
*Mentha piperita* (peppermint), 248–249, 334
*Mentha pulegium* (pennyroyal), 128–129, 332–333
*Menyanthes trifoliata* (bogbean), 93–95, 321
Menzies-Trull, Christopher, 4, 19
   *Artemisia absinthium* (wormwood), 113–115
   *Artemisia vulgaris* (mugwort), 130
   *Centaurium erythraea* (centuary), 140–141
   *Fumaria officinalis* (fumitory), 170
   *Galium aparine* (goosegrass), 178
   *Hyssopus officinalis* (hyssop), 197
   *Lamium album* (white deadnettle), 217
   *Paeonia officinalis* (paeony), 235

# INDEX

*Potentilla erecta* (tomentil), 247–248
*Rubus idaeus* (raspberry), 279–280
*Ruta graveolens* (rue), 285–287
*Stachys officinalis* (wood betony), 313
*Tussilago farfara* (coltsfoot), 322
*Verbena officinalis* (vervain), 332–333
*Viola odorata* (sweet violet), 344
*Mercurialis perennis* (dog's mercury), 331–332
Mesue, John, 7
  *Viola odorata* (sweet violet), 342–343
Methyl eugenol, *Ocimum basilicum* (basil), 228
Migraine
  *Artemisia vulgaris* (mugwort), 130
  *Stachys officinalis* (wood betony), 312–313
Milk thistle (*Silybum marianum*), 313
Miller, Joseph, 3, 15–16
  *Apium graveolens* (wild celery), 84–85
  *Artemisia absinthium* (wormwood), 110, 112–113
  *Botanicum Officinale*, 15
  *Centaurium erythraea* (centaury), 135–137, 140
  *Daucus carota* (wild carrot), 149
  *Fumaria officinalis* (fumitory), 170
  *Hyssopus officinalis* (hyssop), 196
  *Inula helenium* (elecampene), 203, 206
  *Lamium album* (white deadnettle), 216
  *Paeonia officinalis* (paeony), 236–237
  *Rosa damascene* (damask rose), 263
  *Ruta graveolens* (rue), 291
  *Scrophularia nodosa* (figwort), 302
  *Tussilago farfara* (coltsfoot), 319–321
  *Verbena officinalis* (vervain), 332
  *Viola odorata* (sweet violet), 343
Mills, Simon, 4, 19–22
  *Arctium lappa* (burdock), 96
  *Artemisia absinthium* (wormwood), 111, 113
Miscarriages
  *Alchemilla vulgaris* (lady's mantle), 61
  *Arctium lappa* (burdock), 101
Mixed remedies, *Althaea officinalis* (marshmallow), 72
*The Model Family Botanic Guide* (Fox), 17
*A Modern Herbal* (Grieve), 18
Modern sources, 1

Moist conserve, *Rosa damascene* (damask rose), 261–262
Monoterpene(s), *Artemisia vulgaris* (mugwort), 132
Monoterpene glycosides, *Paeonia officinalis* (paeony), 238
Mood alteration, *Inula helenium* (elecampene), 206
*Mother and Child* (Webb), 32–33
Motherwort (*Leonurus cardiaca*), 225
Mouth ulcers, *Rubus idaeus* (raspberry), 275, 280
Mucilage, *Tussilago farfara* (coltsfoot), 323
Mugwort see *Artemisia vulgaris* (mugwort)
Mullein (*Verbascum thapsus*), 204–205, 322
Musa, Antonius
  betony (*Stachys officinalis*), 8
  *Stachys officinalis* (wood betony), 312
Muscular pain, *Centaurium erythraea* (centaury), 142
Musculoskeletal conditions, *Centaurium erythraea* (centaury), 139–140
Myddfai physicians, 2, 9–10
  *Althaea officinalis* (marshmallow), 71
  *Apium graveolens* (wild celery), 85
  *Arctium lappa* (burdock), 95
  *Galium aparine* (goosegrass), 173–175, 177–178
  *Glechoma hederacea* (ground ivy), 185
  *Hyssopus officinalis* (hyssop), 195
  *Inula helenium* (elecampene), 203, 206–207
  *Lamium album* (white deadnettle), 216
  *Red Book of Hergest* (LLyfr Coch Hergest), 9
  *Ruta graveolens* (rue), 290
  *Stachys officinalis* (wood betony), 311
  *Verbena officinalis* (vervain), 331–332
Myocardial contraction, *Scrophularia nodosa* (figwort), 304
*Myrica cerfera* (bayberry), 248
*Myristica fragrans* (nutmeg), 127–128
Myrrh (*Commiphora molmol*), 127, 177, 338–339

*Names of Herbes* (Turner), 11
National Association of Medical Herbalists (NAHM), 18
*The National Botanic Pharmacopoeia*, 3, 18

*Agrimonia eupatoria* (agrimony), 51
*Alchemilla vulgaris* (lady's mantle), 62
*Althaea officinalis* (marshmallow), 74
*Artemisia absinthium* (wormwood), 114
*Galium aparine* (goosegrass), 177–178
*Lamium album* (white deadnettle), 216
*Potentilla erecta* (tomentil), 247–248
*Ruta graveolens* (rue), 290–291
*Scrophularia nodosa* (figwort), 303
*Stachys officinalis* (wood betony), 311–313
*Verbena officinalis* (vervain), 332–333
*Viola odorata* (sweet violet), 343
*Natural History* (Pliny the Elder), 5, 23
Nausea and vomiting, *Artemisia absinthium* (wormwood), 116
Nervines
  *Apium graveolens* (wild celery), 85
  *Verbena officinalis* (vervain), 334
Nervous disorders
  *Artemisia vulgaris* (mugwort), 130–131
  *Hyssopus officinalis* (hyssop), 198
  *Ruta graveolens* (rue), 291–292
  *Stachys officinalis* (wood betony), 312
  *Verbena officinalis* (vervain), 334
Neuralgic pain, *Althaea officinalis* (marshmallow), 74
*A New Herbal* (Turner), 12
Nightmares, *Paeonia officinalis* (paeony), 235–237
Nightshade (*Solanum nigrum*), 319
19th Century, 3, 16–22, 29–35
Nomenclature, 25–26, 42
  *Althaea officinalis* (marshmallow), 70–71
  *Artemisia vulgaris* (mugwort), 123–125
  see also Identification problems
Nosebleeds, *Ruta graveolens* (rue), 287
Nutmeg (*Myristica fragrans*), 127–128

Oak (*Quercus rober*), 277–278
OAS (oral allergy syndrome), *Apium graveolens* (wild celery), 87–88
Obstructive lung disease, *Ruta graveolens* (rue), 292
*Ocimum basilicum* (basil), 221–229, 222f, 224f
  Andreas Vesalius, 224–225
  Apuleius, 225

**367**

# INDEX

constituents, 227b
   methyl eugenol, 228
   phenolic acids, 227
   triterpenes, 227
   volatile oils, 227–228
Culpeper, 221–223
Dioscorides, 221–225
Dodoens, 225
dosage, 227
Galen, 221–223
Grieve, 221
Hill, 225
Ibn Sina, 224–225
identification problems, 223–225
Mattioli, 225
Parkinson, 223, 226
parts used, 221
Pelikan, 226
Pliny, 221–223
quality, 221–223
recommendations, 226–227
   abortions, 223–224
   antibacterial action, 226
   anticatarrhal, 227
   antidepressants, 225
   antioxidants, 226
   antiseptics, 225
   carminative actions, 226–227
   combination therapies, 225
   conception aid, 223
   depression, 225–226
   digestion, 226
   diuretic, 224
   emmenagogue, 223–224
   expectorant, 227
   eyes, 221–223
   flatulence, 224
   grief, 225–226
   gynaecological remedies, 226
   laxative, 224–225
   sight problems, 223–224
   tonic, 225
   topical use, 223, 226
Robinson, 225
safety, 223, 228
   as carcinogen, 228
   emmenagogue, 228
   lactation, 228
   pregnancy, 228
Serapio, 224–225
Williamson, 226
Oedema
   *Ruta graveolens* (rue), 292
   *Stachys officinalis* (wood betony), 311
Oedemata, *Artemisia absinthium* (wormwood), 107–109
Oil of roses, 262
Ointment of roses, 262

*The Old English Herbarium*, 1
   *Artemisia absinthium* (wormwood), 109, 115
   *Artemisia vulgaris* (mugwort), 125, 129
   *Drimia maritima* (squill), 159–160
   *Lamium album* (white deadnettle), 215–216
   *Rosa damascene* (damask rose), 258
   *Rubus idaeus* (raspberry), 277–278
   *Ruta graveolens* (rue), 287–288
   *Stachys officinalis* (wood betony), 309, 311–314
   *Verbena officinalis* (vervain), 331
   *Viola odorata* (sweet violet), 339
*On the Faculties of Foods*, *Althaea officinalis* (marshmallow), 70
Opium antidote, *Artemisia vulgaris* (mugwort), 130–131
Oral allergy syndrome (OAS), *Apium graveolens* (wild celery), 87–88
Oribasius, *Daucus carota* (wild carrot), 147
Osteoarthritis, *Arctium lappa* (burdock), 93

*Paeonia delavayii*, 231
*Paeonia lactiflora*
   recommendations, 233
   combination therapies, 165–167, 233
*Paeonia mascula* (male paeony), 231, 232f
*Paeonia officinalis* (paeony), 231–239
   Apuleius, 235–236
   Bauhin, 235–236
   Chevallier, 235, 237
   constituents, 238b
      gallotannins, 238
      monoterpene glycosides, 238
      phenolic acids, 238
      triterpenoids, 238
      volatile oils, 238
   Cook, 235
   Culpeper, 233–236
   Dioscorides, 231, 233–236
   Dodoens, 233, 235–236
   dosage, 238
   Fuchs, 233–237
   Galen, 234–237
   Gerard, 233
   Hildegard of Bingen, 233–234
   Ibn Sina, 234–235
   identification problems, 231–233
   Mattioli, 233, 235–237
   Menzies-Trull, 235
   Miller, 236–237
   Parkinson, 234–236

   part used, 231, 233–235
   Pelikan, 236
   Pliny, 233–236
   quality, 231
   Quincy, 236–237
   *Rariorum Plantarum Historia*, 233
   recommendations, 237–238
      antispasmodic, 235
      astringent, 233–235
      belly ache, 233–234
      convulsions, 235–237
      digestive system, 234
      eczema, 237
      endometriosis, 237
      epilepsy, 236, 238
      gynaecological conditions, 237
      menopause, 237
      menstrual problems, 235, 237
      nightmares, 235–237
      polycystic ovaries, 237
      psoriasis, 237
      seizures, 237
      topical use, 233–234
      urinary problems, 234–235
   Renaissance, 233
   safety, 238
      pregnancy, 238
   Salernitan herbal, 233–234, 236
   Serapio, 234–237
   Stern, 233
   *Trotula*, 233–234
   Turner, 233, 236
   Wren, 235
*Paeonia spontanea*, 231
Paeony see *Paeonia officinalis* (paeony)
Painful joints, *Scrophularia nodosa* (figwort), 301–302
Palladius, *Apium graveolens* (wild celery), 79
Pansy see *Viola tricolour* (heartsease)
*Pantegni* (Constantine the African), 8
*Paradisi in Sole Paradisus Terrestris* (Parkinson), 14
Paralysis, *Ruta graveolens* (rue), 291
*Parietaria diffusa* (pellitory)
   combination therapies, 333
   Skelton, John, 31–32
Parkinson, John, 2, 14
   *Agrimonia eupatoria* (agrimony), 47–49
   *Alchemilla vulgaris* (lady's mantle), 59, 61
   *Althaea officinalis* (marshmallow), 72–73
   *Apium graveolens* (wild celery), 83–84
   *Artemisia absinthium* (wormwood), 107, 110
   *Artemisia vulgaris* (mugwort), 129

## INDEX

*Centaurium erythraea* (centuary), 139–140
*Eupatorium cannabinum* (hemp agrimony), 49
*Fumaria officinalis* (fumitory), 167
*Glechoma hederacea* (ground ivy), 185–186
*Hyssopus officinalis* (hyssop), 191–193, 195
*Inula helenium* (elecampene), 206
*Lamium album* (white deadnettle), 213, 215
*The National Botanic Pharmacopoeia*, 18
*Ocimum basilicum* (basil), 223, 226
*Paeonia officinalis* (paeony), 234–236
*Paradisi in Sole Paradisus Terrestris*, 14
*Potentilla erecta* (tomentil), 243–246
*Rosa damascena* (damask rose), 255, 257–258, 260–261
*Rubus fruticosa* (bramble), 275
*Rubus idaeus* (raspberry), 275
*Ruta graveolens* (rue), 290
*Scrophularia nodosa* (figwort), 297, 299, 301–302
*Stachys officinalis* (wood betony), 312–314
*Theatrum Botanicum*, 14
*Tussilago farfara* (coltsfoot), 319
*Verbena officinalis* (vervain), 327, 332
*Viola odorata* (sweet violet), 342
*Viola tricolour* (heartsease), 344–345
Parsley root *(Petroselinon crispum)*, 177–178
*Peganum harmala* (white-flowered harmal), 289
Pelikan, Wilhelm, 3, 18, 37–38
*Agrimonia eupatoria* (agrimony), 53
*Alchemilla vulgaris* (lady's mantle), 63
*Althaea officinalis* (marshmallow), 75–76
*Apium graveolens* (wild celery), 86
*Artemisia absinthium* (wormwood), 116
*Centaurium erythraea* (centuary), 140–141
*Daucus carota* (wild carrot), 151
*Fumaria officinalis* (fumitory), 169
*Glechoma hederacea* (ground ivy), 181, 183
*Healing Plants*, 18
*Hyssopus officinalis* (hyssop), 197–198
*Lamium album* (white deadnettle), 217–218
*Ocimum basilicum* (basil), 226
*Paeonia officinalis* (paeony), 236

*Rosa damascene* (damask rose), 265–266
*Ruta graveolens* (rue), 289
*Scrophularia nodosa* (figwort), 299–300
*The Secrets of Metals*, 18
Pellitory *see Parietaria diffusa* (pellitory)
Pennyroyal *(Mentha pulegium)*, 128–129, 332–333
Peppermint *(Mentha piperita)*, 248–249, 334
Peptides, macrocyclic
*Viola odorata* (sweet violet), 347
*Viola tricolour* (heartsease), 347
Perfume, *Viola odorata* (sweet violet), 343–344
Pernicious humours, *Fumaria officinalis* (fumitory), 167–169
Pestilence, *Potentilla erecta* (tomentil), 245
*Petroselinon crispum* (parsley root), 177–178
*Petroselinon hortense* (petroselinon), 81
*Pharmacopoeia Londinensis*
*Althaea officinalis* (marshmallow), 73
*Rosa damascene* (damask rose), 261
*Pharmacopoeia Officinalis & Extemporanea* (Quincy), 15
Phenolic acids
*Agrimonia eupatoria* (agrimony), 54
*Althaea officinalis* (marshmallow), 76
*Arctium lappa* (burdock), 101
*Artemisia absinthium* (wormwood), 117
*Centaurium erythraea* (centuary), 143
*Glechoma hederacea* (ground ivy), 181, 188
*Hyssopus officinalis* (hyssop), 198
*Lamium album* (white deadnettle), 218
*Ocimum basilicum* (basil), 227
*Paeonia officinalis* (paeony), 238
*Rosa damascene* (damask rose), 268
*Stachys officinalis* (wood betony), 315
*Viola tricolour* (heartsease) constituents, 347
Phenylethanoid glycosides, *Stachys officinalis* (wood betony), 315
Phenylpropanoid glycosides, *Lamium album* (white deadnettle), 219
Phenylpropanoids
*Fumaria officinalis* (fumitory), 171
*Lamium album* (white deadnettle), 218–219

*Scrophularia nodosa* (figwort), 304
*Stachys officinalis* (wood betony), 315
*Verbena officinalis* (vervain), 333–335
Phenylpropanols, *Viola odorata* (sweet violet), 347
Phenypropanoids, *Artemisia absinthium* (wormwood), 117
Phthalides, *Apium graveolens* (wild celery), 87
*Physica* (Hildegard of Bingen), 1
*A Physicall Directory (A Translation of the London Dispensatory)* (Culpeper), 14–15
*Phytoclacca americana* (poke root), 331–332
Phytoecdysteroids *Lamium album* (white deadnettle), 219
Phytophotodermatitis
*Apium graveolens* (wild celery), 88
*Ruta graveolens* (rue), 293–294
*Picrasma excelsa* (quassia), 177–178
Piles, *Scrophularia nodosa* (figwort), 302
*Plantago* (plantain), Skelton, John, 31–32
Plant descriptions, 41
Plants Database, nomenclature, 41
Pliny the Elder, 1, 5
*Alchemilla vulgaris* (lady's mantle), 57–59
*Althaea officinalis* (marshmallow), 69, 71–72
*Apium graveolens* (wild celery), 79, 81–82
*Arctium lappa* (burdock), 96
*Artemisia absinthium* (wormwood), 109, 112–113, 115
*Artemisia vulgaris* (mugwort), 123, 129
*Centaurium erythraea* (centuary), 137
*Daucus carota* (wild carrot), 145, 147, 149–150
*Drimia maritima* (squill), 157, 159–161
*Galium aparine* (goosegrass), 173, 177
*Hyssopus officinalis* (hyssop), 193
*Inula helenium* (elecampene), 201, 203, 206
*Lamium album* (white deadnettle), 213–215
*Natural History*, 5, 23
*Ocimum basilicum* (basil), 221–223
*Paeonia officinalis* (paeony), 233–236
*Potentilla erecta* (tomentil), 243

**369**

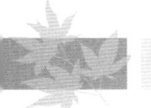

# INDEX

*Rosa damascene* (damask rose), 255, 258–259
*Rubus fruticosa* (bramble), 275
*Rubus idaeus* (raspberry), 273, 275
*Ruta graveolens* (rue), 287–288, 290–291
*Scrophularia nodosa* (figwort), 300–301
*Stachys officinalis* (wood betony), 311–312
*Tussilago farfara* (coltsfoot), 319
*Verbena officinalis* (vervain), 327
*Viola odorata* (sweet violet), 342–343
Pneumonia, *Galium aparine* (goosegrass), 173–175
Poison antidotes
  *Rosa damascene* (damask rose), 261
  *Ruta graveolens* (rue), 289–290
  *Stachys officinalis* (wood betony), 314
Poison resistance, *Potentilla erecta* (tomentil), 245
Poke root *(Phytoclacca amerciana)*, 331–332
Polyacetylenes, *Arctium lappa* (burdock), 101
Polycystic ovaries, *Paeonia officinalis* (paeony), 237
*Polygonium bistorta* (bistort), 127–128
Polyphenolic acids, *Galium aparine* (goosegrass), 179
Polyphenols
  *Agrimonia eupatoria* (agrimony), 53
  *Artemisia vulgaris* (mugwort), 132
Polysaccharides
  *Althaea officinalis* (marshmallow), 76
  *Arctium lappa* (burdock), 101
  *Drimia maritima* (squill), 162
  *Inula helenium* (elecampene), 207
  *Viola odorata* (sweet violet), 346
  *Viola tricolour* (heartsease), 347
Porphyria, *Artemisia absinthium* (wormwood), 118
Porphyrins, *Daucus carota* (wild carrot), 151
*Potentilla alba* (white cinquefoil), 241
*Potentilla anglica*, 241
*Potentilla anserina* (silverweed), 241
*Potentilla erecta* (tomentil), 241–252, 242f, 244f
  Apuleius, 247–248
  Bauhin, 243–245, 247
  British Herbal Pharmacopoeia, 248–249
  Carmichael, 245
  Chevallier, 249
  constituents, 250b

condensed tannins, 249–250
hydrolyzable tannins, 250
tannins, 241, 250
triterpenoid saponins, 250
Cullen, 248
Culpeper, 244–248
Dalechamps, 243–248
de l'Obel, Matthias, 247
Dioscorides, 241–248
Dodoens, 243–245, 247–248
dosage, 250
Fuchs, 243–244
Galen, 245, 247–248
Gerard, 245–246
Grieve, 247–248
Hildegard of Bingen, 245
Mattioli, 243
Menzies-Trull, 247–248
*National Botanic Pharmacopoiea*, 247–248
Parkinson, 243–246
part used, 241
Pliny, 243
Quincy, 245
recommendations, 243–245, 249–250
  arthritic pain, 245–246, 250
  astringency, 241–248
  biliousness, 244
  colitis, 249
  combination therapies, 246–248
  Crohn's disease, 249
  diarrhoea, 243–244, 249–250
  disease resistance, 245
  dysentery, 243–245, 249
  fevers, 245
  fluxes of the blood, 248
  gout, 246–247
  haemorrhoids, 247–248
  hip disease, 246
  infections, 245
  irritable bowel syndrome, 249
  jaundice, 243–245
  leucorrhoea, 247–248
  menorrhagia, 245–246
  menstrual problems, 246, 250
  pestilence, 245
  poison resistance, 245
  rectal bleeding, 249
  rheumatic disorders, 246–247
  toothache, 247–248
  topical uses, 247–248
  ulcerated throat, 247–248
  ulcerative colitis, 249
Renaissance, 243
Robinson, 248
safety, 250
  long-term use, 250
Salernitan herbal, 247–248

*Stirpium Adversaria Nova*, 247
*Theatrum Botanicum*, 247
Theophrastus, 243
Tragus, 243
Turner, 243–248
Weiss, 241, 248–249
*Potentilla reptans* (creeping cinquefoil), 241
*Potter's Cyclopedia* (Wren), 17–18
Pregnancy
  *Apium graveolens* (wild celery), 87
  *Artemisia absinthium* (wormwood), 118
  *Artemisia vulgaris* (mugwort), 133
  *Centaurium erythraea* (centuary), 143
  *Daucus carota* (wild carrot), 152
  *Drimia maritima* (squill), 163
  *Glechoma hederacea* (ground ivy), 188
  *Inula helenium* (elecampene), 207
  *Ocimum basilicum* (basil), 228
  *Paeonia officinalis* (paeony), 238
  *Rubus idaeus* (raspberry), 278–280
  *Ruta graveolens* (rue), 283–285, 293
  *Stachys officinalis* (wood betony), 311–312
  *Tussilago farfara* (coltsfoot), 323
  *Verbena officinalis* (vervain), 335
Premature birth prevention, *Artemisia vulgaris* (mugwort), 128
Premenstrual sore breasts, *Galium aparine* (goosegrass), 177
Premenstrual syndrome, *Ruta graveolens* (rue), 292
Pre-metric units, dosages, 42–44
Priest, Albert and Lilian, 3, 19, 32–33
  *Althaea officinalis* (marshmallow), 75
  *Galium aparine* (goosegrass), 175, 177
  *Inula helenium* (elecampene), 203–204, 206
  *Stachys officinalis* (wood betony), 313
  *Tussilago farfara* (coltsfoot), 322
  *Verbena officinalis* (vervain), 331–333
*Primitive Physic* (Wesley), 32
*Primula veris* (cowslip), 205
Proscillaridin, *Drimia maritima* (squill), 161
*Prunus virginiana* (cherry), 321
Pseudo-Apuleius *see* Apuleius
Psoriasis
  *Fumaria officinalis* (fumitory), 169
  *Paeonia officinalis* (paeony), 237
  *Scrophularia nodosa* (figwort), 304

Psoriatic arthritis, *Scrophularia nodosa* (figwort), 304
Purgatives
    Galen of Pergamon, 24–25
    *Rosa damascene* (damask rose), 258, 260–261
Pyrrolizidine alkaloids
    metabolism, 323–324
    safe limits, 324
    *Tussilago farfara* (coltsfoot), 321–323

*Qanun (Canon of Medicine)* (Ibn Sina), 6–7
Quality, 41
Quartan, *Lamium album* (white deadnettle), 215
Quassia (*Picrasma excelsa*), 177–178
Quercetin, *Rubus idaeus* (raspberry), 276
*Quercus rober* (oak), 277–278
Quincy, John, 2, 15
    *Agrimonia eupatoria* (agrimony), 51
    *Alchemilla vulgaris* (lady's mantle), 61
    *Althaea officinalis* (marshmallow), 73
    *Apium graveolens* (wild celery), 84–85
    *Arctium lappa* (burdock), 93–95
    *Artemisia absinthium* (wormwood), 110, 112–113, 115
    *Artemisia vulgaris* (mugwort), 130
    *British Pharmacopoeia*, 15
    *Centaurium erythraea* (centuary), 139–141
    *Compleat English Dispensatory*, 15
    *Daucus carota* (wild carrot), 150
    *The Edinburgh New Dispensatory*, 15
    *Glechoma hederacea* (ground ivy), 186–187
    *Hyssopus officinalis* (hyssop), 196
    *Inula helenium* (elecampene), 203
    *Lamium album* (white deadnettle), 216
    *The London Dispensatory*, 15
    *Paeonia officinalis* (paeony), 236–237
    *Pharmacopoeia Officinalis & Extemporanea*, 15
    *Potentilla erecta* (tomentil), 245
    *Rosa damascene* (damask rose), 263
    *Rubus idaeus* (raspberry), 276–278
    *Ruta graveolens* (rue), 291
    *Scrophularia nodosa* (figwort), 302
    *Stachys officinalis* (wood betony), 311
    *Tussilago farfara* (coltsfoot), 319–321
    *Verbena officinalis* (vervain), 327, 331–332
    *Viola odorata* (sweet violet), 343

*Rariorum Plantarum Historia*, *Paeonia officinalis* (paeony), 233
Raspberry *see Rubus idaeus* (raspberry)
Raspberry cordial, 276
Raspberry vinegar, 276
Rectal bleeding, *Potentilla erecta* (tomentil), 249
*Red Book of Hergest (LLyfr Coch Hergest)*, 9
Relaxants, *Verbena officinalis* (vervain), 333–334
Religious uses, *Verbena officinalis* (vervain), 329
Renaissance, 2
    *Agrimonia eupatoria* (agrimony), 47–49
    *Apium graveolens* (wild celery), 79–81, 83–84
    *Arctium lappa* (burdock), 95–96
    *Artemisia vulgaris* (mugwort), 129
    *Galium aparine* (goosegrass), 178
    *Glechoma hederacea* (ground ivy), 185
    *Paeonia officinalis* (paeony), 233
    *Potentilla erecta* (tomentil), 243
    *Rosa damascene* (damask rose), 255
    *Scrophularia nodosa* (figwort), 299, 302
    *Verbena officinalis* (vervain), 332
    *Viola odorata* (sweet violet), 342
Reproductive system
    *Daucus carota* (wild carrot), 149–150, 152
    *Stachys officinalis* (wood betony), 311
Respiratory system
    *Althaea officinalis* (marshmallow), 76
    *Hyssopus officinalis* (hyssop), 195–196, 198
    *Inula helenium* (elecampene), 201–206
    *Rubus idaeus* (raspberry), 280
    *Stachys officinalis* (wood betony), 313–314
    *Tussilago farfara* (coltsfoot), 319, 322
    *Verbena officinalis* (vervain), 334
    *Viola odorata* (sweet violet), 339–341
    *Viola tricolour* (heartsease), 344–346
    *see also* Lung conditions
Rheumatic disorders
    *Daucus carota* (wild carrot), 152
    *Potentilla erecta* (tomentil), 246–247
Rheumatic pain, *Artemisia absinthium* (wormwood), 115
Rheumatism

*Galium aparine* (goosegrass), 173–175
*Ruta graveolens* (rue), 292
*Viola tricolour* (heartsease), 346
*Rhus aromatica*, 177
Riddle, J
    *Centaurium erythraea* (centuary), 141
    *Daucus carota* (wild carrot), 149–150
Ringworm
    *Galium aparine* (goosegrass), 175
    *Scrophularia nodosa* (figwort), 302
Robinson, M
    *Althaea officinalis* (marshmallow), 74
    *Centaurium erythraea* (centuary), 140
    *Drimia maritima* (squill), 161
    *Fumaria officinalis* (fumitory), 169
    *Hyssopus officinalis* (hyssop), 196–197
    *Ocimum basilicum* (basil), 225
    *Potentilla erecta* (tomentil), 248
    *Ruta graveolens* (rue), 287–288
Rome ancient, weights and measures, 42t
*Rosa alba*, 255
*Rosa centifolia*, 255–257
*Rosa damascene* (damask rose), 253–270, 254f, 256f
    Barker, 264
    Bauhin, 257, 260
    Beck, 258
    *British Herbal Pharmacopoeia*, 264
    *British Pharmacopoeia*, 264
    Chevallier, 264
    constituents, 268b
        anthocyanins, 268
        flavonoids, 268
        flavonol glycosides, 268
        phenolic acids, 268
        volatile oil, 268
    Cook, 263
    Cullen, 263
    Culpeper, 260–262
    Dioscorides, 255, 257–259
    Dodoens, 255–257, 260–261
    dosage, 267–268
    Galen, 255, 258–259
    Gerard, 260–262
    Grieve, 264
    Grohman, 265
    heritage, 255–257
    Hildegard of Bingen, 257–259
    Hill, 263
    Ibn Sina, 259
    identity, 255–257
    Mattioli, 255, 257, 260

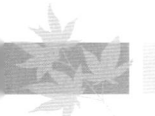

# INDEX

Miller, 263
mythology, 265–266
*Old English Herbarium*, 258
Parkinson, 255, 257–258, 260–261
part used, 253–255, 257, 261
Pelikan, 265–266
*Pharmacopoeia Londinensis*, 261
Pliny, 255, 258–259
preparations, 261–263
    cordial powders, 262
    dry conserve, 262
    honey of roses, 261–262
    infusion of roses, 262
    moist conserve, 261–262
    oil of roses, 262
    ointment of roses, 262
    rose petals, 262
    rose water, 262
    sugar of roses, 262
    syrup, 262
    vinegar of roses, 262
quality, 253–255
Quincy, 263
recommendations, 257–258, 260–261, 264–265, 267–268
    abscesses, 259
    ancients, 257–258
    antiperspirant, 257–258
    astringent, 261, 263
    combination therapies, 264–265
    constipation, 267
    cough, 263
    debility, 264
    deodorants, 257–258
    diarrhoea, 258, 264, 267
    diuretic, 267
    18th Century, 263–264
    erysipelas, 261
    fever, 259, 267
    headaches, 259, 267
    heart disease, 261, 267
    joint ache, 267
    kidneys, 261
    lassitude, 264
    laxative, 260, 263–264
    leucorrhoea, 267
    liver, 261, 267
    Medieval age, 258–259
    melancholy, 267
    menorrhagia, 267
    menstrual problems, 263
    poison antidote, 261
    purgative, 258, 260–261
    sore mouth, 267
    St Anthony's fire, 261
    stomach, 267
    topical use, 267
    vitamin deficiency, 264, 267
    vomiting, 267
Renaissance, 255
safety, 268
Salernitan herbal, 259
Serapio, 259
symbolism, 265–266
    beauty, 265
    goddesses, 265
    loves, 265
*Trotula*, 259
Turner, 257–258, 260
Weiss, 264
*Rosa gallica*, 253, 255
*Rosa moschata*, 253
*Rosa sempervirens*, 253, 258
Rose petals, 262
Rose water, 262
*Rosmarinus officinalis* (rosemary), 313, 321
*Rubus caesius* (dewberry), 271
*Rubus fruticosa* (bramble), 271, 275
    Turner, 275
    Culpeper, 275
    Dodoens, 275
    Fuchs, 275
    Galen, 275
    Mattioli, 275
    Parkinson, 275
    parts used, 275
    Pliny, 275
    recommendations, 275
        digestive tract, 275
        topical uses, 275
    Turner, 275
*Rubus idaeus* (raspberry), 271–282, 272f, 274f
    Aristotle, 271–273
    Bauhin, 275
    *British Herbal Pharmacopoeia*, 277
    Coffin, 277–278
    constituents, 280b
        antioxidants, 276
        ellagitannins, 276
        flavonoids, 276
        flavonol glycosides, 280
        hydrolyzable tannins, 280
        lambertianin C, 276
        quercetin, 276
        sanguiin H6, 276
        tannins, 280
        vitamin C, 276
    Cook, 277–278
    Cullen, 276
    Dioscorides, 273–274
    Dodoens, 275
    dosage, 278–280
    Fox, 277
    Gerard, 273, 275, 277–278
    Grieve, 276
    Hildegard of Bingen, 275–276
    Hoffman, 277
    identity, 271–273
    Mattioli, 273, 275
    Menzies-Trull, 279–280
    *Old English Herbarium*, 277–278
    Parkinson, 275
    part used, 271
    Pliny, 273, 275
    quality, 271
    Quincy, 276–278
    raspberry cordial, 276
    raspberry vinegar, 276
    recommendations, 274, 280
        asthma, 276
        astringent, 271, 276–277
        bacterial infections, 276
        birth preparation, 280
        canker, 277
        combination therapies, 141, 276–278, 313, 332–333
        cough, 276
        croup, 276
        diarrhoea, 277, 280
        dysentery, 277
        gastrointestinal system, 275–277
        kidney stones, 275
        laryngitis, 277
        menstrual problems, 278
        mouth ulcers, 275, 280
        pregnancy, 278
        respiratory system, 280
        stomatitis, 277
        tonsilitis, 277
        topical uses, 277
        uterus, 278
        whooping cough, 276
    safety, 279–280
        pregnancy, 279–280
    Salernitan herbal, 275–276
    self-prescription, 278
    Skelton, 277
    Theophrastus, 271–273
    Thomson, 277–280
    Turner, 273, 275
    Wellman, 273
    Wren, 277
Rue *see Ruta graveolens* (rue)
Ruellius, *Artemisia vulgaris* (mugwort), 125–127
*Rumex crispus* (dock), 93–95, 169, 302
Rush, Benjamin, 30
    *Medical Inquiries and Observations*, 30
*Ruta angustifolia*, 283
*Ruta chalepensis*, 283
*Ruta graveolens* (rue), 283–295, 284f, 286f

Apuleius, 288, 291
Bartram, 285–287
Bauhin, 290, 292
*British Herbal Pharmacopoeia*, 285–288, 291
*British Pharmaceutical Codex*, 291
Chevallier, 285–287
constituents, 293b
    alkaloids, 293
    flavonoids, 293
    furocoumarins, 293
    volatile oils, 293
Cullen, 290–291
Culpeper, 290–291
Dioscorides, 287–292
Dodoens, 290
dosage, 285, 292–293
Galen, 289
Gerard, 289–291
Grieve, 287–291
Hildegard of Bingen, 288
Hill, 291
Hoffman, 285–287, 290–291
Ibn Sina, 287–290
Macer, 291
Mattioli, 289–290
Menzies-Trull, 285–287
Miller, 291
Myddfai physicians, 290
*National Botanic Pharmacopoeia*, 290–291
*Old English Herbarium*, 287–288
Parkinson, 290
part used, 283–285
Pelikan, 289
Pliny, 287–288, 290–291
pseudo-Apuleius herbal, 287
quality, 283–287
Quincy, 291
recommendations, 283–285, 292–293
    abortifacient, 283–285
    amenorrhoea, 292
    anthelmintic, 290–292
    antispasmodic, 292
    arteriosclerosis, 285–287
    arthritis, 292
    asthma, 291
    bronchitis, 293
    classical medicine, 287–289
    combination therapies, 285–289
    emmenagogue, 285–288
    epilepsy, 291, 293
    eye weakness, 288
    hip pain, 292
    infectious diseases, 289
    kidney disease, 290
    lung problems, 291
    nervous complaints, 291–292
    neuralgic pain, 292
    nosebleeds, 287
    obstructive lung disease, 292
    oedema, 292
    paralysis, 291
    poison antidote, 289–290
    premenstrual syndrome, 292
    rheumatism, 292
    scabies, 292
    skin diseases, 293
    spasmolytic, 290–292
    topical uses, 287–288, 292
    typhus, 290
Robinson, 287–288
safety, 293–294
    children, 293
    dosage, 293
    embryo development, 285
    phytophotodermatitis, 293–294
    pregnancy, 283–285, 293
    topical uses, 293
    toxicity, 288–289
Serapio, 287–288, 290
topical uses, 293
Turner, 289–292
Weiss, 285–287
Williamson, 285–287, 290–292
Wood, 285

Safety, 42
Saffron *(Crocus sativus)*, 338–339
Salernitan herbal, 2, 8–9, 26
    *Alchemilla vulgaris* (lady's mantle), 59
    *Althaea officinalis* (marshmallow), 71
    *Arctium lappa* (burdock), 97
    *Artemisia absinthium* (wormwood), 105–107, 113
    *Artemisia vulgaris* (mugwort), 127–130
    compounds, 26
    *Daucus carota* (wild carrot), 149–150
    *Drimia maritima* (squill), 159
    *Fumaria officinalis* (fumitory), 167, 169–171
    *Glechoma hederacea* (ground ivy), 183–185
    *Hyssopus officinalis* (hyssop), 195
    *Inula helenium* (elecampene), 205–206
    *Paeonia officinalis* (paeony), 233–234, 236
    *Potentilla erecta* (tormentil), 247–248
    *Rosa damascene* (damask rose), 259
    *Rubus idaeus* (raspberry), 275–276
    *Scrophularia nodosa* (figwort), 301
    'simples', 26
    *Stachys officinalis* (wood betony), 309, 311–313
    *Verbena officinalis* (vervain), 331–332
    *Viola odorata* (sweet violet), 339
*Sambuccus niger* (elderflower), 175, 313, 319
Sanguiin H6, *Rubus idaeus* (raspberry), 276
*Sanguisorba officinalis* (greater burnet), 313
Saponins, *Viola tricolour* (heartsease), 347
Scabies
    *Lamium album* (white deadnettle), 216
    *Ruta graveolens* (rue), 292
Scar formation, *Inula helenium* (elecampene), 207
Sciatica, *Centaurium erythraea* (centaury), 139
*The Science and Practice of Medicine* (Skelton), 31–32
Scolefield, James, 31
Scorpion stings, *Viola odorata* (sweet violet), 338–339
*Scrivias (Know the Way)* (Hildegard of Bingen), 9
Scrofula
    *Scrophularia nodosa* (figwort), 301–303
    *Verbena officinalis* (vervain), 331–332
*Scrophularia aquatica*, 297
*Scrophularia auriculata* (water figwort), 297
*Scrophularia marilandica*, 297
*Scrophularia ningpoiensis*, 297
*Scrophularia nodosa* (figwort), 297–306, 298f, 300f
    *The American Dispensatory*, 304
    Bauhin, 301–302
    *British Herbal Pharmacopoeia*, 303–304
    Chevallier, 303
    constituents, 304b
        flavonoids, 304
        iridoid glycosides, 304
        phenylpropanoids, 304
    Cook, 302
    Culpeper, 299, 302
    Dioscorides, 297–301
    Dodoens, 299, 301–303
    dosage, 304
    Fuchs, 299–301
    Gerard, 297, 299, 301–302
    Grieve, 301
    identification problems, 297–300
    Mattioli, 300–302
    Miller, 302

# INDEX

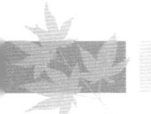

*National Botanic Pharmacopoeia*, 303
Parkinson, 297, 299, 301–302
part used, 297
Pelikan, 299–300
Pliny, 300–301
quality, 297
Quincy, 302
recommendations, 303–304
    arthritis, 303–304
    bruises, 301–302
    burns, 301–303
    combination therapies, 302–304
    eczema, 302, 304
    face wash, 301
    haemorrhoids, 303
    healing wounds, 303
    inflammation, 302
    injuries, 301–302
    kidney problems, 302
    lymphadenitis, 304
    menstrual problems, 302
    painful joints, 301–302
    piles, 302
    psoriasis, 304
    psoriatic arthritis, 304
    ringworm, 302
    scrofula, 301–303
    skin diseases, 302
    swellings, 300–301
    topical use, 300–302
    tuberculosis, 302
    tumours, 301–302
    ulcers, 303–304
    wounds, 304
Renaissance, 299, 302
safety, 304–305
    cardioactive glycosides, 304
    myocardial contraction, 304
    triterpene glycosides, 304
Salernitan herbal, 301
Scudder, 303
Turner, 299, 301
Wren, 303
Scudder, J M
    *Galium aparine* (goosegrass), 177
    *Scrophularia nodosa* (figwort), 303
*Scutellaria galericulata* (English skullcap), 313
*Scutellaria lateriflora* (skullcap), 313–314
Secoiridoid glycosides, *Centaurium erythraea* (centaury), 142–143
*The Secrets of Metals* (Pelikan), 18
Seizures *see* Convulsions
Self-prescription, *Rubus idaeus* (raspberry), 278
Senkirkine, *Tussilago farfara* (coltsfoot), 323
*Senna alexandrina* (senna), 285–287

Serapio the Younger (Ibn Wafid), 1–2, 7–8
    *Althaea officinalis* (marshmallow), 71
    *Artemisia absinthium* (wormwood), 109–110, 112–114
    *Centaurium erythraea* (centaury), 139–140
    *Daucus carota* (wild carrot), 147
    *Fumaria officinalis* (fumitory), 167
    *Inula helenium* (elecampane), 203, 206
    *Liber Aggregatus in Medicinus Simplicibus*, 7
    *Liber Aggregatus in Simplicibus Medicinis*, 1
    *Ocimum basilicum* (basil), 224–225
    *Paeonia officinalis* (paeony), 234–237
    *Rosa damascene* (damask rose), 259
    *Ruta graveolens* (rue), 287–288, 290
    *Stachys officinalis* (wood betony), 312–313
Sesquiterpene lactones
    *Artemisia absinthium* (wormwood), 117
    *Inula helenium* (elecampane), 208
Sesquiterpenes
    *Artemisia vulgaris* (mugwort), 132
    *Tussilago farfara* (coltsfoot), 323
Seth, Simeon, 7
    *Syntagme de Alimentorium Facultatibus*, 7
Sight problems *see* Eye conditions
Silica content, *Agrimonia eupatoria* (agrimony), 53
Silicosis, *Tussilago farfara* (coltsfoot), 322
Silverweed *(Potentilla anserina)*, 241
*Silybum marianum* (milk thistle), 313
'Simples', The Salernitan herbal, 26
Skelton, John, 29–32
    *Parietaria diffusa* (pellitory), 31–32
    *Plantago* (plantain), 31–32
    *Rubus idaeus* (raspberry), 277
    *The Science and Practice of Medicine*, 31–32
Skin ageing, *Alchemilla vulgaris* (lady's mantle), 63
Skin conditions
    *Arctium lappa* (burdock), 93, 100–101
    *Fumaria officinalis* (fumitory), 167–171
    *Galium aparine* (goosegrass), 178–179
    *Ruta graveolens* (rue), 293
    *Scrophularia nodosa* (figwort), 302

*Viola odorata* (sweet violet), 339–341
*Viola tricolour* (heartsease), 346
*Skleton's Botanic Reader* (Coffin), 16–17
Skullcap *(Scutellaria lateriflora)*, 313–314
Slippery elm *(Ulmus fulva)*, 129
*Solarum nigrum* (nightshade), 319
Sore mouth, *Rosa damascene* (damask rose), 267
Sore throats
    *Artemisia absinthium* (wormwood), 115
    *Hyssopus officinalis* (hyssop), 193, 198
Soul, nature of, 30
Southernwood *(Artemisia abrotanum)*, 128
Spasmolytic, *Ruta graveolens* (rue), 290–292
Spirituality
    *Artemisia vulgaris* (mugwort), 130–131
    Goethe, Johann Wolfgang von, 37–38
Spleen
    *Artemisia absinthium* (wormwood), 107–109
    *Stachys officinalis* (wood betony), 309
Spotted deadnettle *(Lamium maculatum)*, 213
Spurge laurel *(Daphne laureola)*, 331–332
Squill *see Drimia maritima* (squill)
*Stachys officinalis* (wood betony), 307–316, 308f, 310f
    Antonius Musa, 309
    anxiety, 314
    Bartholin, 312–313
    Bauhin, 309, 311, 313–314
    *British Herbal Pharmacopoeia*, 313
    Chevallier, 309–312
    Coffin, 313
    constituents, 315b
        flavonoids, 315
        phenolic acids, 315
        phenylethanoid glycosides, 315
        phenylpropanoids, 315
        tannins, 315
        volatile oils, 314–315
    Cullen, 312–313
    Culpeper, 311–312
    Dalechamps, 309, 311–312
    Dioscorides, 309, 311–314
    Dodoens, 312
    dosage, 309–311, 315
    Fox, 313
    Fuchs, 311–312

# INDEX

Galen, 311–312, 314
Gerard, 312
*Herbal of Apuleius Platonicus*, 309
Hill, 312–313
Hoffman, 313
Hool, 313
Mattioli, 312
Menzies-Trull, 313
Musa, 8, 312
Myddfai physicians, 311
*National Botanic Pharmacopoeia*, 311–313
*Old English Herbarium*, 309, 311–314
Parkinson, 312–314
part used, 307
Pliny, 311–312
Priest, 313
quality, 307–309
Quincy, 311
recommendations, 314–315
  abdominal pain, 311
  anxiety, 314
  biliousness, 309–311
  bladder problems, 311
  cephalic action, 313
  cholangitis, 314
  chronic cholecystitis, 314
  colic, 309–311
  combination therapies, 313, 321
  depression, 314
  diuretics, 311
  dyspepsia, 314
  emmenagogic, 311–312
  epilepsy, 312
  eye problems, 314
  fatigue, 312
  headache, 312–314
  heartburn, 309–311
  kidney problems, 311
  liver disease, 309
  malarial fevers, 313–314
  memory loss, 313
  menstrual problems, 311–312
  migraine, 312–313
  nervous system, 312
  oedema, 311
  poison antidote, 314
  reproductive system, 311
  respiratory conditions, 313–314
  spleen, 309
  stomach cramps, 309–311
  stomach disease, 309
  topical use, 313–314
  trauma, 312
  tuberculosis, 313
  urinary system, 311
  wounds, 312, 314

safety, 315
  pregnancy, 311–312
Salernitan herbal, 309, 311–313
Serapio, 312–313
Turner, 312
Tyler, 314
Wood, 313
*Stachys palustris* (marsh woundwort), 307
*Stachys sylvatica* (hedge woundwort), 307
*Standard Guide to Non-Poisonous Herbal Medicien* (Webb), 32–33
Stannard, J, *Drimia maritima* (squill), 159–160
St Anthony's fire
  *Rosa damascene* (damask rose), 261
  *Tussilago farfara* (coltsfoot), 319
Steiner, Rudolf, 37–38
  *Artemisia absinthium* (wormwood), 116
*Stellaria media* (chickweed), 129
Stern, J S, *Paeonia officinalis* (paeony), 233
Steroidal saponins, *Drimia maritima* (squill), 161
Sterols, *Centaurium erythraea* (centuary), 143
Stevens, John, 31
  *Artemisia vulgaris* (mugwort), 128–129
*Stillingia sylvatica*, 302
Stinging nettle *(Urtica dioica)*, 85–86
Stings, *Centaurium erythraea* (centuary), 142
*Stirpium Adversaria Nova*, *Potentilla erecta* (tomentil), 247
*Stirpium historiae pentades sex sive librui XXX* (Dodoens), 12
Stomach cramps, *Stachys officinalis* (wood betony), 309–311
Stomach disorders
  *Hyssopus officinalis* (hyssop), 195–196
  *Inula helenium* (elecampene), 205
  *Rosa damascene* (damask rose), 267
  *Stachys officinalis* (wood betony), 309
Stomatitis, *Rubus idaeus* (raspberry), 277
Sturtevant, E L, *Apium graveolens* (wild celery), 79
Sugar of roses, 262
Sweet violet *see Viola odorata* (sweet violet)
Swellings
  *Althaea officinalis* (marshmallow), 69

*Scrophularia nodosa* (figwort), 300–301
Swollen breasts, *Apium graveolens* (wild celery), 84
Swollen glands
  *Galium aparine* (goosegrass), 179
  *Verbena officinalis* (vervain), 331
*Symphyticum officinale* (comfrey), 203–204
*Syntagme de Alimentorium Facultatibus* (Seth), 7
Syrup, *Rosa damascene* (damask rose), 262
*Syzygium aromaticum* (cloves), 225, 276

Tannins
  *Agrimonia eupatoria* (agrimony), 54
  *Alchemilla vulgaris* (lady's mantle), 62, 64
  condensed *see* Condensed tannins
  *Lamium album* (white deadnettle), 219
  *Potentilla erecta* (tomentil), 241, 250
  *Rubus idaeus* (raspberry), 230
  *Stachys officinalis* (wood betony), 315
  *Tussilago farfara* (coltsfoot), 323
  *Viola tricolour* (heartsease), 347
*Taraxacum officinale* (dandelion), 165–167
Tea tree *(Melaleuca alternifolia)*, 177
Tendon diseases, *Centaurium erythraea* (centuary), 139
Tertian fever, *Viola odorata* (sweet violet), 339
*Teucrium chamaedrys* (germander), 139
*Teucrium scorodonia* (wood sage), 313–314
*Theatrum Botanicum* (Parkinson), 14
  *Potentilla erecta* (tomentil) 247
Theophrastus, 23
  *Althaea officinalis* (marshmallow), 67–69
  *Apium graveolens* (wild celery), 79
  *Daucus carota* (wild carrot), 147
  *Drimia maritima* (squill), 157
  *Potentilla erecta* (tomentil), 243
  *Rubus idaeus* (raspberry), 271–273
Thomson, Samuel, 29
  bloodletting, 29
  cayenne *(Capsicum annum)*, 29
  heat, importance of, 29
  lobelia *(Lobelia inflata)*, 29
  *Rubus idaeus* (raspberry), 277–280
Thread worms, *Daucus carota* (wild carrot), 152
*Thymus longicaulis*, 333
*Thymus vulgaris* (thyme), 128–129, 321
Thyroxine supplements, *Apium graveolens* (wild celery), 87

**375**

# INDEX

*Tilia* (lime), 334
Tinnitus, *Glechoma hederacea* (ground ivy), 183–186
Tobacco, *Tussilago farfara* (coltsfoot), 321
Tomentil *see Potentilla erecta* (tomentil)
Tonics
    *Agrimonia eupatoria* (agrimony), 52, 54
    *Inula helenium* (elecampene), 205, 207
    *Ocimum basilicum* (basil), 225
Tonsilitis, *Rubus idaeus* (raspberry), 277
Toothache, *Potentilla erecta* (tomentil), 247–248
Topical uses
    *Agrimonia eupatoria* (agrimony), 50–51
    *Althaea officinalis* (marshmallow), 76
    *Apium graveolens* (wild celery), 86
    *Arctium lappa* (burdock), 101
    *Artemisia absinthium* (wormwood), 115–116
    *Centaurium erythraea* (centaury), 142
    *Daucus carota* (wild carrot), 152
    *Drimia maritima* (squill), 157, 159
    *Fumaria officinalis* (fumitory), 170–171
    *Galium aparine* (goosegrass), 175, 177
    *Glechoma hederacea* (ground ivy), 188
    *Hyssopus officinalis* (hyssop), 198
    *Inula helenium* (elecampene), 206–207
    *Ocimum basilicum* (basil), 223, 226
    *Paeonia officinalis* (paeony), 233–234
    *Potentilla erecta* (tomentil), 247–248
    *Rosa damascene* (damask rose), 267
    *Rubus fruticosa* (bramble), 275
    *Rubus idaeus* (raspberry), 277
    *Ruta graveolens* (rue), 287–288, 292–293
    *Scrophularia nodosa* (figwort), 300–302
    *Stachys officinalis* (wood betony), 313–314
    *Verbena officinalis* (vervain), 334
Tragus
    *Alchemilla vulgaris* (lady's mantle), 59
    *Inula helenium* (elecampene), 203
    *Lamium album* (white deadnettle), 213
    *Potentilla erecta* (tomentil), 243

Trauma, *Stachys officinalis* (wood betony), 312
*A Treatise on Midwifery* (Coffin), 16–17
Treben, Maria, *Alchemilla vulgaris* (lady's mantle), 62
Triterpene(s)
    *Agrimonia eupatoria* (agrimony), 54
    *Alchemilla vulgaris* (lady's mantle), 64
    *Glechoma hederacea* (ground ivy), 181, 183, 188
    *Lamium album* (white deadnettle), 218
    *Ocimum basilicum* (basil), 227
    *Tussilago farfara* (coltsfoot), 323
    *Verbena officinalis* (vervain), 333–334
Triterpene glycosides, *Scrophularia nodosa* (figwort), 304
Triterpenoid saponins, *Potentilla erecta* (tomentil), 250
Triterpenoids, *Paeonia officinalis* (paeony), 238
Trotula, 8–9
    *Artemisia vulgaris* (mugwort), 127–128, 130
    *Hyssopus officinalis* (hyssop), 195
    *Paeonia officinalis* (paeony), 233–234
    *Rosa damascene* (damask rose), 259
    *Viola odorata* (sweet violet), 339
Tuberculosis
    *Inula helenium* (elecampene), 203–204
    *Scrophularia nodosa* (figwort), 302
    *Stachys officinalis* (wood betony), 313
Tumours *see* Cancer
Turner, William, 2, 11–12, 27
    *Althaea officinalis* (marshmallow), 67, 71
    *Apium graveolens* (wild celery), 81–82
    *Arctium lappa* (burdock), 96–97
    *Artemisia absinthium* (wormwood), 110
    *Artemisia vulgaris* (mugwort), 123–125
    *Centaurium erythraea* (centaury), 139–140
    *Daucus carota* (wild carrot), 149
    *Drimia maritima* (squill), 157–159
    *Inula helenium* (elecampene), 203, 205–206
    *Lamium album* (white deadnettle), 213–215
    *Libellus de Re Herbaria*, 11
    *Names of Herbes*, 11
    *A New Herball*, 12

*Paeonia officinalis* (paeony), 233, 236
*Potentilla erecta* (tomentil), 243–248
*Rosa damascene* (damask rose), 257–258, 260
*Rubus idaeus* (raspberry), 273, 275
*Ruta graveolens* (rue), 289–292
*Scrophularia nodosa* (figwort), 299, 301
*Stachys officinalis* (wood betony), 312
*Tussilago farfara* (coltsfoot), 319
*Verbena officinalis* (vervain), 331
*Tussilago farfara* (coltsfoot), 317–326, 318f, 320f
    associations, 317–319
    Bauhin, 317–319
    British Herbal Pharmacopoeia, 322
    constituents, 322b–323b
        chromones, 323
        flavonoids, 323
        mucilage, 323
        pyrrolizidine alkaloids, 321–323
        senkirkine, 323
        sesquiterpenes, 323
        tannins, 323
        triterpenes, 323
    Culpeper, 317–319
    Dioscorides, 319
    Dodoens, 317–319
    dosage, 322–323
    Ellingwood, 321
    Fox, 319, 321
    Galen, 319
    Gerard, 317–319
    Grieve, 319, 321
    Hildegard of Bingen, 319
    Hill, 319
    Hoffman, 322
    identification, 317, 325
    Marzell, 321
    Menzies-Trull, 322
    Miller, 319–321
    names, 317–319
    Parkinson, 319
    parts used, 317
    Pliny, 319
    Priest, 322
    quality, 317
    Quincy, 319–321
    recipes, 321
    recommendations, 319–323
        abscesses, 319
        antiinflammatory, 322
        antispasmodic, 322
        asthma, 321
        bronchitis, 321
        combination therapies, 205, 319, 321–322, 331–332

cough, 319, 321
coughs, 322
emphysema, 322
inflammations, 322
respiratory system, 319, 322
silicosis, 322
St Anthony's fire, 319
safety, 323–325
   children, 323
   drug interactions, 324
   duration of use, 323–324
   lactation, 323
   pregnancy, 323
tobacco, 321
Turner, 319
Weiss, 319, 321–322
Wood, 322
20th Century, 3
21st Century, 3–4
Tyler, V, *Stachys officinalis* (wood betony), 314
Typhus, *Ruta graveolens* (rue), 290

Ulcerative colitis, *Potentilla erecta* (tomentil), 249
Ulcers
   *Centaurium erythraea* (centaury), 137
   *Galium aparine* (goosegrass), 175
   *Inula helenium* (elecampane), 206–207
   *Potentilla erecta* (tomentil), 247–248
   *Scrophularia nodosa* (figwort), 303–304
*Ulmus fulva* (slippery elm), 129
Unexplained infertility, *Artemisia vulgaris* (mugwort), 131
*Urginea maritima* see *Drimia maritima* (squill)
Urinary stones, *Artemisia vulgaris* (mugwort), 129
Urinary tract conditions
   *Althaea officinalis* (marshmallow), 76
   *Apium graveolens* (wild celery), 86
   *Artemisia vulgaris* (mugwort), 129
   *Daucus carota* (wild carrot), 149, 152
   *Paeonia officinalis* (paeony), 234–235
   *Stachys officinalis* (wood betony), 311
   *Verbena officinalis* (vervain), 334
   *Viola odorata* (sweet violet), 344
   *Viola tricolour* (heartsease), 346
Urinary tract infections
   *Agrimonia eupatoria* (agrimony), 54
   *Galium aparine* (goosegrass), 177, 179

Urination
   *Glechoma hederacea* (ground ivy), 185
   *Inula helenium* (elecampane), 206
Ursolic acid, *Glechoma hederacea* (ground ivy), 183
*Urtica diocia* (stinging nettle), 85–86
Urtication, *Lamium album* (white deadnettle), 217
*The Useful Family Herbal* (Hill), 16
Uterus, *Rubus idaeus* (raspberry), 278

Vaginal discharge, *Artemisia absinthium* (wormwood), 113
*Valeriana officinalis*, 313
*The Vegetable System* (Hill), 16
Vegetarianism, *Verbena officinalis* (vervain), 335
Venereal disease, *Viola tricolour* (heartsease), 345
*Verbascum thapsis* (mullein), 204–205, 322
*Verbena hastata*, 327
*Verbena officinalis* (vervain), 327–336, 328f, 330f
   Bartram, 332–333
   Bauhin, 329
   *British Herbal Pharmacopoeia*, 332–333
   Chevallier, 331–333
   Coffin, 331–333
   constituents, 334b
      flavonoids, 333–334
      iridoid glycosides, 333–334
      phenylpropanoids, 333–335
      triterpenes, 333–334
   Cook, 332–333
   Cullen, 327
   Culpeper, 331–332
   Dalechamps, 332
   Dioscorides, 327
   dosage, 334
   Fuchs, 332
   Galen, 329
   Gerard, 327, 329, 331
   Grieve, 331–333
   Hill, 332
   Hoffman, 332–333
   Macer, 331
   Menzies-Trull, 332–333
   Miller, 332
   Myddfai physicians, 331–332
   *National Botanic Pharmacopoeia*, 332–333
   *Old English Herbarium*, 331
   Parkinson, 327, 332
   Pliny, 327
   Priest, 331–333
   quality, 327–329

   Quincy, 327, 331–332
   recommendations, 329, 332–334
      antiinflammatory, 333
      bladder stones, 331
      combination therapies, 331–333
      convalescence, 334
      digestion, 334
      dysmenorrhoea, 334
      gall bladder, 332–333
      gout, 332
      jaundice, 332–333
      lung conditions, 332–333
      magical uses, 332
      nervine agent, 334
      nervous disorders, 334
      relaxant, 333–334
      religious uses, 329
      respiratory system, 334
      scrofula, 331–332
      swollen glands, 331
      topical uses, 334
      urinary tract, 334
   Renaissance, 332
   safety, 335
      pregnancy, 335
      vegetarianism, 335
   Salernitan Herbal, 331–332
   Turner, 331
Vervain see *Verbena officinalis* (vervain)
Viaticum (Constantine the African), 8
Vinegar of roses, 262
*Viola alba* (white violet), 337
*Viola odorata* (sweet violet), 338–344, 338f, 340f
   Bauhin, 339–343
   *The British Herbal Pharmacopoeia*, 338
   Chevallier, 343, 344
   constituents, 346b–347b
      macrocyclic peptides, 347
      phenylpropanols, 347
      polysaccharides, 346
      volatile oils, 346
   Cullen, 343
   Culpeper, 342–343
   Dalechamps, 339–343
   Dioscorides, 338–339, 342–343
   Dodoens, 342–343
   dosage, 339–341, 344
   Fuchs, 342–343
   Galen, 342–343
   Gerard, 342–343
   Grieve, 343–344
   Hildegard of Bingen, 339
   *Hippocratic Corpus*, 339
   Hoffman, 333, 344
   Ibn Sina, 339–341
   Macer, 339
   Mattioli, 339–341

# INDEX

medieval herbals, 339
Menzies-Trull, 344
Mesue, 342–343
Miller, 343
*National Botanic Pharmacopoeia*, 343
*Old English Herbarium*, 339
Parkinson, 342
part used, 337
Pliny, 342–343
quality, 337
Quincy, 343
recommendations, 338, 344
    antiinflammatory, 344
    antiseptic, 344
    bilious conditions, 344
    bronchitis, 344
    cancer, 343–344
    catarrh, 344
    colds, 344
    colouring agent, 343–344
    combination therapies, 127–128, 338–339
    cough, 344
    18th Century, 343
    expectorant, 344
    eyes, 338–339
    fever, 342
    gastrointestinal system, 339–341
    head pain, 339
    inflammations, 342
    laxative, 342–344
    menstrual problems, 338–339
    perfume, 343–344
    respiratory system, 339–341
    scorpion stings, 338–339
    skin eruptions, 339–341
    tertian fever, 339
    urinary conditions, 344
Renaissance, 342
safety, 347–348
    glucose-6-dehydrogenase deficiency, 347
Salernitan herbal, 339
*Tortula*, 339
Weiss, 344
*Viola palustris* (marsh violet), 337
*Viola reichenbachiana* (early dog-violet), 337
*Viola riviniana* (common dog-violet), 337
*Viola tricolour* (heartsease), 338f, 341f, 344–348
    Bauhin, 345
    *The British Herbal Pharmacopoeia*, 346
    Chevallier, 346
    constituents, 347b
        carotenoids, 347
        flavonoids, 347

flavonol diglycosides, 347
flavonol glycosides, 347
macrocyclic peptides, 347
phenolic acids, 347
polysaccharides, 347
saponins, 347
tannins, 347
Culpeper, 344–345
Dodoens, 345
dosage, 346–347
Fuchs, 345
Gerard, 345
Grieve, 345
Hoffman, 346
Mattioli, 345
nomenclature, 345
Parkinson, 344–345
part used, 337–338
quality, 337–338
recommendations, 345–346
    antibacterial action, 346
    anticonvulsant, 345–346
    arthritis, 346
    asthma, 345–346
    convulsions, 346
    diuresis, 346
    eczema, 346
    respiratory system, 344–346
    rheumatism, 346
    skin conditions, 346
    urinary conditions, 346
    venereal disease, 345
safety *see Viola odorata* (sweet violet)
Weiss, 346
Wren, 345–346
Viscous humours, *Centaurium erythraea* (centaury), 140–141
Vitamin C, *Rubus idaeus* (raspberry), 276
Vitamin deficiency, *Rosa damascene* (damask rose), 264, 267
Volatile oils
    *Agrimonia eupatoria* (agrimony), 54
    *Apium graveolens* (wild celery), 86–87
    *Arctium lappa* (burdock), 101
    *Artemisia absinthium* (wormwood), 117
    *Artemisia vulgaris* (mugwort), 132
    *Daucus carota* (wild carrot), 153
    *Galium aparine* (goosegrass), 179
    *Glechoma hederacea* (ground ivy), 181, 188
    *Hyssopus officinalis* (hyssop), 197–198
    *Inula helenium* (elecampene), 207
    *Lamium album* (white deadnettle), 218
    *Ocimum basilicum* (basil), 227–228

*Paeonia officinalis* (paeony), 238
*Rosa damascene* (damask rose), 268
*Ruta graveolens* (rue), 293
*Stachys officinalis* (wood betony), 314–315
*Viola odorata* (sweet violet), 346
Volumes, system of, 43t
Vomiting
    *Alchemilla vulgaris* (lady's mantle), 63
    *Althaea officinalis* (marshmallow), 69–70
    *Rosa damascene* (damask rose), 267

Water agrimony *(Bidens tripartita)*, 47–49
Water figwort *(Scrophularia auriculata)*, 297
Webb, Sarah, 32–33
    *Diseases of Women*, 32–33
    *Menopause or Change of Life in Women*, 32–33
    *Mother and Child*, 32–33
    *Standard Guide to Non-Poisonous Herbal Medicien*, 32–33
Webb, William, 32–33
Weights, system of, 43t
Weiss, Rudolf, 3, 18
    *Althaea officinalis* (marshmallow), 75
    *Daucus carota* (wild carrot), 151
    *Fumaria officinalis* (fumitory), 170
    *Hyssopus officinalis* (hyssop), 197
    *Lamium album* (white deadnettle), 216–217
    *Potentilla erecta* (tomentil), 241, 248–249
    *Rosa damascene* (damask rose), 264
    *Ruta graveolens* (rue), 285–287
    *Tussilago farfara* (coltsfoot), 319, 321–322
    *Viola odorata* (sweet violet), 344
    *Viola tricolour* (heartsease), 346
Wesley, John, 32
White cinquefoil *(Potentilla alba)*, 241
White deadnettle *see Lamium album* (white deadnettle)
White-flowered harmal *(Peganum harmala)*, 289
White violet *(Viola alba)*, 337
Whooping cough, *Rubus idaeus* (raspberry), 276
Wild carrot *see Daucus carota* (wild carrot)
Wild celery *see Apium graveolens* (wild celery)
Williamson, Elizabeth, 3, 19
    *Alchemilla vulgaris* (lady's mantle), 62

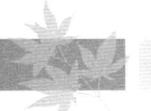

# INDEX

*Arctium lappa* (burdock), 98
*Ocimum basilicum* (basil), 226
*Ruta graveolens* (rue), 285–287, 290–292
Witch hazel *(Hamamelis virginiana)*, 247–248
Woman's Herbal Book of Health, *Artemisia vulgaris* (mugwort), 130
Womb laxity, *Arctium lappa* (burdock), 100
'Women's herb', *Alchemilla vulgaris* (lady's mantle), 59–61
Wood avens *(Geum urbanum)*, 277, 313
Wood betony *see Stachys officinalis* (wood betony)
Wood, Matthew, 4, 22
    *Althaea officinalis* (marshmallow), 76
    *Centaurium erythraea* (centuary), 140
    *Glechoma hederacea* (ground ivy), 187
    *Hyssopus officinalis* (hyssop), 197

*Lamium album* (white deadnettle), 217
*Ruta graveolens* (rue), 285
*Stachys officinalis* (wood betony), 313
*Tussilago farfara* (coltsfoot), 322
Wood sage *(Teucrium scorodonia)*, 313–314
Wormwood *see Artemisia absinthium* (wormwood)
Wounds
    *Agrimonia eupatoria* (agrimony), 53–54
    *Alchemilla vulgaris* (lady's mantle), 59–61, 63
    *Althaea officinalis* (marshmallow), 69
    *Centaurium erythraea* (centuary), 137–139, 142
    *Galium aparine* (goosegrass), 175
    *Lamium album* (white deadnettle), 218
    *Scrophularia nodosa* (figwort), 303–304

*Stachys officinalis* (wood betony), 312, 314
Wren, Richard Cranford, 3, 17–18
    *Althaea officinalis* (marshmallow), 74
    *Arctium lappa* (burdock), 95
    *Paeonia officinalis* (paeony), 235
    Potter's Cyclopedia, 17–18
    *Rubus idaeus* (raspberry), 277
    *Scrophularia nodosa* (figwort), 303
    *Viola tricolour* (heartsease), 345–346

Xanthones, *Centaurium erythraea* (centuary), 143

Yarrow *(Achillea millefolium)*, 187, 204–205, 217, 246
Yellow deadnettle *(Lamium galeobdolon)*, 211, 213

*Zingiber officinale* (ginger), 98, 112–113, 177–178, 246, 248